Textbook of Homosexuality and Mental Health

Textbook of Homosexuality and Mental Health

Edited by
Robert P. Cabaj, M.D.
Terry S. Stein, M.D.

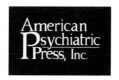

Washington, DC
London, England

Copyright © 1996 American Psychiatric Press, Inc.
ALL RIGHTS RESERVED
Manufactured in the United States of America on acid-free paper
99 98 97 96   4 3 2

American Psychiatric Press, Inc.
1400 K Street, N.W., Washington, DC   20005

Library of Congress Cataloging-in-Publication Data
Textbook of homosexuality and mental health / edited by Robert P.
 Cabaj, Terry S. Stein.
    p.   cm.
  Includes bibliographical references and index.
  ISBN 0-88048-716-X
  1. Gays—Mental health.   2. Bisexuals—Mental health.
3. Psychotherapy.   4. Homosexuality.   5. Bisexuality.   I. Cabaj,
Robert P., 1948–   .   II. Stein, Terry S., 1945–   .
RC451.4.G39G656   1996
616.89′008′664—dc20   95-47271
                                                               CIP

British Library Cataloguing in Publication Data
A CIP record is available from the British Library.

Contents

■ Section I
Homosexuality and Mental Health:
Establishing the Professional Foundation

■ Section II
Understanding Homosexuality and Bisexuality: Demographic,
Cultural, Genetic, Biological, and Psychological Perspectives

■ **Section V**

*Finding Support and Achieving Growth: Psychotherapy
With Gay Men, Lesbians, and Bisexuals*

■ **Section VI**
*Differences and Diversity: Multicultural
Identities and Communities*

■ **Section IX**
Special Topics/Special Concerns: Clinical Implications
of Sexuality and Sexual Orientation

Contributors

D. Lanette Atkins, M.D., D.V.M., is the Medical Director of New Hope Midlands Psychiatric Residential Treatment Center in West Columbia, South Carolina, and Clinical Assistant Professor of Psychiatry for the Department of Neuropsychiatry and Behavioral Science, University of South Carolina School of Medicine, Columbia, South Carolina.

Amy Banks, M.D., is a Clinical Instructor in Psychiatry at Harvard Medical School and McLean Hospital. She is the Psychiatrist-in-Charge of the Women's Treatment Network at McLean Hospital and a psychiatrist at The Fenway Community Health Center in Boston, Massachusetts.

Raymond M. Berger, Ph.D., author of *Gay and Gray: The Older Homosexual Man,* is Professor (Ret.), California State University, Long Beach, California.

Laura S. Brown, Ph.D., A.B.P.P., has practiced feminist clinical and forensic psychology in Seattle, Washington, since 1979 and is Clinical Professor of Psychology at the University of Washington. Her extensive writings have focused on theory, ethics, and practice in feminist therapy, and she has taught at the pre- and postdoctoral levels on matters of ethics and boundaries in psychotherapy, with a special emphasis on the dilemmas faced by lesbian psychotherapists. She is a Diplomate in Clinical Psychology of the American Board of Professional Psychology and a Fellow of both the American Psychological Association and the American Psychological Society.

Bonnie K. Burg, L.C.S.W., B.C.D., is in private practice in Chicago, Illinois. Formerly Clinical Assistant Professor at the University of Illinois at Chicago, she is now a lecturer in the Psychiatry Department at the University of Chicago at the Evelyn Hooker Center for the Study of Gay and Lesbian Mental Health.

William Byne, M.D., Ph.D., is Director of the Neuroanatomy Laboratory of Neuropsychiatric Disease in the Department of Psychiatry at the Mount Sinai School of Medicine in New York and a Research Psychiatrist with Pilgrim State Psychiatric Hospital in Brentwood, New York. His research focuses on correlations between brain structure and brain function in health as well as in psychiatric illness.

Robert P. Cabaj, M.D., is an Associate Clinical Professor of Psychiatry at the University of California, San Francisco, Medical Director of Mental Health Services for the County of San Mateo, California, and in private practice in San Francisco. A Past President of both the Association of Gay and Lesbian Psychiatrists and the Gay and Lesbian Medical Association, he has worked extensively on many components of the American Psychiatric Association. He writes and lectures widely on gay, lesbian, and bisexual issues; the mental health aspects of HIV and AIDS; substance abuse; and the delivery of mental health services to underserved populations.

Vivienne Cass, Ph.D., is a clinical psychologist in private practice in Perth, Western Australia. She has published several articles and book chapters on the topic of lesbian and gay identity formation.

Raymond W. Chan is a doctoral student in developmental psychology at the University of Virginia, Charlottesville, Virginia. His research interests include the study of ethnicity and sexual orientation in couples and families.

Yim H. Chan, M.D., is Assistant Clinical Professor in the Department of Psychiatry at the University of California, San Francisco, San Francisco, California, Associate Medical Director of the Geriatric Psychiatric Unit at Davies Medical Center, San Francisco, and in private practice in San Francisco. His interests include cross-cultural issues among the Asian Pacific Islanders.

Bertram J. Cohler, Ph.D., is the William Rainey Harper Professor of Social Sciences, University of Chicago, and on the faculty of the Institute for Psychoanalysis in Chicago, Illinois.

Eli Coleman, Ph.D., is a professor and director of the Program in Human Sexuality, Department of Family Practice and Community Health, University of Minnesota Medical School in Minneapolis, Minnesota. Dr. Coleman is author of numerous articles about sexual orientation, gender dysphoria, chemical dependency, family intimacy, and the psychological and pharmacological treatment of sexual disorders. He was editor of *Psychotherapy with Homosexual Men and Women: Integrated Identity Approaches for Clinical Practice* in 1988 and is the founding and current editor of the *Journal of Psychology and Human Sexuality.*

Anthony R. D'Augelli, Ph.D., is Professor of Human Development in the Department of Human Development and Family Studies at the Pennsylvania State University, University Park, Pennsylvania. A community psychologist, he has completed several research reports on lesbian, gay, and bisexual youth. He is also coeditor, with Charlotte J. Patterson, Ph.D., of *Lesbian, Gay, and Bisexual Identities Across the Lifespan.*

Jennifer I. Downey, M.D., is Associate Clinical Professor of Psychiatry at Columbia University College of Physicians and Surgeons/New York State Psychiatric Institute, Consultant to the Department of Obstetrics and Gynecology at Columbia, and a member of the faculty of the Columbia Center for Psychoanalytic Training and Research, New York, New York.

Jack Drescher, M.D., a Fellow of the American Psychiatric Association and the American Academy of Psychoanalysis, is a member of the Group for the Advancement of Psychiatry's Committee on Human Sexuality. He is a Faculty Member at the William Alanson White Psychoanalytic Institute, New York, New York. He is also a Clinical Assistant Professor of Psychiatry at SUNY-Downstate in Brooklyn, New York. He is board member of Gay and Lesbian Psychiatrists of New York, and a founding board member of both Gay and Lesbian Analysts and New York Gay and Lesbian Physicians. He is author of the forthcoming book, *Psychoanalytic Psychotherapy and the Gay Man.* He maintains a private practice in New York City.

Oliva M. Espín, Ph.D., is a Professor of Women's Studies at San Diego State University and part-time faculty at the California School of Professional Psychology, San Diego, California. She is a Past President of Division 44 of the American Psychological Association, the Society for the Psychological Study of Gay and Lesbian Issues, at the Department of Psychology, University of California, San Diego. From Cuban origins, she writes, lectures, and has a therapeutic practice focused on Latina lesbians.

Kristine L. Falco, Psy.D., is a clinical psychologist who lives in Portland, Oregon, where she maintains a psychotherapy practice. She provides consultation, writes, trains, and lectures widely on the topics of lesbian psychology and medical psychology.

Eugene W. Farber, Ph.D., is Assistant Professor of Psychiatry and Behavioral Sciences and Clinical Psychologist at the Grady Health System Infectious Disease Program, Emory University School of Medicine, Atlanta, Georgia.

Ronald C. Fox, Ph.D., is a Psychotherapist in private practice in San Francisco, California. He is Cochair of the Task Force on Bisexual Issues in Psychology of the Society for the Psychological Study of Lesbian and Gay Issues, American Psychological Association Division 44. He is the author of an empirical study of bisexual identity development and is currently working on a volume on bisexuality research and an annotated historical bibliography on bisexuality in the social sciences.

Richard C. Friedman, M.D., is Professor of Research Psychology at the Derner Institute, Adelphi University, and Lecturer in Psychiatry at Columbia University College of Physicians and Surgeons, New York, New York. He is a member of the faculty of the Columbia Center for Psychoanalytic Training and Research and the author of *Male Homosexuality: A Contemporary Psychoanalytic Perspective.*

Robert Galatzer-Levy, M.D., is a lecturer in the Department of Psychiatry, University of Chicago, and is on the faculty of the Institute for Psychoanalysis in Chicago, Illinois, where he is a Training and Supervising Analyst.

Nanette K. Gartrell, M.D., is Associate Clinical Professor of Psychiatry at the University of California, San Francisco, California, where she teaches ethics and feminist theory. She is the editor of the recently published book, *Bringing Ethics Alive.*

Francisco J. González, M.D., is a Clinical Instructor in Psychiatry, Department of Psychiatry, University of California, San Francisco. He is a team leader on the HIV-focused inpatient psychiatric unit at San Francisco General Hospital, San Francisco, California. He has researched Latino gay men at risk for HIV infection at the Center for AIDS Prevention, San Francisco, California. He was born in Cuba and moved to the United States at age 4.

Douglas C. Haldeman, Ph.D., is a psychologist in private practice in Seattle, Washington. Dr. Haldeman has been a frequent writer and lecturer on a variety of lesbian and gay mental health issues and is currently developing guidelines for psychotherapists working with lesbians and gay men. He serves on the American Psychological Association's Committee on Lesbian and Gay Concerns, as well as the faculties of the University of Washington and Seattle University, Seattle, Washington.

Graeme Hanson, M.D., is Director of Training in Child and Adolescent Psychiatry, and Clinical Professor, Psychiatry and Pediatrics, Langley Porter Psychiatric Institute, University of California, San Francisco.

Lawrence Hartmann, M.D., is Past President of the American Psychiatric Association. He teaches child, adolescent, and adult psychiatry at Harvard Medical School and practices in Cambridge, Massachusetts. He has written on many topics, including biopsychosocial integration, humane values, the present and future of psychiatry, language and psychiatry, torture, apartheid, human rights, psychotherapy, and play.

Norman B. Hartstein, M.D., is a psychiatrist with the Southern California Permanente Medical Group in Los Angeles, California, and Assistant Clinical Professor of Child Psychiatry at the School of Medicine of the University of California at Los Angeles.

Sarah E. Herbert, M.D., is Assistant Professor in the Department of Psychiatry and Behavioral Sciences at Emory University School of Medicine in Atlanta, Georgia. She is Director of the Psychiatry Obstetrics Consultation/Liaison Service at Grady Memorial Hospital.

Gilbert Herdt, Ph.D., an anthropologist, is Professor of Human Development at the University of Chicago, Illinois. He has conducted research on the Sambia of New Guinea and gay and lesbian youth, their families, and culture in the United States and has published 12 books and many articles.

Gregory M. Herek, Ph.D., is a Research Psychologist at the University of California at Davis. He has published extensively on topics related to heterosexism and antigay violence. He is the editor of *Hate Crimes: Confronting Violence Against Lesbians and Gay Men,* and *AIDS, Identity, and Community.*

Daniel W. Hicks, M.D., is a board-certified psychiatrist and Fellow of the American Psychiatric Association. He has been a psychiatrist with the HIV program at Walter Reed Army Medical Center in Washington, D.C., since 1989.

Marjorie J. Hill, Ph.D., is a public health advocate and has been an activist in the lesbian, gay, and progressive communities for more than 15 years. A licensed clinical psychologist, she has worked extensively with lesbian and gay families, couples, and individuals. Dr. Hill currently serves as vice chair of the New York State Workers' Compensation Board, and she is on the boards of the Black Leadership Commission on AIDS and Gay Men's Health Crisis in New York City.

Evelyn Hooker, Ph.D., is a research psychologist, now living in retirement in Santa Monica, California. An inspiration and friend for many gay, lesbian, and bisexual clinicians and researchers, she pioneered the study of homosexuality and gay men with ground-breaking work in the 1950s. She continues to advise, and consult with, many researchers and clinicians and has enriched the documentation of the efforts to study gay men and lesbians.

Billy E. Jones, M.D., M.S., is a Senior Psychiatrist with 25 years of experience in health and mental health management, policy, training, and treatment. He is the former Commissioner, New York City Department of Mental Health, Mental Retardation and Alcoholism Services, and President, New York City Health and Hospitals Corporation. He has been active in health and mental health issues affecting the African American and gay and lesbian communities. He is a founder of the New York City Minority Task Force on AIDS and is on the board of the National Lesbian and Gay Health Association.

Richard A. Isay, M.D., is Clinical Professor of Psychiatry, Cornell Medical College, and on the faculty of the Columbia Center for Psychoanalytic Training and Research. He is currently also Vice President of the National Lesbian and Gay Health Association.

James J. Kelly, Ph.D., is Director and Professor of the Department of Social Work, California State University, Long Beach, and consultant to the Department of Psychiatry at the University of California, Los Angeles Medical Center.

Robert M. Kertzner, M.D., is Assistant Clinical Professor of Psychiatry, Columbia University, New York, and Principal Investigator of "Psychological Adaptation to Mid-life in Gay Men and Lesbians" at the HIV Center for Clinical and Behavioral Studies, New York State Psychiatric Institute and Columbia University, New York.

Martha Kirkpatrick, M.D., is in private practice in West Los Angeles, California. She is also a Clinical Professor of Psychiatry at UCLA School of Medicine, a member of the senior faculty of the Los Angeles Psychoanalytic Institute, and a Training and Supervising Analyst at the Institute of Contemporary Psychoanalysis, Los Angeles, California.

Rochelle L. Klinger, M.D., is an Associate Professor of Psychiatry and Director of the Medical Psychiatry Program at the Medical College of Virginia/Virginia Commonwealth University in Richmond, Virginia. She served as a member of the American Psychiatric Association Committee on Gay, Lesbian, and Bisexual Issues from 1989 to 1995, and as chairperson from 1993 to 1995. She is Vice President of the Association of Gay and Lesbian Psychiatrists.

James Krajeski, M.D., M.P.A., works as an independent consultant in the field of disability evaluation. He was in private practice for several years, working extensively with gay men and lesbians.

Kewchang Lee, M.D., is completing the Residency Training Program in Psychiatry at the University of California, San Francisco, in June 1996. He is Chief Resident in Psychiatry at the San Francisco Veterans Affairs Medical Center, and is an American Psychiatric Association/Center for Mental Health Services Minority Fellow.

Maggie Magee, M.S.W., is a member and on the faculty of the Los Angeles Institute and Society for Psychoanalytic Studies. She is in private practice in West Los Angeles, California.

Judd Marmor, M.D., is Franz Alexander Professor Emeritus of Psychiatry, University of Southern California, Los Angeles, California, and Past President of both the American Psychiatric Association and the American Academy of Psychoanalysis.

David R. Matteson, Ph.D., teaches psychology and counseling at Governors State University, University Park, Illinois. He has consulted on bisexuality and AIDS for the Centers for Disease Control (CDC) and recently completed a CDC-funded study of Asian American men who engage in bisexual behavior.

Andrew M. Mattison, M.S.W., Ph.D., is in private practice of psychology in San Diego, California. He is also Head, Psychosocial Resources, HIV Neurobehavioral Research Center, San Diego, California; Associate Clinical Professor of Psychiatry and Family and Preventive Medicine, School of Medicine, University of California, San Diego; and coauthor of *The Male Couple*.

J. Stephen McDaniel, M.D., is Associate Professor of Psychiatry and Behavioral Sciences, Medical Director of Mental Health Services at the Grady Health System Infectious Disease Program, and Project Director of the Emory Center for AIDS/HIV Mental Health Services, Emory University School of Medicine, Atlanta, Georgia.

David P. McWhirter, M.D., is Medical Director and Chief of Staff, San Diego County Psychiatric Hospital, San Diego, California, Associate Clinical Professor of Psychiatry, School of Medicine, University of California, San Diego, and coauthor of *The Male Couple.*

Stuart Michaels, Ph.D., is a researcher at the University of Chicago, Chicago, Illinois. He was the project manager for the National Health and Social Life Survey and a coauthor of *The Social Organization of Sexuality: Sexual Practices in the United States.* A former chairperson of the Sociologists' Lesbian and Gay Caucus, he continues to do population-based research on sexuality and issues related to sexual identity in Chicago, Illinois.

Diana C. Miller, M.D., is in private practice in West Los Angeles, California. She is also an Assistant Clinical Professor of Psychiatry at UCLA School of Medicine and a member of the Los Angeles Institute and Society for Psychoanalytic Studies.

Gene A. Nakajima, M.D., is a Robert Wood Johnson Clinical Scholar in the Department of Medicine and Psychiatry, University of California, Los Angeles.

David G. Ostrow, M.D., Ph.D., is Associate Professor of Psychiatry and Behavioral Medicine at the Medical College of Wisconsin, and Research Scientist at the Center for AIDS Intervention Research, Milwaukee, Wisconsin. Until recently, he was the primary psychiatrist responsible for the mental health care of persons living with AIDS/HIV in Southeastern Wisconsin. He has been living with HIV himself since 1982 and dedicates his chapter to the caregivers with HIV who have dealt with intolerable social and political reactions while providing hope and care to millions of others.

William F. Owen, Jr., M.D., has a large private practice, specializing in general internal medicine and HIV care of gay and bisexual men, in the Castro District of San Francisco, California. He is a founder of Bay Area Physicians for Human Rights (BAPHR).

Charlotte J. Patterson, Ph.D., is Associate Professor of Psychology at the University of Virginia. She is coeditor of *Lesbian, Gay, and Bisexual Identities: Psychological Perspectives* and edited a special issue of *Developmental Psychology* on sexual orientation and human development.

Richard C. Pillard, M.D., Professor of Psychiatry, Boston University School of Medicine, Boston, Massachusetts, is a clinician and researcher, and a member of the American Psychiatric Association, the International Academy of Sex Research, and the Society for the Scientific Study of Sex. He was active in the effort to remove homosexuality from the American Psychological Association's *Diagnostic and Statistical Manual* and received the first Winfield Scott Award from the National Lesbian and Gay Health Foundation.

David W. Purcell, J.D., Ph.D., is a Postdoctoral Fellow and Instructor, Department of Psychiatry and Behavioral Sciences, Emory University School of Medicine, Atlanta, Georgia. He received his law degree from the University of Michigan, Ann Arbor, Michigan, in 1986 and practiced law for 3 years in Atlanta, Georgia. He received his Ph.D. in clinical psychology from Emory University, Atlanta, Georgia, in 1995.

B. R. Simon Rosser, Ph.D., is an Associate Professor and coordinates the sexual orientation and HIV prevention services at the Program in Human Sexuality, Department of Family Practice and Community Health, University of Minnesota Medical School in Minneapolis, Minnesota. His research includes two books and more than 40 research articles about male homosexuality in New Zealand, Australia, and the United States.

David Seil, M.D., is a psychiatrist in private practice in Boston, Massachusetts.

Charles Silverstein, Ph.D., is a Clinical Instructor, NYU Medical Center, and is in private practice in New York City. He is editor of *Gays, Lesbians, and Their Therapists: Studies in Psychotherapy* and founding editor of the *Journal of Homosexuality.*

Terry S. Stein, M.D., is Professor of Psychiatry at Michigan State University, East Lansing, Michigan, and Director of the Michigan State University AIDS Education Project. He is Past President of the Association of Gay and Lesbian Psychiatrists and Past Chair of the Committee on Gay, Lesbian, and Bisexual Issues and of the Council on National Affairs of the American Psychiatric Association. He has edited several volumes on mental health issues for lesbians and gay men and written extensively about homosexuality, psychotherapy with lesbians and gay men, gender issues in psychiatry, and medical education.

Mary B. Summerville, Ph.D., is a clinical psychologist in private practice in Atlanta, Georgia.

Margery Sved, M.D., is Clinical Associate Professor of Psychiatry, University of North Carolina, and Division Director of Adult Psychiatry, Dorothea Dix State Hospital, Raleigh, North Carolina. She is a Past President of the Association of Gay and Lesbian Psychiatrists.

Terry N. Tafoya, Ph.D., Taos Pueblo/Warm Springs, was trained as a traditional Native American storyteller and has used Native ritual and ceremony in his work as clinical faculty and senior staff of the Interpersonal Psychotherapy Clinic, Seattle, Washington, part of the University of Washington's Medical School, Seattle, Washington. As Professor of Psychology, he directed the Transcultural Psychological Counseling Program at Evergreen State College, Seattle, Washington. He has served on the faculty of the Kinsey Institute, Indiana University, Bloomington, Indiana, as well as the national teaching faculty of the American Psychological Association. He is known internationally for his work and publications in HIV/AIDS, cross-cultural mental health, human sexuality, and substance abuse prevention.

Mark H. Townsend, M.D., is an Assistant Professor of Psychiatry at Louisiana State University School of Medicine, New Orleans.

Mollie M. Wallick, Ph.D., is Professor of Psychiatry at Louisiana State University School of Medicine in New Orleans, where she is Student–Faculty Liaison for Gay and Lesbian Issues.

Foreword

Lawrence Hartmann, M.D.

This textbook seems to me a potentially important major step forward in education about homosexuality. It brings together new knowledge and new ways of questioning and of combining knowledge in a complex and fascinating biopsychosocial field still cluttered with public ignorance and prejudice.

That so much has been, and is being, learned about homosexuality in the past few decades in the United States is, in significant part, one of many productive results of a shift in American thinking. Many social, political, and scientific themes have contributed to the shift, including the struggle for black civil rights in the 1950s and 1960s and the rethinking of social justice in the 1960s. Some more specifically relevant pioneering and cumulative landmarks include the study of Kinsey et al. (1948), which helped establish that homosexuality can be studied scientifically and that homosexual behavior is far more common than had been thought; Evelyn Hooker's studies (1957, 1958) demonstrating the psychological health of gay people; the Stonewall riot of 1969, in which a persecuted minority, somewhat to its own surprise, stood up for itself; and the American Psychiatric Association's 1973 official and properly considered decision to stop labeling homosexuality a diagnosis or disorder. These actions, and many others, helped change a climate.

After years of being generally scapegoated, and sneered or giggled at, and of being largely seen as too risky and shadowy for scientific study, homosexuality has been allowed out, and has energetically come out, into the light of day and of free scientific inquiry. Scientific writing about homosexuality in many disciplines has been strikingly more energetic and far ranging in the past 40 years than in the 50 years—or even 500 years—before that. There used to be nearly nothing to read about the topic; now there is perhaps more than any one person can read.

This textbook usefully brings together in one place several dozen disciplined essays, studies, and summaries. The very list of its chapter titles, even leaving out those on AIDS, would have been more or less inconceivable a few decades ago.

Many of the chapters are written by current experts in their field. Some of the authors are young; others have half a century or more of expertise. Because I hope that the reader will come to this book and go on from it, with some sense of what has come before it, I would like to list—personally, perhaps idiosyncratically—a few of the thinkers, authors, and journals that have over many years provided me with useful building blocks for understanding homosexuality (even though I will inevitably omit or slight others I have learned from). My thanks go to Ulrichs, Hirschfeld, Ellis, Carpenter, Freud, Gide, Proust, G. Stein, Auden, Isherwood, Kinsey, Cory, Churchill, Ford and Beach, Hooker, Marmor, Stoller, Money, Green, Saghir and Robbins, Bell and Weinberg and Williams, Pomeroy, Goodman, Kameny, Gould, Duberman, Vicinus, Monette, Katz, *The Archives of Sexual Behavior, The Journal of Homosexuality, The Journal of Gay and Lesbian Psychotherapy,* Spiegel, Freedman, Spitzer, Tripp, Kirkpatrick, Boswell, Shilts, Miller, LeVay, Hamer, Pillard, Bailey, Friedman, Lewes, Chauncey, Kessler, Krajeski, Hanley-Hackenbruck, T. Stein, Cabaj, Hanson, and Isay. I have a list of villains too, in this field, but they will fade with time.

In my early adult life, when the nation's leading newspaper, *The New York Times,* would not even mention homosexuality, I remember that even to study homosexuality was considered quite dubious and probably a sign of bad social, moral, or scientific character. There was pervasive pressure to condemn rather than to study, and those who had studied without condemning (such as Ulrichs, Hirschfeld, Ellis, Carpenter, even Freud) were often themselves condemned. That some researchers currently studying various aspects of homosexuality are openly homosexual, others openly heterosexual, and others of unspecified or unpublicized sexuality, seems to me a healthy mix. It combines the potentially different issues, enthusiasms, sensibilities, points of view, and balance of insiders and outsiders. This is parallel to what has been useful in the study of dozens of other areas—for example, women, blacks, Catholics, Jews, Russians, Americans, businessmen, presidents, and so on.

Psychoanalysis, which dominated American psychiatry in the mid-20th century, to its discredit harmed both itself and homosexuality by wandering away from its reasonable early agnosticism about homosexuality. Freud, respectful of much that he did not know, including possible biological factors, and skeptical of the wisdom of labeling such figures as Leonardo and Michelangelo, among others, as ill, declared homosexuality not to be an illness. He also, alas, called it some kind of arrest of development—a view that was accepted as universal law, and developed and made rigid, by some later analysts, causing considerable trouble. But some kind of arrest or not, Freud recommended that homosexual people be allowed to be psychoanalysts. In this recommendation he was outmaneuvered by Ernest Jones' contrary decision, and psychoanalysis then entered several decades of relative neglect and ignorance of homosexuality, characterized by pathologizing and pseudoscientific psychodynamic single-cause reductionism. In the middle of the 20th century, American psychoanalytic and psychiatric thinking about homosexuality had largely settled, with too little and too narrow evidence, on homosexuality as illness or at least as arrested development.

Partly as a result of that, recent thinking on homosexuality has often, to its own disadvantage, thrown out psychoanalytic and dynamic understanding altogether. The psychodynamic approach does have a large place in understanding the biopsychosocial complexity of the many varieties of homosexualities, and in understanding many aspects of the development and psychology of people who have homosexual thoughts, feelings, fantasies, or behavior. The recent work of Isay (1989) is exemplary. This usefulness of psychoanalytic understanding will remain even if, as now seems likely, a large percentage of the factors contributing to the development of homosexuality in many or all gay men or lesbians turns out to be determined by genetic or prenatal hormonal factors, or if some key bits of brain anatomy in at least some gay men and lesbians turn out to be different from comparable brain areas in some heterosexuals and bisexuals. Recent data make it clear that it is a cloistered abuse of the place of psychodynamic thinking to declare—as some of its devotees still do—that psychoanalysis, or one of the developmental stage conflicts it describes, is the *central and adequate* explanation of homosexuality, or that the presence of psychodynamic issues justifies calling homosexuality a diagnosis.

A brief note on this final point: should homosexuality be considered a diagnosis? It should not. This question has repeatedly been debated, and the conclusions since 1973 have been far more useful, as well as accurate, than those before. The philosophic and linguistic power and limits of the contextually influenced, value-influenced, and often imprecise word "diagnosis" require understanding. To discuss the proper meaning of "diagnosis"—an interesting old issue in medicine and in philosophy—would take us far too long for this preface. It seems to me and many others that it is scientifically more modest, accurate, and parsimonious, as well as medically and socially less harmful, to consider homosexuality a cluster of ways of being, doing, fantasizing, or feeling rather than to insist it is *per se* pathological and call it a diagnosis.

A good reason for psychiatrists and other trained mental health professionals now to be major contributors to this book and central to current biopsychosocial research on, and reassessment of, homosexuality, is not just that psychiatrists and their colleagues are relatively well trained and educated in the biopsychosocial integration that is essential for reasonable and balanced thinking about homosexuality, but also that most of psychiatry was, in the mid-20th century, wrong about homosexuality—and harmful to many gay men, lesbians, and bisexuals as well as to science.

Some useful research and education about homosexuality from many relevant disciplines and points of view have recently been appearing in America. Despite wide hostility to, and ignorance and prejudice about, homosexuality in much of the public (and dramatically in many politicians and some religious groups), the current era is relatively favorable for research on homosexuality and dissemination of knowledge about it. Yet while emerging from an era that thought all gay men, lesbians, and bisexuals ill, we are facing continuing problems, some of them fashionable or new, influencing research and balanced judgment. At least two of these, overlapping and mutually supportive, seem worth mentioning.

1. Biological reductionism: The idea or implication that something complex can be explained adequately or solely by reference to anatomy, genetics, hormones, or physiology, and that psychological or social levels of description of phenomena do not really count, or are not quite as true. People like to simplify, and biological reductionism is currently a dominant fashion and problem in psychiatric and biopsychosocial studies. Such reductionism, such a narrow vision of biopsychosocial complexity, simplifies and ignores ample complex psychological, social, and historical data that we already have about homosexuality. Such reductionism tends to exaggerate the importance of what is easiest to measure and quantify, and cannot study or explain homosexuality in anything like a full or balanced manner in history and across groups and cultures and species. Several of the main recent contributors to biological research on homosexuality have, to their credit, acknowledged the intrinsically merely partial validity of anatomical or physiological comments on homosexuality (Burr 1993). Yet people still like to simplify. The contributions of many disciplines are, and will have to be, brought to bear and integrated, because homosexuality across time, cultures, and species is a cluster of phenomena, intrinsically biopsychosocial, varied, and complex. Even to use one word, "homosexuality" (or "homosexual"), is to imply or wish for more unity and precision than is really warranted. There are deeply different varieties and shades of gray or lavender. I sometimes use the word "homosexualities," but I think at present this is perhaps a lost cause.

2. *Political correctness:*   This is the bending of one's thoughts, words, and actions to some group's political or social agenda. Currently, in the United States, "political correctness" is often applied to a rather rigid and righteous agenda of protecting some perceived rights and sensitivities of minorities and underdogs. Political correctness may seem quaint, but it is real and influences science and the use of science. Having been bruised in the past by religious, political, and social pressures on scientific or common-sense clear thinking about homosexuality, many students of homosexuality feel considerable pressure to encourage research and conclusions that will—even if premature or one-sided— seem good or useful to the arbiters of political correctness. Honest free inquiry, and free speech about it, with awareness of context, will in the long run help society make good choices. Science should always be wary of what is seen as politically correct or what seems in the short run to be politically convenient. For instance, a good many people, in and out of science, are now leaping on recent good biological studies (e.g., of twins, siblings, brain anatomy, or genes) to say that homosexuality is all the result of inborn factors. Many consider such a statement politically correct or convenient for some agendas, such as for acquiring civil liberties or equalities now still to a large extent irrationally denied. But data can have unpredictable uses and will not in themselves fix social values or customs. To say that homosexuality is all inborn is to simplify and misread the data, embodying an understandable but unjustifiable

leap. Consider for instance the 52% (Bailey and Pillard 1993)—or whatever the quite high percentage turns out to be—of identical twins who are discordant for gayness; and the gay men whose hypothalami do not look gay.

Homosexuality in the current real world has many mental health aspects and implications, which this book will discuss at some length. Many but probably not all are intertwined with, and partly due to, social intolerance and homophobia—areas worth large and long study, but areas considered far less sensible to study until it dawned on people that gay men, lesbians, and bisexuals could be good and healthy and productive people. I favor tolerance and enjoyment of variety, and I think nature does too. Because I am comfortable and feel ethical about intolerance toward intolerance, I consider social intolerance toward homosexuals less and less compatible with basic American or any other decent values; and I consider homophobia, although widespread and widely taught, and denied, to be pathological and even quite danger-ous, as it repeatedly harnesses untruths and fears to its cause. It will come as no surprise that I do not, in my considered view of the data, think homosexuality is contagious, or a real threat to family values or order or morality or civilization—but I know that many people, were they to read this, would think those words show me to be clearly im-moral if not unfathomably puzzling or stupid.

There are too many reasonable explanations of contributions to homophobia to list them all here, but they include fear of people who are different; fear and hypocrisy about sexuality (not rare), as well as insecurity about one's own gender and sexuality; the need for scape-goats; and denial of all these fears and insecurities. However, one deep fear of homosexuality is probably based on a demand that we reproduce ourselves as a culture and a species. That fear, I am sure, led to some of the several but by no means universal early religious writings con-demning homosexuality. Since overpopulation is now clearly a greater threat to our species than underpopulation, I think time and education are on the side of abolishing or even reversing some of that old fear. Some of the formidable layers of irrational cultural arrangements built partly on that fear over centuries may take additional time and educa-tion to reverse.

I do sympathize with the difficult human task of ever accepting major shifts in concepts from what we were taught as children, or what our elders and ancestors or ancestral civilizations seem to believe and act on. One such shift—and it is not a pure or linear or smooth or unprepared or universal shift but rather a powerful general direction—is in how we see homosexuality: from sin, to crime, to illness, to difference. The difference has many mental health aspects as this book makes clear. But the conceptual shift from sin to crime to illness to difference is large.

I hope that this book, and our current generation of scientists and clinicians, including the biopsychosocial integrators of our generation, can help that conceptual shift become solid.

References

Bailey J, Pillard R: Heritable factors influence sexual orientation in women. Arch Gen Psychiatry 50:217–223, 1993

Burr C: Homosexuality and biology. Atlantic, March:52, 1993

Hooker E: The adjustment of the male overt homosexual. Journal of Projective Techniques 21:18, 1957

Hooker E: Male homosexuality in the Rorschach. Journal of Projective Techniques 21:33, 1958

Isay R: Being Homosexual. New York, Farrar Strous Giroux, 1989

Kinsey A, Pomeroy W, Martin C: Sexual Behavior in the Human Male. Philadelphia, PA, WB Saunders, 1948

Introduction

Robert P. Cabaj, M.D.
Terry S. Stein, M.D.

The astonishing growth in the study of homosexuality and the rapid expansion of the literature on gay men, lesbians, and bisexuals at times leave scholars perplexed about how to integrate the new materials and leave many people new to the study of homosexuality overwhelmed about where to begin. Mental health and medical professionals, students, and trainees and interested individuals face an immense task in collecting relevant material on homosexuality and have thus far had few references that can condense and make the material accessible. This book brings together the range of the material and variety of perspectives concerning homosexuality and mental health.

A Changing Social and Scientific Context

The need for a comprehensive review of homosexuality and mental health arises after decades of change in attitudes about homosexuality in America. Although homoerotic desire and behavior have existed throughout history in all societies and cultures, they have been described, experienced, understood, and responded to in various ways. The words "homosexuality," "heterosexuality," "gay men," "lesbians," and "bisexuals" are modern terms with associated modern concepts.

Before 1970 the available literature about homosexuality or gay men, lesbians, and bisexuals was sparse; now, there is more material than any one person can read.

Because the concept of a gay and lesbian identity is a recent development, gay and lesbian people were rarely described in historical reviews, and the history of attempts by these people to gain civil and legal rights in Europe and the United States is often unknown even to gay people themselves. Duberman et al. (1989) reconstruct this history in *Hidden from History: Reclaiming the Gay and Lesbian Past*. Boswell has made a profound impact on the study of the historical role of homosexuality and societal tolerance with the publication of his studies, *Christianity, Social Tolerance, and Homosexuality* (1980) and *Same-Sex Unions in Premodern Europe* (1994). Many other authors have focused on aspects of gay and lesbian history, including Katz (1976), Porter and Weeks (1991), and Nardi et al. (1994). Marcus (1992) documented the long and difficult struggle for gay and lesbian equal rights in the United States. A vast literature has been published in the last two decades examining the evolving role of homosexuality in virtually every field of study and within almost all aspects of society. During the past decade, the academic field of gay and lesbian studies has been one of the most vital and energetic fields of discourse.

The change in social and scientific attitudes toward homosexuality and gay, lesbian, and bisexual people in America is demarcated by the 1969 Stonewall riots in New York City when a group of gay men, lesbians, bisexuals, and transsexuals resisted a routine police arrest at a gay bar and ignited the power of an emergent gay pride and the fight for gay civil rights (Duberman 1991). The struggle for gay liberation also produced its own literature and helped move along the many scientific, social, legal, and political changes described in this book.

Miller (1989) and Signorile (1993) describe what it is like to be gay, lesbian, or bisexual in America today. Signorile also discusses the politics of coming out in America, including the concept of "outing" (making the sexual orientation of people known publicly even without their permission); his work is a counterbalance to the more conservative approach to the description of gay lives offered by Kirk and Madsen (1989). The special topic of homosexuality and the military (see Chapter 46 in this volume by Purcell and Hicks) has received widespread attention through the works of both Shilts (1993) and Berube (1990) and has been a focus of the struggle for the civil rights of gay men, lesbians, and bisexuals in America.

Purpose of This Book:
A Mental Health Perspective

The editors of *Textbook of Homosexuality and Mental Health* bring together a collection of chapters that present an overview of all the current and updated information on homosexuality from a mental health and medical perspective, written by experts in the field. Although the book is a large collection covering a wide range of material related to gay men, lesbians, bisexuals, and transsexuals, the material is written in an accessible style, with logical groupings of topics and with chapters that can stand alone as comprehensive overviews of a particular subject. Because the topic of homosexuality is so large and complex, some material has been condensed and some may even have been overlooked, but this edition nonetheless is comprehensive.

In addition to meeting the need for an accessible and comprehensive reference book on homosexuality and mental health for the clinician and the general public, this volume updates available resources by incorporating the findings from new studies and research on the medical, biological, genetic, sociological, cultural, and psychological aspects of homosexuality, as well as from recent studies of psychotherapy and medical treatment. Legal, political, and social changes, especially in the United States, regarding gender issues, minority concerns, civil rights, and the right to health care also necessitate a revision of our perspectives on homosexuality in the mental health field.

Until the early 1970s, the scientific, medical, sociological, psychological, and psychiatric literature on homosexuality was limited and most often assumed that homosexuality was abnormal or pathological. As the authors of several chapters in this volume discuss, there were exceptions to the view of homosexuality as pathology, and these exceptions—most especially the early psychological research of Hooker (1957), the famous prevalence studies of the sexual behaviors of men and women from the Kinsey Institute (Kinsey et al. 1948, 1954), and interestingly enough the writings and comments of Freud (Freud 1951; Lewes 1988)—led to the creation in the late 1960s of scientific review panels supported by the federal government that focused on sexuality and homosexuality (see Chapter 2 by Krajeski and Chapter 32 by Marmor).

The findings of these panels served as the incentives for the American Psychiatric Association, in 1972, to review the listing of homosexuality as a mental illness in the second edition of their diagnostic manual (American Psychiatric Association 1968). In 1973, on the basis of this scientific review and encouraged by a broader political movement as well, the board of trustees of the American Psychiatric Association concluded there was no basis for considering homosexuality to be a mental illness and removed it from the manual (American Psychiatric Association 1980). Simultaneously, the American Psychiatric Association issued a position paper on homosexuality and civil rights (American Psychiatric Association 1974) that stands to this day urging full civil rights and freedoms for gay men, lesbians, and bisexuals (see Chapter 2 by Krajeski). Bayer (1987) reviews the history of this diagnostic change, adding a political aspect.

The scientific decision to no longer consider homosexuality a mental illness (defended by a majority of psychiatrists in a referendum in 1974) contributed to the current exponential growth in the literature on homosexuality. When it was no longer viewed as deviant, an illness, or psychopathological, homosexuality could be studied more objectively with fewer biases and with the application of perspectives learned from other areas of psychological and medical study. For example, understanding of the psychology of prejudice and management of differences led to the study of homophobia and heterosexism (as described in Chapter 7 by Herek in this volume) and to the recognition that much of the suffering and presumed psychopathology that had been observed by clinicians in gay men, lesbians, and bisexuals were symptoms of internalized and societal homophobia, not of homosexuality itself.

As another example, the use of multifactorial statistical analysis by Bell et al. (1981) in *Sexual Preferences: Its Development in Men and Women* helped to point out the deficiencies in older studies and to determine that no clear evidence existed that specific patterns of family upbringing or identifiable parental and environmental factors play a determining role in the origins of homosexuality. Similarly, advances in microbiology and other scientific fields have enabled additional investigation of possible genetic, neurological, and biological contributions to the development of sexual orientation.

The publication of other important scientific, sociological, and legal works followed the change in views about homosexuality. The pivotal book, *Society and the Healthy Homosexual* (Weinberg 1972), was followed by *The Gay Mystique* (Fisher 1972), *Male Homosexuals: Their Problems and Adaptations* (Weinberg and Williams 1974), and *The Homosexual Matrix* (Tripp 1975), which all served to expand earlier perspectives. The first edition of *The Joy of Gay Sex* (Silverstein and White 1977) opened new horizons for directness and frankness about same-gender sexual activity.

The amount of readily available, popular literature has continued to grow with volumes on a large number of topics, including the concept of sexual orientation itself (McWhirter et al. 1990; Money 1988); homosexuality and ethics (Batchelor 1980); homosexuality and the law (Editors of the Harvard Law Review 1989); the biology of sexual behavior (Hamer and Copeland 1994); cross-cultural perspectives on homosexuality (Herdt 1981; Whitam and Mathy 1986); public policy and homosexuality (Gonsiorek and Weinrich 1991); social constructionism and sexual orientation (Greenberg 1988); deconstruction of the meanings of being in the closet or hiding one's sexual orientation from others (Sedgwick 1990); growing up gay in America (Herdt 1992; Herdt and Boxer 1993; Schulman 1994); progression through the life cycle for gay men, lesbians, and bisexuals (D'Augelli and Patterson 1995); bisexuality (Weinberg et al. 1994); and the perspective of gay men, lesbians, and bisexuals in psychotherapy, both from the negative impact of psychotherapy based on the belief that homosexuality is pathological (Duberman 1991) and the positive impact when homosexuality is seen as a normal variant of human sexual expression (Silverstein 1991).

This volume was written and edited from the perspective that homosexuality is not an illness and is not psychopathological. This perspective does allow a review of proponents of other viewpoints (such as in Chapter 1 by Silverstein and Chapter 11 by Drescher) and an analysis of the psychodynamic contributions to the expression of homosexuality and the comfort an individual and society may have with homosexuality. The writers in this volume reflect the view that homosexuality is a normal but less frequent expression of human sexual desire and behavior, based on the results of extensive empirical studies and consistent with current mental health practice; as such, the book will not please those practitioners who continue to stigmatize lesbians, gay men, and bisexuals and still treat homosexuality as a type of mental disorder or illness.

Why compile a comprehensive review of homosexuality from a mental health and medical perspective? Rightly or wrongly, homosexuality, since it was first defined by a physician, has been seen and "treated" by physicians, especially psychiatrists, and by psychologists as described in Chapter 1 by Silverstein and Chapter 2 by Krajeski.

The psychiatric, medical, psychological, and sociological fields have contributed to the harmful and prejudicial reports and speculations about homosexuality and to the treatments of gay men, lesbians, and bisexuals, as well as to the major advances in understanding and acceptance of homosexuality and the lives and identities of gay men, lesbians, bisexuals, and transsexuals. It is fair that this book is written by and for health care providers but written in a way that makes it accessible to all interested individuals.

Approaching the Book

This book is organized into sections, and the chapters in each section are meant to complement each other while still providing enough information to be useful if read on their own. Every chapter includes a separate reference list to help with easy study and exploration of material in greater depth.

Section I describes the professional and historical foundations for homosexuality and mental health. Section II explores the demographic, cultural, genetic, biological, and psychological dimensions of homosexuality and bisexuality as well as homophobia and heterosexism. Section III discusses issues for gay men, lesbians, and bisexuals across the life cycle—from childhood to old age—including a model for understanding the development of gay, lesbian, and bisexual identities. Section IV moves beyond individual development to examine gay and lesbian couples and family constellations.

Section V examines the multiple issues involved in psychotherapy with lesbians, gay men, and bisexuals, including individual and couples psychotherapy. Some special and specific issues also are described, including a review of a unique subset of gay men and lesbians, patients with pathological homophobic internalization and self-hatred that interfere with therapy; a discussion of the impact of the sexual orientation of the therapist on psychotherapy; an overview of the controversial topic of efforts to change sexual orientation; and a description of what it is like to be a heterosexual therapist working with and advocating for gay men and lesbians.

Section VI surveys issues related to multicultural diversity among gay men, lesbians, and bisexuals, using several ethnic and cultural populations to illustrate the myriad issues confronting gay and lesbian people of color. Section VII presents the specific issues involved in teaching within the mental health field about homosexuality and the concerns of gay men, lesbians, bisexuals, and transsexuals. Section VIII covers working with gay male, lesbian, and bisexual patients in specific clinical situations, both medical and psychiatric.

Section IX covers subjects that weave through all the previous chapters but can also stand alone as separate areas of study, including gay male and lesbian sexuality, transsexualism, ethical issues, legal concerns, and religion and homosexuality. In addition, this section presents clinical issues for gay men, lesbians, and bisexuals involving such concerns as domestic violence and hate crimes; substance use and abuse; depression and suicide; and the impact of HIV and AIDS.

The volume concludes with an epilogue abstracted from an interview with Dr. Evelyn Hooker, the psychologist and researcher whose groundbreaking and revolutionary study of gay men in the 1950s set the stage for the many changes and new thinking described in this book.

Many topics that are discussed in this volume remain controversial and require additional study, including the multifactorial biological and psychosocial contributions to sexual orientation; greater delineation of the pathways of development during childhood and adolescence of a gay and lesbian identity; additional clarification of the psychological impact on lesbians, gay men, and bisexuals of stigma, discrimination, and violence directed against them; enhanced description of problems within gay, lesbian, and bisexual communities such as domestic violence and substance abuse; delineation of the negative consequences of continued efforts to redirect or convert homosexuality to heterosexuality; and specification of the effects of persistent negative focus on gay men and lesbians in political campaigns to fuel fear and prejudice. Understanding of these issues will increase as a result of additional study consisting of longitudinal and prospective empirical research. Only through careful analysis of data from systematic studies will the full extent of many of these problems be appreciated.

For now, the editors invite the readers of this volume to explore the current state of the field, to learn from the many and varied contributions to the topic provided in the chapters in this book, and to raise new questions about homosexuality and the full range of sexual orientations based on this new information. Most important, this book is a resource for providing high-quality, unbiased mental health care for lesbian, gay male, bisexual, and transsexual patients and for better understanding the complex experience of sexual orientation in ourselves, our colleagues, our friends, and our families.

Thanks and Appreciation

This volume would not have been possible without the contributions of the many authors and contributors, who wrote and rewrote material while also attending to their busy schedules of clinical, administrative, educational, and research work. The staff who helped with the tasks of collecting and editing the material, especially Linda Belman, Debbie Kolk, and Paul Causey; our work colleagues, especially Beverly Abbott, who provided understanding and support; and the editors at the American Psychiatric Press helped make this book possible.

The enthusiasm and excitement of many colleagues and friends—gay, lesbian, bisexual, as well as heterosexual—for this collection and for the impact they hope it will have helped propel the editors through many dark editorial storms. The editors thank the individuals who offered help and contributions for earlier concepts of this book, including Andy Boxer, Marshall Forstein, Scott Goldsmith, Cynthia Gomez, Richard Green, Peggy Hanley-Hackenbruck, Gary Mihalik, Mark McClung, and Laura Roebuck. The conscientious and careful reviewers—Bertram Cohler, Carol Cohen, Anthony D'Augelli, Linda Garnets, John Gonsiorek, Martha Kirkpatrick, Stephen McDaniel, Charlotte Patterson, Charles Silverstein, and Lowell Tong—gave generously of their time, offered extensive advice and suggestions, and helped move this volume along; they all receive the profound appreciation of the editors. And finally, Bob Cabaj extends his greatest thanks to his close friend, Kewchang Lee, and Terry Stein extends his greatest thanks to his life partner, Christopher Carmichael, for their understanding, patience, support, and love during the writing and editing of this volume.

References

American Psychiatric Association: Diagnostic and Statistical Manual of Mental Disorders, 2nd Edition. Washington, DC, American Psychiatric Association, 1968

American Psychiatric Association: Position statement on homosexuality and civil rights. Am J Psychiatry 131:497, 1974

American Psychiatric Association: Diagnostic and Statistical Manual of Mental Disorders, 3rd Edition. Washington, DC, American Psychiatric Association, 1980

Batchelor E (ed): Homosexuality and Ethics. New York, Pilgrim Press, 1980

Bayer R: Homosexuality and American Psychiatry: The Politics of Diagnosis, with a New Afterword on AIDS and Homosexuality. Princeton, NJ, Princeton University Press, 1987

Bell AP, Weinberg MS, Hammersmith SK: Sexual Preference: Its Development in Men and Women. Bloomington, IN, Indiana University Press, 1981

Berube A: Coming Out Under Fire: The History of Gay Men and Women in World War Two. New York, The Free Press, 1990

Boswell J: Christianity, Social Tolerance, and Homosexuality: Gay People in Western Europe from the Beginning of the Christian Era to the Fourteenth Century. Chicago, IL, University of Chicago Press, 1980

Boswell J: Same-Sex Unions in Premodern Europe. New York, Villard Books, 1994

D'Augelli AR, Patterson CJ (eds): Lesbian, Gay, and Bisexual Identities Over the Lifespan: Psychological Perspectives. New York, Oxford University Press, 1995

Duberman MB: Cures: A Gay Man's Odyssey. New York, Dutton, 1991

Duberman MB: Stonewall. New York, Plume, 1993

Duberman MB, Vicinus M, Chauncey G (eds): Hidden from History: Reclaiming the Gay and Lesbian Past. New York, New American Library, 1989

Editors of the Harvard Law Review: Sexual Orientation and the Law. Cambridge, MA, Harvard University Press, 1989

Fisher P: The Gay Mystique: The Myth and Reality of Male Homosexuality. New York, Stein & Day, 1972

Freud S: Letter to an American mother. Am J Psychiatry 102:786, 1951

Gonsiorek JC, Weinrich JD (eds): Homosexuality: Research Implications for Public Policy. Newbury Park, CA, Sage, 1991

Greenberg DE: The Construction of Homosexuality. Chicago, IL, University of Chicago Press, 1988

Hamer D, Copeland P: The Science of Desire: The Search for the Gay Gene and the Biology of Behavior. New York, Simon & Schuster, 1994

Herdt GH: Guardians of the Flute: Idioms of Masculinity. New York, Columbia University Press, 1981

Herdt GH (ed): Gay Culture in America: Essays from the Field. Boston, MA, Beacon Press, 1992

Herdt GH, Boxer A: Children of Horizons: How Gay and Lesbian Teens Are Leading a New Way Out of the Closet. Boston, MA, Beacon Press, 1993

Hooker E: The adjustment of the male overt homosexual. Journal of Projective Techniques 21:18–31, 1957

Katz J: Gay American History: Lesbians and Gay Men in the U.S.A., 1st Edition. New York, Thomas Y. Crowell, 1976

Kinsey A, Pomeroy W, Martin C: Sexual Behavior in the Human Male. Philadelphia, PA, WB Saunders, 1948

Kinsey A, Pomeroy W, Martin C, et al: Sexual Behavior in the Human Female. Philadelphia, PA, WB Saunders, 1954

Kirk M, Madsen H: After the Ball: How America Will Conquer Its Fear and Hatred of Gays in the 90s. New York, Doubleday, 1989

Lewes K: The Psychoanalytic Theory of Male Homosexuality. New York, Simon & Schuster, 1988

Marcus E: Making History: The Struggle for Gay and Lesbian Equal Rights, 1945–1990: An Oral History. New York, HarperCollins, 1992

McWhirter DP, Sanders SA, Reinisch JM (eds): Homosexuality/Heterosexuality: Concepts of Sexual Orientation. New York, Oxford University Press, 1990

Miller N: In Search of Gay America: Women and Men in a Time of Change. New York, Atlantic Monthly Press, 1989

Money J: Gay, Straight, and In-Between: The Sexology of Erotic Orientation. New York, Oxford University Press, 1988

Nardi PM, Sanders D, Marmor J: Growing Up Before Stonewall: Life Stories of Some Gay Men. New York, Routledge, 1994

Porter K, Weeks J (eds): Between the Acts: Lives of Homosexual Men 1885–1967. New York, Routledge, 1991

Schulman S: My American History: Lesbian and Gay Life During the Reagan/Bush Years. New York, Routledge, 1994

Sedgwick EK: Epistemology of the Closet. Berkeley, CA, University of California Press, 1990

Shilts R: Conduct Unbecoming: Gays and Lesbians in the U.S. Military. New York, St. Martin's Press, 1993

Signorile M: Queer in America: Sex, the Media, and Closets of Power. New York, Random House, 1993

Silverstein C (ed): Gays, Lesbians, and Their Therapists: Studies in Psychotherapy. New York, WW Norton, 1991

Silverstein C, White E: The Joy of Gay Sex: An Intimate Guide for Gay Men to the Pleasures of a Gay Lifestyle, 1st Edition. New York, Crown, 1977

Tripp CA: The Homosexual Matrix. New York, McGraw-Hill, 1975

Weinberg G: Society and the Healthy Homosexual. New York, St. Martin's Press, 1972

Weinberg MS, Williams CJ: Male Homosexuals: Their Problems and Adaptation. New York, Penguin Books, 1974

Weinberg MS, Williams CJ, Pryor DP: Dual Attraction: Understanding Bisexuality. New York, Oxford University Press, 1994

Whitam KF, Mathy RM: Male Homosexuality in Four Societies: Brazil, Guatemala, the Philippines, and the United States. New York, Praeger, 1986

SECTION I

Homosexuality and Mental Health

Establishing the Professional Foundation

History of Treatment

Charles Silverstein, Ph.D.

There has always been a close fit between social norms and medical diagnosis and treatment. The treatment of homosexuality is a case in point. In no other diagnostic area can one find greater confusion between social mores and scientific judgment. Homosexuality, which traveled from sin to sickness, was illegal and immoral almost everywhere in the United States until recent years. Until recently, homosexuals might have committed suicide because they were doomed to a life of depression and misery. These people suffered because they were taught to suffer, first by their society at large and then by the scientific community, which declared that homosexuality was a medical illness in an attempt to explain the perceived immorality of homosexual behavior.

The Treatment of Homosexuality as a Disease

Until 1973, when the American Psychiatric Association officially removed homosexuality from its list of mental disorders, the body politic feared homosexual behavior. It did everything possible to prevent homosexuality, control it, and when nothing else worked, punish it. As perceptions of the "causes" of homosexuality reflected the fears of society, so the treatments reflected the appropriate punishments for the transgressions. The psychiatric and psychological establishment had previously invented theories to explain the genesis of homosexual behavior. Freud (1922/1955, 1923/1962) suggested psychodynamic factors. Rado (1940), objecting to Freud's acceptance of bisexuality, originated the phobic theory of homosexuality, and from his work, the Adaptation School of Psychoanalysis was born (Rado 1949). Main subscribers to his work include Bieber et al. (1962), Socarides (1978), and Hatterer (1970), all of whom, in the name of goodness, attempted to cure gay people of their sexual orientation.

The behaviorist school in psychology also attempted to convert [gay people] into heterosexuals. Some of their treatments were caustic. Three forms of aversion therapy were used. Feldman and MacCulloch (1971) used *electrical aversion therapy,* in which an electric shock was administered to the male patient if he responded erotically to a picture of a nude man (Feldman 1977). Cautela (1967) and Barlow et al. (1969) used a procedure called "covert sensitization," in which disgust and images of vomit were thought to "cure" homosexual desire. The third type of aversion therapy used the drug apomorphine (McConaghy et al. 1972), which induces nausea in the patient. Gay liberationists viewed these aversive procedures as punishment, not treatment.

Davison (1968), who later rejected his early work, called his system "Playboy therapy," in which a gay man masturbated to pictures of naked women. A good review of the aversion therapy literature is provided by Bancroft (1974), who himself contributed significantly to the aversion therapy literature. Masters and Johnson (1979) also attempted to change the sexual orientation of gay people.

Perhaps the most bizarre attempt to reorient the sexual orientation of a gay man was performed by Heath (1972). In his "study," Heath implanted electrodes into the brain of a gay man. The patient was then placed in a room with a woman prostitute, who attempted to seduce him; at the same time, Heath stimulated the pleasure centers in the brain of the man. This attempt at reorientation was not a success.

Underlying these attempts by psychiatry and psychology to change sexual orientation is a basic philosophical belief: an assumption that human behavior and sexual orientation are potentially malleable. Of those gay people who volunteered for "the cure," few were able to claim a change in their sexual orientation. Thus, these homosexuals could be seen as "failures," and invariably, researchers blamed the patients themselves for not being sufficiently motivated. Never did they seriously consider the possibility that sexual orientation unfolds naturally like the buds of a flower, rather than as the result of subterranean psychical forces.

The Positive Approach to Psychotherapy With Gay People

The formation of gay counseling centers signified one of the most significant steps toward providing an alternative form of treatment for gay people. In the early 1970s, gay counseling centers were formed in New York, Philadelphia, Pittsburgh, Boston, Seattle, and Minneapolis. Some were staffed only by peer counselors, and others were staffed by both peers and professionals. All provided low-cost service to gay people who were experiencing emotional distress but did not want to change their sexual orientation. Thus, these clinics' services were distinguished from the pathology-focused psychotherapy offered in other clinics. Whereas previously the professional community had been obsessed with the etiology and cure of homosexuality, the gay counseling centers ignored these issues and treated the person.

The gay community centers also provided a place where gay professionals could learn more about the emotional problems of gay people and meet with other gay professionals. Many gay psychiatrists, psychologists, and social workers who worked in these centers authored a new literature on gay-affirmative psychotherapy.

The foundations for these gay counseling centers came from two sources. The first was the gay liberation movement. The second, and more important source for the purposes of this chapter, was the rise of sex research as a scientific discipline, as represented by work such as that of Kinsey and his colleagues (1948, 1953). Kinsey provided the first meaningful studies of sexual behavior ever completed in the United States by documenting the actual sexual experiences of men and women. These researchers published their material to a chorus of anger from traditional religious and psychiatric groups, who reacted, for example, to findings such as one-third of the adult male population had had some homosexual activity to orgasm since puberty.

Out of Kinsey's institute came other sex researchers, such as Simon and Gagnon (1967), Sonenschein (1966, 1968), and Bell (1972, 1978, 1981). Most of these early sex researchers acknowledged the contribution of Hooker (1957). Not as well recognized is Gundlach's early research on lesbians.

Sex research, unfettered by psychoanalytic theory, became a new discipline, and two new journals appeared, *The Journal of Sex Research* and *Archives of Sexual Behavior*. Both are multidisciplinary and publish statistical and clinical papers about all facets of human sexuality. In 1976, the first issue of the *Journal of Homosexuality* was published, giving rise to an ever-increasing collection of published papers on psychotherapy with gay people. This journal also devoted whole issues to descriptions of therapeutic approaches to working with gay people (Coleman 1987; Gonsiorek 1982; Ross 1988). Books by Hetrick and Stein (1984) and Stein and Cohen (1986) rounded out the list of resources available for professionals who rejected the medical model of homosexuality.

The publication of papers and books demonstrating an alternative approach to treating gay men and women was instrumental in teaching the professional community about the therapeutic needs of the gay community. At first, gay professionals used the term "gay-affirmative psychotherapy," described by Malyon (1982) this way:

> This theoretical position regards homosexuality as a nonpathological human potential. But while the traditional goal of psychotherapy with homosexual males has been conversion (to heterosexuality), gay-affirmative strategies regard fixed homoerotic predilections as sexual and affectional capacities which are to be valued and facilitated. (p. 62)

According to Malyon, gay-affirmative psychotherapy should accept homosexuality as a fixed human potential and attempt to alleviate the harmful effects of internalized homophobia.

The literature on psychotherapy with gay people since the removal of homosexuality from the list of diagnoses of mental illnesses in 1973 can be divided into three areas. The first is concerned with the effect of external stressors. These stressors include homophobia (Herek 1984a, 1989), relationships to families (Myers 1982; Silverstein 1977), parenting children (Kirkpatrick 1987; Loulan 1986; Martin 1989), civil and legal rights, "coming out" (Coleman 1982), problems of adolescents (Hetrick and Martin 1987; Martin and Hetrick 1988), impediments to successful love relationships (Burch 1986; Peplau and Amaro

1982; Silverstein 1981), discrimination (Herek 1984b), and the recent epidemic of the acquired immunodeficiency syndrome (AIDS). This material defines various sources of stress and suggests ways to alleviate it. Presumably, if the external stressors were eliminated, psychotherapy for problems in these areas would become moot (to say nothing of making people's lives more productive).

Coping with a discriminatory world is the central theme in all of the literature cited above, and the role of the therapist is often that of an advocate. The gay or lesbian therapist may be open about his or her own sexual identity in the belief that coming out is an important part of the healing process for both therapist and patient. There are, however, differences of opinion on how open the therapist should be regarding his or her own life, including sexual orientation (see Chapter 30 by Cabaj). Those professionals employed in public institutions are rightly worried that disclosures of their sexual orientation will result in discrimination against them by supervisory staff.

In a second area of the literature, attempts are made to define internal psychological processes that are associated with emotional pain for gay people, both male and female. The largest number of papers published in this area are about the effects of low self-esteem and self-hate, or what has been called "internalized homophobia" (Herek 1984a; Malyon 1982; Smith 1988). Other topics include affective disorders, sexual problems (Hall 1987; Reece 1987), merger in lesbian relationships (Burch 1986), identity formation (DeCecco 1981; DeCecco and Shiveley 1983/1984), and borderline conditions (Silverstein 1988).

A few writers have tried to bridge the gap between a gay-affirmative model and traditional psychoanalytic therapy (Hencken 1982), suggesting that one can use the techniques of analytic therapy yet reject analytic beliefs about normal (meaning heterosexual) development. Isay (1985), writing in traditional psychoanalytic journals, described heterosexual bias in the treatment of gay people, and later (1987), supporting Silverstein (1981), suggested that psychoanalysis ignored the special relationship between the gay son and his father. Mainstream psychoanalysis has not been sympathetic to these ideas. In general, this literature more closely approximates the general psychotherapy literature, and a larger number of the authors write from a psychodynamic point of view. The role of the therapist is also more traditional than one finds in gay-affirmative psychotherapy.

The final area of emphasis is on psychotherapy technique. One of the earliest papers on this topic, written by Johnsgard and Schumacher

(1970), described the use of group psychotherapy with gay men. Fensterheim (1972), long known for his work in assertiveness training, used these techniques effectively with gay people. In general, behavior therapists were the earliest to report using psychological techniques to aid sexual functioning in gay men. Some, such as Davison (1976, 1977), addressed the ethical as well as the therapeutic concerns.

This newer literature is distinctly different from the older psychoanalytic writings, which focused obsessively on the etiology and cure of homosexuality. The new forms of treatment reject concepts of etiology with their emphasis on abnormality. Newer therapeutic techniques assume that same-sex desire is an acceptable variation of human sexuality and that attempts to identify the "cause" of homosexuality can lead to political, social, and legal efforts to repress it.

In terms of current psychotherapeutic approaches to working with gay people, a significant controversy persists regarding sexual addiction (Carnes 1983) or sexual compulsion (Mattison 1985; Quadland 1985). Using drug addiction as the paradigm, proponents of these approaches treat "compulsive sexuality," consisting of behaviors such as compulsive masturbation, frequent sex, failure of monogamy, and guilt over sexual acts, with an Alcoholics Anonymous 12-step program.

The conceptual soundness and therapeutic rationale for this treatment program have been questioned by others (Levine and Troiden 1988), who find the conceptual framework one dimensional, the treatment puritanical, and the potential judgment by the therapists suspect. These critics argue that advocates of treatment for sexual compulsions are influenced as much by the moral code as by concern for their patients. The claim by advocates that patients request this help is reminiscent of homosexual men who, before the 1973 American Psychiatric Association decision, asked to be cured of their homosexuality. What those men and the patients volunteering to be cured of their compulsive sexuality have in common is that they have been taught to be ashamed of their sexual desires.

Biomedical Treatments of Homosexuality

Storm clouds are brewing in the treatment literature. Although it may seem that the battle over the diagnosis and treatment of homosexuality is over, that is an illusion. Although the antigay psychoanalytic establishment has been significantly silenced, a new threat to gay people has arisen resulting from the work of biomedical researchers in the United States and Germany. These researchers, working within a biomedical model, have introduced a whole range of theories and treatments that can be used either to prevent the development of homosexuality or to eliminate it in adults. Three techniques for identifying the cause of, and then eliminating, homosexuality have been described: surgical techniques, use of hormones, and prenatal research. Each derives from the belief that biology is destiny.

◼ Surgical Techniques

Steinach in 1917 was the first to use a surgical technique to attempt to cure homosexuality (Schmidt 1984). First, he performed a unilateral castration on a homosexual man, then transplanted testicular tissue from a heterosexual man into the castrated patient. He did this in the belief, prevalent in those times, that homosexuality was a form of hermaphrodism. Steinach was in step with the belief that homosexuality represented a "third sex," an idea originated by Ulrichs (Steakley 1975) and popularized by Hirschfeld (1948). According to Schmidt (1984), at least 11 men were operated on from 1916 to 1921. Complete castration was not performed in the belief that after transplantation of the "normal" testicular tissue, the man would be cured, marry, father children, and lead a heterosexual life. The experiments were a failure.

In 1962 a new surgical technique was introduced by Roeder. He produced a right-side lesion in the tuber cinereum of the brain of a 51-year-old man diagnosed as a pedophilic homosexual. Since then, 75 men considered sexually abnormal have been subjected to hypothalamotomies (Rieber and Sigusch 1979; Schmidt and Schorsch 1981). Most of the men were either imprisoned or involuntarily committed to a mental institution. Most had been diagnosed as either pedophiles or hypersexed; however, the criteria for diagnoses remained unclear. Rieber and Sigusch (1979) claimed that "normal" homosexual men were also operated on. They also showed that one of Roeder's patients was operated on because, at the age of 37, he masturbated daily. They concluded that the procedure was used as an inexpensive alternative to psychotherapy in the West German prison system.

The surgeons claimed that their patients had requested the operations; therefore, no coercion was involved. However, it is likely that the prisoners hoped that by agreeing to the procedures, they would be given their freedom. There is disagreement over the effects of the surgery. The surgeons make no clear claims for success, and there is no evidence that sexual orientation was changed. A 3-year follow-up on 10 patients showed that 3 refused to participate in the evaluation, 1 died, and 3 had "examination findings normal in every respect" (Muller, quoted in Schmidt and Schorsch 1981, p. 319)—whatever that means. The last two patients were found not to have changed their sexual behavior adequately, and *both were surgically castrated*. Sex researchers in Germany demanded that the government declare a moratorium on the use of these surgical techniques in Germany (Sigusch et al. 1982). Publicity over the inhuman nature of these experiments has stopped them, at least temporarily (Reiber and Sigusch 1979).

■ Hormones and Prenatal Research

For a review of research on peripheral hormone treatment and of the newer interest in prenatal hormones, see Chapter 9 by Byne. To summarize this work briefly, researchers have interpreted homosexuality as inadequate masculinity in men and hypermasculinity in women. From this unidimensional notion came the suggestion that one could cure a man of his homosexuality by injecting him with an androgen, thought of as the male hormone. Thus, the gay man would be restored to a proper androgen–estrogen balance and hence live a heterosexual life.

Dürner et al. (1987) even advocated altering the hormonal environment of the fetus. These researchers made it quite clear that they were attempting to eradicate homosexuality. Earlier, Dürner (1983) stated,

> It was concluded from these data that . . . it might become possible in the future—at least in some cases—to correct *abnormal sex hormone levels* during brain differentiation in order *to prevent the development of homosexuality*. However, this should be done, if at all, only if it is *urgently desired by the pregnant mother*. (p. 577, emphasis added)

Meyer-Bahlburg and his colleagues at the Psychiatric Institute in New York also worked toward identifying the prenatal hormonal influences on sexual orientation and gender behavior, although they reject the use of their information to alter sexual orientation (Downey et al. 1982; Meyer-Bahlburg 1977, 1979, 1984).

Conclusion

In this chapter the author argues that many forms of therapeutic treatment imposed on gay people represent punishment inflicted on people who have transgressed sexual rules of our society. The purpose of that punishment is twofold: first, to punish the transgressor and, second, to prevent others from participating in nonconformist sexual activities. *The efficacy of the treatment has rarely been the criterion governing its use.* Steinach tried to cure homosexuality through surgery in 1917. In the 1970s and 1980s, surgeons in Germany performed brain surgery on homosexual men. Although the experiments were a failure, this surgery was stopped for moral and ethical reasons, not because of its ineffectiveness.

Psychologists and psychiatrists attempted to cure homosexuals of their sexual affliction by various means. Aversion therapy ended only because it was no longer fashionable in the egalitarian 1970s. Psychoanalysis has had an even longer life, and after years of failing to "cure" homosexuality, most psychoanalysts still maintain that homosexuality is a pathology that is curable with years of treatment (Nicolosi 1991). Because our society has laid a veneer of guilt on everyone's sexual desires, any form of treatment will find a ready supply of volunteers. A central problem with much biomedical research is that it largely eschews discussion of the moral and ethical implications of its findings; thereby, with respect to sex research, it reinforces society's fear of uncontrolled sexual desire. It is for this reason that DeCecco (1987) feared that the medical research community would come to consider homosexuality to be a type of pathology.

Psychotherapists are now a positive force in the lives of gay people, and loving relationships between gay men and between lesbians are reinforced by gay-affirmative therapists. At the same time, some biomedical researchers have shifted the focus from a psychological pathology to a physical one and have even suggested techniques to prevent the birth of children who might ultimately become gay.

How society will respond to biomedical research is unknown. It may use it to reinforce traditional notions of sexuality, gender, and the family. One hopes—at least this writer hopes—that the knowledge will be used to further appreciation for diversity among people.

References

Bancroft J: Deviant Sexual Behavior: Modifications and Assessment. London, Oxford University Press, 1974

Barlow DH, Leitenberg H, Agras WS: Experimental control of sexual deviations through manipulation of the noxious scene in covert sensitization. J Abnorm Psychol 74:596–601, 1969

Bell A: Human sexuality—a response. Int J Psychiatry 10:99–102, 1972

Bell AP, Weinberg MM: Homosexualities: A Study of Diversity Among Men and Women. New York, Simon and Shuster, 1978

Bell AP, Weinberg M, Hammersmith S: Sexual Preference: Its Development in Men and Women. Bloomington, IN, Indiana University Press, 1981

Bieber I, Dain HJ, Dince PR, et al: Homosexuality: A Psychoanalytic Study. New York, Basic Books, 1962

Burch B: Psychotherapy and the dynamics of merger in lesbian couples, in Contemporary Perspectives on Psychotherapy with Lesbians and Gay Men. Edited by Stein T, Cohen C. New York, Plenum, 1986, pp 57–73

Carnes P: Out of the Shadows: Understanding Sexual Addiction. Minneapolis, MN, CompCare Publications, 1983

Cautela J: Covert sensitization. Psychol Rep 20:459–468, 1967

Coleman E: Developmental stages of the coming-out process, in Homosexuality and Psychotherapy: A Practitioner's Handbook of Affirmative Models. Edited by Gonsiorek J. New York, Haworth, 1982, pp 31–44

Coleman E (ed): Psychotherapy with Homosexual Men and Women: Integrated Identity Approaches for Clinical Practice. New York, Haworth, 1987

Davison GC: Elimination of a sadistic fantasy by a client-controlled counterconditioning technique. J Abnorm Psychol 73:84–90, 1968

Davison GC: Homosexuality: the ethical challenge. J Consult Clin Psychol 44:157–162, 1976

Davison GC: Homosexuality: The ethical challenge: paper 1. J Homosex 2:195–204, 1977

DeCecco JP: Definition and meaning of sexual orientation. J Homosex 6:51–59, 1981

DeCecco JP: Homosexuality's brief recovery: from sickness to health and back again. J Sex Res 23:106–114, 1987

DeCecco JP, Shiveley MG: From sexual identity to sexual relationships: a contextual shift. J Homosex 9:1–26, 1983/1984

Downey J, Becker JV, Ehrhardt AA, et al: Behavioral, psychophysiological, and hormonal correlates in lesbian and heterosexual women, in Abstracts, International Academy of Sex Research, 8th Annual Meeting, Copenhagen, Denmark, August 21–26, 1982, p 9

Dürner G: Letter to the editor. Arch Sex Behav 12:577–582, 1983

Dürner G, Gotz F, Rohde W, et al: Sexual differentiation of gonadotrophin secretion, sexual orientation, and gender role behavior. J Steroid Biochem 27:1081–1087, 1987

Feldman MP, MacCulloch MJ: Homosexual Behavior: Therapy and Assessment. New York, Pergamon Press, 1971

Feldman P: Helping homosexuals with problems: a commentary and a personal view. J Homosex 2:241–250, 1977

Fensterheim H: The initial interview, in Clinical Behavior Therapy. Edited by Lazarus AA. New York, Brunner-Mazel, 1972, pp 22–40

Freud S: Some neurotic mechanisms in jealousy, paranoia and homosexuality (1922), in Standard Edition of the Complete Psychological Works of Sigmund Freud, Vol 18. Translated and edited by Strachey J. London, Hogarth Press, 1955, pp 223–232

Freud S: The ego and the id (1923), in Standard Edition of the Complete Psychological Works of Sigmund Freud, Vol 19. Translated and edited by Strachey J. London, Hogarth Press, 1962, pp 3–66

Gonsiorek JC (ed): Homosexuality and Psychotherapy: A Practitioner's Handbook of Affirmative Models. New York, Haworth, 1982

Hall M: Sex therapy with lesbian couples: a four stage approach, in Psychotherapy with Homosexual Men and Women: Integrated Identity Approaches for Clinical Practice. Edited by Coleman E. New York, Haworth, 1987, pp 137–156

Hatterer L: Changing Homosexuality in the Male. New York, McGraw-Hill, 1970

Heath RG: Pleasure and brain activity in man. J Nerv Ment Dis 154:3–18, 1972

Hencken JD: Homosexuality and psychoanalysis: toward a mutual understanding, in Homosexuality: Research Implications for Public Policy. Edited by Paul W, Weinrich JD. Newbury Park, CA, Sage, 1982

Herek GM: Beyond "homophobia": a social psychological perspective on attitudes toward lesbians and gay men. J Homosex 10:1–21, 1984a

Herek GM: Attitudes toward lesbians and gay men: a factor analytic study. J Homosex 10:39–51, 1984b

Herek G: Heterosexuals' attitudes toward lesbians and gay men: correlates and gender differences. J Sex Res 4:451–477, 1989

Hetrick E, Martin AD: Developmental issues and their resolution for gay and lesbian adolescents, in Psychotherapy with Homosexual Men and Women: Integrated Identity Approaches for Clinical Practice. Edited by Coleman E. New York, Haworth, 1987, pp 25–44

Hetrick E, Stein T (eds): Innovations in Psychotherapy with Homosexuals. Washington, DC, American Psychiatric Press, 1984

Hirschfeld M: Sexual Anomalies. New York, Emerson Books, 1948

Hooker EA: The adjustment of the male overt homosexual. Journal of Projective Techniques 21:17–31, 1957

Isay R: On the analytic therapy of homosexual men. Psychoanal Study Child 40:235–254, 1985

Isay R: Fathers and their homosexually inclined sons in childhood. Psychoanal Study Child 42:275–294, 1987

Johnsgard KW, Schumacher RM: The experience of intimacy in group psychotherapy with male homosexuals. Psychotherapy: Research and Practice 7:173–176, 1970

Kinsey AC, Pomeroy WB, Martin CE: Sexual Behavior in the Human Male. Philadelphia, PA, WB Saunders, 1948

Kinsey AC, Pomeroy WB, Martin CE, et al: Sexual Behavior in the Human Female. Philadelphia, PA, WB Saunders, 1953

Kirkpatrick M: Clinical implications of lesbian mother studies, in Psychotherapy with Homosexual Men and Women: Integrated Identity Approaches for Clinical Practice. Edited by Coleman E. New York, Haworth, 1987, pp 201–212

Levine MP, Troiden RR: The myth of sexual compulsivity. J Sex Res 25:347–364, 1988

Loulan J: Psychotherapy with lesbian mothers, in Contemporary Perspectives on Psychotherapy with Lesbians and Gay Men. Edited by Stein T, Cohen C. New York, Plenum, 1986, pp 181–208

Malyon A: Psychotherapeutic implications of internalized homophobia in gay men, in Homosexuality and Psychotherapy: A Practitioner's Handbook of Affirmative Models. Edited by Gonsiorek JC. New York, Haworth, 1982, pp 59–70

Martin A: Lesbian parenting: a personal odyssey, in Gender in Transition. Edited by Offerman-Zuckerberg J. New York, Plenum, 1989

Martin AD, Hetrick ES: The stigmatization of the gay and lesbian adolescent, in Psychopathology and Psychotherapy in Homosexuality. Edited by Ross MW. New York, Haworth, 1988, pp 163–184

Masters WH, Johnson VE: Homosexuality in Perspective. Boston, MA, Little Brown, 1979

Mattison AM: Group treatment of sexually compulsive gay and bisexual men. Paper presented at the annual meeting of the Eastern Region of the Society for the Scientific Study of Sex, Philadelphia, PA, April 1985

McConaghy N, Proctor D, Barr R: Subjective and penile plethysmography responses to aversion therapy for homosexuality: a partial replication. Arch Sex Behav 2:65–78, 1972

Meyer-Bahlburg HFL: Sex hormones and male homosexuality in comparative perspective. Arch Sex Behav 6:297–326, 1977

Meyer-Bahlburg HFL: Sex hormones and female behavior. Arch Sex Behav 8:101–120, 1979

Meyer-Bahlburg HFL: Psychoendocrine research on sexual orientation: current status and future options. Prog Brain Res 61:375–398, 1984

Myers MF: Counseling the parents of young homosexual male patients, in Homosexuality and Psychotherapy: A Practitioner's Handbook of Affirmative Models. Edited by Gonsiorek JC. New York, Haworth, 1982, pp 131–144

Nicolosi J: Reparative Therapy of Male Homosexuality: A New Clinical Approach. Northvale, NJ, Jason Aronson, 1991

Peplau LA, Amaro H: Understanding lesbian relationships, in Homosexuality and Psychotherapy: A Practitioner's Handbook of Affirmative Models. Edited by Gonsiorek JC. New York, Haworth, 1982, pp 233–248

Quadland MC: Compulsive sexual behavior: definition of a problem and an approach to treatment. J Sex Marital Ther 11:121–132, 1985

Rado S: A critical examination of the concept of bisexuality. Psychosom Med 2:459–467, 1940

Rado S: An adaptational view of sexual behavior, in Psychosexual Development in Health and Disease. Edited by Hoch PH, Zubin J. New York, Grune and Stratton, 1949

Reece R: Causes and treatment of sexual desire discrepancies in male couples, in Psychotherapy with Homosexual Men and Women: Integrated Identity Approaches for Clinical Practice. Edited by Coleman E. New York, Haworth, 1987, pp 157–172

Rieber I, Sigusch V: Guest editorial: psychosurgery on sex offenders and sexual "deviants" in West Germany. Arch Sex Behav 8:523–527, 1979

Ross MW (ed): Psychopathology and Psychotherapy in Homosexuality. New York, Haworth, 1988

Schmidt G: Allies and persecutors: science and medicine in the homosexual issue. J Homosex 10:127–140, 1984

Schmidt G, Schorsch E: Psychosurgery of sexually deviant patients: review and analysis of new empirical findings. Arch Sex Behav 10:301–323, 1981

Sigusch V, Schorsch E, Dannecker M, et al: Official statement by the German Society for Sex Research (Deutsche Gesellschaft fur Sexualforschung e. V.) on the research of Prof. Dr. Gunter Dürner on the subject of homosexuality (guest editorial). Arch Sex Behav 11:445–449, 1982

Silverstein C: A Family Matter: A Parents' Guide to Homosexuality. New York, McGraw-Hill, 1977

Silverstein C: Man to Man: Gay Couples in America. New York, William Morrow, 1981

Silverstein C: The borderline personality and gay people. J Homosex 15:185–212, 1988

Simon W, Gagnon J: Homosexuality: the development of a sociological perspective. J Health Soc Behav 8:177–185, 1967

Smith J: Psychopathology, homosexuality, and homophobia, in Psychopathology and Psychotherapy in Homosexuality. Edited by Ross MW. New York, Haworth, 1988, pp 59–74

Socarides C: Homosexuality. New York, Jason Aronson, 1978

Sonenschein D: Homosexuality as a subject of anthropological inquiry. Anthropological Quarterly 39:73–82, 1966

Sonenschein D: The ethnography of male homosexual relationships. J Sex Res 4, 69–83, 1968

Steakley JD: The Homosexual Emancipation Movement in Germany. New York, Arno Press, 1975

Stein T, Cohen C (eds): Contemporary Perspectives on Psychotherapy with Lesbians and Gay Men. New York, Plenum, 1986

2

Homosexuality and the Mental Health Professions

A Contemporary History

James Krajeski, M.D., M.P.A.

Whereas, homosexuality per se implies no impairment in judgment, stability, reliability, or general social or vocational capabilities, therefore, be it resolved that the American Psychiatric Association [APA] deplores all public and private discrimination against homosexuals in such areas as employment, housing, public accommodation, and licensing, and declares that no burden of proof of such judgment, capacity, or reliability shall be placed upon homosexuals greater than that imposed on any other persons. Further the [APA] supports and urges the enactment of civil rights legislation at the local, state, and federal level that would offer homosexual citizens the same protection now guaranteed to others on the basis of race, creed, color, etc. Further the [APA] supports and urges the repeal of all discriminatory legislation singling out homosexual acts by consenting adults in private. (American Psychiatric Association 1974)

This statement, adopted by the American Psychiatric Association in 1973, evidenced a bold and decisive advance in psychiatric thinking. The position has stood the test of time and remains today as a cornerstone of the American Psychiatric Association's policies regarding homosexuality.

Background

The American Psychiatric Association's position statement is the middle chapter of a saga that began much earlier in the 20th century. As the century unfolded, homosexuality—like many aspects of human existence—provided rich fodder for the ever-expanding theories of American psychiatry and psychology. Because homosexuality was largely viewed in society as a bad outcome, from the theorists' viewpoint it seemed reasonable to assume that there should be pathology to explain it.

Although homosexuality invariably came to be viewed as a defect and a deviation from normal, by no means was there agreement about the exact nature of the presumed pathology. Weinberg and Bell's (1972) comprehensive review of mid-20th-century research and professional literature illustrates the wide variety of viewpoints (also see Chapter 11 by Drescher). Although there was debate about the role of biology in the origin of homosexuality, much of the focus was on psychodynamic formulations. Diverse explanations for homosexuality included immaturity; developmental arrests and conflicts; faulty parenting; and unresolved issues of aggression, dependency, power, or submission. Mental health professionals commonly labeled gay men and lesbians as perverts, deviants, and inverts. These descriptive words were powerful stamps of pathology that gay men and lesbians were to wear as their "scarlet letters."

Even those who were at least somewhat supportive of homosexuality reflected the bias of the larger world. Freud is often quoted from his famous 1935 letter to an American mother as declaring that homosexuality cannot be classified as a mental illness (Freud 1951). Yet in this letter he adds the twist of pathology by declaring that this variation of sexual function is the result of an arrest of sexual development.

The war years of the 1940s created a troublesome relationship between mental health professionals and homosexuality as psychiatrists, in particular, became involved in screening for homosexuality in the military (Berube 1990) (see Chapter 46 by Purcell and Hicks). Although some psychiatrists saw the label of illness as preferable to considering gay men and lesbians to be criminals or moral degenerates, the illness label did not preclude society from also considering them to be criminal and degenerate. Excluding gay men and lesbians from the military on the basis of a presumed psychiatric disorder simply added another justification for stigmatizing these men and women.

By the 1950s many of the dominant names in psychology and psychiatry had come to hold extreme and distorted views of homosexuality. Psychologist Albert Ellis (1965) observed,

> Although I once believed that exclusive homosexuals are seriously neurotic, considerable experience with treating many of them (and in being friendly with a number whom I have not seen for psychotherapy) has convinced me that I was wrong: most fixed homosexuals, I am convinced, are borderline psychotic or outrightly psychotic. (pp. 81–82)

Edmund Bergler (1956), a psychoanalyst, declared,

> though I have no bias . . . homosexuals are essentially disagreeable people. . . . Like all psychic masochists, they are subservient when confronted with a stronger person, merciless when in power, unscrupulous about trampling on a weaker person . . . you seldom find an intact ego . . . among them. (p. 26)

These views were by no means atypical and reflected the flawed state of knowledge and experience of the "experts" of the time.

By the 1960s, certain portentous events were coming together that would provide the sparks for change. Over the years, some gay men and lesbians had become more open about their sexual orientation and more politically active. Gay-oriented organizations began to emerge from hiding. In 1969 a police raid on Stonewall, a gay bar in New York City, proved to be the sentinel event heralding the beginning of the gay liberation movement. Rather than submitting to police action, the patrons of the Stonewall fought back. The Stonewall rebellion became the symbol of release from oppression for gay people.

Within the mental health field, significant changes were also unfolding in the 1950s and 1960s. Psychiatry's exclusive focus on mental illness was beginning to change as clinicians recognized a need to define what was normal (Offer and Sabshin 1966). Szasz (1961) challenged the validity of traditional concepts of mental illness in his popular and provocative book, *The Myth of Mental Illness*. Marmor (1965), who was later to become president of the American Psychiatric Association, presented a synthesis of these themes as they applied to homosexuality. His edited volume on homosexuality explored in substantive ways the concepts of illness and the state of research on homosexuality and raised the question of psychiatry's knowledge base about homosexuality.

The foundation for the view that homosexuality is an illness rested largely on unsupported theories and flawed clinical studies (Gonsiorek 1991). Biases that favored heterosexuality were common in psychological research on homosexuality (Morin 1977). Notable design defects in clinical studies included sampling biases, lack of control subjects, investigator biases, and lack of follow-up on study populations. When researchers began to use standardized instruments and nonpatient populations to look at issues of psychopathology, a different picture emerged.

Hooker published a pivotal work in 1957. Comparing nonclinical samples of gay and nongay men on Rorschach testing protocols, Hooker found no significant difference in psychological adjustment between the two groups. Beginning in the 1960s, many other studies that used standardized psychological instruments began to provide a firm research basis for the finding that homosexuality does not equate with psychopathology (Freedman 1971; Gonsiorek 1982, 1991; Meredith and Reister 1980).

Diagnostic Metamorphosis—From Pathology to Normalcy

The history of homosexuality and mental health is intimately intertwined with the issue of diagnosis. Although in 1917 the American Psychiatric Association adopted a plan for uniform statistics in hospitals for mental disease, subsequently various nomenclatures for diagnosis of mental illness were independently devised by various organizations in the United States (American Psychiatric Association 1952). In the 1930s, an effort was made to standardize all the medical nomenclature. *A Standard Classified Nomenclature of Disease* (National Conference on Nomenclature of Disease 1933) was developed in collaboration with major medical organizations, hospitals, and government agencies. This first edition contained an American Psychiatric Association-approved section on mental disorders that did not mention homosexuality. However, a separate section approved by the American Neurologic Association contained a category of psychopathic personality (sexual perversion).

In 1935 a second edition of the *Standard Classified Nomenclature of Disease* (National Conference on Nomenclature of Disease 1935) contained an expanded section on mental disorders, again approved by the American Psychiatric Association. This time homosexuality was specifically included under psychopathic personality with pathological sexuality.

Apart from the standard classified nomenclature, by the end of the 1940s at least three psychiatric nomenclatures were in general use, none of which was in line with the then-existing International Statistical Classification (American Psychiatric Association 1952). The American Psychiatric Association set about ending this confusing situation by developing a unified national standard. The American Psychiatric Association's first *Diagnostic and Statistical Manual of Mental Disorders* (DSM) was published in 1952. This initial edition of the DSM contained a generic category of sexual deviation as a subset of sociopathic personality disturbance. Homosexuality was mentioned as an example of a sexual deviation along with transvestitism, pedophilia, fetishism, and sexual sadism. This volume succeeded in becoming the diagnostic standard in the United States.

In 1968 a second edition of DSM (American Psychiatric Association 1968) was published. DSM-II listed homosexuality separately as a sexual deviation under the category of personality disorders and certain other nonpsychotic mental disorders. Once again homosexuality shared its status with fetishism, pedophilia, transvestitism, and exhibitionism.

The revision process described in the first two editions of DSM was relatively primitive by current standards. Although there was some collaboration with outside organizations, for the most part the American Psychiatric Association's Committee on Standards and Nomenclature "attempted to put down what it judges to be generally agreed upon by well-informed psychiatrists today" (Gruenberg 1968, p. viii). A draft was circulated in limited numbers—for example, DSM-II was circulated to 120 psychiatrists—and comments were reviewed and reconciled (Gruenberg 1968). Even if the process had been more scientifically sound, in 1952 when the first edition of DSM appeared, a review of the literature would have yielded few sound data about homosexuality. At that time, apart from theoretical formulations, essentially only case reports and anecdotal information about homosexuality were available. When this lack of data is combined with the fact that neither DSM nor DSM-II contained a definition of what constituted a mental disorder or normality, it is apparent that tradition rather than science was behind the inclusion of homosexuality in the diagnostic nomenclature.

Despite the criticisms that might be levied about the manner in which homosexuality came to be a part of the diagnostic nomenclature, the crucial facts are that it was a diagnosis and that it represented the official view that homosexuality was a type of pathology. Because of its control over the diagnostic nomenclature, the American Psychiatric Association became the focus of efforts by gay activists to change the classification of homosexuality. Bayer (1987) described the disruption of the American Psychiatric Association's 1970 annual meeting by gay activists and subsequent events as psychiatrists became mired in controversy over the removal of homosexuality as a disease category.

Framing the Debate

In February 1973 the Northern New England Psychiatric Society, a District Branch of the American Psychiatric Association, called for an end to discrimination against homosexuals and to legal restrictions on sexual acts between consenting adults (District Branch urges revised labeling for homosexuality, March 21, 1973). At the American Psychiatric Association's annual meeting in May 1973, the District Branch submitted a resolution to the Assembly of District Branches to remove homosexuality from the diagnostic nomenclature. Multiple objections were raised, and the resolution was withdrawn for reworking without being voted on (Glasscote 1973a).

At the same meeting a lively presentation of opinions on homosexuality demonstrated the diversity of views at the time. Arguing that homosexuality is not a proper diagnosis, psychiatrist Robert Stoller (1973) declared that the attitude of psychiatry toward homosexuality puts psychiatry in the "role of agent of social control" (p. 3), rather than a healing art and science (Glasscote 1973b). Spitzer (1973), responding to the need to formulate a definition of mental disorder, contended that mental disorders should meet one of two criteria: 1) subjective distress or 2) generalized impairment in social effectiveness or functioning. He argued that homosexuality did not meet either of these criteria because many homosexuals are satisfied with their sexual orientation and do not demonstrate impaired social effectiveness or functioning.

Bieber (1973) expressed the concern that dropping the term "homosexuality" would interfere with "effective prophylaxis." Both Bieber

(1973) and Socarides (1973) cited their clinical research to defend the concept of homosexuality as a psychiatric disorder. They offered differing psychoanalytic explanations of how individuals come to be homosexual as the result of disordered psychosexual development. Marmor (1973) in a sharply worded statement said

> I consider the kind of evidence that Socarides marshals from his clinical practice as essentially meaningless. . . . If our judgment about the mental health of heterosexuals were based only on those whom we see in our clinical practices we would have to conclude that all heterosexuals are also mentally ill. (p. 1211)

Gay activist and writer Ron Gold (1973) gave a personal account of the effects of psychiatry's labels on gay men and women, perhaps best illustrated by the title of his presentation, "Stop It, You're Making Me Sick!" Gold charged that psychiatry "has been the cornerstone of a system of oppression" (p. 1211).

The struggle continued within the American Psychiatric Association over the issue of whether homosexuality was a mental disorder as various components debated the topic. An ad hoc committee to study the definition of homosexuality was established to consider whether homosexuality should be dropped from the list of mental disorders. The resulting recommendation to eliminate the diagnosis of homosexuality from the nomenclature wended its way through the complex American Psychiatric Association structure, eventually being approved by the Council on Research and Development, the Reference Committee, and the Assembly of District Branches (Monroe 1974).

Clarification of the definition of a mental disorder became an important point in the debate. A background report (Spitzer 1974) submitted to the Board of Trustees in 1973 offered the rationale that "clearly homosexuality, per se, does not meet the requirements for a psychiatric disorder since . . . many homosexuals are quite satisfied with their sexual orientation and demonstrate no generalized impairment in social effectiveness or functioning" (p. 11). In what would later be labeled a compromise between two opposing views (Spitzer 1981), the report offered a rationale for the creation of a new diagnostic category, sexual orientation disturbance. This category was to apply to homosexual individuals who were either bothered by, in conflict with, or wished to change their sexual orientation. These individuals were believed to have a mental disorder on the basis of the criterion of subjective distress (Spitzer 1974). At its December 1973 meeting, the Board of Trustees gave its final approval to remove homosexuality from the diagnostic nomenclature and replace it with the diagnosis of Sexual Orientation Disturbance. In a vote behind closed doors, 13 Trustees voted in favor of the change and 2 abstained (Hite 1974).

The American Psychiatric Association had become sensitized to the potential and actual discrimination that resulted from psychiatric labeling. Consequently, at the same time that the issue of homosexuality as a mental disorder was being discussed, the Council on Professions and Associations proposed a position statement urging the repeal of all discriminatory legislation directed at "homosexuals" (Robbins 1974). This statement (reproduced at the beginning of this chapter) was approved by the Board of Trustees at the same meeting in which they removed homosexuality from the diagnostic nomenclature.

◼ Referendum

In an unusual step, the opponents of the action by the Board of Trustees used the American Psychiatric Association's referendum process to attempt to overturn the action of the board. Although the petitioners were decrying the board's action as evidence of a sacrifice of scientific standards, the petitioners themselves opened the process to more extensive criticism. Green (1974) wrote that the referendum "makes a mockery of our specialty and flaunts this mockery in full public view. . . . Decisions [such] as these should be based on a careful, lengthy review of available facts by expert committees on nomenclature and research. This has been done" (p. 2).

The arguments on both sides of the issue paralleled those that had already been aired. In the final vote the decision of the Board of Trustees was upheld by the membership by a majority of 58%. It is noteworthy that this action of the American Psychiatric Association is often misrepresented to make it appear that homosexuality was deleted from the DSM simply by a popular vote. In fact, the decision was made through a formal process similar to that which the American Psychiatric Association continues to use when it makes decisions on scientific issues.

In January 1975 the American Psychological Association's governing Council of Representatives adopted a statement supporting the removal of homosexuality from the nomenclature (Conger 1975). The

Council also adopted a statement opposing discrimination against gay men and lesbians that was nearly identical to that of the American Psychiatric Association. In addition, the American Psychological Association urged "all mental health professionals to take the lead in removing the stigma of mental illness that has long been associated with homosexual orientations" (Conger 1975, p. 633).

Ego-Dystonic Homosexuality

In 1980, with the publication of DSM-III (American Psychiatric Association 1980), the category of sexual orientation disturbance, which had replaced homosexuality in DSM-II, was renamed ego dystonic homosexuality. However, with the proposed revision of DSM-III in the mid-1980s, this category too engendered considerable controversy.

With each revision of DSM, the American Psychiatric Association developed a more extensive and credible review process. The revision of DSM-III involved the creation of advisory bodies on broad diagnostic categories. In the fall of 1985 the Advisory Committee on Sexual Dysfunctions recommended that there be no change in the category of ego dystonic homosexuality, a decision formulated without consultation with the American Psychiatric Association's Committee on Gay, Lesbian, and Bisexual Issues (J. Krajeski, letter to R. Spitzer, April 9, 1986). In fact, the issues had not been reviewed originally in any detail by the Advisory Committee on Sexual Dysfunctions (R. Spitzer, letter to T. Stein, R. Cabaj, J. Krajeski, et al., December 30, 1985). The announcement that the status quo would prevail sparked dissent from both psychologists and psychiatrists.

The dissent led the American Psychiatric Association to hold a December 1985 meeting with representatives of the American Psychological Association and of gay constituents within the American Psychiatric Association. No changes were recommended as a result of the meeting. However, as controversies over other DSM diagnoses intensified, efforts by gay and lesbian members of the American Psychiatric Association and the American Psychological Association generated sufficient pressure for a second rehearing of the ego dystonic homosexuality controversy.

On June 24, 1986, Terry Stein, M.D., Robert Cabaj, M.D., James Krajeski, M.D., and Alan Malyon, Ph.D., met with members of the Advisory Committee on Psychosexual Disorders, the Work Group to Revise DSM-III, the Ad Hoc Committee of the Assembly, and the Board on DSM-III-R. This meeting offered a more substantive airing of the issues. Arguments in favor of retaining the diagnosis centered primarily on the belief that the diagnosis was clinically useful and that it was necessary for research and statistical purposes.

The opposing arguments noted, however, that empirical data do not support the diagnosis, that it is inappropriate to label culturally induced homophobia as a mental disorder, that the diagnosis was rarely used clinically, and that few articles in the scientific literature use the concept (American Psychiatric Association 1987; P. Cabaj et al., unpublished observations, June 24, 1986).

The Ad Hoc Committee was convinced by the arguments and recommended the elimination of the diagnosis of ego dystonic homosexuality. The only remnant left in DSM-III-R was "persistent and marked distress about one's sexual orientation," which was listed as one example of sexual disorder not otherwise specified. All the examples in this category addressed distress over some aspect of sexuality. Four days later the Board of Trustees approved the draft revision.

What was remarkable about this episode was that for the first time openly gay psychiatrists and psychologists played a significant role in bringing about the changes. Not content with the initial cursory review and rejection, they mobilized their arguments and forces within their respective professional organizations to ensure that there was a substantial and fair hearing of the issues. By succeeding in eliminating ego dystonic homosexuality as a diagnosis, they rid the mental health profession of a diagnostic relic that had indirectly, if not directly, perpetuated the mental illness model of homosexuality. The diagnostic change was one more crucial step in a paradigm shift that would impel mental health professionals to turn their focus to more relevant models and concepts in understanding gay men and lesbians.

Assimilation of Gay Men and Lesbians

■ Psychology

The first organized lobbying efforts on behalf of gay and lesbian psychologists were initiated in 1973 with the Association of Gay Psychologists' Caucus meeting at the annual meeting of the American Psychological Association (American Psychological Association 1979). In 1974 the American Psychological Association established a Task Force on the Status of Lesbian and Gay Male Psychologists, which provided a final report in 1979. A Committee on Gay Concerns was then established within the American Psychological Association in 1980. The name was changed to the Committee on Lesbian and Gay Concerns in 1985. In 1984 the American Psychological Association approved the establishment of the Society for the Psychological Study of Lesbian and Gay Issues as Division 44 (Committee on Lesbian and Gay Concerns 1991).

◼ Psychiatry

Gay and lesbian psychiatrists met informally for many years during the course of the annual meetings of the American Psychiatric Association. In 1978 at the annual meeting, a formal structure was adopted for the Gay, Lesbian, and Bisexual Caucus of the American Psychiatric Association ("Spiegel visits business meeting: structure voted" 1978), which is now named the Association of Gay and Lesbian Psychiatrists.

Within the official American Psychiatric Association structure, a Task Force on Gay, Lesbian, and Bisexual Issues was established in 1978. This group was given formal status as a standing committee in 1981. In 1982 the Assembly of District Branches approved the addition of gay and lesbian representatives to be elected from a group initially designated as the Caucus of Homosexually Identified Psychiatrists, but subsequently renamed the Caucus of Lesbian, Gay and Bisexual psychiatrists.

◼ Social Work

The Delegate Assembly of the National Association of Social Workers (NASW) adopted its first Public Policy Statement on Gay Issues in 1977. In 1979 a Task Force on Lesbian and Gay Issues was appointed. In June 1982 the NASW Board of Directors established the National Committee on Lesbian and Gay Issues, which became a by-laws–mandated committee in 1993 (NASW Fact Sheet, March 21, 1994).

■ Results of Assimilation

The assimilation of gay men and lesbians into professional organizations has several important ramifications. Well-functioning gay and lesbian mental health professionals provide role models to dispel stereotypes far more effectively than abstract descriptions in books and lectures might do. Most important, the assimilation of gay men and lesbians gives members of these groups access similar to that enjoyed by other members. Gay-related issues can be introduced and spearheaded by those most invested in, and often those most familiar with, the issues.

As a result, mental health organizations have adopted numerous position statements on issues important to gay men and lesbians. Assimilation also has fostered legislative, judicial, and public policy actions by the mental health organizations supporting gay-affirmative positions at local, state, and national levels. Still, many issues are not addressed. The subject of bisexuality is often ignored, and the needs of gay, lesbian, and bisexual minority individuals and persons from special populations such as adolescents and the elderly are often given less attention than desirable. Yet overall, mechanisms are in place that can permit these issues to be addressed, providing a crucial legacy within the mental health field to gay men, lesbians, and bisexuals.

Conclusion

The brief history presented in this chapter addresses only major trends and events of the 20th century relevant to homosexuality and mental health. What it does not convey is the very personal effect that these events had on the everyday lives of millions of individuals. The label of illness sanctioned discrimination whether or not it was intended to do so. The repercussions from the old views of homosexuality as illness persist to this day, as those who oppose equality for gay men and lesbians still frequently revert to an illness model to justify discrimination.

The history of homosexuality and mental health has much to say about the mental health field in general. It exposes many of the flaws inherent in a diagnostic system. It highlights the difficulties in differentiating scientific views of mental health or illness from religious and moral views of society. However, it also demonstrates strengths, as we see mental health organizations capable of adapting to changing knowledge. The same organizations that contributed to the stigmatization of gay men and lesbians became instrumental in the struggle to end discrimination and prejudice, to provide education and support, and to validate the lives and experiences of gay men and lesbians. The chronicle of these sweeping changes of the past century presents a truly remarkable history.

References

American Psychiatric Association: Diagnostic and Statistical Manual of Mental Disorders. Washington, DC, American Psychiatric Association, 1952

American Psychiatric Association: Diagnostic and Statistical Manual of Mental Disorders, 2nd Edition. Washington, DC, American Psychiatric Association, 1968

American Psychiatric Association: Diagnostic and Statistical Manual of Mental Disorders, 3rd Edition. Washington, DC, American Psychiatric Association, 1980

American Psychiatric Association: Diagnostic and Statistical Manual of Mental Disorders, 3rd Edition, Revised. Washington, DC, American Psychiatric Association, 1987

American Psychiatric Association: Position statement on homosexuality and civil rights. Am J Psychiatry 131:497, 1974

American Psychological Association: Removing the Stigma: Final Report of the Board of Social and Ethical Responsibility for Psychology's Task Force on the Status of Lesbian and Gay Male Psychologists. Washington, DC, American Psychological Association, 1979

Bayer R: Homosexuality and American Psychiatry. Princeton, NJ, Princeton University Press, 1987

Bergler E: Homosexuality: Disease or Way of Life? New York, Collier Books, 1956

Berube A: Coming Out Under Fire. New York, Free Press, 1990

Bieber I: Homosexuality—an adaptive consequence of disorder in psychosexual development. Am J Psychiatry 130:1209–1211, 1973

Committee on Lesbian and Gay Concerns: American Psychological Association Policy Statements on Lesbian and Gay Issues. Washington, DC, American Psychological Association, 1991

Conger JJ: Proceedings of the American Psychological Association, Incorporated, for the year 1974: minutes of the annual meeting of the Council of Representatives. Am Psychol 30:620–651, 1975

District Branch urges revised labeling for homosexuality. Psychiatric News, March 21, 1973, p 1

Ellis A: Homosexuality: Its Causes and Cure. New York, Lyle Stuart, 1965

Freedman M: Homosexuality and Psychological Functioning. Belmont, CA, Brooks/Cole, 1971

Freud S: Historical notes: a letter from Freud (1935). Am J Psychiatry 107:786–787, 1951

Spiegel visits business meeting: structure voted. Gay, Lesbian and Bisexual Caucus of the American Psychiatric Association Newsletter, June 1978, pp 1–2

Glasscote RM: Homosexuality and American Psychiatric Association—the issues are joined. Psychiatric News, June 6, 1973a, pp 18–19

Glasscote RM: Homosexuality issue—disorder or lifestyle? Psychiatric News, June 20, 1973b, pp 3, 27

Gold R: Stop it, you're making me sick! Am J Psychiatry 130:1211–1212, 1973

Gonsiorek JC: Results of psychological testing on homosexual populations, in Homosexuality Social, Psychological, and Biological Issues. Edited by Weinrich PW, Gonsiorek JC, Hotvedt ME. Beverly Hills, CA, Sage, 1982, pp 71–88

Gonsiorek JC: The empirical basis for the demise of the illness model of homosexuality, in Homosexuality Research Implications for Public Policy. Edited by Gonsiorek JC, Weinrich JD. Newbury Park, CA, Sage, 1991, pp 115–136

Green R: Letter to the editor. Psychiatric News, April 3, 1974, p 2

Gruenberg EM: Foreword, in Diagnostic and Statistical Manual of Mental Disorders, 2nd Edition. Washington, DC, American Psychiatric Association, 1968, pp vii–x

Hite C: American Psychiatric Association rules homosexuality not necessarily a disorder. Psychiatric News, January 2, 1974, p 1, 6, 16

Hooker E: The adjustment of the male overt homosexual. Journal of Projective Techniques 21:18–31, 1957

Marmor J (ed): Sexual Inversion the Multiple Roots of Homosexuality. New York, Basic Books, 1965

Marmor J: Homosexuality and cultural value systems. Am J Psychiatry 130:1208–1209, 1973

Meredith RL, Reister RW: Psychotherapy, responsibility and homosexuality: clinical examination of socially deviant behavior. Professional Psychology 11:174–193, 1980

Monroe RR: The Council on Research and Development. Am J Psychiatry 131:486–487, 1974

Morin SF: Heterosexual bias in psychological research on lesbianism and male homosexuality. Am Psychol 32:629–637, 1977

National Conference on Nomenclature of Disease: A Standard Classified Nomenclature of Disease. New York, Commonwealth Fund, 1993

National Conference on Nomenclature of Disease: Standard Classified Nomenclature of Disease, 2nd Edition. Chicago, IL, American Medical Association, 1935

Offer D, Sabshin M: Normality Theoretical and Clinical Concepts of Mental Health. New York, Basic Books, 1966

Robbins LL: The Council on Professions and Associations. Am J Psychiatry 131:490–491, 1974

Socarides CW: Homosexuality: findings derived from 15 years of clinical research. Am J Psychiatry 130:1212–1213, 1973

Spitzer RL: A proposal about homosexuality and the American Psychiatric Association nomenclature: homosexuality as an irregular form of sexual behavior and sexual orientation disturbance as a psychiatric disorder. Am J Psychiatry 130:1214–1216, 1973

Spitzer RL: Homosexuality decision—a background paper. Psychiatric News, January 16, 1974, pp 11–12

Spitzer RL: The diagnostic status of homosexuality in DSM-III: a reformulation of the issues. Am J Psychiatry 138:210–215, 1981

Stoller RJ: Criteria for psychiatric diagnosis. Am J Psychiatry 130: 1207–1209, 1973

Szasz TS: The Myth of Mental Illness. New York, Harper & Row, 1961

Weinberg MS, Bell AP: Homosexuality: An Annotated Bibliography. New York, Harper & Row, 1972

Gay, Lesbian, and Bisexual Mental Health Professionals and Their Colleagues

Robert P. Cabaj, M.D.

The profound changes over the past decade in the way mental health and medical professionals view homosexuality came about as a result of the extraordinary efforts of many individuals. Many professional disciplines, including psychiatry, other medical fields, psychology, nursing, social work, and law, played a role and continue to assist in this ongoing process. Chapters 1 and 2 present a history of the efforts to change professional approaches to homosexuality and to improve the treatment of gay men and lesbians; in this chapter the author describes some of the individuals and organizations involved but primarily explores what it is like to be an openly gay, lesbian, or bisexual professional today.

Individual Efforts in the Evolution of Modern Thinking on Homosexuality

Heterosexual professionals share the stage with gay, lesbian, and bisexual colleagues in facilitating the changes in thinking on homosexuality.

33

Attempts to instill positive attitudes about homosexuals, when initiated by gay people, are often dismissed as political or self-serving by those who wish to see gay people as mentally ill or undeserving of the protection of civil rights. Heterosexual colleagues speaking out on gay issues have thus stimulated and helped make possible many of the advances in thinking.

Sigmund Freud set a positive tone for the recognition of civil rights for gay men, lesbians, and bisexuals when he supported the acceptance of colleagues who happened to be homosexual into medical and psychiatric societies (Freud 1921/1977). Sexual orientation by itself, he believed, in no way impaired judgment or caused problems in delivering medical or psychiatric care by a homosexual colleague (Freud 1903). Although his thinking on homosexuality was not entirely clear, he did believe in innate bisexuality and in a biological contribution to sexual orientation (see Chapter 11 by Drescher).

Despite Freud's opinions, European psychoanalysts and psychoanalytic organizations were not welcoming of or friendly to homosexuals in the early years of psychiatry. Many American psychiatrists, especially the psychoanalytic leaders, were hostile and promoted the notion that homosexuality was a mental disorder. Changing that point of view would have been more difficult without the help of Judd Marmor, M.D. As he describes in Chapter 32 and as supported by the statements from the psychologist, Evelyn Hooker, Ph.D., in the epilogue, Marmor championed new thinking about homosexuality and new approaches to the treatment of gay men and lesbians. Many other heterosexual and gay psychiatrists, including a psychiatrist disguised as "Dr. X" at a 1972 American Psychiatric Association meeting, reveal that there were, indeed, gay and lesbian psychiatrists who played important roles in helping to change attitudes about homosexuality.

Hooker can be credited with initiating the acceptance of changes in thinking about homosexuality within the mental health field, and psychologists have continued to take the lead in writing and promoting new psychotherapeutic approaches. Many psychologists, sociologists, and sociobiologists have written extensively about issues of concern to gay men, lesbians, and bisexuals and have helped with many of the social and civil rights advances for these persons. In addition, social workers, nurses, nonpsychiatric medical professionals, mental health counselors, teachers, researchers, and historians have contributed significantly to changing attitudes about homosexuality; formulating better clinical treatment for gay men, lesbians, and bisexuals; and fighting political battles for the civil rights of sexual minorities.

Local and national organizations also have contributed to the evolution of new thinking about homosexuality and bisexuality and to new approaches to treatment of lesbians, gay men, and bisexuals. Strong leadership has been shown by the Association of Gay and Lesbian Psychiatrists; Division 44 of the American Psychological Association—the Society for the Scientific Study of Lesbian and Gay Concerns; the Gay and Lesbian Medical Association (formerly known as the American Association of Physicians for Human Rights); the Lesbian, Gay, and Bisexual People in Medicine Committee of the American Medical Student Association; the National Association of Lesbian and Gay Alcoholism Professionals; the National Lesbian and Gay Health Association; the National Gay and Lesbian Task Force; and the Human Rights Campaign Fund.

New research, studies, ideas, and treatment recommendations about homosexuality and gay men, lesbians, bisexuals, and transgendered people are enjoying wider acceptance in the established and traditional professional literature. However, resistance to accepting such material in established journals and growth in available studies led to the establishment of new professional journals devoted to the field, including the *Journal of Homosexuality,* the *Journal of Gay and Lesbian Psychotherapy,* and a proposed journal on gay and lesbian health issues.

Despite ongoing resistance, progress continues in helping professionals and the public to become more aware of new ideas and findings regarding homosexuality. Hopefully, a collaborative effort by heterosexual, gay, lesbian, and bisexual colleagues will guide future research, education, gay-sensitive and gay-affirmative treatment approaches, planning for gay and lesbian treatment centers, and political and civil rights efforts in these areas.

Coming Out as a Medical and Mental Health Professional

Many gay, lesbian, and bisexual professionals in powerful roles did not, and do not, voluntarily come out as gay, lesbian, or bisexual, depriving many other professionals of the opportunity to learn from their peers and denying their own capacity to serve as role models for the public. As a result of continued societal homophobia and internalized homophobia, many professionals do not feel able to come out. Sometimes "closeted" professionals even take positions harmful to gay people. For example, Harry Stack Sullivan felt that he could not be public about his homosexuality, and in the 1940s, he helped establish the attempts by the United States military to screen out homosexuals during the induction interview and physical.

Lesbian, gay, and bisexual mental health and medical providers may face many issues if they are open about sexual orientation. The process of coming out, or being public about one's sexual orientation, is a major developmental process for anyone with a sexual orientation other than heterosexual (see Chapter 14 by Cass). Lesbian, gay, and bisexual professionals need to negotiate how to come out both personally and professionally.

The personal process, recognizing a sexual orientation that is different from the majority and then accepting and deciding to act on that recognition, is not necessarily linked to age or career development. Although most gay men and lesbians are aware of their sexual orientation in childhood or adolescence, any one individual may not become fully aware or accepting of a nonheterosexual sexual orientation until later in life. Many mental health and medical professionals put education and career development ahead of personal and social development and may not become consciously aware of differences in sexual orientation until later in life. A provider in training may thus simultaneously be developing an identity as a professional and as a lesbian, gay, or bisexual person.

Coming out is an individual and personalized process, progressing through several stages via a route that is neither uniform nor standard. One of the simplest models of coming out consists of the three stages of *must not*, *must*, and *choice* (Hanley-Hackenbruck 1988). After an individual does recognize a differing sexual orientation, he or she negotiates the individual process of self-acceptance, often going through the *must not* stage of denial, refusing to accept what is becoming more apparent, thereby reflecting the societal disapproval of homosexuality. After learning to accept the difference and developing a self-identity that includes a gay, lesbian, or bisexual sexual orientation (the *must* stage), the individual can make choices about how to act on his or her difference and about who will get to share the knowledge of the difference (the *choice* stage).

The extent of coming out is largely the result of a personal choice; individuals must be able to negotiate various steps as described. The phenomenon of *outing* (i.e., someone else announces an individual's sexual orientation without his or her permission) does not respect this choice or respect the individual. Proponents of outing believe it is beneficial to have as many out gay, lesbian, and bisexual people as possible to demonstrate how many homosexual people there really are and to try and influence public opinion in a positive way. After being forced out of the closet, such an individual, however, may not be able to handle the public exposure, may not have developed the psychological tools to handle being out, and is generally not able, at least initially, to serve as a positive role model.

The individual's internal psychological matrix will interact with career and life choices throughout the career of the gay, lesbian, and bisexual professional. The complex balance between the level of internalized homophobia, the acceptance from family and friends of coming out, and the community and professional support the individual has will affect when an individual feels able to come out. If all the components of the system are not supportive of a gay, lesbian, or bisexual sexual orientation, the level of comfort in coming out professionally for a particular individual will be significantly diminished. Conversely, having less internalized homophobia, supportive family and friends, and a strong connection with a gay, lesbian, or bisexual network may make it much easier to be out as a gay, lesbian, or bisexual professional.

When entering a professional training program, an individual who is cognizant of a gay, lesbian, or bisexual sexual orientation faces decisions about who should know and what role sexual orientation should have in career choices. As discussed in Chapter 39 by Atkins and Townsend, applicants to professional training programs will need to decide whether they will self-disclose to people who have power in the selection process, risking the consequences of covert homophobia. If selected without being publicly out, such individuals need to consider whether they will come out to classmates and work colleagues during their training. When beginning a position, practice, or career, gay, lesbian, and bisexual individuals need to choose whether to be open about their sexual orientation with colleagues or with potential patients and clients, risking ostracization or diminished referrals. Many professionals believe they can be out in one or more parts of their lives (e.g., with colleagues, patients, friends, or family) and not have those parts affect one another.

Possible benefits to being more publicly out include serving as a role model for other professionals or providers in training; being in a position to confront bias or prejudice at work sites or in professional organizations; helping to support other gay, lesbian, and bisexual colleagues; and, in turn, seeking support or help as needed if problems occur as a result of being out. In areas with a large gay, lesbian, and bisexual community, the openly gay provider might find a steady patient referral base or find employment in a position involving work with lesbians, gay men, and bisexuals.

Psychological benefits also may result from being open and not compartmentalizing various aspects of one's life. Being open professionally and socially may result in a more integrated identity and help reduce anxiety, fear, or paranoia about possible discovery or exposure. A lesbian, gay, or bisexual sexual identity fully integrated with a professional identity can result in improved professional and social fulfillment.

The adverse consequences of coming out, however, are not minimal. Professional and societal homophobia is real and can affect any lesbian, gay, or bisexual provider. The bias can come from patients who might not be comfortable in seeing a gay, lesbian, or bisexual provider or it may come from colleagues and professional organizations. For example, Matthews et al. (1986) surveyed 930 physicians in San Diego County about their attitude toward homosexuality. In this study, 30% of the respondents would not admit a highly qualified applicant to medical school if they knew that the applicant was gay or lesbian; 40% would discourage a gay or lesbian medical student from entering a psychiatric or pediatric residency; 40% would stop referring to a colleague who was found out to be gay or lesbian, regardless of past referral history with that colleague; and 40% reported being uncomfortable caring for a gay or lesbian patient. A 1990 survey (McGrory et al. 1990) of third-year New York medical students did not reveal such negative attitudes, but the students estimated that more than 25% of their peers and 50% of their faculty did have such negative attitudes about gay men and lesbians.

Coming out may jeopardize career or academic advancement, depending on the location and the attitudes of the directors of programs and people in the decision-making roles. Geography also may play a role. For example, coming out in a large city may provide some anonymity regarding patient referrals, whereas being open in a small town or rural area may preclude such confidentiality. Work settings also may influence coming out. A provider who depends solely on private practice may be more concerned about referrals, whereas a provider working in a public health setting or in an administrative position may feel protected from that concern. A provider working in a school system or with children and adolescents in other settings may feel more constrained in coming out, because of societal homophobia, which often mistakenly links homosexuality and child molestation.

The degree of openness about their sexual orientation for many gay, lesbian, and bisexual professionals can reflect a wish to teach or do research about homosexuality or to provide direct clinical care for gay men, lesbians, bisexuals, and transgendered people. Career paths such as these, hopefully, indicate an emerging trend that will allow more professionals to come out, enhance personal self-esteem, be a role model for others, and serve as providers for care of the gay, lesbian, bisexual, and transgendered patient.

In summary, although the possible negative consequences of coming out are real, a gay, lesbian, or bisexual professional also may find that coming out enhances a career and contributes to a more integrated personal life and personality. The greatest benefit, however, may be one to society itself or at least to homophobic individuals. As Herek indicates in Chapter 7, homophobia and heterosexism are reduced in individuals who personally know more than two gay, lesbian, or bisexual people. Therefore, openly gay, lesbian, and bisexual professionals, merely by being open about their sexual orientation, mount a major assault on homophobia and the many harmful effects it has on society.

References

Freud S: Interview. Die Zeit, Vienna, p 5, October 27, 1903

Freud S: Letter to Ernst Jones, 1921. Reprinted in Body Politic, Toronto, Canada, p 9, May, 1977

Hanley-Hackenbruck P: "Coming-out" and psychotherapy. Psychiatric Annals 18:29–32, 1988

Matthews W, Booth MW, Turner J, et al: Physicians attitudes toward homosexuality: survey of a California county medical society. West J Med 144:106–110, 1986

McGrory BJ, McDowell DM, Muskin PR: Medical students' attitudes toward AIDS, homosexual, and intravenous drug-abusing patients: a re-evaluation in New York City. Psychosomatics 31:426–433, 1990

SECTION II

Understanding Homosexuality and Bisexuality

Demographic, Cultural, Genetic, Biological, and Psychological Perspectives

The Prevalence of Homosexuality in the United States

Stuart Michaels, Ph.D.

Estimates of the prevalence of homosexuality in the United States have generated a great deal of interest and controversy. Media attention to homosexuality in general, and to the issue of prevalence in particular, has increased as a result of a number of factors, including the HIV/AIDS crisis and political struggles over civil rights for lesbians and gay men. Debate has been recently reinvigorated by the appearance of prevalence estimates from a number of probability surveys of sexual behavior in this country and in Europe. These surveys, largely a response to the AIDS crisis, have produced estimates of the prevalence of various measures of homosexuality much lower than those from the famous Kinsey studies (Kinsey et al. 1948, 1953).

Determining the prevalence of homosexuality is not as simple as might first appear. Although recent large-scale, sophisticated population surveys of sexuality (Billy et al. 1993; Catania et al. 1992; Laumann et al. 1994; Spira et al. 1993; Wellings et al. 1994) represent a major advance in the production of prevalence data, a great deal of confusion remains about surveys, what questions they can answer, and how to interpret the results they provide. Much of this confusion has nothing to do with surveys themselves but rather with the lack of conceptual clarity about the nature and definition of homosexuality. This is often confounded by methodological problems in surveys, which have led some (particularly in the gay and lesbian community) to the wholesale rejection of the results of these surveys because they do not fit with their preconceptions (e.g., that 10% of the population is gay). However, rejection of empirical evidence that does not fit preexisting beliefs is dangerous. Instead, the results of these surveys should be studied carefully for what they can tell us about the world. This chapter clarifies some of these conceptual issues, reviews prior prevalence data, and examines in detail some key results of the most comprehensive scientific survey of sexual behavior in the United States to date (Laumann et al. 1994).

Concepts and Terms: Practice Versus the Person and Homosexuality Versus the Homosexual

Much of the confusion regarding prevalence arises from the blurring of a crucial distinction between specific same-gender sexual experiences (both behavior and feelings) and the categorization of persons as homosexual. The meaning and implications of the presence or absence of certain types of sexual behavior or desire are the subject of intense theoretical debate (Stein 1992) and are discussed in Chapter 6 by Stein. However, when doing population surveys, it makes the most sense to focus on specific experiences that can be inquired about through clear, direct interview questions without labeling a person as homosexual or heterosexual. An additional advantage is that, by analytically separating the various elements of homosexuality such as behavior and feelings, one can investigate their interrelationship. For these reasons, "homosexuality," "homosexual" (as an adjective rather than a noun), and "same-gender" are the primary terms used in this chapter. They are meant to be descriptive, and the reader should avoid inferring more than that, such as a biological model, male gender connotations, or theories of etiology. Terms such as "gay," "lesbian," "bisexual," and "heterosexual" are generally avoided, especially as nouns or descriptors of persons rather than practices. "Gay" and "lesbian" seem too closely tied to the idea of a modern gay culture and community and the social roles or identities that exist therein, although these terms are often used as equivalent to "homosexual" in expressions such as "gay sex."

In a discussion of prevalence, it is important to avoid confusing homosexuality with the notion of the homosexual. The latter is closely tied to the search for a single estimate of the number or proportion of (true or real) homosexual individuals. However, the presumptions built into this approach merit careful consideration. It presumes that two clearly delineated, distinguishable groups exist: homosexual persons and nonhomosexual persons. Furthermore, it presumes that the distinguishing quality or trait used to classify people is homogeneous across individuals and stable over time, both in individuals' lives and across historical periods. Typically, researchers have used indicators such as the presence or absence of any homosexual experience or exclusive homosexual experience. Although nothing is inherently wrong with this approach, the danger arises when one moves, often quite subtly, from this sort of simple and arbitrary operation of grouping to the conceptual distinction between homosexual and nonhomosexual individuals as types of persons and then quickly to the inference of all sorts of other psychological, social, and sexual associations for individuals in one group or the other. In response to recent surveys, the media and others have treated measures of homosexual behavior (e.g., any same-gender partners in specific time periods or ever), desire (e.g., any attraction to persons of one's own gender), and identity (e.g., any self-identification as homosexual) as if they were equivalent to each other and also to the conceptual entity, the "homosexual or gay population." Therefore, in interpreting research results, it is very important to be attentive to what is actually being measured and reported.

The Kinsey Research and 10%

For 40 years, the major data on the prevalence of homosexual activity in the United States were the two volumes written by Kinsey and his colleagues after World War II, *Sexual Behavior in the Human Male* (Kinsey et al. 1948) and *Sexual Behavior in the Human Female* (Kinsey et al. 1953). Kinsey's work is cited as the basis for the widely accepted notion that 10% of the population is homosexual, although Kinsey never reported this and explicitly argued against this type of categorization. These volumes were the result of an important pioneering effort to study the distribution of sexual behavior in a broad cross-section of the

American population. Kinsey was a zoologist who applied the same sampling approach to humans that he had used in studying insects. He assumed it was impossible to randomly select people and then interview them about their sexual experiences. Therefore, all of the respondents were volunteers actively solicited by the researchers (Gebhard and Johnson 1979; Kinsey et al. 1948).

The Kinsey studies primarily emphasized behavior, especially sexual practices that led to orgasm. Kinsey rejected the notion that people were divided into the categories heterosexual, homosexual, or bisexual. Instead, he believed that everyone was capable of both homosexual and heterosexual responses and that individuals should be described in terms of the distribution of their total experiences along a seven-point "heterosexual-homosexual" continuum, from 0 to 6. Within this framework, Kinsey tabulated and presented his data on homosexual experience, and what he found was extremely surprising to the public at the time. Of the more than 4,000 white men who were studied, 37% had had "at least some overt homosexual experience to the point of orgasm between adolescence and old age"; 25% had had "more than incidental homosexual experience or reactions for at least 3 years between the ages of 16 and 55" (values of 2 through 6); 10% were "more or less exclusively homosexual for at least 3 years between the ages of 16 and 55" (values of 5 and 6); and 4% were "exclusively homosexual throughout their lives, after the onset of adolescence" (values of 6) (Kinsey et al. 1948, pp. 650–651). In the research on sexual behavior in women, Kinsey did not provide as extensive a summary of the data but did state that the rates were much lower for women, about one-half to one-third of those for men. For example, only 13% of the women had ever had a sexual experience to orgasm with another woman, in contrast to 37% of men (Kinsey et al. 1953).

The work of Kinsey et al. had a profound influence on the thinking about homosexuality and the move to treat it as nonpathological. This was, in large part, because of his nonmedical, nonclinical approach as a population biologist interested in variation within species. Unfortunately, in subsequent discussions, Kinsey's sympathetic thinking about homosexuality has become associated with the rates of homosexual behavior that he reported. Although there is no necessary relationship between prevalence and normality or health in any moral or biological sense, behaviors engaged in by more than one-third of the male population are at least common. This finding has often been used to argue for the normality and acceptability of homosexuality.

The Kinsey research had a number of design characteristics that tended to inflate the amount of homosexuality found, particularly among men. Primary among these are the inclusion of men from all-male institutions such as prisons and reform schools, the inclusion of men from gay social networks, and the use of volunteers (who are likely to have been more comfortable with their sexuality and more sexually active and experienced than those who were unwilling to be interviewed). On the other hand, there are indications that the interviewing techniques of Kinsey et al. and the use of a small group of highly trained interviewers (Kinsey himself interviewed more than half the men) may have helped reduce some of the typical underreporting of homosexuality, as well as other stigmatized behaviors such as masturbation. In addition, the researchers included adolescent experiences in ways that have often been subsequently ignored. For example, the 10% rate for white men refers to predominant homosexual behavior for 3 years or more between the ages of 16 and 55 years. Thus, adolescent experiences with other boys and experiences before marriage were included along with much longer-standing and extensive experiences that would be expected in a developing or life-long homosexual identity.

Kinsey made no estimates of the proportion of the population that should be considered homosexual. Those most familiar with the data have, when pressed, made more cautious estimates than the 10% that has become widespread in the media recently. Gebhard, one of Kinsey's main collaborators and the director of the Institute for Sex Research that Kinsey founded, constructed a reasoned estimate that "about 4% of the white college-educated adult males are predominantly homosexual" and that "in the total adult female population, the incidence of predominantly homosexual individuals is between 1 and 2%, probably nearer 1" (Gebhard 1972, pp. 27–28). Similarly, Gagnon and Simon (1973) reanalyzed the Kinsey data to show that much of the reported homosexual behavior occurred in adolescence.

Research on Sexual Behavior and Homosexuality After Kinsey

Surprisingly, it took a long time for researchers to attempt to replicate and improve on the work of Kinsey et al., particularly given that its major statistical problem (the lack of a probability-based sample) was authoritatively identified within a few years of the publication of the first volume (Cochran et al. 1954). Only under the press of AIDS did governments, social scientists, and private foundations begin to become acutely aware of the lack of adequate information about sexual behavior (Institute of Medicine 1986). The AIDS epidemic also highlighted the importance of knowledge specifically about male-male sex. Information on the number of men who are homosexually active, their sexual practices, the number of partners they have, and the proportion who have sex with both men and women was needed to help project the future course of the epidemic and to target interventions to prevent its spread further. This need led to an extremely careful and sophisticated analysis of behavioral data on sex between men from a 1970 Kinsey Institute study (Fay et al. 1989). At about the same time, a small amount of data became available from the addition of a few sex questions to the General Social Survey (GSS), an annual survey fielded by the National Opinion Research Center. These data provided some corroboration of the results of the 1970 study. A review and comparison of 1988 through 1990 data from the GSS, the 1970 Kinsey Institute study, and a 1989 study of male-male sexual behavior in Dallas were published by Rogers and Turner (1991). They concluded that "roughly 5 to 7% of American men *report* some same-gender sexual contact in adulthood . . . that reported prevalence is somewhat higher for men living in urbanized areas. . . . These survey estimates . . . are best treated as lower bounds on the actual prevalence of such contact" (Rogers and Turner 1991, pp. 513–514; emphasis in original).

In response to the growing AIDS crisis, major government-initiated surveys of adult sexual behavior have been carried out in a number of countries, including France, Great Britain, and the United States. Conservative governments in Great Britain and the United States withdrew support for their national surveys, which were completed with private foundation support. These surveys all used probability samples and, in France and Great Britain, were based on large national samples (20,055 and 18,876 persons, respectively); the American study (Laumann et al. 1994) had a smaller sample (3,432 persons). The French study was done by telephone, whereas the English and American studies were done by interviews in households. Although these surveys were done independently by different teams of researchers, they share a number of traits. All used modern survey research methods and organizations to draw high-quality representative samples of the adult populations in their respective countries. These were not primarily studies of homosexuality; rather, they investigated the distribution of a range of sexual behaviors in as broad a cross-section of the adult population as was feasible with available limited resources. Although motivated by the AIDS crisis, the studies focused not on high-risk populations but on the distribution of specific behaviors in the entire adult population. This is the preferable design for estimating the prevalence of homosexuality in the population. However, because the rate of reported homosexual experience is relatively low, this design is not optimal for generating large probability samples of homosexually active persons; these samples are too small to allow for extensive analysis.

Measurement of Homosexuality in Survey Research

■ Definition of Homosexuality in Survey Research

Survey research uses a standardized questionnaire to interview a representative sample of a clearly defined population. The great advantage and power of this approach derive from being able to generalize in a precise and cost-efficient way from a sample to a much larger population. The use of probability sampling also largely removes the unmeasurable biases that may be introduced by any sort of purposive or convenience samples.

The problems of conceptualization previously discussed apply in the survey research interview just as they did in the Kinsey interviews. It makes more sense to inquire about specific behaviors and experiences than to inquire about vague concepts such as whether persons are homosexual or heterosexual. Respondents need to be convinced that the research is legitimate, that all answers will be treated with the utmost confidentiality, and that they themselves will not be identifiable. The way that questions are asked also is important. Although there is a lack of accumulated research in this area, certain obvious principles can be followed. Questions should be asked in a way that is clear and unambiguous, and a nonjudgmental attitude must be communicated so that respondents will answer as honestly as possible. A number of techniques are used to accomplish these goals. First, professional interviewers are trained to convey a sympathetic but neutral and non-judgmental attitude. The language and phrasing of questions are constructed to help legitimize all answers. For example, the terms "homosexual" and "heterosexual" should be avoided when asking about sexual behavior. Instead, questions should be asked about sexual experience with both men and women. Questions can be asked that assume that a behavior is likely to have occurred, as in "How old were you the first time you had sex with a (person of the same gender as the respondent)?" In face-to-face interviews, the reporting of some stigmatized behaviors has been shown to increase with the use of techniques such as self-administered questionnaires that the respondents complete and return in a sealed envelope (Bradburn 1983).

Recent Surveys

The major focus of recent large-scale national sex surveys has been on behavior (ACSF Investigators 1992; Johnson et al. 1992; Laumann et al. 1994; Spira et al. 1993; Wellings et al. 1994), with most of the data on homosexuality based on responses to questions about sexual partners and practices. Questions about behavior are always, explicitly or implicitly, relative to a specific time frame. Typically, questions were asked about the gender of sexual partners in time frames such as the last week, month, year, or several years, since a particular age (e.g., since age 16 or 18 years), or ever. These are not equivalent to the notion of an underlying sexual orientation but give rise to four possibilities: no sexual partners or activity in a given period, only same-gender partners, both same-gender and opposite-gender partners, and only opposite-gender partners. Recent surveys have focused primarily on the existence of any same-gender experience, because same-gender experience is rare and the simplest distinction seems to be between persons who report any such experience and those who report none. In addition to addressing behavior or experience, surveys might also ask about other dimensions of homosexuality such as desire (i.e., attraction to same-gender individuals) and identity (i.e., self-definition as homosexual, gay, lesbian, or bisexual). There are others as well, for example, the publicness or openness of a nonheterosexual identity and the degree of integration into gay, lesbian, or bisexual social worlds. These all have implicit time dimensions as they are subject to change over the life course.

■ National Health and Social Life Survey and the Interrelationship of Dimensions of Homosexuality

Although the recent survey data on homosexuality are limited, it is still possible to investigate the interrelationships between at least some analytically separate dimensions of homosexuality. In the National Health and Social Life Survey (NHSLS), the most comprehensive probability-based survey of sexual behavior ever done in the United States (Laumann et al. 1994), questions pertaining to homosexuality covered three dimensions: behavior, desire, and identity. Behavior mainly refers to same-gender sexual experience or partners since age 18 years. Desire was measured by combining responses to two items in the survey: sexual attraction to same-gender individuals and appeal of having sex with someone of the same gender. Although homosexual identity is a complex phenomenon, in the NHSLS study, it referred simply to a self-definition as homosexual or bisexual (or a variant such as gay or lesbian). Desire and identity were asked about in the present tense, although in a global way.

If these three dimensions are considered as either present or absent in a given period for a given individual, there are eight possible combinations of homosexual behavior, desire, and identity (including the absence of any of these). Most discussions assume that if any one of these is observed, the other two also will be present, but this is only a single possibility. In the NHSLS, some persons reported one of the three dimensions of homosexuality but not the other two. For example, there were both men and women who reported sexual experience with persons of their own gender but no same-gender desire or identity. This could occur in many conceivable scenarios, including situational homosexuality in the absence of opposite-gender partners such as occurs in prisons or other single-gender institutions. In addition, in the United States and in many cultures and groups, men who play the "masculine" or "active" role in sex with other men (i.e., the inserting partner in fellatio or anal intercourse) have not historically been considered homosexual and may not think of themselves as homosexual (Almaquer 1991; Alonso and Koreck 1989; Carrier 1980; Chauncey 1994). On the other hand, it was not surprising to find persons who were aware of sexual feelings toward individuals of their own gender or who found the idea of having sex with someone of their own gender appealing but who have never actually had this experience and who do not consider themselves to be either homosexual or bisexual.

Identity is conceptually distinct from either desire or behavior. Conceivably, there are individuals who have either had homosexual sex or experienced some level of homosexual desire but who do not consider themselves homosexual or bisexual. It is harder to conceive of persons who would say that they are homosexual or bisexual but who do not experience homosexual desire, because a self-definition as homosexual or bisexual usually develops over time and depends on at least antecedent conscious desire. However, strong identification with gay or lesbian culture or politics (e.g., the "political lesbian" or "woman-identified woman") might be an example. Homosexual culture and politics today often seem to emphasize a general opposition to "straightness" or "normality" rather than specific sexual practices and desires; this might lead some to identify themselves as "gay" or "queer" independently of feelings and experience.

Figure 4–1 illustrates the relative proportions of women and men reporting the various combinations of the three basic dimensions of homosexuality (behavior, desire, and identity) in the NHSLS. The pie charts reflect the responses of the 9% of women and 10% of the men who reported any homosexual behavior, desire, or identity as adults, that is, since turning age 18 years. These three different dimensions of homosexuality are far from completely overlapping. A substantial proportion of those who reported any adult homosexuality reported only one aspect, either behavior or desire: 13% of the women and 22% of the men reported only homosexual experience, and 59% of the women and 44% of the men reported only desire. Thirteen percent of the women and 6% of the men reported both same-gender sexual experience and some level of same-gender desire but did not self-identify as homosexual or bisexual; most considered themselves heterosexual (with a very small number saying "something else"). In contrast, homosexual identity is not a dimension that can be said to exist independently of the other two; rather, it seems to entail them both. Practically all of the persons who thought of themselves as homosexual or bisexual also reported homosexual experiences and feelings. This group represented 15% of the women and 24% of the men who reported any same-gender sexuality. This pattern is compatible with the view of a homosexual or bisexual identity as the outcome of a well-ordered temporal process, such as a developmental process of "coming out." However, the behavioral measures used here from the NHSLS refer to any homosexual ex-

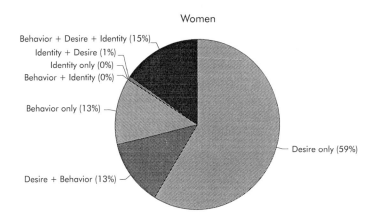

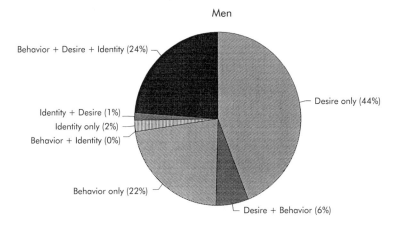

Figure 4–1. Interrelationship of same-gender sexual behavior, desire, and identity in women (top; $n = 150$, $N = 1,749$) and men (bottom; $n = 143$, $N = 1,410$), age 18–59 years, in the United States who reported any adult same-gender sexuality. Results are based on data from the National Health and Social Life Survey in 1992 (Laumann et al. 1994). Behavior referred to same-gender sexual experience or partners since age 18 years. Desire and identity were asked about in the present. Desire was measured by combining responses to two items in the survey: sexual attraction to persons of one's own gender and appeal of having sex with a person of the same gender. Identity referred to self-definition as homosexual or bisexual (or a variant such as gay or lesbian).

perience since age 18, whereas the questions about desire and identity were asked in the present tense. The survey provided no retrospective information about sexual desire and self-identification, which are not necessarily static and may change over time.

Analysis of data from the NHSLS demonstrates the importance of a more multidimensional approach to our thinking about homosexuality. It should also serve to warn against moving from any single measure of homosexuality to the idea of homosexual, bisexual, gay, or lesbian as a separate category of people. Consider the various wedges of the pie charts and ask whether all the persons in it should be considered homosexual or bisexual. Although it may be tempting to argue for self-identification as a necessary and sufficient condition for inclusion and labeling, consider also whether there are any wedges that would not contain some persons who might be called homosexual or bisexual for certain purposes. These empirical data should help underscore the importance and difficulty of precise definition of homosexuality and its degree of variation in the population.

Prevalence of Various Measures of Homosexuality in the United States

■ The Prevalence of Homosexuality in Women and Men

Figure 4–2 presents the prevalence of various dimensions of homosexuality (behavior, desire, and identity) in American adults, age 18–59 years. The bar charts shown are based on data from the NHSLS (Laumann et al. 1994) and the GSS (Davis and Smith 1993). Men and women differed dramatically on most of these measures, with the rates in men often almost twice those in women. Not surprisingly, the longer the time period, the higher the rates of reporting of same-gender sexual experience.

About 1% of the women and about 3% of the men reported a same-gender partner in the past year. The rates increased to about 4% in women and about 5% in men when experience since age 18 years was included. When the question was expanded to include any same-gender sexual experience since puberty, the rate in men almost doubled to 10%, whereas the rate in women increased only to 5%. This suggests a substantial group of men who reported having had same-gender sexual experience during adolescence but not since age 18.

The remaining sets of bars in Figure 4–2 refer to mental (cognitive/affective) state rather than behavior. Desire again refers to being sexually attracted to persons of one's own gender or finding the idea of having sex with someone of the same sex appealing. The rates of reporting homosexual desire in both women and men are about 8%, noticeably higher than the respective rates of behavior, especially more recent behavior. The last set of bars reflects the proportions of women and men who reported that they considered themselves to be either

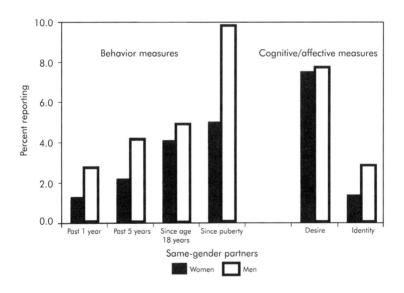

Figure 4–2. Prevalence of same-gender sexual behavior, desire, and identity in women (shaded bars) and men (open bars), age 18–59 years, in the United States. Results for percent reporting same-gender sexual partners in the past year, past 5 years, and since age 18 years are based on combined data from the General Social Surveys of 1988–1991 and 1993 (Davis and Smith 1993) and the National Health and Social Life Survey (NHSLS) of 1992 (Laumann et al. 1994); those for percent reporting same-gender sexual partners since puberty or same-gender sexual desire or self-identity are based on data from the NHSLS. Exact percentages and minimum *N*s for each bar can be found in Table 4–1.

homosexual or bisexual. The rate in men, almost 3%, is double that in women. Although these rates are similar to those for reporting a same-gender partner in the last year, these are not identical groups. About one-third of the women and men who have had same-gender partners in the past year did not consider themselves homosexual or bisexual. About one-quarter of the men and one-third of the women who considered themselves homosexual or bisexual had not had a same-gender partner in the past year.

■ Prevalence of Homosexuality in Social and Demographic Groups

Many discussions of homosexuality seem to assume that it is randomly distributed in the population; certainly the way that the 10% estimate is often used implies this. In fact, reported rates of homosexuality vary by many social and demographic variables, such as age, marital status, education, religion, race, and urbanization of place of residence.

Table 4–1 presents the reported prevalence of homosexual behavior in four different time periods (the past year, the past 5 years, since turning 18, and since puberty) and of two nonbehavior (cognitive/affective) measures, desire and identity, in women and men in several social and demographic groups. The overall rates in women and men are also illustrated in Figure 4–2 and discussed in the previous section. The results for the first three behavior variables are based on data from five waves of the GSS of 1988, 1989, 1990, 1991, and 1993 (Davis and Smith 1993) and those from the NHSLS of 1992. Those for experience since puberty, desire, and identity (self-identification) are based only on NHSLS data, because these dimensions were not included in the GSS. All of the social and demographic variables analyzed have at least some effect on the prevalence of homosexual behavior; some have powerful and dramatic effects.

A few general caveats about the data in Table 4–1 should be stated. The variations in rates in different groups demonstrate correlation but not necessarily causation and result from complex processes involving a number of different variables operating simultaneously. For example, the temporal order of influence may vary, as gender and race clearly predate sexual experiences. However, variables such as education and even religion may be at least partially the result of sexuality, and the observed differences may be the result of reciprocal or interactive pro-

Table 4–1. Prevalence of same-gender sexual behavior, desire, and identity in women and men in social and demographic groups in the United States

| | Behavior | | | | | | | | Desire | | Identity | |
| | Past year[a] | | Past 5 years[a] | | Since age 18 years[a] | | Since puberty[b] | | Attraction or appeal[b] | | Homosexual or bisexual[b] | |
Group	Women	Men	Women	Men	Women	Men	Women	Men	Women	Men	Women	Men
Overall[c]	1.3	2.7	2.2	4.1	4.1	4.9	5.0	9.8	7.5	7.7	1.4	2.8
Age in years												
18–29	1.6	3.0	2.5	4.3	4.2	4.4	4.7	7.3	6.7	9.1	1.6	2.9
30–39	1.8	3.5	3.2	5.4	5.3	6.6	6.1	11.4	9.2	7.2	1.8	4.2
40–49	0.8	2.1	1.3	3.0	3.6	3.9	5.0	11.7	8.3	8.6	1.3	2.2
50–59	0.4	1.4	0.9	2.5	2.2	4.2	3.5	9.0	4.6	4.0	0.4	0.5
Marital status												
Never married	3.6	6.6	4.8	9.2	8.2	9.5	6.8	14.6	10.4	13.9	3.7	7.1
Married	0.2	1.0	0.8	1.7	2.1	2.4	3.4	7.0	5.2	4.7	0.1	0.6
Divorced/ widowed/ separated	1.3	1.0	2.7	2.2	4.5	4.9	6.3	8.9	9.6	3.9	1.9	1.0
Education												
Less than high school	0.9	3.1	2.2	3.0	4.9	4.5	3.7	6.8	3.3	5.8	0.4	1.6
High school graduate	0.8	1.4	1.4	2.7	2.7	2.7	2.9	7.9	5.3	5.5	0.4	1.8
Some college	1.1	3.0	2.0	4.6	3.8	5.3	5.4	11.3	7.3	8.9	1.2	3.8
College graduate	2.5	3.5	3.5	5.4	5.8	6.9	7.9	11.1	12.8	9.4	3.6	3.3

Table 4-1. Prevalence of same-gender sexual behavior, desire, and identity in women and men in social and demographic groups in the United States (*continued*)

Group	Behavior								Desire		Identity	
	Past year[a]		Past 5 years[a]		Since age 18 years[a]		Since puberty[b]		Attraction or appeal[b]		Homosexual or bisexual[b]	
	Women	Men	Women	Men	Women	Men	Women	Men	Women	Men	Women	Men
Religion												
Protestant type 1[d]	1.7	3.0	2.2	5.0	4.0	5.3	2.8	10.2	5.2	8.3	0.5	3.1
Protestant type 2[d]	0.6	1.8	1.7	2.5	3.5	3.3	3.8	7.2	5.5	5.6	0.3	0.7
Catholic	0.7	1.7	1.2	2.3	2.5	2.8	5.0	8.8	8.4	5.3	1.7	2.1
Jewish	2.7	4.5	2.0	8.7	6.7	5.0	10.3	15.4	10.3	11.5	3.4	7.7
Other	4.2	3.4	9.8	7.5	11.6	10.9	18.9	14.6	16.2	19.5	5.4	7.5
None	4.0	5.9	5.7	8.1	9.7	10.7	11.8	15.5	15.8	12.9	4.6	6.2
Religious attendance per year												
None	2.7	4.4	3.1	6.7	6.6	8.8	5.7	14.7	7.4	7.6	2.2	4.7
1–2	1.7	2.5	3.8	4.0	5.6	4.5	8.1	7.9	10.1	9.6	3.1	2.6
3–39	1.1	2.5	1.8	4.2	3.8	4.4	4.8	8.4	8.0	7.9	1.1	2.9
40 or more	0.7	1.9	1.3	2.2	2.6	3.4	3.2	10.5	5.5	5.1	0.3	1.5
Race												
White	1.2	2.7	1.9	4.0	3.7	5.0	5.1	10.3	7.6	7.6	1.5	3.0
Black	1.3	3.6	2.9	5.4	5.4	5.0	4.5	9.5	7.3	7.0	0.4	1.9
Other	2.1	1.4	5.9	1.3	7.4	3.3	5.6	4.2	7.1	9.4	1.6	1.1

Place of residence[e]												
Top 12 CCs	2.1	10.2	3.3	14.3	6.2	16.4	6.5	15.8	9.7	16.7	2.6	9.2
Next 88 CCs	1.2	3.6	2.5	5.2	5.5	5.7	8.2	11.4	7.8	11.4	1.6	3.5
Suburbs top 12 CCs	1.2	2.7	1.9	5.4	4.3	5.9	6.2	13.0	9.0	10.3	1.9	4.2
Suburbs next 88 CCs	1.3	1.6	1.7	3.5	3.6	3.4	5.2	6.6	9.8	4.5	1.6	1.3
Other urban areas	0.8	1.8	1.7	2.5	2.9	4.1	3.7	10.4	6.9	5.3	1.1	1.9
Rural areas	0.6	1.0	1.0	0.9	2.8	1.5	2.6	3.1	2.1	7.5	0.0	1.3
Minimum N	3,255	4,054	1,983	2,512	3,530	3,649	1,394	1,727	1,394	1,727	1,362	1,692

[a]Results (as percent reporting same-gender sexual partners in the past year, past 5 years, or since age 18 years) are based on combined data from the General Social Surveys of 1988–1991 and 1993 (Davis and Smith 1993) and the National Health and Social Life Survey (NHSLS) of 1992 (Laumann et al. 1994).

[b]Results (as percent reporting same-gender sexual partners since puberty or same-gender sexual desire or self-identity) are based on data from the NHSLS of 1992.

[c]Overall rates are also graphically presented in Figure 4–1.

[d]Protestant type 1 refers to liberal and moderate denominations, such as Episcopalian, Lutheran, Methodist, Presbyterian, and United Church of Christ. Protestant type 2 refers to conservative denominations, such as Baptist, Church of Christ, Jehovah's Witness, Mormon, and Pentecostal (Laumann et al. 1994).

[e]Central cities (CCs) of 12 largest Standard Metropolitan Statistical Areas (SMSAs). CCs of the remainder of 100 largest SMSAs. Suburbs of 12 largest SMSAs. Suburbs of remaining 100 largest SMSAs. Other urban areas are counties with towns of 10,000 or more. Rural areas are counties having no towns of 10,000 or more (see Davis and Smith 1993 for further detail).

cesses. It is also impossible to distinguish differences in reporting from differences in actual behavior. Some of the higher rates of reporting may be the results of the group members' greater level of comfort in revealing homosexual experiences. A number of the categories with elevated rates, such as younger age and higher levels of education, are associated with social liberalism. Even for religion and religious attendance, the categories associated with higher rates of homosexuality (i.e., Jewish persons, Protestant type 1 [liberal/moderate] persons, persons reporting no religion, and those reporting no attendance) are associated with secularism and sexual and social liberalism. However, it is plausible that higher levels of social acceptance of homosexuality in these groups also lead to higher rates of activity and experience. In fact, it is practically impossible to separate the two processes, and it seems likely that there is some effect of both on many of these rates.

Age appears to have, at least partially, a cohort effect. Those between the ages of 30 and 39 years at the time of the interview (birth years 1952–1962) had the highest rates of homosexuality by most measures. The strong relationship between marital status and measures of homosexuality is probably largely a result of the legal prohibition of same-gender marriages. Not surprisingly, the rates of homosexuality were highest among those who had never married at the time of the survey. In addition to the effect of education previously described, graduation from college had marked effects on the rates of homosexuality in women. The differences between white and black categories were neither strong nor consistent. Black men and women had somewhat higher rates of same-gender sexual behavior in the last year, last 5 years, and since age 18 years but lower rates of same-gender desire, identity, and lifetime (since puberty) experience. Those living in large urban settings reported higher rates of homosexuality than those in smaller cities and suburban and rural areas; the differences were more dramatic in men than in women. One explanation for this would be the migration of homosexually inclined persons to the more congenial environment of the larger cities, with their higher levels of tolerance and anonymity and their visible gay enclaves and communities. However, it is also possible that larger cities and their environs provide more opportunities for same-gender sex and thereby produce higher rates. This explanation is supported by elevated rates of homosexuality in persons who resided in more urbanized areas before age 17 years, which would have predated most migration independent of the family as a whole (Laumann et al. 1994). Most likely, both migration and increased opportunity contribute to the observed differences.

These results demonstrate a high degree of social organization of homosexuality. Homosexuality does not appear to be evenly distributed in American society. Similar patterns of variability in prevalence exist in other Western industrial countries such as England and France (Spira et al. 1993; Wellings et al. 1994). Unfortunately, many discussions of contemporary homosexuality ignore this variation. However, it may help explain some of the outrage and disbelief expressed in the organized gay community after recent surveys reported low average rates of homosexual behavior. For many persons residing in large cities, in or around gay enclaves, or in social networks with many openly gay men and lesbians, the proportion of men who identify themselves as gay is likely to be much closer to or even higher than 10%. Although the proportion of women who identify themselves as lesbian or bisexual in such environments does not appear as high as 10%, it is still much higher than elsewhere in society and, within certain settings could well be even higher. Furthermore, it follows that the proportion of persons who engage in homosexual behavior would be higher still. The degree of social variability described here should alert us to the importance of the social environment and the complexities of describing the prevalence of homosexuality.

Conclusion

Homosexuality is often treated as if it were a unitary phenomenon that can be used to unambiguously differentiate persons into discrete categories. However, data from surveys of sexual behavior indicate that the distinction between the heterosexual person and the homosexual person is often imprecise. These data also illustrate that homosexual behavior, desire, and identity are not completely overlapping. In particular, such feelings and behavior often exist independently of each other and of a homosexual self-identity.

The prevalence of homosexuality in the population varies, depending on a number of factors: the particular dimension of homosexuality being reported and the social and demographic characteristics being examined, including gender, age, marital status, education, religion and religious attendance, race, and relative urbanization of place of residence. The rates of the various dimensions of homosexuality are consistently lower in probability samples of the population than those reported by Kinsey et al. (1948; 1953). However, many of the basic patterns identified by the latter researchers remain the same, for example, higher rates of homosexual behavior in men than in women, higher rates in adolescents (especially males) than in adults, and variations between many social and demographic groups. Given the high degree of stigma attached to homosexuality in society, these data no doubt represent some degree of underreporting of actual experiences. However, recent estimates are based on high-quality representative samples of large sections of the population and, therefore, provide a major advance beyond the limitations of the Kinsey research and a new baseline for further research and analysis in determining the prevalence of homosexuality in American society.

References

ACSF (Analyse des Comportements Sexuels en France) Investigators: AIDS and sexual behaviour in France. Nature 360:407–409, 1992

Almaquer T: Chicano men: a cartography of homosexual identity and behavior. Differences 3:75–100, 1991

Alonso AM, Koreck MT: Silences: "Hispanics," AIDS, and sexual practices. Differences 1:101–124, 1989

Billy JOG, Tanfer K, Grady WR, et al: The sexual behavior of men in the United States. Fam Plann Perspect 25:52–60, 1993

Bradburn NM: Response effects, in The Handbook of Survey Research. Edited by Rossi PH, Wright JD, Anderson AB. New York, Academic Press, 1983, pp 289–328

Carrier JM: Homosexual behavior in cross-cultural perspective, in Homosexual Behavior: A Modern Reappraisal. Edited by Marmor J. New York, Basic Books, 1980, pp 100–122

Catania JA, Coates TJ, Stall R, et al: Prevalence of AIDS-related risk factors and condom use in the United States. Science 258:1101–1106, 1992

Chauncey G: Gay New York: Gender, Urban Culture, and the Making of the Gay Male World, 1890–1940. New York, Basic Books, 1994

Cochran WG, Mosteller F, Tukey JW: Statistical Problems of the Kinsey Report on Sexual Behavior in the Human Male. Washington, DC, American Statistical Association, 1954

Davis JA, Smith TW: General Social Surveys, 1972–1993: Cumulative Codebook. Chicago, IL, National Opinion Research Center, 1993

Fay RE, Turner CF, Klassen AD, et al: Prevalence and patterns of same-gender sexual contact among men. Science 243:338–348, 1989

Gagnon JH, Simon W: Sexual Conduct: The Social Sources of Human Sexuality. Chicago, IL, Aldine, 1973

Gebhard PH: Incidence of overt homosexuality in the United States and western Europe, in National Institute of Mental Health Task Force on Homosexuality: Final Report and Background Papers. Edited by Livingood JM. Rockville, MD, National Institute of Mental Health, 1972, pp 22–29

Gebhard PH, Johnson AB: The Kinsey Data: Marginal Tabulations of the 1938–1963 Interviews Conducted by the Institute of Sex Research. Philadelphia, PA, WB Saunders, 1979

Institute of Medicine: Confronting AIDS: Directions for Public Health, Health Care, and Research. Washington, DC, National Academy Press, 1986

Johnson AM, Wadsworth J, Wellings K, et al: Sexual lifestyles and HIV risk. Nature 360:410–412, 1992

Kinsey AC, Pomeroy WB, Martin CE: Sexual Behavior in the Human Male. Philadelphia, PA, WB Saunders, 1948

Kinsey AC, Pomeroy WB, Martin CE, et al: Sexual Behavior in the Human Female. Philadelphia, WB Saunders, 1953

Laumann EO, Gagnon JH, Michael RT, et al: The Social Organization of Sexuality: Sexual Practices in the United States. Chicago, IL, University of Chicago Press, 1994

Rogers SM, Turner CF: Male-male sexual contact in the U.S.A.: findings from five sample surveys, 1970–1990. J Sex Res 28:491–519, 1991

Stein E (ed): Forms of Desire: Sexual Orientation and the Social Constructionist Controversy. New York, Routledge, 1992

Spira A, Bajos N, Bejin A, et al: Les Comportements Sexuels en France. Paris, La Documentation Française, 1993

Wellings K, Field J, Johnson A, et al: Sexual Behaviour in Britain: The National Survey of Sexual Attitudes and Lifestyles. London, Penguin, 1994

5

Issues in the Cross-Cultural Study of Homosexuality

Gilbert Herdt, Ph.D.

Since the time of the American Psychiatric Association's decision to remove homosexuality from its list of diagnoses, few issues have generated more controversy in psychiatry and the social sciences than the question of the "normality" of homosexuality. From before Freud's (1905/1962) late 19th-century discussions of same-sex desire as an "inversion" characteristic of "psychic hermaphrodites," to the large-scale survey studies of Kinsey et al. (1948) in the mid-20th century that normalized the idea that same-sex practices were frequent in the population but usually transitional, and up to the present explosion of study in anthropology, social history, and

The following material is reprinted in a slightly modified form from Herdt G: "Cross-Cultural Forms of Homosexuality and the Concept 'Gay.'" *Psychiatric Annals* 18:37–39, 1988, and a special issue of the *Journal of Homosexuality*, "Bisexual and Homosexual Identity: Critical Theoretical Issues" (Winter 1983, Spring 1984, Vol. 9); it was published in the *Journal of Homosexuality* 10:53–62, under the title "A Comment on Cultural Attributes and Fluidity of Bisexuality."

studies of gay men and lesbians demonstrating the significance of same-sex roles, institutions, and subcultures, the study of homosexuality has often been driven by the effort to posit its ultimate causes. Today, scholars in the field generally believe that the question of causation is unanswerable, and they concentrate instead on identifying the forms, functions, and meanings of same-sex relations across time and space and within the perspective of the socially constructed life-course as lived by the actors in society.

Cross-cultural study of sexual development is relatively new and difficult because of the uneven anthropological and historical research on sexuality in non-Western societies. Many recent studies reviewed below have greatly contributed to our understanding of the expressions of human sexual behavior. Only now, however, are these data being integrated and analyzed in the light of contemporary study. The effort at systematic analysis is the most precarious regarding sexual development in children and adolescents across cultures, because our data are so sparse. This chapter is only a partial contribution toward this end. It reviews recent work on homosexuality in terms of currently received classification models. Comparative study of homoerotic practices provides new insights into a general understanding of sexual development, largely because these studies have raised our understanding of cultural influences on the expression of sexual desires and contacts in radically different cultures. In the second part of this chapter the author reconsiders the meanings of bisexuality in both Western and non-Western settings. Bisexuality provides a linking framework for study of these classificatory models of homosexuality around the world and our own assumptions and expressions of diverse sexual responses during development.

Advances in the past 10 years have fundamentally altered the understanding of same-sex erotic behavior in the social and health sciences. We must be aware of the fundamental unpacking of the construct of homosexuality as a Western, typically culture-bound concept, in the sense that it implies a certain social role and identity that radiate largely from the 19th century, and these meanings as we now understand them are not present in many other cultures and histories (Herdt 1994). Likewise, the constructs of gay men and lesbians, although reflecting a new positive social identity to supplant the former closet homosexual identity of before, are generally typical of western European and North American culture but not of other parts of the world. Even within the United States, many individuals who engage in same-sex practice do

not self-identify as homosexual, gay, or lesbian, but rather identify themselves in terms of another community or cultural identity. Thus, the effort
to understand the meanings of same-sex behavior must take account of
the local roles, knowledge, and practices of people. In doing so, we are
drawn into the problems of cross-cultural and intracultural variations of
homosexuality and bisexuality in our own society and others.

Strong preconceptions about homosexuality are that it is always
regarded as deviant or perverse, that it is rare or absent from most societies, or that, if it occurs, same-sex behavior is stigmatized or punished
(reviewed in Herdt 1984, 1993a; Mead 1961). At the turn of the century,
Freud (1905/1962) challenged such views by suggesting that homosexual activity occurred in various archaic and tribal societies. Even in Western society, Freud thought, sexual behavior was more heterogeneous
than was believed. Freud's famous phrase "polymorphous perverse" was
meant to indicate the potential of humans to manifest sexual acts with
both genders, such behaviors being subject to social regulation. Kinsey
et al. (1948) provided massive empirical evidence that supported this
idea in their study of American society, demonstrating that homosexual
behavior was more prevalent in American society, with 37% of all U.S.
men experiencing significant homosexual contact sometime in their
lives. The effect of the work was to disengage sex from reproductive
behavior and to indicate how the homosexual-heterosexual dichotomies
are more an idealized cultural model than an empirical fact.

In cross-cultural studies, a similar point was made soon afterward
in the classic study by Ford and Beach (1951), who found that homosexual behavior was socially acceptable and normative for certain people in 64% of the 76 societies studied. Carrier (1980) has gone further
and divided cultures around the world into those that are approving,
disapproving, or neutral with regard to homosexual acts, illustrating
that societies differ greatly in their conceptions of homosexuality. The
North American value system, which negatively stigmatizes same-sex
eroticism, is uncharacteristic of many societies.

Important conceptual refinements in the understanding of sexuality have been made during the same period. One of these refinements
concerns the theoretical separation of phylogenetically universal determinants from socioculturally variable elements (e.g., masculinity
and femininity) in human sexuality (Money and Ehrhard 1972; Stoller
1968). Another refinement—critical for understanding the meaning of
homosexuality—is the difference between sexual identity and sexual
behavior. That someone engages in a particular gendered sexual act

does not necessarily mean that he or she has the characteristics associated with the general category of homosexual, bisexual, or heterosexual (Herdt 1989). Thus, a woman may marry and have children but regard her sexual orientation as lesbian or a man may engage in sexual activity with males but regard himself as heterosexual (Money and Ehrhard 1972; Plummer 1975). We must therefore distinguish homosexuality as a state of being, an essence, from same-sex acts and transient relationships, which may not involve homoerotic sex-object choice and intentionality in the same way (Stoller 1980; Stoller and Herdt 1985).

A recent survey has shown that these conceptual refinements help us to cluster culturally patterned same-sex practices found historically and cross-culturally into four forms as follows (Herdt 1987a).

Age-Structured Same-Sex Practice

Institutionalized same-sex acts between males of unequal ages are common but unevenly distributed throughout the world (Adam 1986). These are customary practices, usually obligatory for older and younger males, which are associated with normative gender development. Age-structured homoeroticism occurred in ancient China, Japan, Islam, and in certain Indo-European traditions, but the most famous example is known from our cultural ancestors, the ancient Greeks (Dover 1978). At least as early as 800 B.C., this form of homosexual practice was known among the Homeric Greeks, especially the Dorians, although it was later widely distributed in the city-states of Athens and Sparta. Originally, this homoeroticism was associated with military prowess and organization. Later it was transferred in the development of noble qualities of honor, citizenship, and spirituality in the male. Ritualized female homosexual contacts also were known among the Greeks.

In the tribal world of contemporary non-Western people, age-structured homosexuality is known from Africa, lowlands South America, the Pacific, and elsewhere, but it has been most studied in New Guinea and the South Seas (Herdt 1984). Here, as among the Sambia of highlands New Guinea, age-structured homoerotic activities are implemented through initiation rites. Sambia boys ages 7–10 years are inducted into ritual and military organizations. The Sambia experience many years of these practices, first as semen recipients and later in adolescence as semen donors. But then, at fatherhood, the Sambia forbid additional boy-inseminating practices (Herdt 1981). These males experience both passive (fellator) and active (fellated) homosexual roles in the course of their lives, yet they, like the Greeks, nonetheless marry and have children (Herdt 1987b). In some New Guinea societies, however, this homoerotic relation with younger males continues throughout life, even into old age (Van Baal 1993). A survey of all South Seas societies has shown that this approved pattern of age-structured boy inseminating occurs in between 10% and 20% of cultures and is probably an ancient practice, the result of ultimata migrations and adaptations for several thousands of years (Herdt 1993a).

Gender-Transformed Same-Sex Practice

A different form of homoerotic practice is based on the adoption and role of the opposite sex in a society. Sometimes this is referred to as "institutionalized cross-dressing" or "transvestitism." Gender transformation often begins in childhood, has recognized customs associated with it, and is acknowledged and supported by the society (Blackwood 1986). The institution of the Berdache among North American Indians is the best-known example. Some 115 Indian tribes recognized the Berdache, in which boys acted and dressed as girls and took the roles of girls, and some in which girls adopted the roles of boys. Berdache could marry, adopt children, acquire property, and participate in most aspects of group life. They were not stigmatized, and in some societies, they were revered for their special qualities and pragmatic socioeconomic contributions to the group (Devereux 1937; Williams 1986).

Role of Class-Specialized Same-Sex Practice

A third form of sexual contact occurs in those societies in which engaging in a same-sex act is based solely on the entitlements of a role or status not widely held in a culture. One of these patterns is divine bisexuality. Those who became shamans among the Chukchi tribe of Siberia were entitled by supernatural authority to engage in homosexual behavior, even though this was generally disapproved of for the wider society. A more recent pattern is known from female factory workers of the 19th-century Canton delta in China. Young Chinese women who lived and worked in silk factories formed erotic and economic bonds with each other and usually did not marry, even though female homosexual contact was disapproved of in the patriarchal culture of China (Blackwood 1986). This example reveals how industrialization, urbanization, and the development of a class system may be antecedents of the homosexual category in the modern period. Indeed, such is suggested by the identification of the role of the artist with homosexuality and the incipient gay culture of 18th- and 19th-century England (McIntosh 1968; Weeks 1985).

Gay and Lesbian—Egalitarian Same-Sex Practices

The rise of the modern period saw the rise of egalitarian ideas of sexual partnerships in Western history. Hierarchical gay and lesbian relations are still common, paralleling the strongly structured forms of canonical heterosexual relation as signified by the sacramental rite of marriage for husband and wife. From the late 19th century until the present, however, the emergence of sexual reform movements led to the creation of modern gay and lesbian communities in many parts of the United States. This movement represented a fusion of public and private, sexual and gender, and sexual and political and a fusion of role and sexual orientation and identity as previously defined. Foucault (1986) showed that social constructions of homosexuality in this sense did not emerge until the medicalization and stigmatization of gender-deviant behavior were disputed by social history. Coupling this sexual category with early homosexual rights movements in Germany, England, and the United States provided the basis for the advocacy of the human right to live a gay lifestyle permanently. Thus, gay has become a sexual orientation (a particular kind of homosexuality), a social identity, and a political movement. Clearly, gay is a new form of homosexual practice, which in its fullest sense is unique in human history.

The psychosocial conditions of being lesbian or gay in current society must therefore be understood in cultural place and historical time. Being gay or lesbian is a commentary on the dualistic tendency of Western society to dichotomize body and mind, masculinity and femininity, and homosexual and heterosexual as discussed below. The modern gay movement both reflects and mediates these dualisms, indicating that social and erotic transformation is a part of human potential, as Freud suggested. The coming-out process of identity development can be seen in relation to this commentary. Gay men and lesbians undergo a profound process of cognitive change within themselves, because the self is at first placed in a heterosexual category, by virtue of growing up in heterosexual environments, but is then placed into a homosexual or gay category that replaces it (Dank 1971). The study of adolescent coming out substantiates this trend further (Herdt 1989). The concomitants of this process are complex and multidimensional, but they obviously depend on the cultural barriers to the expression of homosexuality in society (Hooker 1965; Weeks 1985). The meaning of being gay in popular culture is currently at the forefront of newspaper headlines in part because of its association with AIDS. We can expect that further changes in social attitudes toward homosexuality and bisexuality will depend in part on efforts to combat AIDS and to deal with homophobic responses to it. In sum, homosexuality is not one but many psychosocial forms that can be viewed as symbolic mediations between psychocultural and historical conditions and human potentials for sexual response during life.

Societies vary greatly in their attitudes toward same-sex response. Homosexual acts are probably universal in humans, but institutionalized forms of homosexual activity are not. These depend, to a great extent, on the specific historical problems and outlooks of a culture. Western negativity toward homosexuality must be seen in this light as a special and historically determined stigma, the symbols of which, in religious and political discourse, are inextricably tied to broader socioeconomic issues we are only beginning to understand.

Fluidity of Bisexuality

To delve deeper into the cultural definitions and meanings of homosexuality in human development, we must study bisexuality. The histories of bisexuality and homosexuality in Western history and in sexology are inextricably linked (Money 1987, 1988). The concepts and metaphors of bisexuality reveal an underlying preconception of fluidity; a greater capacity to alter and transmute sexual drive, libido, and related sexual objects to which erotic interest is directed than occurs in either heterosexuality or homosexuality. The outline of forms of homosexuality cross-culturally, discussed above, gives a different framework for reconsidering our preconceptions about bisexuality.

DeCecco and Shively (1983–1984) have reconfigured the study of bisexuality in its historical and cultural contexts. Their essay explicates this view in an approach that combines the historiography of Foucault (1986) with a reanalysis of the ideas of Freud, Kinsey, and others. In seconding their idea, it seems best that we consider same-sex practices in the total context of human sexuality (Herdt 1981, 1993b).

The key contribution of DeCecco and Shively is the multidimensional challenge to the "essentialist" explanations of sexuality in general, and homosexuality in particular. We must wonder with them at the "willingness of historians to make a biological concept the foundation of a historical inquiry that has consisted of describing the circumstances under which this identity existed in the past" (DeCecco and Shively 1983–1984, p. 4).

Why this biological emphasis? DeCecco and Shively see the focus on isolated individuals and the biological motivation of essences as imports by the social sciences from medicine and the natural sciences. They argue that the idea of identity has invariably been anchored to a core or base of biological essence. They propose, instead, the investigation of the whole structure of sexual relationships in a social field of roles and relationships. Although the essentialist model is not specifically analyzed as such, the anthropologist wonders to what extent Western cosmology motivated the overriding preoccupation with biology and individuality in sexual matters. A decisive alternative is needed as a counterpoint, as suggested by DeCecco and Shively (1983–1984): "The structure of sexual relationships, as conceived here, exists as an intersection of both the uniquely personal meanings of the individual partners and a locus in history and society" (p. 15).

This view is fully compatible with an anthropological emphasis on the integration of personality and culture. It contrasts with a strictly behavioral, psychoanalytic, or symbolic interactionist approach. By making the structure of sexual relationships their theoretical focus, DeCecco and Shively offer a unit of study and analysis that is compatible with that currently used in population psychology and biology. This focus on social structure allows for conceptions of change and stability through normative gender-role models created out of both social expectations and private meanings, a prospect attractive to psychological anthropology (Levine 1982).

The essays in this collection, however, do not confront the whole system of "spirit, body, mind, personality, or social relations" that DeCecco and Shively (1983–1984, pp. ix) describe as the ingredients of the idea of sexual identity; DeCecco and Shively, Hoffman (1983–1984), Paul (1983–1984), and Herdt and Boxer (1993) come closest to this goal. The absence of holism in understanding development fosters culture-bound conceptualizations and limits understanding of the impact that a new identity—being gay—has on North American culture and on Western consciousness (Altman 1982; Greenberg and Bystryn 1984).

In the next section the author considers cross-cultural influences on the structures of sexual relationships, particularly from an anthropological perspective, drawing on material from *Ritualized Homosexuality in Melanesia* (Herdt 1984). Reference to data on these age-structured practices is germane to this discussion, for bisexuality looms large in the Melanesian cultures. Indeed, the word *ritualized* conceptualizes homosexuality, heterosexuality, and bisexuality as the total social field of signs and symbols regarding sexuality in the Melanesian world.

The idea of ritual captures several distinctive attributes of the complex symbolism of Melanesian homosexuality. First, homosexual contacts are begun in adolescent initiation rites. Many of these societies, however, prescribe homosexual activity only among young male adults. Second, ritual taboos and strict codes of conduct govern homosexual contacts (e.g., incest taboos comparable to those for heterosexual contact are evident). Third, these practices are supported by the society as a whole or, at the least, by the religious organizations of men. Ritual is therefore inextricably bound up with homosexual behavior and sexual identity (Bateson 1936; Herdt 1982). Other words could be substituted for ritualized (Stoller 1980). Ritual, however, can be viewed as a culturally pervasive mechanism of sexual identity development and behavior. Similar to incest taboos, the analysis of ritual as a universal Melanesian mechanism makes the pervasive coding of sexual behavior and identity through ritual analogous to biological causation argued in medicine. What is widespread or universal (even though socially constructed), some argue, must be biological. At the least, it must be a collective response to inherent biosocial ingredients of the human condition (Whitehead 1981). Therefore, ritual as a concept has provided a convenient mediating variable linking culture, gender identity, and sexual behavior.

The Melanesian data are directly relevant to the essentialist explanation of homosexual and bisexual identity. In a review of the extant data from the 1860s to now, the author has shown the occurrence of the ritual practice of homosexual activity in about 40 different societies (Herdt 1993a). Because this practice exists only in 10%–20% of all

Melanesian societies, we must understand its psychosocial distribution. The geographic distribution of these cultures is not random; the configurations of psychosocial traits associated with these cults of homosexuality are systematically and highly correlated (Lindenbaum 1993). Warfare, antagonism between the sexes, and male initiation rites, for example, are highly elaborated in all of these societies. Furthermore, in virtually all the known groups in the southwest Pacific, the non-Austronesian language phylum prevails. No simple genetic or biochemical factor could possibly be advanced to explain this complex behavioral phenomenon, its distribution, or its absence in societies with similar ecological traits. Historical diffusion and a psychosocial system related to it are ultimate and proximate causes.

There is increasing recognition in anthropology of the politics of gender roles and their personal and cultural implications. For example, the Melanesian data (Herdt 1984) support the developmental formulation of Margaret Mead (1935) concerning the polarity of adult gender roles and the difficulty males experience in achieving the gender identity competence expected of them in situations of warfare, ritual, and hunting. The evidence, however, does not support Mead's idea that the inability to live up to gender norms leads to the formation in a society of the homosexual identity (Paul 1983–1984).

Throughout the DeCecco and Shively collection of essays (1983–1984) the term "fluidity" appears as a metaphor for bisexuality. That researchers use this word so casually in text should give us pause. Fluidity implies the rigidity of the old heterosexual-homosexual dichotomy, which is reviewed in several articles but perceptively analyzed by Murphy (1983–1984). In the next section the author will use the Melanesian data to elucidate this provocative but slippery notion.

First, the meanings of the term "fluidity" and its referents should be clarified. Fluidity denotes that capable of flowing or being easily changed and not fixed or solid. What is it in the bisexual identity that is changeable: sexual orientation, gender role, gender identity, object choice, erotic technique used in sexual contact (e.g., oral and anal intercourse), exclusivity of sexual contact, or the degree of intimacy characterizing a contact or relationship? The author believes some of the ambiguity surrounding the idea of fluidity of sexual orientation described in the DeCecco and Shively collection (1983–1984) revolves around the potential cultural change inherent in the sexual orientation of an individual. Weeks (1977) has pointed to important situation-specific factors that mediate between sexual identity and culture. The emergence of the cultural term "coming out"—with its associated psychosocial attitudes and meanings—generally indicates social expectations of greater fluidity of sexual behavior and identity development among North Americans than have hitherto existed (Herdt 1989). Moreover, why should sexual orientation remain stable during the entire life of an individual when so much else changes, unless of course sexual exclusivity of erotic contact with only one sex is its bedrock? In short, the existence of fluidity as a metaphor in sexology raises new questions about the prominence of bisexuality in scientific and popular culture.

There are four interrelated aspects of sexual development and fluidity to highlight. The first aspect comes from culturally constituted life-cycle transitions that allow relative flexibility of bisexual choices. Societies vary according to their sexual restriction. The variance arises from such factors as the economic division of labor (D'Andrade 1966) and gender stratification (Strathern 1988). Clearly, some societies permit or even encourage universal homosexual or bisexual contact at different stages in the life cycle. Some Melanesian societies may be classified in this way: For a few years their sexual codes direct male activity toward other males and away from females. These prescriptions are congruent with harsh taboos associated with premarital heterosexuality, fear of female pollution from menstrual blood, virginity in women, and adultery. In North American society, we recognize adolescence as a cultural phase of experimentation and rebellion that incorporates strong bonds between young people of the same morphological sex, which may include homosexual play.

The second aspect of fluidity concerns the cultural system of sexual signs and symbols used as contrast features in the stimulation of bisexual erotic response. Phenomenologically, these erotic possibilities would seem to be virtually infinite. Freud's (1925/1961) well-known essay on sexual and erotic differentiation classified erotic features into three domains: physical anatomy (sexual signs), mental traits (masculine and feminine symbols), and object choice (signs and symbols that internally stimulate arousal). The degree of polarity structured into a culture in the three domains determines the degree of sexual restrictiveness. Who may interact with whom? What sexual activity is permitted and during what conditions is it preferred or acceptable? Such questions and the social pressures they indicate ultimately restrict choices of sexual identity. Ritual taboos rigidly structure, for example, older–younger or interethnic interactions between individuals of the same sex, which are thereby more eroticized than in unrestricted societies. Specific forms of anatomy, adornments, and behavioral acts may thus become stimulating and attractive regardless of the sex of the object. Stoller (1979) has explored this erotic terrain. In this regard the concept of fetishization holds promise in deepening our general understanding of the psychological and cultural interplay of a broad spectrum of erotic elements (Herdt 1982). Bisexual fluidity may point to a paradigm of eroticism that suggests a broader field of arousal than is normative in Western societies (Mead 1961).

Linked to sexual arousal is the bewildering question of what constitutes sexual desire. As a concept, sexual desire embodies myriad objects of attraction and states of being. Many individuals have the capacity for erotic response to a wide range of people. Erotic refers to conscious sexual response (the unconscious counterpart is distressingly complex). Some erotic responses involve homosexual desire. The initial arousal of a bisexual's response may hinge on highly specialized sexual scripts and personal traits in the object of attraction as well as on the right situation (Gagnon 1979). The response is not bisexual, the person is. It is rare for a person to be aroused simultaneously by a male and a female, as in a threesome. Erotic desire, in this sense, implies a great deal about the persons involved, their culture, and the direction of their sexual activity (Herdt and Stoller 1990).

The bisexual here poses a dilemma for the gay movement in its effort to institutionalize gay and lesbian lifestyles in Western culture. Yet heterosexual family members and friends may try to persuade bisexuals to be exclusive and exercise their heterosexual option. The matter of choice is key. Traditional social pressures belie the fluidity of self-concepts in intimate ties between friends and sexual partners, as reviewed by Cass (1983–1984). Does the Western abhorrence of anomaly (Plummer 1966) and artificial dichotomies such as heterosexual versus homosexual play a part in pressures on bisexuals to adopt either an exclusively heterosexual or homosexual orientation?

In contrast, in certain Melanesian societies there is no great concern with classifying people into the dichotomous categories of heterosexual or homosexual, because these categories do not exist in their cultures. People exist, and in the course of life, they may engage in sexual contact with the members of the same or opposite sex. They should marry and have children. Yet these societies have highly restrictive sexual codes of their own. The Sambian male, for example, has the opportunity for direct experience of both homosexual and heterosexual relations and the opportunity to compare and evaluate them.

Shared communications about the relative quality of all sexual activities are an ordinary part of male discourse (Herdt 1993b). Nevertheless, homosexuality is secret among Sambians, as it is among most Melanesian groups. Clearly, these features—sexual restrictiveness, verbal comparison of bisexual experiences, and ritual secrecy surrounding homosexuality—affect self-closure. These features, in turn, surely affect the self-concept as it is involved in sexual relationships. According to the evidence, however, the self-esteem of males involved in bisexual relationships in Melanesia is not impaired: their bisexuality is egosyntonic. Neither they nor their fellows lobby for or against their bisexuality, and it bears no stigma.

A final aspect of fluidity concerns the correlation between social and sexual interactions in the person's social network. Many researchers have overlooked the contrast between homosocial and homosexual behavior. Homosociality indicates the extent of same-sex exclusivity of social contacts and interactions. Generally, the more polarized the gender roles and restrictive the sexual code, the more homosociality one expects to find in a society. Although homosociality and homosexuality are independent factors, it is not clear how they are correlated cross-culturally (Read 1986). We expect much homosociality in sexually antagonistic culture areas such as those of Melanesia. Certainly, homosociality does not lead inevitably to genital homosexuality, as is exemplified by male socialization in Ireland (Messenger 1969).

Whither Cross-Cultural Study?

The cross-cultural material on human sexuality reviewed here points to the incompleteness of our understanding of sexual development outside Western society. New classifications of homosexuality help to sort out the variation in context, meanings, and behavioral forms. They are useful heuristics, but they remain analogies and models that inevitably must give way to new findings in the future. Recent work on bisexuality provides a similar reminder of the tentativeness of explanatory principles regarding sexual development in our own cultural tradition. Much new work is needed to go farther.

Ethnographic studies suggest an urgent need for new research on sexual development in children and adolescents across cultures. Current understanding of adolescent sexual development (especially regarding homosexuality) is too centered on Western ideological norms, without awareness of the presence of gay or homosexual youth. This bias in sample construction had distorted the interpretation of variation in our own society. When it is noted that about 3 million adolescents in our society are or will be permanently homosexually identified, the significant developmental variation ignored in past studies becomes more obvious (Herdt 1989). Many of these previous studies emphasized causes rather than outcomes in their research design (Boxer and Cohler 1989). Here, too, a new research effort is required to understand the effects of sexual variation in development on the course of adult functioning. As prior work reviewed above on sexual identity development among gay and lesbian youth in the United States indicates, social movements and positive cultures provide new and supportive settings that enhance positive well-being. This augurs for understanding the relationship between sexuality and well-being or mental health in the broader sense. The answers to such questions in cross-cultural settings remain enticing to investigators of the future.

Cross-cultural study of sexual development reveals the great contribution of social structure and cultural meaning in the expression of individual sexual desires and relationships. Biosocial antecedents and personality factors clearly play a role in this developmental process, but we cannot at present say how much so, in what combination, and with what frequency they exert themselves in sexual development (Ehrhardt 1985). Nonetheless, one can take heart from how much has been learned cross-culturally since the speculations of Freud (1905/1962), while recognizing how much remains speculative. Sexology has come a long way. Future study in psychiatry and the social sciences should build on these past efforts, with an eye to seeing what impact new social and cultural formations have on the mental health outcomes of sexuality.

References

Adam BD: Age, structure, and sexuality: reflections on the anthropological evidence on homosexual relations, in Anthropology and Homosexuality. Edited by Blackwood E. New York, Haworth, 1986, pp 19–34

Altman D: The Homosexualization of America, the Americanization of Homosexuality. New York, St. Martin's Press, 1982

Bateson G: Naven. Cambridge, Cambridge University Press, 1936

Blackwood E (ed): Anthropology and Homosexual Behavior. New York, Haworth, 1986

Boxer AM, Cohler B: The life course of gay and lesbian youth: an immodest proposal for the study of lives, in Gay and Lesbian Youth. Edited by Herdt G. New York, Haworth, 1989, pp 315–355

Carrier JM: Homosexual behavior in cross-cultural perspective, in Homosexual Behavior: A Modern Reappraisal. Edited by Marmor J. New York, Basic Books, 1980, pp 100–122

Cass VC: Homosexual identity: a concept in need of definition. J Homosex 9(2/3):105–126, 1983–1984

D'Andrade RG: Sex differences and cultural institutions, in The development of Sex Difference. Edited by Maccoby EE. Stanford, CA, Stanford University Press, 1966, pp 173–203

Dank B: Coming out in the gay world. Psychiatry 34:180–197, 1971

DeCecco JP, Shively MG: From sexual identity to sexual relationships: a contextual shift. J Homosex 9(2/3):1–26, 1983–1984

Devereux G: Institutionalized homosexuality of the Mohave Indians. Hum Biol 9:498–527, 1937

Dover K: Greek Homosexuality. Cambridge, MA, Harvard University Press, 1978

Ehrhardt AA: The psychobiology of gender, in Gender and the Life Course. Edited by Rossi A. New York, Aldine, 1985, pp 81–96

Ford CS, Beach FA: Patterns of Sexual Behavior. New York, Harper, 1951

Foucault M: The History of Sexuality, Vol 1: An Introduction. Translated by Hurley R. New York, Vintage Books, 1986 (original work published in 1976)

Freud S: Three Essays on the Theory of Sexuality (1905). New York, Basic Books, 1962

Freud S: Some psychical consequences of the anatomical distinction between the sexes (1925), in Standard Edition of the Complete Psychological Works of Sigmund Freud, Vol 19. Translated and edited by Strachey J. London, Hogarth Press, 1961, pp 241–258

Gagnon J: The interaction of gender roles and sexual conduct, in Human Sexuality. Edited by Katchadurian HA. Berkeley, CA, University of California Press, 1979, pp 225–245

Greenberg DF, Bystryn MH: Capitalism, bureaucracy, and male homosexuality. Contemp Crisis 8:33–56, 1984

Herdt G: Guardians of the Flutes: Idioms of Masculinity. New York, McGraw-Hill, 1981

Herdt G: Fetish and fantasy in Sambia initiation, in Rituals of Manhood: Male Initiation in Papua New Guinea. Edited by Herdt G. Berkeley, CA, University California Press, 1982, pp 48–98

Herdt G (ed): Ritualized Homosexuality in Melanesia. Berkeley, CA, University of California Press, 1984

Herdt G: Homosexuality, in Encyclopedia of Religion. New York, MacMillan, 1987a

Herdt G: The Sambia: Ritual and Gender in New Guinea. New York, Holt, Rinehart and Winston, 1987b

Herdt G: Introduction: gay youth, emergent identity, and cultural sense at home and abroad, in Homosexuality and Adolescence. Edited by Herdt G. New York, Harrington Press, 1989

Herdt G (ed): Ritualized homosexual behavior in the male cults of Melanesia, 1862–1983: an introduction, in Ritualized Homosexuality in Melansia. Berkeley, CA, University of California Press, 1993a, pp 1–81

Herdt G (ed): Semen transactions in Sambia culture, in Ritualized Homosexuality in Melanesia, 2nd Edition. Berkeley, CA, University of California Press, 1993b, pp 167–210

Herdt G (ed): Third Sex, Third Gender: Beyond Sexual Dimorphism in Culture and History. New York, Zone Books, 1994

Herdt G, Boxer A: Children of Horizons. Boston, MA, Beacon Press, 1993

Herdt G, Stoller RJ: Intimate Communications: Erotics and the Study of Culture. New York, Columbia University Press, 1990

Hooker E: An empirical study of some relations between sexual patterns and gender identity in male homosexuals, in Sex Research: New Developments. Edited by Money J. New York, Holt, Reinhart and Winston, 1965, pp 24–52

Hoffman RJ: Vices, gods, and virtues: cosmology as a mediating factor in attitude toward male homosexuality. J Homosex 9(2/3):244–270, 1983–1984

Kinsey A, Pomeroy WB, Martin CE, et al: Sexual Behavior in the Human Male. Philadelphia, PA, WB Saunders, 1948

Levine RA: Culture, Behavior and Personality. Chicago, IL, Aldine, 1982

Lindenbaum S: Sociosexual forms in transition in Melanesia, in Ritualized Homosexuality in Melanesia, 2nd Edition. Edited by Herdt G. Berkeley, CA, University of California Press, 1993, pp 221–236

McIntosh M: The homosexual role. Soc Probl 16:182–192, 1968

Mead M: Sex and Temperament in Three Primitive Societies, New York, EP Dutton, 1935

Mead M: Cultural determinants of sexual behavior, in Sex and Internal Secretions. Baltimore, MD, Williams & Wilkins, 1961, pp 1433–1479

Messenger JC: Inis Beag: Isle of Ireland. New York, Holt, Rinehart and Winston, 1969

Money J: Sin, sickness, or society? Am Psychol 42:384–399, 1987

Money J: Gay, Straight and In-Between: The Sexology of Erotic Orientation. New York, Oxford University Press, 1988

Money J, Ehrhard A: Man, Woman, Boy, Girl. Baltimore, MD, Johns Hopkins University Press, 1972

Murphy TF: Freud reconsidered: bisexuality, homosexuality, and moral judgment. J Homosex 9(2/3):65–77, 1983–1984

Paul JP: The bisexual identity: an idea without social recognition. J Homosex 9(2/3):45–63, 1983–1984

Plummer K: Sexual Stigma. London, Routledge and Kegan Paul, 1975

Read KE: Other Voices. Navato, CA, Chandler and Sharp, 1986

Stoller RJ: Sex and Gender. New York, Science House, 1968

Stoller RJ: Sexual Excitement: Dynamics of Erotic Life. New York, Pantheon Books, 1979

Stoller RJ: Problems with the term "homosexuality." J Clin Psychiatry 2:3–25, 1980

Stoller RJ, Herdt G: Theories of origins of homosexuality. Arch Gen Psychiatry, 42:399–404, 1985

Strathern M: The Gender of the Gift. Berkeley, CA, University of California Press, 1988

van Baal J: The dialectics of sex in Marind-anim culture, in Ritualized Homosexuality in Melanesia, 2nd Edition. Edited by Herdt G. Berkeley, CA, University of California Press, 1993, pp 128–166

Weeks J: Coming Out: Homosexual Politicos in Britain, from the Nineteenth Century to the Present. London, Quartet Books, 1977

Weeks J: Sexuality and Discontents. London, Routledge and Kegan Paul, 1985

Whitehead H: The bow and the burden strap: a new look at institution-alized homosexuality in native North America, in Sexual Meanings. Edited by Ortner SB, Whitehead H. Cambridge, UK, Cambridge University Press, 1981, pp 80–115

Williams W: The Spirit and the Flesh. Boston, MA, Beacon, 1986

6

The Essentialist/Social Constructionist Debate About Homosexuality and Its Relevance for Psychotherapy

Terry S. Stein, M.D.

A fervent academic debate in gay and lesbian studies during the past decade concerns the extent to which a social constructionist versus an essentialist approach to conceptualizing human sexuality, and particularly sexual orientation and homosexuality, provides a better understanding of these complex phenomena. Although the debate has occurred primarily within the social sciences and humanities and outside of psychiatry and the other mental health fields, in this chapter the author reviews these two ideas,

This chapter is based in part on Stein T: "Social Constructionism and Essentialism: Theoretical and Clinical Considerations Relevant to Psychotherapy." *Journal of Gay and Lesbian Psychotherapy* (in press).

explains their relevance for mental health, and outlines issues raised by these theories for the clinician working with gay and lesbian patients.

Social Constructionism

The ground-breaking work of Kinsey and colleagues (1948, 1953) on human sexuality anticipated contemporary social constructionist approaches to the study of sexuality. On the basis of findings from surveys of the sexual lives of men and women, Kinsey et al. concluded that division of individuals into simple dichotomous categories based on some sexual characteristic was impossible and argued instead for an appreciation of the diversity and variation in human sexuality. Kinsey et al. (1948) stated that the world cannot

> be divided into sheep and goats. . . . It is a fundamental of taxonomy that nature rarely deals with discrete categories. Only the human mind invents categories and tries to force facts into separate pigeonholes. The living world is a continuum in each and every one of its aspects. (p. 639)

Social constructionism is a belief both in the primary importance of social forces in shaping human behavior and experience and that knowledge is not a reflection of the world but rather a product of discourse.

Gergen and Davis (1985) describe four assumptions that underlie social constructionist theory:

1. Existing categories and ideas arise from language and context and do not serve as a map of the world. For example, commonly accepted concepts, such as gender, emotions, and psychological disorder, should not be taken as objective facts derived from observation but rather as social conventions.
2. Common ideas and categories are artifacts of particular societies at particular times and change across time. Even the most fundamental conceptions, such as ideas of self, identity, romantic love, emotion, reason, and language, should be understood as culturally and historically specific social constructions.
3. The degree to which an idea gains prominence or survives over time should not be understood as a reflection of its empirical ac-

curacy but rather as a function of processes of social interaction. Thus, according to this view, even methods for attaining truth and knowledge, as represented, for example, in scientific rules, can serve primarily as a means for achieving social control rather than for acquiring understanding.

4. Forms of descriptions and explanations serve as expressions of social meaning and action. Gergen and Davis cite the example within psychology of how conceptions about emotion regarding the extent to which individuals experience choice or lack of choice about having their emotions will significantly affect the implications for treating people who suffer from certain emotional states like depression, anxiety, and fear.

The contemporary appearance of social constructionism is linked to the publication of *The Social Construction of Reality* (Berger and Luckmann 1966). In the study of human sexuality, McIntosh (1968) first described social constructionism and defined the distinction between homosexual behavior and the homosexual role. Plummer's (1975) discussion of sexual stigma is another important early contribution to the social constructionist literature. Both McIntosh and Plummer examined homosexuality from the sociological perspective known as labeling theory, which says that the homosexual role and identity came about as a result of stigmatizing and labeling the person who engages in homosexual behavior, thereby creating the notion of the homosexual person.

The seminal work of the French philosopher Foucault, beginning with the publication of *The History of Sexuality, Volume I: An Introduction* (1978), significantly shaped the parameters of the social constructionist debate about sexuality. Foucault argues that there is no inner human sexual drive, rather that the human potential for thinking and acting is shaped by social forces of regulation and categorization into various forms of sexuality at different times in history. According to this view, sexuality is not simply influenced or molded but is actually created by cultural forces.

Numerous other writers have applied social constructionist methods to the analysis of homosexuality as well. Weeks (1977), Katz (1983), and D'Emilio (1986) have documented the emergence of modern gay and lesbian identities and communities in specific historical periods. Altman (1982) and Epstein (1987) have explored the political aspects of the construction of contemporary homosexual identities. Several collections of articles (Altman et al. 1989; Hart and Richardson 1981; Stein 1992) have provided an examination of social constructionist approaches to homosexuality through the lens of psychology, sexology, and the social sciences. Additional writings in anthropology (Herdt 1981, 1992), sociology (Greenberg 1988; Ponse 1978), history (Halperin 1990), and the humanities (Butler 1990) have further elaborated the social constructionist analysis of sexual identity and homosexuality.

The central conclusions from these scholarly discussions from the perspective of social constructionism about the meaning and origins of human sexuality undermine traditional assumptions about the fixity and naturalness of any sexual category, label, or desire. The methods of social constructionism present a new way of questioning and examining notions of sexuality and any other label, theory, or idea. Through these methods, the assumptions underlying the social construction of our discourse about a particular topic can be identified and analyzed, leading not to new answers about the topic but to additional questions at the interface of the disciplines of thought that have contributed to the belief. Such an approach contrasts with the essentialist perspective described below.

Essentialism

The description of essentialism has largely been developed in the writing of the social constructionists and refers to the view that sexual categories and sexual identities represent fixed personal characteristics that are inherent, objective, transcultural, and transhistorical. Essentialism treats sexuality as a biological force underlying genuine gender differences that in turn serve as the basis for sexual categories and identities. In relation to sexual orientation, essentialism argues that differences in sexual desire create categories of persons known as homosexual and heterosexual that are fundamentally the same across time and in different cultures. In writing, there are few self-identified essentialists. Vance (1989) compares this absence of self-identified essentialists to the lack of awareness of heterosexual identity. The dominant system of belief, like the dominant form of sexual identity, can only have form and be named in relation to a competing and alternative system. Thus, historically the definition of heterosexuality took place after the description of homosexuality in the late 19th century; similarly, the adumbration of essentialism occurred only in relation to the elaboration of social constructionist theory. According to this view, the absence of self-proclaimed essentialist writers reflects an unselfconsciousness about an individual's views when they represent the fundamental assumptions of society about the natural status of sexual categories and behaviors.

Essentialist authors include Boswell (1980), Rich (1983), and Dynes (1990). Essentialists adhere to a belief that fundamental differences exist between persons based on their sexuality; these differences may derive from biological factors such as neuroendocrine, anatomical, or genetic features, from early developmental experience, or from unspecified causes. Essentialism suggests the presence of a fixed sexual quality in a person, a lack of choice about the existence of the quality, and an underlying and enduring core basis for categorical descriptions of persons based on the quality.

Comparison of Essentialism and Social Constructionism

Epstein (1987) argues that the distinction between essentialism and social constructionism reflects the earlier debate between nature and nurture as the cause of homosexuality. He describes the essentialist position as seeing sexuality as a "biological force seeking expression in ways that are preordained" (p. 13) and the constructionists as "treating sexuality as a blank slate, capable of bearing whatever meanings are generated by the society in question" (p. 13). Epstein further characterizes essentialism as being consistent with a politics of identity practiced in gay and lesbian communities that demands recognition of being gay as comparable to being a member of other groups defined by a difference such as race or ethnicity. He portrays social constructionism, in contrast, as an intellectual theory that may be viewed as being out of step with gay and lesbian experience and the practice of minority politics.

Troiden (1988) focuses on several additional concepts to contrast essentialism and social constructionism. He describes an emphasis by essentialists on the underlying sexual preferences and feelings of persons, rather than on their sexual behaviors, to define sexual orientation.

Troiden further discusses the interest of essentialists in determining the causes of homosexuality, arising from psychodynamic, hormonal, or prenatal factors, and in predicting adult sexual orientation based on childhood characteristics and behaviors, particularly early gender role nonconformity. He classifies both adherents of the view that homosexuality is pathological (Bieber et al. 1962; Socarides 1978) as well as those who believe that it is a normal variation (Bell et al. 1981; Green 1987; Harry 1982; Whitam and Mathy 1986) as essentialists.

Although currently ascendant in academic circles, social constructionism is viewed by some as politically incorrect because it is characterized as equating a social construction of sexuality with a voluntary choice about sexual orientation. This position is seen as strengthening the socially conservative argument that, if one can choose to be gay or lesbian, then a person can be held responsible for his or her sexual orientation, and efforts can be undertaken to require individuals to choose to be heterosexual. Conversely, it is argued that essentialism represents a belief in the fixed nature of sexual orientation for which a person cannot be held responsible.

Social constructionism and essentialism share a belief in the transcultural and transhistorical existence both of homosexual behavior and of the experience of a homosexual inclination by some individuals (Ruse 1988). In general, they also agree that some individuals in all societies are more or less exclusively homosexual in their orientation. Beyond these fundamental commonalities, the two schools of thought present a wide range of differences in beliefs.

Criticisms of Essentialism and Social Constructionism

The social constructionist position has been defined in part by its criticism of essentialist views of sexuality and sexual orientation. Thus, inherent in social constructionism is a critique of traditional essentialist views of sexuality. Vance (1989) says, "We have all been brought up to think about sexuality in essentialist ways" (p. 14) that rely on an assumption about the natural status of labels used to describe sexuality; in contrast, social constructionism represents an alternative and opposing way of understanding and questioning the language, metaphors, and assumptions that serve to define human sexuality.

Essentialism is criticized by the social constructionists for defining homosexuality based on popular beliefs and values and for reifying a homosexual person as a type of individual based solely on sexual behavior. What is viewed by the essentialist as a natural and objective reason for dividing up people throughout history and in all cultures is considered by the social constructionist to be a constructed notion about sexuality developed by a particular society at a point in history. According to this conceptualization, the differences between people who participated in same-gender sexual relations in ancient Greece, medieval Europe, and modern America are more important than the commonality in their sexual behavior. A typology of persons based on their sexual behavior is viewed as no more natural or real than categories based on eating practices or exercising behaviors.

Richardson (1983) describes essentialist beliefs about homosexuality as developing in three distinct patterns that conceptualize homosexuality as 1) a state of being, associated with the creation of the concept of the homosexual person; 2) a state of sexuality, linking both sexual desire and behavior with the homosexual category; and 3) a state of personal identity, involving the incorporation of the effects of both labeling and political forces into the notion of homosexuality. Richardson argues that theories about homosexuality must consider the separate categories of sexual desire, behavior, and identity and not assume some inherent essential sexuality in the individual.

Another criticism of the essentialist position relates to its role as the dominant ideology serving to maintain existing sexual categories and arrangements. The modern sexual ideologues, according to Padgug (1979), determine the nature of all spheres of operation related to sexuality, including gender, reproduction, the family, and love. He reconceptualizes sexuality as praxis, that is, sexual "meaning and contents are in a continual process of change" (p. 11). Viewing sexuality as praxis in this manner clearly would move the historical perspective of homosexuality from an essentialist to a social constructionist conceptualization.

Vance (1989) outlines three criticisms of social constructionism that need additional development. The first criticism is the notion that social constructionism implies a devaluation of sexual identities. This criticism equates the questioning in social constructionist writing of the cultural meaning of identity with an undermining or destruction of these identities. Vance argues that this criticism trivializes social constructionist thinking.

Vance identifies another criticism of social constructionism as deriving from the belief that it implies—as a result of its emphasis on the cultural construction of identity—that individual sexual identity is completely malleable, comparable to a set of clothing that can be tried on and disposed of at will. She states that this criticism arises from a confusion between the individual and cultural levels of analysis in social constructionism. Specific cultural forces can be identified that influence and shape individual identity, but this does not suggest that the individual or group experiencing a particular identity can simply change or discard this identity at will. Vance states that social constructionism does question traditional assumptions about the rigidity of and inability to change identity, implying that identity may not be as fixed and as immutable as we have believed.

The third criticism of social constructionism identified by Vance is that it assumes discontinuity and rupture across cultures and throughout history in behaviors and in the subjective experience of meaning associated with these behaviors. She believes this criticism arises from a misreading of social constructionism and ignores the fact that the theory neither requires discontinuity or change nor eliminates the possibility of continuity and similarities.

Implications of the Essentialist/Social Constructionist Debate for Clinical Work With Lesbians, Bisexuals, and Gay Men

An important understanding about the nature of sexual orientation and homosexuality has come about as the result of work completed by both essentialist and social constructionist researchers and theoreticians. However, because of the adherence of most mental health clinicians to essentialist ideas about sexuality, the concerns of social constructionists have not found their way into the discourse about approaches to evaluation and treatment of lesbians, bisexuals, and gay men. Tiefer (1992) states, "The major obstacle to a social constructionist approach to sexuality is the domination of theory and research by the biomedical model" (p. 311).

Another explanation for the lack of attention to social constructionist theory within the field of mental health may lie in the deliberate movement away from views of homosexuality that may be understood to imply choice on the part of the individual about the direction of his or her sexual orientation. Psychotherapists working with gay men and lesbians have argued for the need to accept and adapt to a particular inborn sexual orientation. The idea that an individual's sexual orientation might change has been associated with the notion that one should attempt to change it if it is homosexual, an obviously disagreeable thought for those interested in promoting more openness about and tolerance of homosexuality.

The essentialist belief that sexual orientation is the expression of an inherent and largely fixed essence of a person is pervasive within the fields of psychiatry and psychotherapy currently. This belief underlies both theories that view homosexuality as pathological as well as those that describe it as a normal variation, and it serves as a central motivation within the biomedical sciences for attempting to determine the cause of homosexuality, whether it is believed to lie primarily in genetic, hormonal, environmental, or familial factors. The two central essentialist assumptions underlying virtually all contemporary approaches to psychotherapy with lesbians, bisexuals, and gay men today are 1) that sexual orientation is the expression of some inner nature of a person that is determined either before birth or within the first 2 or 3 years of life and 2) that sexual orientation, although it may be denied or repressed because of social or individual forces acting against its expression, especially if it is homosexual, rarely changes across a lifetime.

Few writers have tackled the problem of translating social constructionist theory to the practice of psychotherapy. Hart (1981, 1984), however, emphasized the role of choice in deciding how to act in relation to sexual identity and the need for the therapist to distinguish between those problems for clients related to social sex-role characteristics and those involving sexual orientation. He also describes the need for the therapist to recognize the essentialist beliefs of clients about the immutability of their sexual identity. Richardson (1987) outlined the necessity for the therapist both to explore the meaning and significance of being gay for each individual and to understand that sexual identity and sexual orientation are open to change. At the same time, Richardson cautioned that a wish to change sexual orientation may often arise from guilt about being homosexual and that the therapist, therefore, must fully explore the motivation for change.

Moving beyond the social constructionist ideas about change and variability in relation to sexual orientation, Schippers (1989) describes four pragmatic approaches that represent his response within therapy to constructionism: 1) exploring the meaning of homosexuality for each person in therapy; 2) exploring the possibilities and limitations associated with adopting a homosexual identity; 3) emphasizing the different ways to express an individual's homosexuality; and 4) using feelings within the transference to demonstrate the variability of the emotions that can be associated with being homosexual.

Toward a Synthesis of Essentialist and Social Constructionist Views

Ultimately, clinicians working with lesbians, bisexuals, and gay men (or a person of any sexual orientation) will use both essentialist and social constructionist ideas in their approach to evaluation and treatment. Four sets of contrasting statements—derived from extreme positions representing essentialist and social constructionist schools of thought—are discussed below in terms of their relevance to clinical work.

■ First Set of Statements

"Sexual orientation represents some universal transcultural and transhistorical characteristic (essentialism)" versus "Sexual orientation is different in every society and at different times in history (social constructionism)." Note that the level of argument in these two statements takes place at a cultural level, juxtaposing the universal and the specific character of sexual identity in relation to society. In clinical work, however, we are concerned with the experience of the individual. The importance of this argument in relation to the individual resides in its examination of the role of sexual orientation both in creating connection and universality across time and place (essentialism) and in defining uniqueness, individuality, and cultural specificity within a particular society at a given time (social constructionism). Both dimensions are important to appreciate and elaborate as individuals explore their sexuality during the course of psychotherapy.

Within the context of psychotherapy, the individual can neither be held responsible for larger social forces nor be seen as operating outside of these forces. Although the cultural factors contributing to the patient's experience of sexual orientation may not be a primary focus of psychotherapy, the effects of age, generation, and a multitude of other culturally shaped variables will still significantly influence the individual's experience of sexuality. For example, recognition of the existence of homosexuality in some form in societies throughout history may help some persons appreciate the universality of their experience, whereas appreciation of the differences for middle-aged individuals who "came out" in the 1950s and younger persons coming out in the 1990s could highlight for some persons the specific problems with which persons in each generation have had to contend in relation to their homosexuality within the same society at different times.

Second Set of Statements

"Sexual orientation is innate (essentialism)" versus "Sexual orientation is constructed (social constructionism)." To say that sexual orientation is constructed should not be construed to mean that the individual consciously sets out to build a particular sexual orientation, but rather that sexuality in all its forms is shaped and determined by social forces beyond the control of the individual. Because the psychotherapist must remain close to the experience of the person seeking help, the phylogenetic origin of sexuality will often have little to do with the work to be done in psychotherapy. Whether the origins of sexual orientation reside in universal and innate characteristics or in variable and external cultural factors or in both, gay, lesbian, and bisexual individuals need to come to terms with their experience of sexual desire, behavior, and identity and the societal reactions to these components of sexuality. The individual cannot be viewed as a psychological battlefield on which warring theories fight for ascendance.

Third Set of Statements

"Sexual orientation is fixed (essentialism)" versus "Sexual orientation is mutable (social constructionism)." Within the larger debate, this argument has thus far received the most attention with respect to its implications for psychotherapy and, with the following related argument, has the most relevance for individual psychological experience of sexual orientation. Empirical findings tell us that sexual orientation is neither rigidly fixed—sexual desire, behavior, and identity do change for many persons during their lives—nor easily changed—as demonstrated in the failure of multiple efforts by psychotherapists to alter underlying sexual orientation. Those adhering to a belief in a fixed sexual orientation generally explain these findings by defining the existence of some inner nature that is discovered or acknowledged by individuals in the process of changing their sexuality.

Those believing in a fixed and relatively uniform sexual orientation during an individual's life are rightfully challenged by the social constructionist position in this argument. The enormous variability in the patterns of developing and expressing sexual orientation and of establishing a gay or lesbian identity clearly indicates that a multitude of ways exist to develop and experience sexual orientation, that some persons have different sexual orientations and identities at different points in their lives, and that no unitary definitions exist for homosexuality, bisexuality, or heterosexuality that fit everyone. The implications of these conclusions for work with persons in psychotherapy could be enormous and may have significant political and social ramifications as well.

Several shifts in approaches to psychotherapy might result from adopting a social constructionist position in relation to change of sexual orientation. For example, the belief that all persons who experiment with homosexual behavior or adopt a gay or lesbian identity or lifestyle are fundamentally homosexual would be abandoned in favor of a more flexible view of sexual identity, more consistent with the experiences of many women, who in general seem to experience more fluidity than men in their sexual orientation (see Chapter 23 by Falco; Golden 1987; Hanley-Hackenbruck 1993). Approaches to assessment of sexual orientation also might begin to reflect a more complex view of the actual nature of sexuality and incorporate recognition of differences in past, present, and future (ideal) experiences (Coleman 1987; Klein et al. 1985). The concern that all attempts to convert gay men and lesbians to heterosexuality (Martin 1984) invariably reflect a coercive and anti-homosexual approach could be diminished and focus on those specific instances of conversion treatment that may involve homophobic motivation (Nicolosi 1991; Pattison and Pattison 1980). Finally, greater acceptance of the idea of the mutability of sexual orientation may encourage more attention to the diverse forms of sexual orientation described within ethnic and other cultural groups.

■ Fourth Set of Statements

"Sexual orientation represents a characteristic over which the individual has no choice (essentialism)" versus "Sexual orientation can to some extent be chosen by the individual (social constructionism)." Most psychotherapists and perhaps the majority of the general public as well hold the essentialist assumption that the individual has little choice in determining sexual orientation. This belief is consistent with the experience of most persons, who in no way consciously choose to be gay, lesbian, bisexual, or heterosexual. In addition, the factors that are felt to contribute to the formation of adult sexual orientation, including genes, hormones, familial influences, and even social forces, are rarely under the control of the individual. Given the virtually universal belief in the absence of choice about sexual orientation, it is difficult even to imagine how to think about the degree of choice an individual may have in shaping sexual desire, behavior, and identity. Perhaps (this is a position taken by many social constructionists) it is just such a focus on choice that is needed if we are to maintain any understanding of individual freedom in relation to our sexuality.

Out of fear that others may impose a particular choice about appropriate sexuality, mental health practitioners may argue that we have no choice at all about our sexuality or our identity and fall into a deterministic mode of thinking that lays out a course of development and experience for all persons based on narrow and predictable options available to them as a result of their sexual orientation. Hart (1981, 1984) and Richardson (1987) examine some aspects of the role of choice in working with persons in counseling regarding their concerns about sexual orientation and sexual identity, but they do not consider fully the difficult questions raised by introducing the notion of change in sexual orientation into the therapeutic process.

Some of these questions include the following. To what extent do we foreclose personal options by informing people that they have no choice about their sexual orientation? How do practitioners truncate the full understanding of sexual development and expression by adherence to a belief that we have so little choice about who we are sexually? Do practitioners collude with those who wish to prescribe and legislate proper sexuality when they fail to argue from a position that supports the right for individuals to choose whatever form of sexual identity appeals to them and resort instead to a belief that individuals cannot choose their sexuality?

These questions must be addressed within theory and research to develop an appreciation for the full human potentiality in relation to sexuality. At the same time, within the practice of psychotherapy, therapists must not blame individuals seeking help for those factors that contributed to their sexual development or for their current form of sexuality. Therapists also can help their patients by presenting an attitude of openness about both future sexual patterns and the extent of choice an individual may have in determining these patterns.

Conclusion

The debate between essentialists and social constructionists is relevant to the field of psychotherapy with lesbians, bisexuals, and gay men. The virtual exclusion of much of the social constructionist argument from the biomedical sciences and the mental health field reinforces an intellectual position of unreflective adherence to essentialist assumptions. The essentialist dominance in theory, research, and practice may preclude a debate that has really never taken place within these fields. Because the terms of the debate have not been translated into an applied medical and psychological jargon, the social constructionist propositions sometimes seem confusing. If questions concerning the origins of sexual orientation and the degree of change and choice possible in relation to sexuality are to be fully studied, this debate also must be taken up within the fields of psychiatry and the other mental health disciplines. Neither essentialism nor social constructionism alone holds the answers to these questions, but both offer valuable tools for the examination of our objective and subjective experience of sexuality.

References

Altman D: The Homosexualization of America. Boston, MA, Beacon Press, 1982

Altman D, Vance C, Vicinus M, et al: Homosexuality, Which Homosexuality? London, GMP Publishers, 1989

Bieber I, Dain HJ, Dince PR, et al: Homosexuality: A Psychoanalytical Study. New York, Basic Books, 1962

Bell AP, Weinberg MS, Hammersmith SK: Sexual Preference: Its Development in Men and Women. Bloomington, IN, Indiana University Press, 1981

Berger P, Luckmann T: The Social Construction of Reality. Garden City, NY, Doubleday, 1966

Boswell J: Christianity, Social Tolerance and Homosexuality. Chicago, IL, University of Chicago Press, 1980

Butler J: Gender Trouble: Feminism and the Subversion of Identity. New York, Routledge, 1990

Coleman E: Assessment of sexual orientation. J Homosex 14:9–24, 1987

D'Emilio J: Making and unmaking minorities: the tensions between gay politics and history. New York University Review of Law and Social Change 14:915–922, 1986

Dynes WR, Johansson W, Percy WA (eds): Encyclopedia of Homosexuality. New York, Garland Publishing, 1990

Epstein S: Gay politics, ethnic identity: the limits of social constructionism. Socialist Review 93/94:9–54, 1987

Foucault M: The History of Sexuality, Volume I: An Introduction. Translated by Hurley R. New York, Pantheon, 1978

Gergen K, Davis K (eds): The Social Construction of the Person. New York, Springer, 1985

Golden C: Diversity and variability in women's sexual identities, in Lesbian Psychologies. Edited by Boston Lesbian Psychologies Collective. Urbana, IL, University of Illinois Press, 1987, pp 18–34

Green R: The Sissy Boy Syndrome and the Development of Homosexuality. New Haven, CT, Yale University Press, 1987

Greenberg D: The Construction of Homosexuality. Chicago, IL, University of Chicago Press, 1988

Halperin D: One Hundred Years of Homosexuality and Other Essays on Greek Love. Boston, MA, Routledge, 1990

Hanley-Hackenbruck P: Working with lesbians in psychotherapy, in American Psychiatric Press Review of Psychiatry, Vol 12. Edited by Oldham J, Riba M, Tasman A. Washington, DC, American Psychiatric Press, 1993, pp 59–83

Harry J: Gay Children Grown Up: Gender Culture and Gender Deviance. New York, Praeger, 1982

Hart J: Theoretical explanations in practice, in The Theory and Practice of Homosexuality. Edited by Hart J, Richardson D. London, Routledge and Kegan Paul, 1981, pp 38–67

Hart J: Therapeutic implications of viewing sexual identity in terms of essentialist and constructionist theories. J Homosex 9(4):39–51, 1984

Hart J, Richardson D (eds): The Theory and Practice of Homosexuality. Boston, MA, Routledge, 1981

Herdt GH: Guardians of the Flutes: Idioms of Masculinity. New York, McGraw-Hill, 1981

Herdt GH (ed): Gay Culture in America: Essays from the Field. Boston, MA, Beacon Press, 1992

Katz JN: Gay American Almanac. New York, Harper, 1983

Kinsey AC, Pomeroy WB, Martin CE: Sexual Behavior in the Human Male. Philadelphia, PA, WB Saunders, 1948

Kinsey AC, Pomeroy WB, Martin CE: Sexual Behavior in the Human Female. Philadelphia, PA, WB Saunders, 1953

Klein F, Sepekoff B, Wolf TJ: Sexual orientation: a multi-variable dynamic process. J Homosex 11:35–49, 1985

McIntosh M: The homosexual role. Social Problems 17:262–270, 1968

Martin D: The emperor's new clothes: modern attempts to change sexual orientation, in Innovations in Psychotherapy with Homosexuals. Edited by Hetrick E, Stein T. Washington, DC, American Psychiatric Press, 1984, pp 23–58

Nicolosi J: Reparative Therapy of Male Homosexuality: A New Clinical Approach. Northvale, NJ, Jason Aronson, 1991

Padgug RA: Sexual matters: on conceptualizing sexuality in history, in Radical History Review 20:3–23, Spring/Summer 1979

Pattison EM, Pattison ML: Ex-gays: religiously mediated change in homosexuals. Am J Psychiatry 137:1553–1562, 1980

Plummer K: Sexual Stigma. London, Routledge, 1975

Ponse B: Identities in the Lesbian World: The Social Construction of Self. Westport, CT, Greenwood Press, 1978

Rich A: Compulsory heterosexuality and lesbian existence. Signs: Journal of Women in Culture and Society 5:631–660, 1983

Richardson D: The dilemma of essentiality in homosexual theory. J Homosex 9(2/3):79–90, 1983

Richardson D: Recent challenges to traditional assumptions about homosexuality: some implications for practice. J Homosex 13(4):1–12, 1987

Ruse M: Homosexuality. Oxford, UK, Basil Blackwell, 1988

Schippers J: Homosexual identity, essentialism and constructionism, in Homosexuality, Which Homosexuality? Edited by Altman D, Vance C, Vicinus M, Weeks J. London, GMP Publishers, 1989, pp 139–148

Socarides C: Homosexuality. New York, Jason Aronson, 1978

Stein E (ed): Forms of Desire. New York, Routledge, 1992

Tiefer L: Social constructionism and the study of human sexuality, in Forms of Desire. Edited by Stein E. New York, Routledge, 1992, pp 295–324

Troiden RR: Gay and Lesbian Identity. Dix Hills, NY, General Hall, 1988

Vance CS: Social construction theory: problems in the history of sexuality, in Homosexuality, Which Homosexuality? Edited by Altman D, Vance C, Vicenus M, Weeks J. London, GMP Publishers, 1989, pp 13–34

Weeks J: Coming Out: Homosexual Politicos in Britain from the Nineteenth Century to the Present. London, Quartet Books, 1977

Whitam FL, Mathy RM: Male Homosexuality in Four Societies: Brazil, Guatemala, the Philippines, and the United States. New York, Praeger, 1986

7

Heterosexism and Homophobia

Gregory M. Herek, Ph.D.

Heterosexism and homophobia refer generally to a hostility and prejudice against both homosexual behavior and gay and lesbian people. Of the two terms, "homophobia" was the first to be coined. Weinberg (1972) used the term to characterize heterosexuals' dread of being in close quarters with homosexuals as well as homosexuals' self-loathing. "Heterosexism" has been defined as the ideological system that denies, denigrates, and stigmatizes any nonheterosexual form of behavior, identity, relationship, or community (Herek 1990).

Although the term "homophobia" is commonly used to characterize heterosexuals' antigay prejudice, such usage is avoided here for two reasons. First, empirical research does not support the classification of heterosexuals' antigay attitudes as a phobia in the clinical sense. Indeed, the limited data available suggest that many heterosexuals who express hostility toward gay men and lesbians do not manifest the physiological reactions to homosexuality that are associated with other phobias (Shields and Harriman 1984). Second, the term "homophobia" implicitly conveys the assumption that antigay prejudice is an individual, clinical entity rather than a social phenomenon rooted in cultural ideologies and intergroup relations. As noted below, antigay prejudice is often functional for the heterosexuals who manifest it.

In this chapter, homophobia is used only in Weinberg's (1972) second sense, that is, to describe internalized homophobia or the hostility of gay men or lesbians toward their own homosexuality. Heterosexism—which suggests parallels between antigay sentiment and other forms of prejudice, such as racism, antisemitism, and sexism—is used to characterize heterosexuals' prejudices against lesbians and gay men, as well as the behaviors based on those prejudices.

Heterosexism is manifested both at the cultural and individual levels. Cultural heterosexism, like institutional racism and sexism, pervades societal customs and institutions. It operates through a dual process of invisibility and attack. Homosexuality usually remains culturally invisible; when people who engage in homosexual behavior or who are identified as homosexual become visible, they are subject to attack by society. Examples of cultural heterosexism in the United States include the widespread lack of legal protection from antigay discrimination in employment, housing, and services; the continuing ban against lesbian and gay military personnel; the absence of legal recognition for lesbian and gay committed relationships; and the existence of sodomy laws in nearly one-half of the states (see Chapter 46 by Purcell and Hicks).

Psychological heterosexism is the individual manifestation of cultural heterosexism. It is reflected in heterosexuals' feelings of personal disgust, hostility, or condemnation of homosexuality and of lesbians and gay men. Public opinion data indicate that psychological heterosexism is widespread. Most Americans consistently condemn homosexuality or homosexual behavior as morally wrong or a sin, regard it as unnatural, and express disgust toward it (Herek 1994; Wood 1990). Furthermore, most Americans do not consider homosexuality to be an acceptable alternative lifestyle (Herek, in press; Hugick 1992).

Psychological heterosexism also is expressed behaviorally. Of 113 lesbians and 287 gay men interviewed in a 1989 national telephone survey, 5% of the men and 10% of the women reported having been physically abused or assaulted in the previous year because they were gay. Nearly one-half (47%) reported experiencing some form of discrimination (job, housing, health care, or social) at some time in their life as a result of their sexual orientation (San Francisco Examiner 1989).

Other research also has found that significant numbers of gay men and lesbians have been the targets of verbal abuse, discrimination, or physical assault because of their sexual orientation. In a review of 24 separate questionnaire studies with convenience samples of gay men and lesbians, Berrill (1992) reported that a median of 44% of respondents had been threatened with violence because of their sexual orientation; 33% had been chased or followed; 25% had had objects thrown at them; 13% had been spat on; and 80% had been verbally harassed. Across the studies, a median of 9% of respondents had been assaulted with a weapon; 17% reported simple physical assault; and 19% reported vandalism of property. Berrill's review was restricted to incidents that resulted from the victim's perceived sexual orientation. It is likely that the survey respondents also had experienced the sort of routine criminal victimization that is part of daily life for everyone living in the United States.

Because none of the studies reviewed by Berrill (1992) used probability samples, the percentages he reported cannot be generalized to the entire U.S. gay and lesbian population. The figures, however, have a heuristic value. Although the exact number of gay and lesbian individuals who have experienced violence as a result of their sexual orientation remains unknown, it is clear that an alarming number of such attacks have occurred in the past decade and that they continue to occur today (see Chapter 48 by Klinger and Stein).

Despite widespread antipathy toward gay Americans, however, national surveys during the past two decades reveal a growing willingness to grant basic civil rights to gay people. Americans are increasingly reluctant to condone discrimination on the basis of sexual orientation. The proportion of American adults surveyed by the Gallup organization who say that homosexual men and women should have equal rights in terms of job opportunities has increased steadily during the past 15 years. The same polls indicate that a plurality of Americans now feel that homosexual relations between consenting adults should be legal (Hugick 1992). Data collected by the National Opinion Research Center show increasing support for free speech rights for gay Americans during the past two decades (Herek 1994; Wood 1990). The vast majority of Americans now feel that a person who "admits he is a homosexual" should be able to teach in a college or university or to make a speech in their community and would oppose removing a book in favor of homosexuality from the local public library (Herek 1994; Wood 1990). In summary, although they show increasing willingness to extend basic civil liberties to gay men and lesbians, most heterosexual

Americans continue to condemn homosexuality morally and to reject or feel uncomfortable about gay people personally.

Social Psychological Research on Heterosexism

■ Correlates of Prejudice

Empirical research has demonstrated that heterosexuals' attitudes toward gay men and lesbians consistently are correlated with various psychological, social, and demographic variables. In contrast to heterosexuals with favorable attitudes toward gay people, those with negative attitudes are 1) less likely to have had personal contact with gay men or lesbians; 2) more likely to be strongly religious and to subscribe to a conservative religious ideology; 3) more likely to support traditional gender roles; 4) more likely to believe that sexual orientation is not a matter of personal choice; 5) likely to be older and less well educated; and 6) more likely to have resided in geographic areas (e.g., rural areas or the midwestern or southern United States) where negative attitudes represent the norm (for reviews, see Herek 1984, 1991; Kite 1994).

In addition, heterosexual males tend to manifest higher levels of prejudice than do heterosexual females, especially toward gay men. This sex difference results in part from heterosexual females' greater likelihood of personal contact with openly gay people, which is strongly correlated with greater acceptance of lesbians and gay men (Herek and Capitanio 1995, in press; Herek and Glunt 1993). Such differential opportunities for contact may be a product of the strong link in American culture between masculinity and heterosexuality, which creates considerable social and psychological pressures for males to affirm their masculinity through rejection of that which is not culturally defined as masculine (male homosexuality) and that which is perceived as negating the importance of males (lesbianism). Because heterosexual women are less likely to perceive rejection of homosexuality as integral to their own gender identity, they may experience fewer pressures to be prejudiced and consequently have more opportunities for personal contact with gay people.

■ Functions of Prejudice for the Individual

As with other types of prejudice, different heterosexuals hold negative attitudes toward lesbians and gay men for different reasons. The basis of those reasons is the psychological benefit an individual derives from prejudice. Four principal psychological functions have been identified that underlie heterosexuals' antigay attitudes (Herek 1987, 1992).

First, attitudes serving an *experiential* function assist heterosexuals in making sense of their previous interactions with gay people by fitting them into a larger world view, one that is organized primarily in terms of the individual's own self-interest. Some heterosexuals accept gay people in general on the basis of pleasant interaction experiences with a specific gay man or lesbian. Others hold negative attitudes toward the entire group primarily as a result of their unpleasant experiences with particular gay men or lesbians.

Because only about one-third of American adults personally know someone who is openly gay (Herek and Capitanio, in press; Herek and Glunt 1993), most heterosexuals' attitudes necessarily are not experiential. For them, homosexuality and gay people are primarily symbols. Whereas attitudes toward people with whom one has direct experience function primarily to organize and make sense of those experiences, attitudes toward symbols serve a different function. Such attitudes help people to increase their self-esteem by expressing important aspects of themselves—by declaring (to themselves and to others) what sort of people they are. Affirming who one is often *is* accomplished by distancing oneself from or even attacking people who represent the sort of person one *is not* (or does not want to be).

Three different attitude functions have been identified that serve these symbolic purposes. Attitudes serving a *value-expressive* function enable heterosexuals to affirm their belief in and adherence to important values that are closely related to their concepts of self. When attitudes serve a *social expressive* function, expressing the attitude strengthens one's sense of belonging to a particular group and helps an individual to gain acceptance, approval, or love from other people whom he or she considers important (e.g., peers, family, or neighbors). Finally, attitudes serving an *ego-defensive* function lower an individual's anxiety resulting from his or her unconscious psychological conflicts, such as those surrounding sexuality or gender.

It is important to recognize the nexus between psychological and cultural heterosexism. A particular manifestation of psychological heterosexism can serve one or more of these functions only when the individual's psychological needs converge with the ideology of the culture. Antigay prejudice can be value-expressive only when an individual's concept of self is closely tied to values that also have become socially defined as antithetical to homosexuality. It can be socially expressive only insofar as an individual strongly needs to be accepted by members of a social group that rejects gay people or homosexuality, and it can be defensive only when lesbians and gay men are culturally defined in a way that links them to an individual's psychological conflicts.

■ Heterosexism and Stereotypes

Strongly correlated with heterosexuals' expression of hostility toward lesbians and gay men is their acceptance of negative stereotypes about gay people. As used here, negative stereotypes are exaggerated, fixed, and derogatory beliefs based on membership in a social category or group. Like negative stereotypes about other minority groups, those about lesbians and gay men reflect the internalization of historically evolved cultural ideologies or belief systems that justify the subjugation of minorities. Because these ideologies are ubiquitous in popular culture (e.g., mass media), individuals' stereotypes are continually reinforced.

Some stereotypes reflect ideologies that are specific to a particular out-group. One of the most widespread stereotypes is that a homosexual orientation is inherently and necessarily associated with gender role nonconformity (i.e., lesbians manifest characteristics that are masculine and gay men manifest feminine qualities). This belief is sufficiently strong that people whose behavior and appearance are inconsistent with cultural gender prescriptions are more likely than others to be labeled homosexual. Some empirical research suggests that lesbians and gay men who do not conform to stereotypical expectations may be disliked more intensely by heterosexuals than are gay individuals who meet those expectations (Laner and Laner 1979; Storms 1978).

Other stereotypes reflect cultural ideologies about outsiders in general, typically portraying out-group members as simultaneously threatening and inferior to members of the dominant in-group. Adam (1978) documented some of the themes common to cultural images of gay people, blacks, and Jews. These include being animalistic, hypersexual, overvisible, heretical, and conspiratorial. Yet another ideology ascribes disease (physical and mental) to all three groups. Just as being black or Jewish was equated historically with pathology, so was homosexuality considered a mental illness until recently. It was officially labeled so by the American Psychiatric Association until 1973 (Bayer 1987).

Internalized Homophobia Among Gay Men and Lesbians

Like members of other stigmatized groups, gay people face numerous psychological challenges as a result of society's hostility toward them. One challenge results from the consequences of hiding one's sexual orientation. Lesbians and gay men must traverse a sequence of events through which they recognize their homosexual orientation, develop an identity based on it, and disclose their orientation to others, a process usually termed "coming out" (a shortened form of "coming out of the closet"). Conversely, being "in the closet" or "closeted" refers to passing as heterosexual. Because of cultural heterosexism, people generally are presumed to be heterosexual. Coming out, therefore, is an ongoing process; lesbians and gay men continually must come out as they encounter new people. Different gay people are out of the closet to varying degrees.

Most children internalize society's ideology of sex and gender at an early age. As a result, lesbians and gay men usually experience some degree of negative feeling toward themselves when they first recognize their homosexuality in adolescence or adulthood. This sense of what is usually called "internalized homophobia" often makes the process of identity formation more difficult (Malyon 1982). In the course of coming out, most lesbians and gay men successfully overcome the threats to psychological well-being posed by heterosexism. They manage to reclaim disowned or devalued parts of themselves, developing an identity into which their sexuality is well integrated. Psychological adjustment appears to be highest among men and women who are committed to a gay or lesbian identity and who do not attempt to hide their homosexuality from others. Conversely, people with a homosexual orientation who have not yet come out, who wish that they could become heterosexual, or who are isolated from the gay community may experience greater psychological distress (Bell and Weinberg 1978; Hammersmith and Weinberg 1973; Malyon 1982; Weinberg and Williams 1974).

As a result of heterosexism, many individuals feel compelled to hide their homosexuality or "pass" as heterosexual. Respondents to the *San Francisco Examiner*'s 1989 national survey of lesbians and gay men, for example, waited an average of 4.6 years after knowing they were gay until they came out (which presumably involved disclosing their homosexual orientation to another person). Depending on the area of the country, between 23% and 40% had not told their family that they were gay, and between 37% and 59% had not disclosed their sexual orientation to coworkers (San Francisco Examiner 1989).

Hiding one's sexual orientation can create a painful discrepancy between public and private identities. Because they face unwitting acceptance of themselves by prejudiced heterosexuals, gay people who are passing may feel inauthentic, that they are living a lie, and that others would not accept them if they knew the truth. The need to pass is likely to disrupt longstanding family relationships and friendships if lesbians and gay men feel they must distance themselves from others to avoid revealing their sexual orientation. When contact with heterosexuals cannot be avoided, they may keep their interactions at a superficial level as a self-protective strategy.

Passing also creates considerable strain for gay partnerships. As already noted, even openly gay people are generally deprived of the many tangible supports afforded to married heterosexuals (e.g., insurance benefits and inheritance rights). In addition, those who are passing must actively hide or deny their same-gender relationship to family and friends. Consequently, the problems and stresses common to any relationship must be faced without the social supports typically available to heterosexual lovers or spouses.

When heterosexism is expressed through overt hostility and attacks, it creates additional psychological challenges for lesbians and gay men. Once they come out, lesbians and gay men risk rejection by others, discrimination, and even violence, all of which can have psychological consequences that endure long after their immediate physical effects have dissipated. Being the target of discrimination, for example, often leads to feelings of sadness and anxiety; it also can lead to an increased sense that life is difficult and unfair and to dissatisfaction with one's larger community (Garnets et al. 1990).

Lesbian and gay male victims of hate crimes may face special psychological challenges. Because antigay hate crimes represent an attack on the victim's gay identity and community, they may affect a victim's feelings about herself or himself as a gay individual and toward the gay community. The victim's homosexuality may become directly linked to the heightened sense of vulnerability that normally follows victimization. One's homosexual orientation consequently may be experienced as a source of danger, pain, and punishment rather than intimacy, love, and community. After an attack, internalized homophobia may re-emerge or may be intensified. Attempts to make sense of the attack, coupled with the common need to perceive the world as a just place, may lead to feelings that one has been justifiably punished for being gay. Such characterological self-blame can lead to feelings of depression and helplessness, even in individuals who are otherwise comfortable with their sexual orientation (Garnets et al. 1990).

Furthermore, a lesbian or gay male hate crime survivor may experience increased discrimination or stigma when others learn about her or his sexual orientation as a consequence of the victimization. Such *secondary victimization* (Berrill and Herek 1992), which can further intensify the negative psychological consequences of victimization, is often expressed explicitly by representatives of the criminal justice system, including police officers and judges. The consequences also extend outside the criminal justice system. If their sexual orientation becomes publicly known as the result of a crime, for example, some lesbians and gay men risk losing employment or child custody. Even in jurisdictions where statutory protection is available, many gay people fear that disclosure of their sexual orientation consequent to victimization will result in hostility, harassment, and rejection from others. Secondary victimization may be experienced as an additional assault on one's identity and community and thus become an additional stress. The threat of secondary victimization often acts as a barrier to reporting a crime or seeking medical, psychological, or social services.

A third consequence of heterosexism is its effects on heterosexuals. Because of the stigma attached to homosexuality, many heterosexuals monitor and restrict their own behavior to avoid being labeled as gay; this pattern appears to be especially strong among American males. For example, many men avoid clothing, hobbies, and mannerisms that might be labeled "effeminate." Antigay prejudice also interferes with same-sex friendships. Males with strongly antigay attitudes appear to have fewer intimate nonsexual friendships with other men than do males with tolerant attitudes (Devlin and Cowan 1985).

Reducing Heterosexism

As noted above, heterosexuals in the United States now support civil rights for lesbians and gay men in greater numbers than ever before. Several factors probably account for this shift. First, as lesbians and gay men have become increasingly visible in society, more heterosexuals than in the past have had opportunities for personal contact with an openly gay or lesbian individual. Such contact experiences are strongly associated with more favorable attitudes toward lesbians and gay men as a group (Herek and Glunt 1993). The relationship between contact and favorable attitudes is stronger to the extent that heterosexuals report multiple contacts, more intimate contacts, and contacts that involve direct disclosure of sexual orientation (Herek and Capitanio 1995).

Empirical data also indicate that lesbians and gay men are somewhat selective in revealing their sexual orientation to others. Certain groups of heterosexuals (e.g., women, highly educated individuals, political liberals) are more likely than others to report having contact with gay men or lesbians (Herek and Capitanio 1995). Thus, it is likely that the relationship between interpersonal contact and psychological heterosexism is reciprocal; that is, contact tends to foster greater acceptance by heterosexuals of gay people, and heterosexuals with already positive attitudes (or who belong to a group in which accepting attitudes are common) are more likely than others to experience contact.

A second factor that probably accounts for recent shifts in heterosexuals' attitudes toward gay people is the increased availability of information about homosexuality and the gay and lesbian community. During the 1980s and 1990s, lesbians and gay men have gained public visibility as never before. Consequently, heterosexuals have been confronted with the reality of homosexuality and, in many cases, have received information that challenged their previous stereotypes and prejudices.

A third factor associated with shifts in heterosexuals' attitudes is that, as lesbians and gay men have become more visible, their status in society has changed. Consequently, the psychological functions served by heterosexuals' attitudes toward gay people may have shifted. As gay and lesbian civil liberties have become defined as a human rights issue, it has become increasingly possible for heterosexuals' attitudes toward gay people to represent an endorsement of human rights principles and thereby to serve the value-expressive function described previously.

To the extent that different heterosexuals have different motivations for their heterosexism, a variety of strategies will be required to reduce any particular individual's prejudice. When expressions of homophobia function to reinforce a person's self-concept as good Christians, for example, appeals to other important values such as compassion and love of a neighbor, patriotism, and support for civil rights are more likely to change his or her attitudes than are factual refutations of incorrect stereotypes about homosexual people.

Personal contact with gay people has consistently been found to be one of the strongest correlates of heterosexuals' attitudes. This finding indicates that disclosing one's homosexual orientation to family members, friends, and coworkers often is a potent means for challenging psychological heterosexism. This hypothesis highlights the importance of institutional changes—such as the elimination of sodomy laws, passage of antidiscrimination legislation, and protection from hate crimes—that will enable lesbians and gay men to come out to others with fewer risks.

References

Adam BD: The Survival of Domination: Inferiorization and Everyday Life. New York, Elsevier, 1978

Bayer R: Homosexuality and American Psychiatry: The Politics of Diagnosis, 2nd Edition. Princeton, NJ, Princeton University Press, 1987

Bell AP, Weinberg MS: Homosexualities: A Study of Diversity Among Men and Women. New York, Simon and Schuster, 1978

Berrill KT: Antigay violence and victimization in the United States: an overview, in Hate Crimes: Confronting Violence Against Lesbians and Gay Men. Edited by Herek GM, Berrill KT. Newbury Park, CA, Sage, 1992, pp 19–45

Berrill KT, Herek GM: Primary and secondary victimization in anti-gay hate crimes: official response and public policy, in Hate Crimes: Confronting Violence Against Lesbians and Gay Men. Edited by Herek GM, Berrill KT. Newbury Park, CA, Sage, 1992, pp 289–305

Devlin PK, Cowan GA: Homophobia, perceived fathering, and male intimate relationships. J Pers Assess 49:467–473, 1985

Garnets L, Herek GM, Levy B: Violence and victimization of lesbians and gay men: mental health consequences. Journal of Interpersonal Violence 5:366–383, 1990

Hammersmith SK, Weinberg MS: Homosexual identity: commitment, adjustment, and significant others. Sociometry 36:56–79, 1973

Herek GM: Beyond "homophobia": a social psychological perspective on attitudes toward lesbians and gay men. J Homosex 10:1–21, 1984

Herek GM: Can functions be measured? A new perspective on the functional approach to attitudes. Social Psychology Quarterly 50:285–303, 1987

Herek GM: The context of anti-gay violence: notes on cultural and psychological heterosexism. Journal of Interpersonal Violence 5:316–333, 1990

Herek GM: Stigma, prejudice, and violence against lesbians and gay men, in Homosexuality: Research Implications for Public Policy. Edited by Gonsiorek J, Weinrich J. Newbury Park, CA, Sage, 1991, pp 60–80

Herek GM: Psychological heterosexism and antigay violence: the social psychology of bigotry and bashing, in Hate Crimes: Confronting Violence Against Lesbians and Gay Men. Edited by Herek GM, Berrill KT. Newbury Park, CA, Sage, 1992, pp 149–169

Herek GM: Assessing attitudes toward lesbians and gay men: a review of empirical research with the ATLG scale, in Lesbian and Gay Psychology: Theory, Research, and Clinical Applications. Edited by Greene B, Herek GM. Newbury Park, CA, Sage, 1994, pp 206–228

Herek GM: The HIV epidemic and public attitudes toward lesbians and gay men, in The Impact of the HIV Epidemic on the Lesbian and Gay Community. Edited by Levine MP, Nardi P, Gagnon J. Chicago, IL, University of Chicago Press (in press)

Herek GM, Capitanio JP: Black heterosexuals' attitudes toward lesbians and gay men in the United States. J Sex Res 32:95–105, 1995

Herek GM, Capitanio JP: "Some of my best friends": intergroup contact, concealable stigma, and heterosexuals' attitudes toward gay men and lesbians. Personality and Social Psychology Bulletin (in press)

Herek GM, Glunt EK: Interpersonal contact and heterosexuals' attitudes toward gay men: results from a national survey. J Sex Res 30:239–244, 1993

Hugick L: Public opinion divided on gay rights. Gallup Poll Monthly, June:2–6, 1992

Kite ME: When perceptions meet reality: individual differences in reactions to gay men and lesbians, in Contemporary Perspectives in Lesbian and Gay Psychology, Vol 1. Edited by Greene G, Herek GM. Newbury Park, CA, Sage, 1994, pp 25–53

Laner MR, Laner RH: Personal style or sexual preference: why gay men are disliked. International Review of Modern Sociology 9:215–228, 1979

Malyon AK: Psychotherapeutic implications of internalized homophobia in gay men. J Homosex 7:59–69, 1982

San Francisco Examiner: Results of poll. San Francisco, CA, San Francisco Examiner, June 6, 1989, p A19

Shields SA, Harriman RE: Fear of male homosexuality: cardiac responses of low and high homonegative males. J Homosex 10:53–67, 1984

Storms MD: Attitudes toward homosexuality and femininity in men. J Homosex 3:257–263, 1978

Weinberg G: Society and the Healthy Homosexual. New York, St. Martin's, 1972

Weinberg MS, Williams CJ: Male Homosexuals: Their Problems and Adaptations. New York, Oxford University Press, 1974

Wood FW (ed): An American Profile: Opinions and Behavior 1972–1989. Detroit, MI, Gale Research, 1990

8

Homosexuality From a Familial and Genetic Perspective

Richard C. Pillard, M.D.

T he forces shaping human sexual orientation are largely unknown. We understand something about the development of nonspecific sexuality: prenatal gender differentiation, the sex steroid hormones and their interplay with gonadotropic hormones, the effect of these on brain and gonads, and the family and cultural institutions that support a capacity to respond to another person intimately and sexually. However, with regard to the development of heterosexuality, bisexuality, and homosexuality, hardly anything tangible is known. This chapter reviews evidence suggesting that genes play a role in sexual orientation. Family, twin, and gene linkage studies are reviewed, and their relevance to a genetic theory of sexual orientation is discussed.

Historical Background

Many distinguished sexologists during the past 100 years believed that sexual orientation has a biological or genetic basis. In various forms, this view was shared by von Krafft-Ebing (1901), Ellis (1922), Hirschfeld (1936), and Freud (1959). Ellis (1922) said, "Any theory of the etiology of homosexuality which leaves out . . . the hereditary factor . . . cannot be admitted" (p. 626). His opinion was based on three observation: 1) homosexuality often runs in families; 2) many gay men and lesbian women behave, during childhood, in ways we would now call "gender atypical," and 3) homosexual desire seems in many cases to spring into being spontaneously, that is, it was never taught to, discussed with, or observed by the child.

Ellis reported homosexual relatives in more than one-third of his male homosexual patients although he does not give exact numbers or the degree of relationship. Hirschfeld (1936) presented a family pedigree with 12 homosexual or bisexual individuals (of both sexes) out of 21 ascertained kin. He also noted concordance for homosexuality in six of seven pairs of identical twins. These writers cite others, mostly in the German literature, who reported constellations of siblings and twins with unusual frequencies of a homosexual orientation.

These researchers were unable to go beyond a simple consideration of the possibility that genes predispose to a particular sexual orientation because their understanding of genetics was insufficiently developed—as ours largely remains. von Krafft-Ebing excluded genetic considerations in cases where neither parent exhibited the trait in question because the possibility of recessive traits was unknown to him. (von Krafft-Ebbing wrote at the end of the 19th century; the rediscovery of Mendel's work occurred in the early 20th century.) Additionally, they lacked the statistical models to assess the probability that their findings were attributable to chance alone.

Alfred Kinsey et al. (1948, 1953) proposed criteria that should be fulfilled to substantiate the hereditary basis of homosexuality. The researchers recognized the importance of careful definition of the phenotype, ascertainment of the sexual orientation of all members of a sibship, and use of appropriate statistical comparisons. Kinsey also said that account must be taken of individuals who, during their life, change their position on the heterosexual-homosexual continuum he had defined.

Frequency of Gay, Lesbian, and Bisexual Orientations

The Kinsey researchers provided the first large population survey of human sexual behavior. They defined seven anchor points along a continuum of sexual orientation, definitions that are still widely used by sex researchers (see Chapter 4 by Michaels).

The Kinsey data and those of subsequent researchers (Diamond 1993; Gebhard 1972; Remafedi et al. 1992; Seidman and Rieder 1994) show that most women and men behave heterosexually more or less exclusively throughout their lives. A minority (2%–5% of men and 1%–3% of women) are more or less exclusively homosexual, whereas only a small percentage are bisexual beyond adolescence. Thus it appears that the overall incidence of a predominant homosexual orientation has changed little—certainly it has not increased—in the 45 years since Kinsey's first survey, despite the "sexual revolution" and the greater social acceptance of gays and lesbians.

Bisexuality is controversial. A bisexual, by the above definition, would be one who is attracted to or sexually active with both sexes (Kinsey range 2–4). One might expect bisexuals to be more common than predominant or exclusive homosexuals, yet survey respondents who currently label themselves bisexual (or fall in the mid-Kinsey range 2–4) tend to be few and to be adolescents or younger adults who move toward either end of the Kinsey continuum as they get older. Diamond (1993) concludes that "exclusive or predominantly exclusive homosexual activities are more common than bisexual activities" (p. 291).

A gender difference, however, may exist. Women more often than men describe themselves as bisexual and some women even resist a "lesbian-bisexual-heterosexual" schema saying that it does not adequately capture their perception of their sexuality (see Chapter 10 by Fox).

Of course, other dimensions of sexuality exist that could serve as useful classifiers for research. Some individuals prefer to take a more active or proceptive role in a sexual interaction, whereas others prefer a more passive role. Some prefer younger partners and others, older partners. Particular parts of the body serve as the focus of eroticism for some, particular sexual activities for others. Some are restrictive in their partner preferences and others catholic. Recognizing these and other dimensions of sexuality, it still seems true that the heterosexual-bisexual-homosexual continuum has been recognized across cultures and historical eras.

Family Studies

In 1941, George W. Henry published extensive case material on 40 male and 40 female "sex variants" (mostly homosexual as suggested from the case descriptions, although three of the men were probably transsexual or heterosexual transvestites). Pillard et al. (1981) tabulated the frequency of homosexuality in siblings from the family trees of Henry's studies and concluded that 10.6% of the brothers and 7.7% of the sisters of the sex variants also were homosexual, considerably more than the above surveys would predict from a random draw of the population. A small point but of considerable interest is that of the 12 homosexual or bisexual uncles and aunts in Henry's kindreds, 11 came from the maternal lineage ($P < .006$, two-tailed binomial probability). This same review (Pillard et al. 1981) of the literature on familial homosexuality documents numerous scattered reports suggesting that some families have an aggregation of homosexual members that exceeds chance.

◼ Siblings

To examine the issue of familiality more closely, Pillard et al. (1982; Pillard and Weinrich 1986) recruited predominantly gay and predominantly heterosexual men for a systematic family study. The authors took sexual histories from these probands, then obtained their permission to recruit and interview their siblings. Sibling data were gathered by interviewers blind to the orientation of the proband. The results show that gay male probands had a considerable excess of gay and bisexual brothers but no excess of lesbian sisters (Table 8–1). A similar study of lesbian and heterosexual women showed a trend for the lesbians to have more lesbian sisters and a few more gay brothers (Pillard 1988).

Bailey and Benishey (1993) recruited 79 heterosexual and 84 lesbian women plus 60% of their 395 siblings. They assessed sibling homosexuality using four criteria of different degrees of stringency and found that the lesbian probands had more lesbian sisters on all four.

Table 8–1.   Siblings' Kinsey Scale rating by male proband's Kinsey rating and by sex of sibling

Index subjects' Kinsey ratings	Siblings' Kinsey Scale ratings		
	0–1	**2–6**	**Total**
	Sisters		
0–2	61	6	**67**
3–6	44	4	**48**
Total	**105**	**10**	**115**
	Brothers		
0–2	53	2	**55**
3–6	53	15[*]	**68**
Total	**106**	**17**	**123**

Note.   Male index subjects: predominantly heterosexual (Kinsey 0–2) $n = 50$; predominately gay (Kinsey 3–6) $n = 50$.

[*]Kinsey 3–6 index men have significantly more Kinsey 2–6 brothers ($P < .03$, exact multinomial probability) but not more Kinsey 2–6 sisters ($P > .25$).

For example, of the sisters of the lesbian probands, 15.4% rated themselves as either lesbian or bisexual, whereas only 3.5% of the sisters of heterosexual women rated themselves as lesbian or bisexual. The lesbian probands also had a nonsignificant trend toward more gay male brothers.

After the above studies were done, the authors interviewed a sibship of three brothers and four sisters in which all three brothers were homosexual or bisexual and three of the four sisters were homosexual (unpublished data). The odds that such a sibship could occur by chance depends on the frequency of male and female homosexuality in the population; the more common homosexuality is, the less remarkable a family with multiple homosexual siblings would be. With the use of conservative assumptions, this author calculated the odds at about 1 in 100 million.

◼ Extended Pedigrees

It would be interesting to know if familial homosexuality is confined to siblings or if it can be identified elsewhere in a pedigree. The question is difficult to answer because second- and third-degree relatives are often geographically dispersed and have little motivation to participate in this type of study. In addition, homosexuality in ascendants who lived prior to the 1970s is likely to be a well-guarded secret, even from the family. The ascertainment of extended pedigrees would be a service to this research.

In summary, powerful evidence exists that homosexuality runs in families, and no evidence contradicts it. Familiality is a necessary but by no means a sufficient requisite to substantiate a genetic factor. Two additional kinds of evidence aim in that direction: twin and adoptee, and molecular genetic studies.

Twins and Adoptees

Homosexuality in identical or monozygotic twins has been reported (Green and Stoller 1971; Heston and Shields 1968; Kallmann 1952; Mesnikoff et al. 1963; Parker 1964; Pillard et al. 1981; Puterbaugh 1990; Rainer et al. 1960). A high degree of concordance is invariably found, ranging upward from 50%, but the cited literature also contains reports of twin pairs unquestionably monozygotic and unquestionably discordant for sexual orientation.

Whitam et al. (1993) reported sexual orientation data from 61 twin pairs. Their concordance for homosexuality in the monozygotic pairs was 66%, and for the dizygotic pairs, 30%. Their report also provided interesting clinical details such as the twin pair who, unknown to each other and while living in different cities, photographed older shirtless construction workers and masturbated to the photographs.

Bailey and Pillard (1991) and Bailey et al. (1993b) published studies of gay probands (men in the first study, women in the second) who had an identical or fraternal twin or an adopted brother (or sister). These studies provided data to compare monozygotic twins, fraternal or dizygotic twins, and unrelated adoptees.

For both sexes, the concordance for monozygotic twins was much higher than for dizygotic twins though it fell short of the near 100% expected if genes are all important. The male monozygotic twin concordance was 52%. The dizygotic twin concordance (22%) was the same as the nontwin brother concordance reported by Pillard and Weinrich (1986) (see Table 8–1). Adopted brother concordance (11%) was somewhat higher than the population base rate. Women subjects achieved a similar pattern of concordance rates: 48% for monozygotic twins, 16% for dizygotic twins—the same as Bailey and Benishay (1993) found in nontwin sisters—and 6% for adopted sisters.

The authors used a statistical model to estimate the heritability (i.e., the percentage of variance in the sample presumably accounted for by genes). For both sexes and for a variety of assumptions about population prevalence and response bias, the heritability was greater than 50%. Note that "heritability" is a tricky concept. It is the complement of "environmentality"; if one goes up, the other must go down. For example, a phenotype of mental retardation called phenylketonuria (PKU), associated with light-colored skin and hair, used to be highly heritable in families carrying the gene for an insufficiency of the enzyme phenylalanine hydroxylase. An environmental intervention, feeding a phenylalanine-free diet, prevents brain damage from phenylketonuria and reduces the heritability of the low-IQ phenotype to near zero even though nothing changes in the genes. In addition, an obviously inherited trait like having two arms and two legs will have a heritability of zero, environmental intervention aside, because that characteristic has hardly any variability. Thus, a heritability estimate for a trait like sexual orientation depends on the contribution both of genes and environment in the population being studied.

Classic heritability studies examine animals reared in different controlled environments. Objection can be raised to conclusions from human twin studies that monozygotic twins have not only their genes but their environments in common, at least more in common than dizygotic twins. One test of this objection would be to compare twins raised to be alike (e.g., in dress, schooling, friends, or parental treatment) with twins raised to be different. This comparison has been made, not for sexual orientation but for other traits such as intelligence and dimensions of personality. In general, the dissimilarly raised twins are nevertheless as alike on the measured dimensions as are the similar twins (Plomin et al. 1990). A counterargument is that a hypothetical trait-relevant environment variable might be unaffected by the conscious efforts of parents to individuate their twins.

A stronger case could be made if monozygotic twins separated at birth and raised apart turned out to be concordant for sexual orientation. Eckert et al. (1986) identified two male monozygotic pairs raised apart but reunited as adults in the Minnesota twin study. One pair was remarkably alike, both had an almost exclusive homosexual orientation as well as other similar personality traits. A second pair included one substantially homosexual twin (Kinsey rating 5), and the other, although married and labeling himself heterosexual, had engaged in more than casual homosexual experience (Kinsey rating 2). Eckert et al. (1986) also reported four pairs of female twins, all of whom were discordant. Whitam et al. (1993) added two male pairs raised apart, one pair concordant and one discordant.

Even these rare cases, as persuasive as they seem, are not perfect experiments of nature. The best "experiment" requires random assignment of environments; however, adoption agencies try to do the opposite, to place adoptees in families as like as possible to their biological parents. Who knows whether some subtle feature of the environment, relevant to sexual orientation, is thereby imperfectly controlled? Cross-fostering and half-sibling studies would be useful to address these questions, but they are expensive and logistically complex.

Molecular Genetic Studies

Linkage

Genetic linkage studies become more appealing as the library of gene markers enlarges, currently consisting of about 5,000 markers for the human genome. A marker is a polymorphic stretch of DNA at a known location on a chromosome. Several linkage research strategies exist: one is to identify pedigrees with two or more gay members, collect genetic material, and examine the known DNA markers. Linkage occurs when a matching stretch of DNA is found at the same chromosomal address (locus) in the gay family members (e.g., pairs of brothers). Heterosexual relatives should have different markers at the locus. Thus, linkage of a DNA marker to the trait of sexual orientation is simply a probability statement about the odds of finding the same stretch of DNA in gay family members just by chance.

A study of this type was done by Hamer et al. (1993a) at the National Cancer Institute. They chose as subjects pairs of gay brothers, some of whom had other gay relatives related through the maternal lineage—the enate family pattern we observed in the Henry study. Hamer reasoned that gay brothers in such families might have a relevant gene on the X chromosome, the chromosome inherited from the mother. This strategy would greatly simplify the search for a linked marker because only the X chromosome need be examined, and many markers span it.

Hamer recruited 40 pairs of gay brothers (plus other relatives in some families) from whom he obtained sex histories and blood samples for genetic analysis. The Hamer team found evidence for linkage, specifically 33 of the 40 pairs of brothers had the same alleles at 5 adjacent marker sites at the Xq28 region at the tip of the long arm of the X chromosome. The probability of chance association at each of these 5 loci ranged from < .006 to < .0002, and the cumulative probability of a chance finding was $< 10^{-5}$ (see Risch et al. 1993 for a critique and Hamer et al. 1993b for a response).

Hamer's study is exciting because the statistical odds are strong and because this will be, if replicated, the first evidence of genetic linkage for a complex behavioral trait. Hamer has still not found a "gay gene." The markers in the Xq28 region span a string of dozens or hundreds of genes that must be examined by other techniques to see which ones are influencing sexual orientation. The gene must then be cloned, and its precise function must be determined. That function could be, for example, influencing neuron development in the hypothalamic nucleus INAH3 that LeVay (1991) has reported to be dimorphic with respect to sexual orientation.

■ Allelic Association

Linking a marker to a behavioral trait works well in theory if the candidate gene exerts a large influence on the trait. However, what if a behavioral trait is influenced by several or many genes, called quantitative trait loci (oligogenes or polygenes), each making only a small and perhaps interchangeable contribution to the trait? Small effects by many genes can be detected by a form of linkage analysis called "allelic association. Instead of comparing marker sites in family members, allelic association requires a genome scan of many unrelated individuals (both study subjects and control subjects) to find markers present at slightly but significantly elevated frequencies in the study subjects. The advantage of allelic association is that it is sensitive to detect small differences in marker frequencies at many sites, and importantly, subjects need not be related. The disadvantage is that a large number of study and control subjects must be recruited. Hamer et al. (1993a) needed only 40 pairs of brothers to demonstrate linkage, but detecting quantitative trait loci could require many hundreds of individuals, particularly if the relevant genes are many and each contributes only a small part to the phenotype. (N.B.: In traditional linkage analysis, the marker need not be in linkage disequilibrium with the target gene. A false-negative finding will occur only when, e.g., one gay brother has a recombination event separating marker and target gene. Allelic association requires that the marker be either in the gene or tightly linked to it.) So far, no study of sexual orientation has used this method, but it and other linkage strategies are being developed to detect subtle gene effects (Plomin et al. 1994).

Conclusion

The work reviewed shows that genes probably have an influence on sexual orientation, but the environment is important as well. Note that genetically identical monozygotic twins have different orientations half of the time. Data on childhood gender nonconformity and homosexuality suggest that whatever the environment bestows, it probably does so early in life (Bailey et al. 1993a; Zucker and Green 1992; Zucker et al. 1993). This is one reason that environmental influences are hard to study; they could be present in the prenatal hormone milieu or in long ago and forgotten patterns of family interaction or could occur as extraneous events, opportunities, traumas, or relationships for one individual but not another.

Our data suggest that the *unshared* rather than the shared environment is likely to be most relevant. If shared environment (e.g., the family's socioeconomic level) contributed to the variance, we should observe a lesbian or gay orientation about equally often in adopted as in biological siblings insofar as they all share the same family situation. Studies of other behavioral traits point in the same direction: environmental influences tend to make children in the same family different rather than similar (Plomin et al. 1994).

If genes bias development in a homosexual direction, how do they operate and what evolutionary significance might they have? The paradox is that a gay or lesbian individual must exert a "reproductive tax," yet a homosexual orientation also must have been favorably selected at some point in human evolution because it is far too common to be the result of occasional deleterious mutations that are eventually selected out of a kindred. This question has been addressed by Kirsch and Weinrich (1991).

One possibility is the phenomenon of "kin altruism." The term refers to individuals who help relatives survive and reproduce at the expense of their own reproductive potential (Alcock 1984). An interesting example perhaps illustrating kin altruism was observed in African lions by Packer et al. (1991). A coalition of males (often brothers) lives with a pride of females. Larger coalitions are more effective at patrolling territory and protecting cubs; more cubs per capita survive when the coalition contains more than four males than when it contains only two or three. Therefore, a reproductive advantage exists for males to belong to larger cohorts.

Logically, males living together should sire a more or less equal number of cubs. Packer et al. (1991), however, established cub paternity by DNA fingerprinting, and the surprise is that the larger the male group, the more skewed is individual reproductive success. One or two males sire most of the cubs, some males sire none. Because the males are closely related, however, the genes of a nonreproducing male get passed to the cubs via a brother. Whether kin altruism or some other mechanism can explain the conservation of "gay genes" remains for future research.

Sexual orientation-determining genes are compatible with neuro-anatomic and hormonal theories discussed by Byne in Chapter 9. Genes might operate by promoting or inhibiting the development of particular areas of the brain, which in turn could influence the neuroanatomy and biochemistry of sexual development. However, it may turn out that even the most exact knowledge of sexual orientation development will provide little more than a guess about the outcome in a particular individual. Evidence exists that neural connections in the brain are imprecisely directed. As neurons sprout and grow, there appears to be only a statistical chance of their hooking up at an exact destination. Thus, it may be that, even knowing the specific genes, the particular home environment, and the cultural milieu, the outcome is still partly the result of chance.

The genetic analysis of behavior is a powerful tool to advance our understanding of sexual orientation. The eventual payoff will be to link genes, brain function, psychological development, and human social organization in a multilevel understanding of human sexuality. Various sexual orientations should become a comprehensible part of nature rather than a deviation or perversion of it. To understand the diversity of life is gratefully to recognize our dependence on that diversity.

References

Alcock J: Animal Behavior: An Evolutionary Approach. Sunderland, MA, Sinauer Associates, 1984

Bailey JM, Benishey D: Familial aggregation of female sexual orientation. Am J Psychiatry 150:272–277, 1993

Bailey JM, Pillard RC: A genetic study of male sexual orientation. Arch Gen Psychiatry 48:1089–1096, 1991

Bailey JM, Miller JS, Willerman L: Maternally rated childhood gender nonconformity in homosexuals and heterosexuals. Arch Sex Behav 22:461–469, 1993a

Bailey JM, Pillard RC, Neale MC, et al: Heritable factors influence sexual orientation in women. Arch Gen Psychiatry 50:217–223, 1993b

Diamond M: Homosexuality and bisexuality in different populations. Arch Sex Behav 32:291–310, 1993

Eckert ED, Bouchard TJ, Bohler J, et al: Homosexuality in monozygotic twins reared apart. Br J Psychiatry 148:421–425, 1986

Ellis H: Studies in the Psychology of Sex, Vol II, Sexual Inversion. Philadelphia, PA, FA Davis, 1922, p 626

Freud S: The pathogenesis of a case of homosexuality in a woman, in Collected Papers, Vol 2. Edited by Riviere J. New York, Basic Books, 1959, pp 202–231

Gebhard PH: Incidence of overt homosexuality in the United States and western Europe, in National Institute of Mental Health Task Force on Homosexuality: Final Report and Background Papers (USDHEW Publ No 76–357). Edited by Livingood JM. Washington, DC, U.S. Department of Health, Education, and Welfare, 1972, pp 22–29

Green R, Stoller RJ: Two monozygotic (identical) twin pairs discordant for gender identity. Arch Sex Behav 1:321–327, 1971

Hamer DH, Hu S, Magnuson VL, et al: A linkage between DNA markers on the X chromosome and male sexual orientation. Science 261:321–327, 1993a

Hamer DH, Hu S, Magnuson VL, et al: Response. Science 262:2065, 1993b

Henry GW: Sex Variants: A Study of Homosexual Patterns. New York, Paul B. Hoeber, 1941

Heston LL, Shields J: Homosexuality in twins. Arch Gen Psychiatry 18:149–160, 1968

Hirschfeld M: Homosexuality, in Encyclopaedia Sexualis. Edited by Bloch I, Hirschfeld M. New York, Dingwall-Rock, 1936, pp 321–334

Kallmann FJ: Comparative twin study on the genetic aspects of male homosexuality. J Nerv Mental Dis 115:283–298, 1952

Kinsey AC, Pomeroy WB, Martin CE: Sexual Behavior in the Human Male. Philadelphia, PA, WB Saunders, 1948

Kinsey AC, Pomeroy WB, Martin CE, et al: Sexual Behavior in the Human Female. Philadelphia, PA, WB Saunders, 1953

Kirsch JAW, Weinrich JD: Homosexuality, nature, and biology: is homosexuality natural? Does it matter? in Homosexuality: Research Findings for Public Policy. Edited by Gonsiorek JC, Weinrich JD. Newbury Park, CA, Sage, 1991

LeVay S: A difference in hypothalamic structure between heterosexual and homosexual men. Science 253:1034–1037, 1991

Mesnikoff AM, Rainer JD, Kolb LC, et al: Intrafamilial determinants of divergent sexual behavior in twins. Am J Psychiatry 119:732–738, 1963

Packer C, Gilbert DA, Pusey AE, et al: A molecular genetic analysis of kinship and cooperation in African lions. Nature 351:562–565, 1991

Parker N: Homosexuality in twins: a report on three discordant pairs. Br J Psychiatry 110:489–495, 1964

Pillard RC: Sexual orientation and mental disorders. Psychiatric Annals 18:52–56, 1988

Pillard RC, Poumadere JI, Carretta RA: A family study of sexual orientation. Arch Sex Behav 11:511–520, 1982

Pillard RC, Poumadere JI, Carretta RA: Is homosexuality familial? A review, some data, and a suggestion. Arch Sex Behav 10:465–475, 1981

Pillard RC, Weinrich JD: Evidence of familial nature of male homosexuality. Arch Gen Psychiatry 43:808–812, 1986

Plomin R, DeFries JC, McClearn GE: Behavioral Genetics: A Primer. New York, WH Freeman, 1990, pp 315–319

Plomin R, Owen MJ, McGuffin P: The genetic basis of complex human behaviors. Science 264:1733–1739, 1994

Puterbaugh G: Twins and Homosexuality: A Casebook. New York, Garland, 1990

Rainer JD, Mesnikoff A, Kolb LC, et al: Homosexuality and heterosexuality in identical twins. Psychosom Med 22:251–259, 1960

Remafedi G, Resnick M, Blum R, et al: Demography of sexual orientation in adolescents. Pediatrics 89:714–721, 1992

Risch N, Squires-Wheeler E, Keats BJB: Male sexual orientation and genetic evidence. Science 262:2063–2064, 1993

Seidman SN, Rieder RO: A review of sexual behavior in the United States. Am J Psychiatry 151:330–341, 1994

von Krafft-Ebing R: Psychopathia Sexualis, 3rd Edition. (Translation of 10th German edition.) Chicago, IL, WT Keener, 1901

Whitam FL, Diamond M, Martin J: Homosexual orientation in twins: a report of 61 pairs and three triplet sets. Arch Sex Behav 22:187–206, 1993

Zucker KJ, Green R: Psychosexual disorders in children and adolescents. J Child Psychol Psychiatry 33:107–151, 1992

Zucker KJ, Wild J, Bradley SJ, et al: Physical attractiveness of boys with gender identity disorder. Arch Sex Behav 22:23–36, 1993

9

Biology and Homosexuality

Implications of Neuroendocrinological and Neuroanatomical Studies

William Byne, M.D., Ph.D.

Basic Considerations

The role of biology in sexual orientation has been a topic of recurrent debate in Western medicine for the past century and a half. Because appeals are made to medicine to inform social policy, this debate has been mired in politics since its inception. The goal of this chapter is to examine, from a scientific perspective, the implications of recent biological research pertaining to the origins of sexual orientation. First, however, it is necessary to extricate the scientific concerns from the political.

It is widely believed that social and criminal sanctions against homosexuality and homosexual behavior should be diminished or eliminated if homosexuality is involuntary (Schmalz 1993). By inference, the common but erroneous assumption that "involuntary" means "inborn" leads to the belief that society would be more tolerant of homosexuality if it were proven to be biologically determined. Consequently, research findings consistent with a major biological influence have been interpreted as "good news for gays" (Bailey and Pillard 1991). Conversely, criticism of the biological evidence has been perceived as antigay (Jefferson 1993).

In considering the biological evidence dispassionately, one must realize that the chain of logic from biology and sexual orientation to social policy is often based on misinformation. To begin with, biological evidence is not needed to demonstrate that sexual attractions are not a matter of choice. That is shown clearly in the psychological literature reporting the ineffectiveness of reorientation therapies (Haldeman 1994). Furthermore, "involuntary" does not invariably mean "inborn." For example, the fact that we do not choose our native language does not suggest that it is biologically ordained.

More broadly, we should question whether the issue of choice is an enlightened criterion for a free society to employ in decisions regarding the liberties of its nonconformists. Even if homosexuality were entirely a matter of choice, attempts to extirpate it by social and criminal sanctions would devalue basic human freedoms and diversity.

In the absence of tolerance, biological and psychosocial theories are perhaps equally capable of being put into the service of social prejudice. Historically, both have been employed to the detriment of gay individuals. In addition to psychoanalysis and aversion therapies, physicians have employed hormonal treatments and brain surgery in attempts to "cure" homosexuality (see Chapter 1 by Silverstein). Accordingly, the biological evidence should be evaluated from the perspective that etiological concerns should not inform social policy.

■ Models for Biological Involvement

All psychological phenomena are dependent on the biological activity of the brain. Thus, all that we do, think, perceive, or feel has an ultimate biological substrate. With respect to sexual orientation, the salient question is not, "Is it biological?" but rather, "*How* is biology involved?" Theoretically, biology could be involved in one or more of three basic ways, as described in the following models.

Formative experience models. In the least restrictive sense, biology simply provides the slate of neural circuitry upon which sexual orientation is inscribed by formative experience. Biology might also determine the developmental period during which that experience must occur. For example, some birds must hear their native call during a restricted period of early development in order to learn it (Nottebohm 1972). If they hear and learn the call of another species during that period, that call will become their song for life. They will not be able to unlearn that song or learn another. Although the bird's song is acquired through experience, biology specifies the period during which that experience must occur. (By no means is this example meant to imply that sexual orientation is acquired by mimicry.)

Direct models. In the most restrictive sense, as in the so-called direct models, biological factors such as genes and hormones exert their influence on sexual orientation by directly organizing the neural circuits that mediate sexual orientation. In more complex versions of these models, direct biological effects and social influences might act sequentially to shape sexual orientation. For example, prenatal biological effects could subsequently be reinforced or overridden by experiential factors. Thus, direct models allow for the possibility that biological factors might either determine one's sexual orientation or predispose one to a particular orientation.

Indirect models. Alternatively, biological factors might exert effects on the brain that influence sexual orientation only indirectly. For example, rather than directly organizing the brain for sexual orientation, biological factors might instead influence other personality traits. These biologically influenced traits would then influence the formative experiences that contribute to the social acquisition of sexual orientation. The organization of sexual orientation is mediated by formative experiences in both the indirect and formative experience models, but only in the former does biology organize the brain in a manner that influences the relevant experiences. In contrast to direct effects, which could be either determinative or predisposing, indirect effects could only be predisposing. In addition to acting in sequence with social factors, indirect biological effects would also interact with social factors in shaping sexual orientation. A particular indirect effect might contribute to the development of sexual orientation in some environments while making no contribution in others.

The Dominant Research Paradigm

Most biological research addressing the issue of sexual orientation is premised on the direct model and the assumption that sexual orientation is a sexually dimorphic trait (i.e., a trait with two forms, male and female). Some researchers thus expect particular aspects of an individual's brain or physiology to conform to one of two archetypes: a male type that drives sexual attraction to women and is shared by heterosexual men and lesbians or a female type, shared by heterosexual women and gay men, that drives sexual attraction to men. Research then proceeds by seeking to demonstrate that a variety of presumed sexual dimorphisms (sex differences) are either reversed or incompletely differentiated in homosexual individuals.

The validity of this paradigm is questionable. To begin with, as the author has argued elsewhere (Byne 1995), there is little evidence that the features that are alleged to be sex-reversed in homosexual individuals actually differ between the sexes in humans, although some of them do clearly differ by sex in laboratory rodents. Until the relevant sex differences can be clearly documented in humans, it will not be logically possible to demonstrate that they are sex-reversed in homosexual individuals.

Furthermore, sexual orientation is not simply dimorphic; it has many forms. Just as a computer might be programmed to accomplish a given task by more than one strategy, the conscious and unconscious motivations associated with sexual attraction could differ even among individuals of the same sex and sexual orientation. Myriad experiences (and subjective interpretations of those experiences) could interact to lead different individuals to the same relative degree of sexual attraction to men, women, or both. Because sexual attraction to men, for example, could be driven by various different psychological motives, there is no reason to expect that all individuals attracted to men should share any particular motive, and therefore any particular brain function, that distinguishes them from individuals attracted to women. If a particular orientation does not require a particular brain function, it follows that it does not necessarily require a distinguishing physiology or brain structure.

The notion that gay men are feminized and lesbians masculinized may tell us more about our culture than about the biology of erotic responsiveness. Some Greek myths, as discussed in Plato's *Symposium* (Joyce 1961), held that heterosexual rather than homosexual desire had intersex origins: those with predominately same-sex desires were considered the most manly of men and womanly of women. In contrast, those who desired the opposite sex supposedly mixed masculine and feminine in their being. Classical culture acknowledged the homosexual exploits of archetypally masculine heroes such as Zeus, Hercules, and Julius Caesar (Boswell 1980). In addition, until only a decade ago when the practice was repudiated by missionaries, various tribal Melanesian cultures expected teenage boys to engage in homosexual activities (Money and Ehrhardt 1972). Contrary to being associated with femininity, that homosexual experience was believed necessary for the attainment of strength and virility (Herdt 1984).

Studies of Adult Hormonal Constitution

One of the more obvious differences between men and women is that they have different gonads. Although different, their gonads (testes and ovaries) nevertheless secrete many of the same substances, including estrogens, androgens, and progestins—the so-called sex hormones. From the turn of the century into the 1970s a popular hypothesis held that the amounts of androgens or estrogens in the blood of heterosexual individuals might be typical of the opposite sex or else intermediate between the amounts in the blood of heterosexual men and women. This hypothesis is no longer viewed favorably because an overwhelming majority of studies failed to demonstrate a correlation between sexual orientation and adult hormonal constitution (Meyer-Bahlburg 1984). Moreover, hormonal "therapies" failed to change sexual orientation, and sexual orientation has not been shown to shift in adults as a consequence of alterations in hormone levels resulting from gonadal malignancies, trauma, or surgical removal (Gooren 1990).

The Prenatal Hormonal Hypotheses

■ Direct Model Version

At present the major impetus for speculation concerning a hormonal basis of sexual orientation is the observation that, in rodents, hormonal exposure in early development determines the balance between male and female patterns of mating behaviors displayed in adulthood. Specifically, female rodents that have been exposed to androgens early in development show more male-typical mounting behavior than do normal adult females. Conversely, males deprived of androgens by castration during the same critical period will subsequently mount less and display a female mating posture called "lordosis," or saddle back, when they are mounted (Goy and McEwen 1980). According to the hypothesis of direct prenatal hormonal effects, prenatal hormones influence sexual orientation in humans in the same direct manner by which they influence the mating behaviors displayed by rodents. Specifically, the hypothesis posits that heterosexual men and homosexual women were exposed to high levels of androgens during a critical period of early development, whereas heterosexual women and homosexual men were exposed to low androgen levels at that time. A common direct model hypothesis is that prenatal hormones influence sexual orientation in humans by acting on the same brain circuits that regulate sexually dimorphic copulatory behaviors in laboratory mammals (Dorner et al. 1975; LeVay 1991a; LeVay and Hamer 1994).

Extrapolating from observable behaviors in rodents to psychological phenomena in humans is problematic. According to some researchers and many popular accounts, the neonatally castrated male rat that shows lordosis when mounted by another male is homosexual, as is the female rat that mounts other females. Lordosis, however, is little more than a reflex. A neonatally castrated male will take the same posture if a handler strokes its back. Furthermore, the male that mounts another male is considered to be heterosexual, as is the female that displays lordosis when mounted by another female. In this laboratory paradigm, sexual orientation is defined in terms of specific behaviors and postures. In contrast, sexual orientation in humans is defined not by the motor patterns of copulation but by one's pattern of erotic responsiveness and the sex of one's preferred sex partner.

◼ Indirect Model Version

In laboratory animals, prenatal hormonal exposure is responsible not only for the sexual differentiation of coital behaviors but also for the propensity to engage in a variety of other behaviors (Goy and McEwen 1980). The hypothesis of indirect hormonal effects suggests that one or more of these hormonally influenced propensities might influence the formative experiences that contribute to the development of sexual orientation (see below).

Testing the Prenatal Hormonal Hypotheses

It is obviously not ethical to experimentally manipulate the prenatal hormonal exposure of human fetuses and study the effects on subsequent sexual orientation. Thus, alternative strategies must be employed. These include assessing sexual orientation in individuals with known or suspected prenatal hormonal abnormalities and assessing presumed correlates of prenatal hormonal exposure in known homosexual and heterosexual individuals. These two strategies will be discussed in turn.

■ Orientation Following Documented Prenatal Hormonal Abnormalities

If the direct prenatal hormonal hypothesis were correct, one might expect that a large proportion of men with medical conditions known to involve prenatal androgen deficiency would be homosexual, as would a large proportion of women exposed prenatally to excess androgens. Because androgens are required for the development of the external male genitalia, males exposed to abnormally low levels may be born with female-like genitals. On the other hand, females exposed to high levels may have a clitoris enlarged to the point that it resembles a penis and the labia may be fused to form an empty scrotum. Thus, the sex of affected individuals may not be apparent at birth and plastic surgery may be done to construct normal appearing genitals. The decision to raise them as boys or as girls is sometimes based on the possibilities for surgical genital reconstruction rather than on genetic sex or the presence of testes or ovaries.

Research into the subsequent sexual orientation of such individuals tends to support a formative experience model. Regardless of their genetic sex or the nature of their prenatal hormonal exposure, these individuals usually become heterosexual in accordance with the sex they are assigned—provided that the sex assignment is made unambiguously and early (Meyer-Bahlburg 1993a). Nevertheless, some studies have reported an increase in homosexual fantasies or behavior among women who were exposed to excess androgens as fetuses. As reviewed by Friedman and Downey (1993), however, these findings are not robust and their usefulness for interpretation is limited because of problems with experimental design and execution.

■ Presumed Correlates of Prenatal Hormonal Exposure in Homosexual Individuals

Gonadal and genital stigmata.   Another strategy in attempting to establish a link between prenatal hormonal exposure and sexual orientation has been to examine presumed correlates of such exposure in known homosexual and heterosexual individuals. The most obvious correlates would be abnormalities of testicular or ovarian function and abnormalities in the differentiation of the external genitalia. Such stigmata are rare in homosexual individuals and lend no support to the prenatal hormonal hypothesis. Rodent studies have demonstrated two additional correlates of prenatal androgen exposure that have been hypothesized to be of relevance in humans: (1) sex differences in hormonal feedback mechanisms and (2) sex differences in brain structure. The second of these will be covered below.

Hormonal feedback mechanisms.   In rodents, androgen activity in the developing hypothalamus determines the signal that the adult's brain will relay to the pituitary gland in response to high levels of estrogen in the bloodstream. If rats experience high levels of androgens at a certain early stage of development (as normal males do), the adult brain will respond to estrogen by directing the pituitary to decrease its secretion of luteinizing hormone (LH). If the developing rodent brain has not been exposed to high androgen levels (as in normal females), it will later respond to high estrogen levels by directing the pituitary to secrete more LH—a positive feedback response required for cyclical ovarian function and fertility in females (Goy and McEwen 1980).

Two laboratories published evidence that gay men exhibit feminized positive feedback responses when injected with estrogen (Dorner et al. 1975; Gladue et al. 1984). However, other studies have found no correlation between sexual orientation and the amount of LH secreted in response to estrogen (Gooren 1986; Hendricks et al. 1989).

Moreover, the suggestion that homosexual men might have feminized feedback responses to estrogen injections is highly suspect on theoretical grounds. In humans and other primates the brain mechanism regulating LH appears to be the same in both sexes rather than taking two sexually distinct forms as in rodents (Byne and Parsons 1993). Although men and women do have different patterns of LH secretion, it is because they have different gonads and different levels of androgens and estrogens in their circulations—not because they have differently organized brains. If there is no sex difference in the human feedback mechanism to begin with, then it cannot be argued logically that the mechanism should be feminized in male homosexual individuals.

Neuroanatomical Studies

During the past decade and a half, sex differences have been confirmed in the size of several brain structures in a variety of laboratory animals. These findings have generated speculation concerning the existence of parallel differences in the human brain associated not only with sex but also with sexual orientation.

■ Hypothalamus

Most of the structural sex differences identified to date involve specific cell groups within a broad region of the rodent hypothalamus that participates in regulating a variety of functions, including sexually dimorphic copulatory behaviors. Like the sex differences in copulatory behaviors, several of the structural sex differences in the rodent brain have been demonstrated to develop in response to sex differences in early androgen exposure: high androgen levels at the appropriate time lead to male-typical structures, whereas low levels lead to female-typical structures. Consequently, the behavioral sex differences are thought to be mediated, at least in part, by the structural differences.

The best-studied anatomical sex difference in the rodent brain involves a cell group that straddles the medial preoptic and anterior regions of the hypothalamus. In the rat, where it was initially described (Gorski et al. 1978), this structure is five to eight times larger in males than in females and is called the sexually dimorphic nucleus of the preoptic area (SDN-POA).

Damage to the preoptic region of the brain has been demonstrated to decrease mounting behavior in a variety of laboratory species, whereas electrical stimulation of the region elicits mounting behavior (Slimp et al. 1978). These observations, and the finding that the size of the SDN-POA correlates positively with mounting frequencies in rats (Anderson et al. 1986), have established the belief that the preoptic area participates in regulating male sex behavior.

Interstitial nuclei. Speculation that the SDN-POA may be involved in the regulation of reproductive behavior in male rats has stimulated considerable interest in finding a comparable nucleus in humans. Four candidates have been identified and designated as the interstitial nuclei of the anterior hypothalamus (INAH1, INAH2, INAH3, and INAH4). Measurement of these nuclei by different laboratories has generated inconsistent results (Allen et al. 1989; LeVay 1991a; Swaab and Fliers 1985). Nevertheless, two studies are in agreement in finding INAH3 to be larger in men than in women (Allen et al. 1989; LeVay 1991a). One of these, the highly publicized study conducted by LeVay (1991a), also reported that in homosexual men INAH3 was as small as in women.

LeVay's study has been widely interpreted as strong evidence that the size of the INAH3 determines or influences sexual orientation. The common criticisms that his study is invalid because of inadequate sexual histories and small sample sizes are not very convincing. These factors would have actually decreased rather than increased the probability of obtaining statistically significant results. As reviewed elsewhere (Byne 1994, 1995), a variety of more valid criticisms detract from the study. Only three of these will be considered here.

First, the finding has not been corroborated, and studies based on measurements of human brain structures have a dismal record of replicability (Byne 1995). In light of this track record, Meyer-Bahlburg (1993b) suggested that as a rule of thumb no such study should be accepted until it has been replicated three times over—provided that there are no intervening failures of replication. To date, no report of a difference in the structure of the human brain associated with either sex or sexual orientation has met this criterion.

Second, all of the brains of gay men came from men with the acquired immune deficiency syndrome (AIDS). This is relevant because at the time of death virtually all men with AIDS have decreased testosterone levels as the result of AIDS itself or of the side effects of particular treatments (Croxon et al. 1989). In some laboratory animals, the size of a structure comparable to the SDN-POA of rats varies with the amount of testosterone in the animal's circulation (Commins and Yahr 1994). Thus, it is possible that the effects on the size of the INAH3 that were attributed to sexual orientation were actually the result of the hormonal abnormalities associated with AIDS. The inclusion in this study of a few brains from heterosexual men with AIDS did not constitute an adequate control to rule out this possibility.

Third, much speculation concerning the function of the INAH3 is based on the assumption that it is the homologue of the rat's SDN-POA. However, the function of the rat's SDN-POA has eluded researchers for more than a decade and a half. In fact, the SDN-POA can be totally destroyed without any discernible effect on the mounting behavior of male rats (Arendash and Gorski 1983). While brain damage in the vicinity of the SDN-POA does decrease mounting behavior, the precise site of the effective damage appears to be above the SDN-POA itself. Similarly, it has been claimed that damage to the preoptic area causes male monkeys to become apparently indifferent to sex with female monkeys (LeVay and Hamer 1994). But the data are more complex (Slimp et al. 1978). Although they decreased the frequency of copulatory behavior in male monkeys, preoptic lesions did not eliminate it entirely. Moreover, the lesions actually appeared to increase the frequency with which males would press a lever for access to females.

The suprachiasmatic nucleus (SCN). In contrast to the INAH3, this nucleus has been reported to be larger in homosexual men than in heterosexual individuals (Swaab and Hoffman 1990). This study has yet to be replicated and also relied on the brains of homosexual men with AIDS and is thus subject to many of the same criticisms as LeVay's study of the INAH3. Unlike INAH3, however, the size of the SCN was not found to vary with sex. Furthermore, the SCN is not believed to be directly involved in the regulation of sexual behaviors. Thus, if the dimorphism proves to be replicable, it will not lend support to the notion that sexual orientation reflects the sexually differentiated state of the brain. Alternative explanations will have to be considered.

■ The Brain Commissures

In addition to the hypothalamus, researchers have begun to seek differences in sex and sexual orientation in the brain commissures, the bundles of fibers that interconnect the left and right halves of the brain. These studies and their rationale are critiqued more fully elsewhere (Byne 1995). Briefly, one as yet uncorroborated study, which examined the brains of gay men with AIDS, reported the anterior commissure (AC) to be larger in women and homosexual men than in heterosexual men (Allen et al. 1992). Even though there was a statistical difference between these groups in the average size of the AC, the size of the AC of 27 of 30 homosexual men fell within the range established by 30 heterosexual men. Thus, even if this study proves replicable, the size of the AC alone would tell us nothing about an individual's sexual orientation. Moreover, the only other laboratory to examine the AC for sex differences reported a tendency for it to be larger in men than in women (Demeter et al. 1988).

There has also been speculation that the morphology of the corpus callosum may be sex reversed in homosexual individuals (LeVay 1991b); however, no sex difference has been consistently reported in the callosum, even though approximately three dozen studies have looked for one. Moreover, a meta-analysis conducted on 33 of these studies found no evidence for a main effect of sex on any aspect of callosal morphology (D. Wahlsten and K. M. Bishop, unpublished observations, 1995).

Conclusion and Suggestions for Future Research

Existing research allows us to draw no definitive conclusions regarding the precise role of biology in sexual orientation. Certainly, sexual orientation is not determined by the levels of sex hormones in an adult's circulation, nor is there compelling evidence that hormonal feedback responses distinguish between homosexual and heterosexual individuals. Similarly, the studies of sexual orientation of individuals exposed to aberrant androgen levels as fetuses are inconclusive. Regarding the neuroanatomical studies, technical considerations call their results into question, but even if the results were valid, their interpretation would hinge on a variety of assumptions of questionable validity.

▇ Direct Model

Unfortunately, research continues to be premised almost exclusively on the model of direct biological effects and to rely heavily on animal models. However, because the reproductive strategies of each species are uniquely adapted to its own ecological niche, it makes no sense to expect one species to provide a model for the study of the sexual behavior of any other. Instead, by studying a variety of species we may gain a better understanding of the range over which neural mechanisms may vary so that the reproductive behaviors of each species mesh with the evolutionary demands imposed by its ecological niche.

Considering matters from a phylogenetic perspective, findings in laboratory rodents are a poor basis for constructing theories concerning the biological substrates of human sexuality. These rodents copulate only at the time of the ovarian cycle when the female is fertile. In fact, it is the hormonal changes associated with ovulation that act on the hypothalamus to make the female sexually receptive. In these animals, one would expect the neural circuits that ensure that mating occurs at the appropriate time to be sexually dimorphic. Because these circuits reside, in part, in the hypothalamus, it is not surprising that the anatomy of the hypothalamus is sexually dimorphic in such species. On the other hand, in species such as our own, in which copulation is not restricted to the female's fertile period, there is no stringent evolutionary requirement for such sexually dimorphic neuronal circuitry. As discussed above, copulatory behaviors in animals cannot be equated with sexual orientation, nor is it likely that the brain circuits that regulate these behaviors in rodents are the same circuits involved in sexual orientation.

It remains possible that a biological factor, reliably tagged by an endocrinological, neuroanatomical, or genetic marker, will one day be discovered that will contribute to an understanding of the sexual orientation of some individuals. However, the intermediate mechanisms linking such a marker to sexual orientation will have to be clarified to substantiate a direct biological model. In the interim it will remain possible that even a robust correlation between a particular marker and sexual orientation could be better explained by an alternative model.

■ Formative Experience Model

The encoding of sexual orientation into the brain through formative experiences remains a possible avenue for biological factors to influence sexual orientation. An analogy may be drawn to gender identity (which is distinct from sexual orientation). It now appears that both boys and girls pass through an early developmental period of undifferentiated, overinclusive gender identity—that is, they exclude no aspect of experience as impossible or inappropriate to them on the basis of their sex (Fast 1984). It also appears that there is a sensitive period for the development of a differentiated sense of gender, roughly between the ages of 18 months to 3 years. However, what biological factors are involved and how they act to delimit this sensitive period are still unknown. With regard to sexual orientation, there may be biological factors that similarly set a sensitive period for development or that render the individual particularly sensitive to the impact of formative experiences at different ages. Research into such factors must not fail to explore the psychosexual developmental processes through which gendered stimuli acquire their erotic significance.

■ Indirect Model

Although this model is the most complex and the most methodologically demanding with respect to research, it may prove to be the most fruitful. An indirect model posits that certain biological factors may act on the brain to influence temperaments, traits, dispositions, and so on. These personality characteristics would then influence not only how an individual interacts with and modifies his or her environment, but how the environment is experienced internally. This model goes beyond a simple formative experience model in that it addresses the possibility that formative experiences may be strongly affected by biologically influenced personality variables.

The interaction between biological factors and environment in the development of sexual orientation may be conceptualized in a variety of ways and is not limited to the examples that will be sketched briefly here. One of the more robust findings in the literature of behavioral endocrinology is that the propensity to engage in rough-and-tumble play is influenced by prenatal androgen exposure. This finding has held up across species and laboratories and may even apply to humans (Ehrhardt and Meyer-Bahlburg 1991). Aversion to competitive rough-and-tumble play in boys is thought by many to be moderately predictive of homosexual development (Bell et al. 1981). Direct model theorists suggest that such an aversion is merely the childhood expression of a brain that has been prewired for homosexuality (Isay 1989), perhaps through a genetic or hormonal mechanism (Bell et al. 1981). An indirect model interpretation postulates that the biologically influenced aversion to rough-and-tumble play does not imply prewiring for homosexuality. Instead, this aversion would become a potent factor predisposing to homosexual development in particular environments—for example, where it is stigmatized by family or peers as "sissy" behavior. It would arguably have different consequences in environments where it is accepted, perhaps making no contribution to sexual orientation at all.

Similarly it has been conjectured that temperamental variants (for example, reward dependence, novelty seeking, and harm avoidance) could have an impact on the acquisition of sexual orientation in an interactive way (Byne and Parsons 1993). If so, and if such temperamental variants were genetically influenced, homosexuality would appear to be heritable. This is because heritability refers only to the extent to which a given outcome is linked to genetic factors. Heritability says nothing about the nature of those genetic factors nor about the mechanisms by which they influence a particular outcome. Importantly, genes for homosexuality are not required for homosexuality to be heritable.

Although biological and social factors are likely to interact in shaping sexual orientation, no naturalistic data exist at present to substantiate any interactive model. Indeed, it is the difficulty of conducting research that adequately addresses the possibility of multiple and interactive pathways to sexual orientation that fosters nearly exclusive reliance on the direct model paradigm. Yet, if the reality indeed follows an indirect model, the search for predisposing biological factors will result in misleading and inconclusive findings until their interactions with environmental factors are taken into account and controlled for in adequate longitudinal studies.

References

Allen LS, Gorski RA: Sexual orientation and the size of the anterior commissure in the human brain. Proc Natl Acad Sci USA 89:7199–7202, 1992

Allen LS, Hines M, Shryne JE, et al: Two sexually dimorphic cell groups in the human brain. J Neurosci 9:497–506, 1989

Anderson RH, Fleming DE, Rhees RW, et al: Relationships between sexual activity, plasma testosterone, and the volume of the sexually dimorphic nucleus of the preoptic area in neonatally stress and non-stressed rats. Brain Res 370:1–10, 1986

Arendash GW, Gorski RA: Effects of discrete lesions of the sexually dimorphic nucleus of the preoptic area or other medial preoptic regions on the sexual behavior of male rats. Brain Res Bull 10:147–154, 1983

Bailey MJ, Pillard RC: Are some people born gay? The New York Times, December 17, 1991, p A19

Bell AP, Weinberg MS, Hammersmith SK: Sexual Preference: Its Development in Men and Women, Bloomington, IN, Indiana University Press, 1981

Boswell J: Social Tolerance, Christianity and Homosexuality. Chicago, IL, University of Chicago Press, 1980

Byne W: The biological evidence challenged. Sci Am 270:50–55, 1994

Byne W: Science and belief: psychobiological research on sexual orientation. J Homosex 28:303–344, 1995

Byne W, Parsons B: Sexual orientation: the biological theories reappraised. Arch Gen Psychiatry 50:228–239, 1993

Commins D, Yahr P: Adult testosterone levels influence the morphology of a sexually dimorphic area in the Mongolian gerbil brain. J Comp Neurol 224:132–140, 1994

Croxon TS, Chapman WE, Miller LK, et al: Changes in the hypothalamic-pituitary–gonadal axis in human immunodeficiency virus-infected men. J Clin Endocrinol Metab 68:317–321, 1989

Demeter S, Ringo JL, Doty RW: Morphometric analysis of the human corpus callosum and anterior commissure. Human Neurobiol 6:219–226, 1988

Dorner G, Rhode W, Stahl F, et al: A neuroendocrine predisposition for homosexuality in men. Arch Sex Behav 4:1–8, 1975

Ehrhardt AA, Meyer-Bahlburg HFL: Effects of prenatal sex hormones on gender-related behavior. Science 211:1312–1318, 1991

Fast I: Gender Identity: A Differentiation Model. Hillsdale, NJ, Erlbaum Press, 1984

Friedman RC, Downey J: Neurobiology and sexual orientation: current relationships. J Neuropsychiatry Clin Neurosci 5:131–153, 1993

Gladue BA, Green R, Hellman RE: Neuroendocrine response to estrogen and sexual orientation. Science 225:1496–1499, 1984

Gooren L: The neuroendocrine response of luteinizing hormone to estrogen administration in the human is not sex specific but dependent on the hormonal environment. J Clin Endocrinol Metab 63:589–593, 1986

Gooren L: Biomedical theories of sexual orientation: a critical examination, in Homosexuality/Heterosexuality: Concepts of Sexual Orientation. Edited by McWhirter DP, Sanders SA, Reinisch JM. New York, Oxford University Press, 1990, pp 71–87

Gorski RA, Gordon JH, Shryne JE, et al: Evidence for a morphological sex difference within the medial preoptic area of the rat brain. Brain Res 148:333–346, 1978

Goy RW, McEwen BS: Sexual Differentiation of the Brain. Cambridge, MA, MIT Press, 1980

Haldeman DC: The practice and ethics of sexual orientation conversion therapy. J Consult Clin Psychol 62:221–227, 1994

Hendricks SE, Graber B, Rodriquez-Sierra JF: Neuroendocrine responses to exogenous estrogen. No differences between heterosexual and homosexual men. Psychoneuroendocrinology 14:177–185, 1989

Herdt GH: Semen transactions in Sambia culture, in Ritualized Homosexuality in Melanesia. Edited by Herdt GH. Berkeley, CA, University of California Press, 1984, pp 167–210

Isay R: Being Homosexual: Gay Men and Their Development. New York, Avon Press, 1989

Jefferson DJ: Science besieged: studying the biology of sexual orientation has political fallout. The Wall Street Journal, August 12, 1993, p A1

Joyce M (translator): Symposium, in Plato: The Collected Dialogues. Edited by Hamilton E, Cairns H. Princeton, NJ, Princeton University Press, 1961, pp 526–574

LeVay S: A difference in hypothalamic structure between heterosexual and homosexual men. Science 253:1034–1037, 1991a

LeVay S: Replication will tell (letter). New York Times, October 7, 1991b, p A16

LeVay S, Hamer D: Evidence for a biological influence in male homosexuality. Sci Am 270:44–49, 1994

Meyer-Bahlburg HFL: Psychoendocrine research on sexual orientation: current status and future options. Prog Brain Res 71:375–397, 1984

Meyer-Bahlburg HFL: Gender development in intersex patients. Child and Adolescent Clinics of North America 2:501–512, 1993a

Meyer-Bahlburg HFL: Sexual orientation: new biological data debated. Presented at the 146th Annual Meeting of the American Psychiatric Association, San Francisco, CA, May 27, 1993b

Money J, Ehrhardt AA: Man and Woman, Boy and Girl. Baltimore, MD, Johns Hopkins University Press, 1972

Nottebohm F: The origins of vocal learning. American Naturalist 105:116–140, 1972

Slimp JC, Hart BL, Goy RW: Heterosexual, autosexual and social behavior of adult male rhesus monkeys with medial preoptic anterior hypothalamic lesions. Brain Res 142:105–122, 1978

Schmalz J: Poll finds even split on homosexuality's cause. The New York Times, March 5, 1993, p A14

Swaab DF, Fliers E: A sexually dimorphic nucleus in the human brain. Science 228:1112–1114, 1985

Swaab DF, Hoffman MA: An enlarged suprachiasmatic nucleus in homosexual men. Brain Res 537:141–148, 1990

Bisexuality

An Examination of Theory and Research

Ronald C. Fox, Ph.D.

Greater acknowledgment of bisexuality as a valid sexual orientation and sexual identity has come about as a result of changes in how the term "bisexuality" has been defined in theory, clinical practice, and research. Two factors have contributed significantly to a more affirmative approach to bisexuality: 1) the elimination of homosexuality as a clinical diagnostic category, which led to the development of lesbian and gay identity theory, and 2) the critical

Portions of this chapter are adapted or excerpted from Fox RC: "Bisexual Identities," in *Lesbian, Gay, and Bisexual Identities Over the Lifespan: Psychological Perspectives*. Edited by D'Augelli AR, Patterson CJ. New York, Oxford University Press, 1995, pp. 48–86. Used with permission. Copyright 1995 Oxford University Press.

reexamination of the dichotomous model of sexual orientation, which led to the articulation of a multidimensional model of sexual orientation. This chapter reviews these changes by examining the uses of the concept of bisexuality in several related areas: psychoanalytic theory, lesbian and gay identity theory, sexual orientation theory, research on homosexuality, and finally, theory and research on bisexuality and bisexual identities.

Bisexuality in Psychoanalytic Theory

"Bisexuality" has existed as a concept and descriptive term in the literature since the process of psychosexual development was first conceptualized. Early theorists used the concept of bisexuality to explain homosexuality in terms of evolutionary theory (Ellis 1905/1960; Freud 1905/1960; Krafft-Ebing 1886/1965; Weininger 1908). They believed that the human species evolved from a primitive hermaphroditic state to the gender-differentiated physical form of today and that individual physiological and psychological development parallels this evolutionary process (Ritvo 1990; Sulloway 1979). Like his contemporaries, Freud (1925/1959) used the theory of bisexuality to account for homosexuality, which he saw as an indication of arrested psychosexual development. At the same time, he believed that all individuals have some homosexual feelings:

> The most important of these perversions, homosexuality . . . can be traced back to the constitutional bisexuality of all human beings. . . . Psychoanalysis enables us to point to some trace or other of a homosexual object-choice in everyone. (pp. 71–72)

Freud (1937/1963) later described as bisexual individuals with both homosexual and heterosexual attractions and behavior:

> It is well known that at all times there have been humans who can take as their sexual objects persons of either sex without one trend interfering with the other. We call these people bisexual and accept the fact of their existence without wondering much at it. . . . But we have come to know that all human beings are bisexual in this sense and that their libido is distributed between objects of both sexes, either in a manifest or a latent form. (pp. 261–262)

Most psychoanalysts saw the theory of bisexuality as an essential conceptual reference point for understanding psychosexual development (Stekel 1922/1946), masculinity and femininity (Stoller 1972), psychopathology (Khan and Masud 1974; Kubie 1974), and homosexuality (Alexander 1933; Limentani 1976). Some psychoanalysts disagreed, arguing that individual responses to family influences are more relevant in understanding these subjects (Bieber et al. 1962; Rado 1940, 1949). Many viewed sexual orientation in strictly dichotomous terms and argued with the term "bisexual" as a descriptive category referring to individuals with both homosexual and heterosexual attractions or behavior. For example, Bergler (1956) believed that those who consider themselves bisexual are denying a homosexual orientation:

> Bisexuality—a state that has no existence beyond the word itself—is an out-and-out fraud. . . . The theory claims that a man can be—alternatively or concomitantly—homo and heterosexual. . . . Nobody can dance at two different weddings at the same time. These so-called bisexuals are really homosexuals with an occasional heterosexual excuse. (pp. 80–81)

From this point of view, the diagnostic category homosexuality was appropriate for individuals with any same-gender sexual attractions or behavior. Furthermore, the goal of psychoanalytic psychotherapy was an exclusively heterosexual orientation, which was seen as more easily attainable by individuals with some heterosexual attractions or behavior (Bieber et al. 1962; Hatterer 1970; Socarides 1978).

Bisexuality in Lesbian and Gay Identity Theory

The illness model of homosexuality was not universally accepted in the psychiatric community, and in 1973, the American Psychiatric Association removed homosexuality as a diagnostic category (Bayer 1981). This action facilitated the development of affirmative models of lesbian and gay identity formation (Cass 1979, 1983/1984; Coleman 1981/1982b; Troiden 1988). In these models, the coming out process begins with first homosexual attractions, which are followed by same-gender sexual experiences and relationships, self-identification as gay or lesbian, and disclosure of one's sexual orientation to others. The developmental process culminates in participation in the lesbian and gay community, exclusively same-gender sexual relationships, and an integrated lesbian or gay identity.

As with other developmental models, explanations were offered for deviations from the typical sequence of events. For example, Cass (1979) saw bisexual self-identification as an example of identity foreclosure, delaying or preventing the formation of a positive homosexual identity. From this point of view, persistent heterosexual attractions and behavior are only transitional phenomena some individuals experience as they move toward permanent monosexual lesbian and gay identities.

In contrast, Coleman (1981/1982b) suggested that the developmental stages he articulated for the coming out process also might apply to bisexuals. Troiden (1988) also saw bisexuality as a valid sexual orientation. He believed, however, that the general lack of recognition given to bisexuality and the lack of a supportive community of other bisexual people make it difficult for an individual to sustain a bisexual identity. Cass (1990) has suggested more recently that homosexual, heterosexual, and bisexual identities form along distinct developmental pathways, the components of which are both similar and different. Cass emphasized that, although sexual identities may be long lasting, they are not necessarily fixed. An individual might minimize the relevance of experiences that imply a different sexual identity to maintain an already established homosexual, heterosexual, or bisexual identity or might question this identity, potentially initiating the development of an alternative sexual identity.

Bisexuality and Sexual Orientation Theory

Kinsey et al. (1948, 1952) departed from traditional thinking about sexual orientation and emphasized the inadequacy of a dichotomous model for describing the diversity of human sexual experience:

> Males do not represent two discrete populations, heterosexual and homosexual. The world is not divided into sheep and goats. Not all things are black nor all things white. It is a fundamental of taxonomy that nature rarely deals with discrete categories. Only the human mind invents categories and tries to force facts into separated pigeonholes. The living world is a continuum in each and every one of its aspects. The sooner we learn this concerning human sex-

ual behavior the sooner we shall reach a sound understanding of
the realities of sex. (Kinsey et al. 1948, p. 639)

Other authors viewed heterosexuality and homosexuality as independent aspects of sexual orientation, which they saw as the physical
and affectional preferences of the individual for persons of the same
or other biological sex (Shively and DeCecco 1977; Storms 1980). Sexual orientation was seen as one of four components of sexual identity,
along with biological sex, gender identity, and social sex role (Shively
and DeCecco 1977). The research literature has included a variety of
criteria for defining sexual orientation, including sexual behavior, affectional attachments (close relationships), erotic fantasies, arousal,
erotic preference, and self-identification as bisexual, heterosexual, or
homosexual (Shively et al. 1983/1984).

The Klein Sexual Orientation Grid (Klein et al. 1985) provides a
comprehensive approach to assessing sexual orientation by including
scales for emotional preference, social preference, heterosexual-bisexual-homosexual lifestyle, and self-identification as well as for sexual
attractions, fantasies, and behavior. Individuals are asked to rate themselves on a seven-point heterosexual-bisexual-homosexual scale for
each variable for past, present, and ideal time frames. The Assessment
of Sexual Orientation (Coleman 1987) is an instrument that was designed to facilitate clinical interviews in which the presenting issues
include sexual orientation. The client indicates current relationship
status, sexual orientation self-identification, desired future identification, and level of comfort with present orientation. A series of circles
also are marked (in terms of "up to the present" and "ideal" time
frames) to indicate physical identity, actual and fantasized gender identity, sex-role identity, and sexual, fantasy, and emotional aspects of sexual orientation. Both of these instruments take a multidimensional
approach to sexual orientation that integrates bisexuality as a useful
descriptive category and describes more accurately factors that are involved in an individual's sexual orientation over time.

Bisexuality in Sexuality Research

The discussion of homosexuality in the anthropological literature has
been framed primarily in terms of several categories of homosexual
behavior, such as age-structured, reverse-gendered, and role-specialized

homosexuality, and modern lesbian and gay lifestyles (Herdt 1990) or transgenerational, transgenderal, egalitarian, and class-differentiated homosexuality (Greenberg 1988). In many cultures in which homosexual behavior occurs, some individuals exhibit both homosexual and heterosexual behavior. Anthropologists have not generally characterized such patterns of sexual expression as examples of bisexuality. An exception is found in an early cross-cultural survey of sexual behavior (Ford and Beach 1951):

> When it is realized that 100% of the males in certain societies engage in homosexual as well as heterosexual alliances, and when it is understood that many men and women in our own society are equally capable of relations with partners of the same or opposite sex . . . then it should be clear that one cannot classify homosexual and heterosexual tendencies as being mutually exclusive or even opposed to each other. (p. 242)

Mead (1975) also saw bisexuality as normal, remarking that "even a superficial look at other societies and some groups in our own society should be enough to convince us that a very large number of human beings—probably a majority—are bisexual in their potential capacity for love" (p. 29). She believed that social attitudes about sex and love constrain the expression of bisexual attractions in terms of sexual behavior. Bisexual behavior has been examined in research on sexuality in Melanesia (Davenport 1965; Herdt 1984) and Mexico (Carrier 1985) and in a survey of bisexuality in Australia, India, Indonesia, Latin America, Mexico, the Netherlands, New Zealand, sub-Saharan Africa, Thailand, the United States, and the United Kingdom (Tielman et al. 1991).

One of the most striking findings of Kinsey et al. (1948, 1952) was the significant proportion of individuals who had engaged in adult homosexual behavior. Other researchers since then have reported similar findings but have differed in their interpretations of how concurrent homosexual and heterosexual attractions or behavior relate to sexual orientation. Some authors contend that such individuals are gay or lesbian rather than bisexual (Hunt 1974; Saghir and Robins 1973; Spada 1979). Other researchers have taken a more affirmative approach, including observations of bisexual respondents about their sexual orientation (Hite 1976, 1981; Jay and Young 1979) or contrasting respondents on the basis of both identity and sexual behavior (Playboy Readers' Sex Survey 1983).

Research on the lesbian community has revealed a variety of experiences and attitudes regarding bisexuality (Golden 1987; Ponse 1978; Rust 1992, 1993; D. G. Wolf 1979). Some lesbians have never experienced heterosexual attractions or behavior, whereas others have been involved in sexual relationships with men. Some lesbians are accepting of women who acknowledge ongoing sexual attractions to men or who consider themselves bisexual, but many believe that such women are not "real" lesbians or have not completed the coming out process. Similar reactions toward bisexual men were found in a study of a gay male community (Warren 1974). In research on situational homosexual behavior, most individuals self-identify themselves as either homosexual or heterosexual. Some, however, consider themselves bisexual as shown in studies of sex in prison (Wooden and Parker 1982), male prostitution (Boles and Elifson 1994; Reiss 1961), gay bars (Read 1980), and sex in public places (Humphreys 1970).

Several researchers questioned the dichotomous model of sexual orientation, classifying individuals with heterosexual and homosexual attractions and behavior as bisexual. For example, in their study of male homosexuality, Weinberg and Williams (1974) found that the bisexual men were more involved with heterosexuals and were more concerned with passing as heterosexual. They had more frequent and enjoyable sex with women and were more likely to have been heterosexually married. Weinberg and Williams found no support for the argument that bisexuals are confused about their sexual identities.

In their survey on homosexuality in women and men, Bell and Weinberg (1978) did not differentiate the responses of bisexual and homosexual respondents, even though a substantial proportion of participants rated themselves in the midrange on the Kinsey scale. The criticism was made that considering bisexual and homosexual respondents as a single group obscures information particular to both components and limits the ability of the researchers to generalize about either component from the study results (MacDonald 1983). In a later study of sexual preference, Bell et al. (1981) classified respondents rating themselves in the midrange of the Kinsey scale as bisexual. On the basis of their findings, they speculated that in contrast to their exclusively homosexual respondents, "among the bisexuals, adult sexual preference is much less strongly tied to pre-adult sexual feelings" (p. 200).

A study of lesbian and gay male psychologists also included a substantial proportion of respondents who considered themselves bisexual (Kooden et al. 1979). Although the general responses of all groups were similar, the bisexual psychologists appeared to lack the social support networks of the gay and lesbian psychologists. They were more likely to be heterosexually married and less likely to be involved in the gay movement. Like the closeted gay and lesbian psychologists, the bisexual psychologists "did not report having the positive experiences that were reported by the gay respondents who were generally open" (p. 68).

Research on Bisexuality

Early theory and research on bisexuality addressed questions about bisexuality and psychological adjustment, bisexual identity and sexual behavior, and homosexuality and bisexuality in heterosexual marriages. Several typologies of bisexuality have been developed, and more recent research has focused on factors involved in the development of positive bisexual identities.

■ Psychological Adjustment

Research demonstrating that homosexuality is not associated with psychopathology was an important factor in the decision of the American Psychiatric Association to remove homosexuality as a diagnostic category. Nevertheless, the dichotomous model of sexual orientation remained and supported the belief that bisexuals were psychologically maladjusted. Two psychiatrists (Klein 1978; Wolff 1979) challenged the position that sexual relationships with both women and men indicate immaturity and psychopathology. Wolff (1979) supported the concept of an inherent bisexuality and believed that bisexuality is an intrinsic factor in psychosexual development (Wolff 1971): "We certainly are bisexual creatures, and this innate disposition is reinforced by the indelible memory of childhood attachments, which know no limitation of sex" (pp. 45–46). Klein (1978) maintained that bisexuality is as normal an outcome of the developmental process as are heterosexuality or homosexuality and that awareness and expression of both heterosexual and homosexual attractions can enhance the experience of intimacy and personal fulfillment of the individual. Furthermore, research has found no evidence of psychopathology or psychological maladjustment in bisexual women and men (Harris 1977; Harwell 1976; LaTorre and Wendenberg 1983; Markus 1981; Masters and Johnson 1979; Nurius 1983; M. W. Ross 1983; Weinberg and Williams 1974; Zinik 1984).

Some research has found that self-identified bisexuals are characterized by high self-esteem (Galland 1975; Rubenstein 1982), self-confidence and autonomy (Galland 1975), a positive self-concept independent of social norms (Twining 1983), assertiveness (Bode 1976), and cognitive flexibility (Zinik 1984).

■ Identity and Sexual Behavior

Researchers who viewed heterosexuality and homosexuality as irreconcilable opposites believed that individuals who self-identify as bisexual or whose sexual attractions or behavior are not exclusively heterosexual or homosexual are in denial about a gay or lesbian sexual orientation (Fast and Wells 1975; Miller 1979; H. L. Ross 1971; Schafer 1976). Other researchers proceeded from a more neutral perspective. For example, Blumstein and Schwartz (1976a, 1976b, 1977) found that a variety of sexual behaviors was associated with bisexual, lesbian, and gay identities. Although some self-identified bisexual respondents had sexual relationships with both men and women during a particular period, others did not. Furthermore, although most respondents who considered themselves lesbian or gay had exclusively homosexual relationships, some also had heterosexual relationships. Other researchers have also found a variety of sexual behaviors among self-identified gay, lesbian, bisexual, and heterosexual individuals (Doll et al. 1992; Lever et al. 1992; Reinisch et al. 1990; Stokes et al. 1993). Furthermore, for many individuals, gender is not necessarily a deciding factor in their choice of a sexual or relationship partner (Ross and Paul 1992).

Sexual identity may be related to factors other than current sexual behavior, such as whether a person is in a heterosexual or homosexual relationship, fear of being known as gay or bisexual, or political reasons such as loyalty to the gay or lesbian communities (Blumstein and Schwartz 1976a, 1976b, 1977; Golden 1987, 1994; Rust 1992, 1993). Some individuals move from a heterosexual identity to a bisexual identity, whereas others first consider themselves lesbian or gay before they consider themselves bisexual (Fox 1995b; Golden 1987; Rust 1992, 1993). These findings suggest that sexual attractions, fantasy, and behavior and self-identification may vary over time for lesbian, gay, and heterosexual individuals as well as for bisexual individuals.

On the other hand, most self-identified bisexuals fall in the midrange of the Kinsey scale for ideal sexual behavior but tend to fall at either the heterosexual or homosexual ends of the scale for actual behavior (Fox 1995b; George 1993; Klein et al. 1985; Reinhardt 1985). Actual sexual behavior appears to be constrained by the structure and dynamics of current relationships in which individuals may be engaged. Although sexual identity does change for some individuals, continuity in identity clearly exists for many individuals, whether or not their bisexual attractions are expressed in terms of sexual behavior or relationships during a particular period.

■ Homosexuality and Bisexuality in Heterosexual Marriages

The traditional psychiatric position was that the expression of homosexual attractions by heterosexually married individuals is an indication of psychopathology (Allen 1961; Bieber 1969; Hatterer 1970; Imielinski 1969). Others also have portrayed mixed-orientation marriages as problematic, with separation as the typical outcome for the husband in coming out as a gay man (Bozett 1982; Hill 1987; Maddox 1982; Miller 1979; H. L. Ross 1971).

Several authors have taken a more neutral approach, focusing on adjustments that couples have made to continue their marriages (Gochros 1989; Latham and White 1978; Nahas and Turley 1979; M. W. Ross 1983; Whitney 1990). Others identified characteristics of successful marriages of bisexual men (Brownfain 1985; Coleman 1981/1982a, 1985b; D. Dixon 1985; Matteson 1985; T. J. Wolf 1985) and bisexual women (Coleman 1985a; J. K. Dixon 1985; Reinhardt 1985). These characteristics include open communication between partners, acceptance of and discussion about the homosexual feelings of the bisexual partner, commitment to making the relationship work, the spouse's maintenance of a sense of worth outside the context of the relationship, and, in some cases, agreement to some degree of open relationship. The impact of the husband's disclosure of sexual orientation on his spouse and the marital relationship also has been examined (Buxton 1994; Gochros 1989; Hays and Samuels 1989).

■ Typologies of Bisexuality

Several typologies of bisexuality have been elaborated, based on the extent and timing of past and present heterosexual and homosexual behavior. Klein (1978) differentiated transitional, historical, sequential, and concurrent bisexuality. For some individuals, bisexuality does represent a stage in the process of coming out as lesbian or gay (transitional bisexuality), whereas for others a gay or lesbian identity is a step in the process of coming out bisexual. Some individuals, whose sexual lives are presently heterosexual or homosexual, have experienced both same- and opposite-gender sexual attractions or behavior in the past (historical bisexuality). Other individuals have had relationships with both women and men, but with only one person during any period of time (sequential bisexuality), whereas others have had relationships with both men and women at the same time (concurrent bisexuality). Similar typologies have been developed by other authors (Berkey et al. 1990; Boulton and Coxon 1991; Weinberg et al. 1994). Other factors relevant to a consideration of bisexuality also have been identified (Doll et al. 1991), including the social context in which a person lives (heterosexual, homosexual, or both), the relationships in which an individual is involved, and how open a person is with others about being bisexual.

Bisexuality also has been described in terms of the circumstances in which homosexual behavior takes place (M. W. Ross 1991). For example, a person may be hiding a homosexual orientation or exploring homosexuality or may be in transition to a gay or lesbian identity (defense bisexuality). When a society provides no alternatives to marriage, homosexual behavior may take place away from the family environment (married bisexuality). Homosexual behavior may be prescribed for some or all members of a society, as in Melanesia (ritual bisexuality). For some people, gender is not a criterion for sexual attraction or partner selection (equal bisexuality). In some cultures, a male who takes only the inserter role in anal intercourse with another male is considered heterosexual ("Latin" bisexuality). Homosexual behavior may be circumstantial, taking place once or a few times (experimental bisexuality) or only when there are no heterosexual outlets (secondary bisexuality). Homosexual behavior also may occur as part of male or female prostitution (technical bisexuality).

Bisexual Identity Development

Several authors have discussed bisexual identity development based on results of their empirical research. Twining (1983) examined issues involved in the coming out process for bisexual women and concluded that "an initial formulation of a conceptual theory of bisexual identity development seems to call for a task model rather than a phase or stage model" (p. 158). In contrast, based on the results of their 1983, 1984/1985, and 1988 studies, Weinberg et al. (1994) outlined the stages they believed were involved in the development of bisexual identities: initial confusion, finding and applying the label, settling into the identity, and an additional stage, continued uncertainty, which they saw as a common experience of many bisexuals. They saw bisexuality as an "add-on" to an already established heterosexual identity.

Rust (1992, 1993) and Fox (1995a, 1995b) have emphasized that multiple factors are at work in the development of bisexual identities and that dichotomous and linear conceptual approaches to sexual identity formation do not adequately describe the coming out experiences of many individuals. Gender, age, social class, ethnicity, sexual and emotional attractions, fantasies, and behavior affect the experience and presentation of bisexual identities. Furthermore, although many men and women develop a bisexual identity after first considering themselves heterosexual, others arrive at a bisexual identity from an established lesbian or gay identity. This suggests that sexual identity is not as immutable for all individuals as some theorists and researchers have assumed.

The following sections summarize the results of an examination of research findings on typical milestone events involved in bisexual, lesbian, and gay identity development (Fox 1995a). Consideration of the average ages at which developmental milestones occur as well as gender and age differences for these events allows for a fuller understanding of the process of coming out bisexual.

■ Heterosexual Attractions and Behavior

Bisexual women and men have their first heterosexual attractions on average in their early teens. This is somewhat earlier than for lesbians and gay men who have had heterosexual attractions. Bisexual women have their first sexual experiences with men in their middle teens, somewhat earlier than bisexual men have their first sexual experiences with women. This is about the same as for lesbians and gay men who have had sexual experiences with persons of the other gender.

■ Homosexual Attractions and Behavior

Bisexual men have their first homosexual attractions on average in their early to middle teens, whereas bisexual women have their first homosexual attractions in their middle to late teens. Bisexual men have their first same-gender sexual experiences in their middle to late teens, whereas bisexual women have their first same-gender sexual experiences in their early twenties. These events occur somewhat later than for gay men and lesbians. The earlier ages of first homosexual attractions and behavior for bisexual men compared with bisexual women are strikingly parallel to the earlier ages for gay men compared with lesbians.

■ Sexual Orientation Self-Identification

Bisexual men and women first self-identify themselves as bisexual on average in their early to middle twenties. This is later than the ages of first homosexual self-identification of gay men and lesbians. For bisexual men and women who have considered themselves gay or lesbian, the men identify themselves as gay in their early twenties, which is earlier than the women self-identify as lesbian. This parallels the earlier homosexual self-identification of gay men compared with lesbians.

■ Self-Disclosure of Sexual Orientation

Bisexual women and men typically first disclose their sexual orientation to another person in their twenties, at about the same time they first self-identify as bisexual, and this is about the same as for lesbians and gay men. Bisexual women and men are most likely to have disclosed their sexual orientation to their friends and relationship partners or a therapist and less likely to have disclosed to family members or to people at work or at school. This is the same pattern as for lesbians and gay men, although the proportions of bisexuals disclosing their sexual orientation to persons other than friends and relationship partners are less than for lesbians and gay men.

◼ Gender and Age Differences in the Coming-Out Process

The timing and sequence of developmental milestone events reveal different normative patterns for bisexual women and men. Most bisexual women experience their first homosexual attractions and behavior after their first heterosexual attractions and behavior. They also adopt a bisexual identity sooner after their first homosexual attractions than bisexual men. In contrast, a greater proportion of bisexual men experience their first homosexual attractions and behavior before or at about the same age as their first heterosexual behavior. Most bisexual men experience concurrent heterosexual and homosexual attractions and behavior at an earlier age than bisexual women and for a longer period of time before their first bisexual self-identification.

Significant differences exist in the ages at which younger and older individuals have experienced these developmental milestone events, suggesting that the entire coming-out process is occurring earlier for younger bisexual women and men. Similar age differences have been found between younger and older gay men and lesbians for these developmental milestone events. These trends are a reflection of more affirmative attitudes toward homosexuality and bisexuality, greater access to accurate information about sexuality and sexual orientation, and the development of visible and supportive lesbian, gay, and bisexual communities.

◼ Coming Out Issues

Several issues that bisexual women and men typically face in coming out have been identified (Coleman 1981/1982a; Little 1989; Lourea 1985; Matteson 1987; Morse 1989; Nichols 1988, 1989; Paul 1983/1984, 1985; Schuster 1987; Twining 1983; Weise 1992; T. J. Wolf 1987, 1992). These issues include uncertainty—how to interpret concurrent sexual attractions to both women and men, alienation—feeling different from heterosexuals and from gay men and lesbians, isolation—not knowing other bisexual women or men and feeling the lack of a sense of community, self-acceptance—dealing with external and internalized homophobia and biphobia, and apprehension about the impact of disclosing their bisexuality in existing or new relationships. Autobiographical accounts provide insight into these issues by illustrating how bisexual individuals in diverse circumstances have experienced and successfully moved through the coming-out process (Geller 1990; Hutchins and Kaahumanu 1991; Kohn and Matusow 1980; Norris and Read 1985; Ochs and Deihl 1995; Off Pink Collective 1988; Weise 1992; Wolff 1979).

An important difference historically between coming out bisexual and coming out lesbian or gay has been the relative lack of access of bisexual women and men to a community of similar others. As a result, bisexual men and women have often looked to the gay and lesbian communities for support and understanding regarding their homosexual interests and sexual minority status. In the 1970s and early 1980s, bisexual groups were organized in several urban areas (Barr 1985; Mishaan 1985; Rubenstein and Slater 1985). Since then, a dramatic growth has occurred in the number of local, regional, national, and international bisexual groups and organizations (Ochs 1995; Tucker 1995). This more extensive and diverse bisexual support network represents a major change in the degree to which bisexual women and men will have access to the experience of community during the coming-out process and on an ongoing basis.

Discussion

The elimination of homosexuality as a clinical diagnostic category served to encourage the development of theory and research on the development of positive lesbian and gay identities. Thinking about sexual orientation and sexual identity, however, remained based on the assumption of monosexuality or exclusivity of heterosexual or homosexual "object choice." Through the lens of this dichotomous model, bisexuality appeared anomalous, and individuals who claimed a bisexual identity were seen as psychologically and socially maladjusted, just as lesbians and gay men were considered maladjusted from the point of view of the illness model. At the same time, research on human sexuality demonstrated that a substantial proportion of individuals have experienced both heterosexual and homosexual attractions and behavior. Furthermore, research found no indication of psychopathology in bisexual women and men, just as prior research had found no evidence of psychopathology in lesbians and gay men.

Affirmative approaches to bisexuality challenge several assumptions about sexual orientation: that exclusive heterosexuality and homosexuality are the only normal outcomes of the developmental process, that heterosexuality and homosexuality are mutually exclusive, that gender is the primary criterion for sexual partner selection, and that sexual orientation is immutable. Bisexual identity development has not been conceptualized as a linear process with a fixed outcome, as in theories of heterosexual, lesbian, and gay identity development, but rather as a complex and open-ended process. For some individuals, sexual identity remains constant, whereas for others, sexual identity varies in response to changes in sexual and emotional attractions, behavior, and relationships and the social and political contexts in which these occur.

Like lesbians and gay men, bisexual women and men need to acknowledge and validate their homosexual attractions and relationships to achieve positive and integrated sexual identities. Bisexual men and women, however, need to acknowledge and validate both the homosexual and the heterosexual components of their identities, regardless of the degree to which either or both of these occur in sexual behavior or relationships. The development of a multidimensional approach to sexual orientation has been essential in more accurately conceptualizing bisexuality and understanding the life experiences of bisexual women and men. Furthermore, recent theory and research on bisexuality and bisexual identities have contributed significantly to our knowledge about sexual orientation and sexual identity development as well as the relationships between lesbian, gay, and bisexual issues.

References

Alexander F: Bisexual conflict in homosexuality. Psychoanal Q 2:197–201, 1933

Allen C: When homosexuals marry, in The Third Sex. Edited by Rubin I. New York, New Book, 1961, pp 58–62

Barr G: Chicago Bi-Ways: an informal history. J Homosex 11:231–234, 1985

Bayer R: Homosexuality and American Psychiatry: The Politics of Diagnosis. New York, Basic Books, 1981

Bell AP, Weinberg MS: Homosexualities: A Study of Diversity Among Men and Women. New York, Simon and Schuster, 1978

Bell AP, Weinberg MS, Hammersmith SK: Sexual Preference: Its Development in Men and Women. Bloomington, IN, Indiana University Press, 1981

Bergler E: Homosexuality: Disease or Way of Life. New York, Collier, 1956

Berkey B, Perelman-Hall T, Kurdeck LA: Multi-dimensional scale of sexuality. J Homosex 19:67–87, 1990

Bieber I: The married male homosexual. Med Aspects Hum Sex 3:76–84, 1969

Bieber I, Dain HJ, Dince PR, et al: Homosexuality: A Psychoanalytic Study. New York, Random House, 1962

Blumstein PW, Schwartz P: Bisexuality in men. Urban Life 5(3):339–358, 1976a

Blumstein PW, Schwartz P: Bisexuality in women. Arch Sex Behav 5(2):171–181, 1976b

Blumstein PW, Schwartz P: Bisexuality: some social psychological issues. Journal of Social Issues 33(2):30–45, 1977

Bode J: View from Another Closet: Exploring Bisexuality in Women. New York, Hawthorne Books, 1976

Boles J, Elifson, KW: Sexual identity and HIV: the male prostitute. J Sex Res 31:39–46, 1994

Boulton M, Coxon T: Bisexuality in the United Kingdom, in Bisexuality and HIV/AIDS: A Global Perspective. Edited by Tielman RAP, Carballo M, Hendriks AC. Buffalo, NY, Prometheus Books, 1991, pp 65–72

Bozett FW: Heterogeneous couples in heterosexual marriages: gay men and straight women. Journal of Marital and Family Therapy 8(1):81–89, 1982

Brownfain JJ: A study of the married bisexual male: paradox and resolution. J Homosex 11:173–188, 1985

Buxton AP: The Other Side of the Closet: The Coming Out Crisis for Straight Spouses and Families. New York, Wiley, 1994

Carrier JM: Mexican male bisexuality. J Homosex 11(1/2):75–86, 1985

Cass VC: Homosexual identity formation: a theoretical model. J Homosex 4:219–235, 1979

Cass VC: Homosexual identity: a concept in need of definition. J Homosex 9:105–126, 1983/1984

Cass VC: The implications of homosexual identity formation for the Kinsey model and scale of sexual preference, in Homosexuality/Heterosexuality: Concepts of Sexual Orientation. Edited by McWhirter DP, Sanders SA, Reinisch JM. New York, Oxford University Press, 1990, pp 239–266

Coleman E: Bisexual and gay men in heterosexual marriage: conflicts and resolutions in therapy. J Homosex 7:93–104, 1981/1982a

Coleman E: Developmental stages of the coming out process. J Homosex 7:31–44, 1981/1982b

Coleman E: Bisexual women in marriages. J Homosex 11:87–100, 1985a

Coleman E: Integration of male bisexuality and marriage. J Homosex 11:189–208, 1985b

Coleman E: Assessment of sexual orientation. J Homosex 14:9–24, 1987

Davenport W: Sexual patterns and their regulation in a society of the Southwest Pacific, in Sex and Behavior. Edited by Beach FA. New York, Wiley, 1965, pp 164–207

Dixon D: Perceived sexual satisfaction and marital happiness of bisexual and heterosexual swinging husbands. J Homosex 11:209–222, 1985

Dixon JK: Sexuality and relationship changes in married females following the commencement of bisexual activity. J Homosex 11:115–134, 1985

Doll L, Peterson J, Magana JR, et al: Male bisexuality and AIDS in the United States, in Bisexuality and HIV/AIDS: A Global Perspective. Edited by Tielman RAP, Carballo M, Hendriks AC. Buffalo, NY, Prometheus Books, 1991, pp 27–40

Doll L, Petersen LR, White CR, et al: The Blood Donor Study Group: homosexually and nonhomosexually identified men who have sex with men: a behavioral comparison. J Sex Res 29:1–14, 1992

Ellis H: Studies in the Psychology of Sex (1905). New York, Random House, 1960

Fast J, Wells H: Bisexual Living. New York, Pocket Books, 1975

Ford CS, Beach FA: Patterns of Sexual Behavior. New York, Harper and Row, 1951

Fox RC: Bisexual identities, in Lesbian, Gay, and Bisexual Identities over the Lifespan: Psychological Perspectives. Edited by D'Augelli AR, Patterson CJ. New York, Oxford University Press, 1995a, pp 48–86

Fox RC: Coming Out Bisexual: Identity, Behavior, and Sexual Orientation Self-disclosure. (Doctoral dissertation, California Institute of Integral Studies, 1993). Dissertation Abstracts International 55(12): 5565B, 1995b

Freud S: An autobiographical study (1925), in Standard Edition of the Complete Psychological Works of Sigmund Freud, Vol 20. Translated and edited by Strachey J. London, Hogarth Press, 1959, pp 1–74

Freud S: Three Essays on the Theory of Sexuality (1905). New York, Basic Books, 1960

Freud S: Analysis terminable and interminable (1937), in Therapy and Technique. Edited by Rieff P. New York, Collier, 1963, pp 233–272

Galland VR: Bisexual Women. (Doctoral dissertation, California School of Professional Psychology, San Francisco, 1975). Dissertation Abstracts International 36(6):3037B, 1975

Geller T: Bisexuality: A Reader and Sourcebook. Ojai, CA, Times Change Press, 1990

George S: Women and Bisexuality. London, Scarlet Press, 1993

Gochros JS: When Husbands Come Out of the Closet. New York, Harrington Park Press, 1989

Golden C: Diversity and variability in women's sexual identities, in Lesbian Psychologies: Explorations and Challenges. Edited by The Boston Lesbian Psychologies Collective. Urbana, IL, University of Illinois Press, 1987, pp 18–34

Golden C: Our politics and choices: the feminist movement and sexual orientation, in Lesbian and Gay Psychology: Theory, Research, and Clinical Applications. Edited by Greene B, Herek GM. Thousand Oaks, CA, Sage, 1994, pp 54–70

Greenberg DF: The Construction of Homosexuality. Chicago, IL, University of Chicago Press, 1988

Harris DAI: Social-Psychological Characteristics of Ambisexuals. (Doctoral dissertation, University of Tennessee, 1977). Dissertation Abstracts International 39(2):574A, 1977

Harwell JL: Bisexuality: Persistent Lifestyle or Transitional State? (Doctoral dissertation, United States International University, 1976). Dissertation Abstracts International 37(4):2449A, 1976

Hatterer LJ: Changing Homosexuality in the Male: Treatment for Men Troubled by Homosexuality. New York, Dell Publishing, 1970

Hays D, Samuels A: Heterosexual women's perceptions of their marriages to bisexual or homosexual men. J Homosex 18:81–100, 1989

Herdt GH: A comment on cultural attributes and fluidity of bisexuality. J Homosex 10:53–62, 1984

Herdt GH: Developmental discontinuities and sexual orientation across cultures, in Homosexuality/Heterosexuality: Concepts of Sexual Orientation. Edited by McWhirter DP, Sanders SA, Reinisch JM. New York, Oxford University Press, 1990, pp 208–236

Hill I: The Bisexual Spouse: Different Dimensions in Human Sexuality. New York, Harper & Row, 1987

Hite S: The Hite Report: A Nationwide Study of Female Sexuality. New York, Dell, 1976

Hite S: The Hite Report on Male Sexuality. New York, Ballantine, 1981

Humphreys L: Tearoom Trade: Impersonal Sex in Public Places. Chicago, IL, Aldine, 1970

Hunt M: Sexual Behavior in the 1970s. New York, Dell, 1974

Hutchins L, Kaahumanu L (eds): Bi Any Other Name: Bisexual People Speak Out. Boston, MA, Alyson, 1991

Imielinski K: Homosexuality in males with particular reference to marriage. Psychother Psychosom 17:126–132, 1969

Jay K, Young A: The Gay Report: Lesbians and Gay Men Speak Out About Sexual Experiences and Lifestyles. New York, Summit Books, 1979

Khan M, Masud R: Ego orgasm and bisexual love. International Review of Psychoanalysis 1:143–149, 1974

Kinsey AC, Pomeroy WB, Martin CE: Sexual Behavior in the Human Male. Philadelphia, PA, WB Saunders, 1948

Kinsey AC, Pomeroy WB, Martin CE, et al: Sexual Behavior in the Human Female. New York, Pocket Books, 1952

Klein F: The Bisexual Option: A Concept of One Hundred Percent Intimacy. New York, Arbor House, 1978

Klein F, Sepekoff B, Wolf TJ: Sexual orientation: a multi-variable dynamic process. J Homosex 11:35–50, 1985

Kohn B, Matusow A: Barry and Alice: Portrait of a Bisexual Marriage. Englewood Cliffs, NJ, Prentice-Hall, 1980

Kooden HD, Morin SF, Riddle DI, et al: Removing the Stigma: Final Report of the Board of Social and Ethical Responsibility for Psychology's Task Force on the Status of Lesbian and Gay Male Psychologists. Washington, DC, American Psychological Association, 1979

Krafft-Ebing R: Psychopathia Sexualis: A Medico-forensic Study (1886). New York, GP Putnam, 1965

Kubie LS: The drive to become both sexes. Psychoanal Q 43:349–426, 1974

Latham JD, White GD: Coping with homosexual expression within heterosexual marriages: five case studies. J Sex Marital Ther 4:198–212, 1978

LaTorre RA, Wendenberg K: Psychological characteristics of bisexual, heterosexual, and homosexual women. J Homosex 9:87–97, 1983

Limentani A: Object choice and actual bisexuality. Int J Psychoanal Psychother 5:205–218, 1976

Little DR: Contemporary Female Bisexuality: A Psychological Phenomenon (Doctoral dissertation, The Union for Experimenting Colleges and Universities, 1989). Dissertation Abstracts International 50(11):5379B, 1989

Lourea D: Psycho-social issues related to counseling bisexuals. J Homosex 11:51–62, 1985

MacDonald AP Jr: A little bit of lavender goes a long way: a critique of research on sexual orientation. J Sex Res 19:94–100, 1983

Maddox B: Married and Gay: An Intimate Look at a Different Relationship. New York, Harcourt Brace Jovanovich, 1982

Markus EB: An Examination of Psychological Adjustment and Sexual Preference in the Female. (Doctoral dissertation, University of Missouri, Kansas City, 1980). Dissertation Abstracts International 41(10):4338A, 1981

Masters WH, Johnson VE: Homosexuality in Perspective. Boston, MA, Little, Brown, 1979

Matteson DR: Bisexual men in marriage: is a positive homosexual identity and stable marriage possible? J Homosex 11:149–172, 1985

Matteson DR: Counseling bisexual men, in The Handbook of Counseling and Psychotherapy with Men. Edited by Scher M, Stevens M, Good G, et al. Beverly Hills, CA, Sage, 1987, pp 232–249

Mead M: Bisexuality: what's it all about? Redbook:January 6–7, 1975

Miller B: Gay fathers and their children. Family Coord 28:544–552, 1979

Mishaan C: The bisexual scene in New York City. J Homosex 11:223–226, 1985

Morse CR: Exploring the Bisexual Alternative: A View from Another Closet (Master's thesis, University of Arizona). Master's Abstracts 28(2):320, 1989

Nahas R, Turley M: The New Couple: Women and Gay Men. New York, Seaview Books, 1979

Nichols M: Bisexuality in women: myths, realities, and implications for therapy, in Women and Sex Therapy: Closing the Circle. Edited by Cole E, Rothblum E. New York, Harrington Park Press, 1988, pp 235–252

Nichols M: Sex therapy with lesbians, gay men, and bisexuals, in Principles and Practice of Sex Therapy: Update for the 1990s, 2nd Edition. Edited by Leiblum SR, Rosen RC. New York, Guilford, 1989, pp 269–297

Norris S, Read E: Out in the Open: People Talking About Being Gay or Bisexual. London, Pan Books, 1985

Nurius PS: Mental health implications of sexual orientation. J Sex Res 19:119–136, 1983

Ochs R (ed): Bisexual Resource Guide. Cambridge, MA, Bisexual Resource Center, 1995

Ochs R, Deihl M: Moving beyond binary thinking, in Homophobia: How We All Pay the Price. Edited by Blumenfeld W, 1995, pp 67–75

Off Pink Collective: Bisexual Lives. London, Off Pink Publishing, 1988

Paul JP: The bisexual identity: an idea without social recognition. J Homosex 9:45–64, 1983/1984

Paul JP: Bisexuality: reassessing our paradigms of sexuality. J Homosex 11:21–34, 1985

Playboy Readers' Sex Survey (part three). Playboy Magazine, May 1983, pp 126–128, 136, 210–220

Ponse B: Identities in the Lesbian World: The Social Construction of Self. Westport, CT, Greenwood Press, 1978

Rado S: A critical examination of the concept of bisexuality. Psychosom Med II(4):459–467, 1940

Rado S: An adaptational view of sexual behavior. American Psychopathological Association Proceedings 38:159–189, 1949

Read KE: Other Voices: The Style of a Male Homosexual Tavern. Novato, CA, Chandler and Sharp, 1980

Reinhardt RU: Bisexual Women in Heterosexual Relationships: A Study of Psychological and Sociological Patterns. (Doctoral dissertation, The Professional School of Psychological Studies, 1985). Research Abstracts International 11(3):67, 1985

Reinisch JM, Ziemba-Davis M, Sanders SA: Sexual behavior and AIDS: lessons from art and sex research, in AIDS and Sex: An Integrated Biomedical and Biobehavioral Approach. Edited by Voeller B, Reinisch JM, Gottlieb M. New York, Oxford University Press, 1990

Reiss AJ: The social integration of queers and peers. Soc Probl 9:102–120, 1961

Ritvo LB: Darwin's Influence on Freud: A Tale of Two Sciences. New Haven, CT, Yale University Press, 1990

Ross HL: Modes of adjustment of married homosexuals. Soc Probl 18:385–393, 1971

Ross MW: The Married Homosexual Man: A Psychological Study. London, Routledge and Kegan Paul, 1983

Ross MW: A taxonomy of global behavior, in Bisexuality and HIV/AIDS: A Global Perspective. Edited by Tielman RAP, Carballo M, Hendriks AC. Buffalo, NY, Prometheus Books, 1991, pp 21–26

Ross MW, Paul JP: Beyond gender: the basis of sexual attraction in bisexual men and women. Psychol Rep 71:1283–1290, 1992

Rubenstein M: An in-depth study of bisexuality and its relationship to self-esteem. Unpublished doctoral dissertation, The Institute for Advanced Study of Human Sexuality, San Francisco, CA, 1982

Rubenstein M, Slater CA: A profile of the San Francisco Bisexual Center. J Homosex 11:227–230, 1985

Rust PC: The politics of sexual identity: sexual attraction and behavior among lesbian and bisexual women. Soc Probl 39:366–386, 1992

Rust PC: "Coming out" in the age of social constructionism: sexual identity formation among lesbian and bisexual women. Gender and Society 7(1):50–77, 1993

Saghir MT, Robins E: Male and Female Homosexuality: A Comprehensive Investigation. Baltimore, MD, Williams & Wilkins, 1973

Schafer S: Sexual and social problems of lesbians. J Sex Res 12:50–79, 1976

Schuster R: Sexuality as a continuum: the bisexual identity, in Lesbian Psychologies: Explorations and Challenges. Edited by The Boston Lesbian Psychologies Collective. Urbana, IL, University of Illinois Press, 1987, pp 56–71

Shively M, DeCecco J: Components of sexual identity. J Homosex 3:41–48, 1977

Shively MG, Jones C, DeCecco JP: Research on sexual orientation: definitions and methods. J Homosex 9:127–136, 1983/1984

Socarides CW: Homosexuality. New York, Jason Aronson, 1978

Spada J: The Spada Report: The Newest Survey of Gay Male Sexuality. New York, New American Library, 1979

Stekel W: Bi-sexual Love (1922). New York, Emerson Books, 1946

Stokes JP, McKirnan DJ, Burzette RG: Sexual behavior, condom use, disclosure of sexuality, and stability of sexual orientation in bisexual men. J Sex Res 30:203–213, 1993

Stoller RJ: The 'bedrock' of masculinity and femininity: bisexuality. Arch Gen Psychiatry 26:207–212, 1972

Storms MD: Theories of sexual orientation. J Pers Soc Psychol 38:783–792, 1980

Sulloway FJ: Freud, Biologist of the Mind: Beyond the Psychoanalytic Legend. New York, Basic Books, 1979

Tielman RAP, Carballo M, Hendriks AC (eds): Bisexuality and HIV/AIDS: A Global Perspective. Buffalo, NY, Prometheus Books, 1991

Troiden RR: Gay and Lesbian Identity: A Sociological Analysis. Dix Hills, NY, General Hall, 1988

Tucker N (ed): Bisexual Politics: Theories, Queeries and Visions. New York, Haworth, 1995

Twining A: Bisexual Women: Identity in Adult Development. (Doctoral dissertation, Boston University School of Education, 1983). Dissertation Abstracts International 44(5):1340A, 1983

Warren CAB: Identity and Community in the Gay World. New York, Wiley, 1974

Weinberg MS, Williams CJ: Male Homosexuals: Their Problems and Adaptations. New York, Oxford University Press, 1974

Weinberg MS, Williams CJ, Pryor DW: Dual Attraction: Understanding Bisexuality. New York, Oxford University Press, 1994

Weininger O: Sex and Character. London, W Heinemann, 1908

Weise ER (ed): Closer to Home: Bisexuality and Feminism. Seattle, WA, Seal Press, 1992

Whitney C: Uncommon Lives: Gay Men and Straight Women. New York, Plume Books, 1990

Wolf DG: The Lesbian Community. Berkeley, CA, University of California Press, 1979

Wolf TJ: Marriages of bisexual men. J Homosex 11:135–148, 1985

Wolf TJ: Group counseling for bisexual men. Journal for Specialists in Group Work 11:162–165, 1987

Wolf TJ: Bisexuality: a counseling perspective, in Counseling Gay Men and Lesbians: Journey to the End of the Rainbow. Edited by Dworkin SH, Gutierrez FJ. Alexandria, VA, American Association for Counseling and Development, 1992, pp 175–187
Wolff C: Love Between Women. New York, St. Martin's Press, 1971
Wolff C: Bisexuality: A Study. London, Quartet Books, 1979
Wooden W, Parker J: Men Behind Bars: Sexual Exploitation in Prison. New York, Plenum Press, 1982
Zinik GA: The Relationship Between Sexual Orientation and Eroticism, Cognitive Flexibility, and Negative Affect. (Doctoral dissertation, University of California, Santa Barbara, 1983). Dissertation Abstracts International 45(8):2707B, 1984

Psychoanalytic Subjectivity and Male Homosexuality

Jack Drescher, M.D.

Psychoanalytic attitudes toward male homosexuality have changed over the last hundred years. Early analysts were part of a culture of scientific enlightenment, seeing homosexuals as victims of unconscious forces beyond their control who should not be persecuted (or prosecuted). The psychoanalyst Sandor Ferenczi persuaded the police of Budapest to stop arresting a female transvestite on grounds that she suffered from a mental disorder (Stanton 1991). Freud believed homosexuals should not be excluded from analytic training and signed a public appeal to decriminalize homosexuality in Austria and Germany (Lewes 1988).

This tolerant psychoanalytic attitude was later replaced by one that sought to pathologize all expressions of same-sex relationships. Mitchell (1981) criticizes those analysts who have

> a proverbial axe to grind in relationship to homosexuality, viewing it as something out of the ordinary, posing unique technical problems and requiring a departure from the traditional analytic pro-

cess. This misleading impression is partly responsible for the extremely negative attitude toward psychoanalysis found in many sectors of the gay community. (p. 63)

The exclusion of lesbian and gay candidates from analytic training until contemporary times reinforced this impression (Drescher 1995). Despite recent changes in discriminatory policies, there remains a reluctance within psychoanalytic institutions to openly discuss how discriminatory policies evolved and are rationalized. Although psychoanalysis preceded the culture in its acceptance of homosexuality, it subsequently came to oppose the larger culture's growing acceptance of homosexuality. The work within psychoanalysis of Marmor (1980), Mitchell (1981), Friedman (1988), Lewes (1988), Isay (1989), and Schafer (1995) reversed that trend. The views of these authors parallel an increased tolerance and acceptance of homosexuality in the larger culture.

Psychoanalytic theories dominated academic psychiatry for many years and had an impact unmatched by any other specialization within psychiatry. Psychoanalytic ideas found their way into literature, theater, film, and other artistic forms. The general public may never have read Freud, but they have heard of the Oedipus complex and the theory that male homosexuality is caused by a certain kind of parenting. No discussion of homosexuality can ignore the history of the influence psychoanalysts exerted on the subject and the impact of their theories on the larger culture.

In this chapter, the author reviews some of the history of psychoanalytic thinking about male homosexuality. The subject of female homosexuality is covered elsewhere (see Chapter 12 by Magee and Miller in this volume). Questions about human sexuality are inseparable from the time and culture in which they are posed. Psychoanalytic theorists in recent years have become increasingly curious about how the theories of the analyst and patient generate subjective narratives that affect clinical outcomes. Observer bias is a problem that has an affect on all of the scientific disciplines. It is difficult, if not impossible, to shield psychoanalytic inquiry from this phenomenon. The result has been a variety of psychoanalytic attitudes toward homosexuality (Drescher, in press) that often take the form of a political or moral debate rather than a scientific discussion. This debate is inseparable from how the culture itself contends with the issue of homosexuality.

Freud

Freud (1905/1953) did not see homosexuality as a special problem, and his ideas on this subject were an integral part of his broader theory of human psychology: "Psychoanalytic research is most decidedly opposed to any attempt at separating off homosexuals from the rest of mankind as a group of special character . . . it has found that all human beings are capable of making a homosexual object-choice and have in fact made one in their unconscious" (p. 145). His first (topographical) theory of the mind, presented in "The Interpretation of Dreams" (1900/1953), argued that sexual instincts and the resistances to them not only caused hysterical symptoms (Breuer and Freud 1895/1955) but were also responsible for normal dreams. In "Three Essays on the Theory of Sexuality" (1905/1953), Freud expanded the domain of psychoanalysis when he linked hysteria and dreams to a range of sexual perversions. The latter were defined as sexual aims other than heterosexual genital intercourse. Freud (1905/1953) defined libido as "'a sexual instinct,' on the analogy of the instinct of nutrition, that is of hunger" (p. 135). Hysterical symptoms and dreams were compromises between perverse instincts and repressive psychic forces attempting to keep instincts out of consciousness. An absence of intrapsychic conflict in persons with perversions permitted their instincts to be openly expressed in their behavior. Freud concluded, with mathematical elegance, that "neuroses are . . . the negative of perversions" (1905/1953, p. 165). Freud's subsequent structural model of the mind attributed repressive abilities to the ego. The hypothesized absence of intrapsychic conflict in persons with perversions led later psychoanalytic theorists to presume that homosexuals, like borderline and psychotic patients, lacked the ego strengths necessary for analytic treatment and training.

Freud (1905/1953) argued both for and against innate factors causing homosexuality. Though he favored psychological explanations, he admitted that "We are therefore forced to a suspicion that the choice between 'innate' and 'acquired' is not an exclusive one or that it does not cover all the issues involved in inversion" (p. 140) and "It may be questioned whether the various accidental influences would be sufficient to explain the acquisition of inversion without the cooperation of something in the subject himself. As we have already shown, the existence of this last factor is not to be denied" (p. 141).

Freud believed in constitutional bisexuality. Referring to neuroanatomical models of his time, he said "a certain degree of anatomical hermaphroditism occurs normally" (p. 141), but he then rejected the metaphor stating that "inversion and somatic hermaphroditism are on the whole independent of each other" (p. 142). Bisexuality rested on the assumption that sexual object and aim are separable: libido is equally capable of attaching (cathecting) itself to members of the same sex as it is to those of the opposite sex. Homosexuality offered Freud a compelling way to make a case for instinct theory.

Freud described developmental or psychosexual stages of libidinal expression that culminated in the oedipal conflict. The oral phase included pleasurable activities such as eating and thumb-sucking. As development continued, libido tended toward gratification in the anal area via expulsion and withholding of feces or physical stimulation of the anus. Next, libidinal gratification was achieved through the genitals. Adult sexuality was defined as genital-genital intercourse. Because this was not anatomically possible in same-sex relations, Freud placed homosexuality below heterosexuality in his developmental hierarchy. Libidinal gratifications (pleasures) obtained orally or anally were more "primitive" or "less developed" than genital ones. As a result, homosexuality was believed to be caused by either libidinal arrest (a person had failed to reach the final psychosexual stage of genitality because of some blockage) or regression (the person had reached the genital stage but because of trauma had reverted to an earlier stage). Genital sexuality had to ultimately lead to the Oedipus complex, the sine qua non of Freud's psychoanalysis.

In the developing male child, both parents were potential sources of libidinal gratification. The child had the potential for identifying with either parent and taking the other parent as an object. More commonly, the boy was attracted to his mother and experienced his father as a competitor. Attraction to the father and competition with the mother constituted the negative Oedipus complex. The positive resolution of the Oedipus complex required that the boy abandon his desires for his mother and his competition with his father. Detachment of libido from mother was aided by castration anxiety fueled by a growing awareness that not everyone has a penis. The boy had to renounce the triangulated relationship with his parents and pursue his own life with a suitable heterosexual partner of his own. Detaching his libidinal cathexes led to identifications. As Freud (1924/1961) stated, "The authority of the father or the parents is introjected into the ego, and there it forms the nucleus of the super-ego, which takes over the severity of the father and perpetuates his prohibition against incest, and so secures the ego from the return of the libidinal object-cathexis" (pp. 176–177). Completion of this identification led to latency. Influenced by Darwin, Freud (1905/1953) believed a boy had to go through all psychosexual stages to become a reproductive, heterosexual adult:

> The final outcome of the sexual development lies in what is known as the normal sexual life of the adult, in which the pursuit of pleasure comes under the sway of the reproductive function and in which the component instincts, under the primacy of a single erotogenic zone, form a firm organization directed towards a sexual aim attached to some extraneous sexual object. (p. 197)

Because Freud wrote no major paper that confined itself to the subject of male homosexuality, one must sift through many works to come up with his composite view of the subject. Lewes (1988) did such an exhaustive study. He suggests that Freud had four theories of male homosexuality; two are presented here.

According to the first theory, the young boy had a normal erotic bond to his mother, but she was too involved with him. This close relationship was overstimulating to the child's psychosexual development. It led to an excess of libidinal investment in his genitals that caused him to overvalue his own penis. Because he assumed that his mother also had a penis, he became fearful of losing his own penis when he learned she did not. The thought of a penisless mother evoked his castration anxiety. This caused the severing of the erotic tie with his mother, and he sought a compromise in his sexual object: a boy with a feminine appearance. Thus, the homosexual man tries to find the mother with a penis he once believed she possessed to reduce his castration anxiety.

The second theory presumed the absence or unavailability of the boy's father. A concurrent overly close mother-son relationship overstimulated the boy, leading to an overvaluing of his penis. In this case, there was no rupture of the erotic tie due to castration anxiety. Because of maternal overinvolvement, he refused to give up his erotic tie to her, as one would expect of a heterosexual child. The heterosexual child, in giving up the tie with mother, identified with father and sought an object like mother. To preserve his relationship with mother, the future homosexual boy unconsciously identified with her and selected sexual objects that resembled himself. This was Freud's (1910/1957) explanation of da Vinci's homosexuality. Thus, Freud (1914/1957) linked homosexuality to narcissism:

> We have discovered, especially clearly in people whose libidinal development has suffered some disturbance, such as perverts and homosexuals, that in their later choice of love-objects they have taken as a model not their mother but their own selves. They are plainly seeking *themselves* as a love-object, and are exhibiting a type of object-choice which must be termed "narcissistic." (p. 88; Freud's italics)

Freud did not consider overt homosexuality an illness. Because it did not involve intrapsychic conflict or symptom formation, he was pessimistic about a cure. In 1936, he wrote a "Letter to an American Mother" who was seeking treatment for her homosexual son:

> Homosexuality is assuredly no advantage, but it is nothing to be ashamed of, no vice, no degradation; it cannot be classified as an illness; we consider it to be a variation of the sexual function, produced by a certain arrest of sexual development. . . . By asking me if I can help, you mean, I suppose, if I can abolish homosexuality and make normal heterosexuality take its place. The answer is, in a general way, we cannot promise to achieve it. In a certain number of cases we succeed in developing the blighted germs of heterosexual tendencies which are present in every homosexual, in the majority of cases it is no more possible. (E. Freud 1960, pp. 423–424)

Freud's attitudes about homosexuality sometimes seem contradictory. In "'Civilized' Sexual Morality and Modern Nervous Illness" (1908/1959), he anticipates future writings on homophobia: "It is one of the obvious social injustices that the standard of civilization should demand from everyone the same conduct of sexual life—conduct which can be followed without any difficulty by some people, thanks to their organization, but which imposes the heaviest psychical sacrifices on others" (p. 192). These views coexist with others that seem more intolerant:

> Since normal intercourse has been so relentlessly persecuted by morality—and also, on account of the possibilities of infection, by hygiene—what are known as the perverse forms of intercourse between the two sexes, in which other parts of the body take over the role of the genitals, have undoubtedly increased in social impor-

tance. These activities cannot, however, be regarded as being as harmless as analogous extensions [of the sexual aim] in love relationships. They are ethically objectionable, for they degrade the relationships of love between two human beings from a serious matter to a convenient game, attended by no risk and no spiritual participation. (p. 200)

Freud was both ahead of his time and a product of his times. He believed one had to construct a sexual (and gender) identity but also believed evolutionary and social forces favored heterosexual constructions:

Psycho-analysis considers that a choice of an object independently of its sex—freedom to range equally over male and female objects—as it is found in childhood, in primitive states of society and early periods of history, is the original basis from which, as a result of restriction in one direction or the other, both the normal and the inverted types develop. Thus from the point of view of psychoanalysis the exclusive sexual interest felt by men for women is also a problem that needs elucidating and is not a self-evident fact based upon an attraction that is ultimately of a chemical nature. (Freud 1905/1953, pp. 145–146)

Rado

Sandor Rado had an important influence on psychoanalytic theories about homosexuality. Like Freud, he did not address homosexuality as a special problem, and his thoughts on that subject were part of a larger theoretical model. Writing and teaching in the 1940s, he took issue with many aspects of Freudian theory. He criticized classical metapsychology for relying too heavily on unprovable inferences. He proposed concepts he believed were closer to observable clinical data and drew heavily on physiological and evolutionary models of his time. He saw an individual's psychodynamics as a reaction to cultural experiences to which he or she had to adapt. Given the complexity of the human mind, one could make compromises that were psychologically adaptive in one context and inappropriate in another. Rado's (1969) view of psychological dysfunction could be captured in the statement, "Man is the only animal that does not learn from experience; he rationalizes away his mistakes" (p. 52).

Rado refuted Freud's models of drives and bisexuality. His hypotheses about homosexuality were consistent with his adaptive, reproductive evolutionary model:

> The male-female sexual pattern is dictated by anatomy. . . . [B]y means of the institution of marriage, the male-female sexual pattern is culturally ingrained and perpetuated in every individual from earliest childhood. . . . [Homosexual] pairs satisfy their repudiated yet irresistible male-female desire by means of shared illusions and actual approximations; such is the hold on the individual of a cultural institution based on biological foundations. . . . Why is the so-called homosexual forced to escape from the male-female pair into a homogeneous pair? . . . [T]he familiar campaign of deterrence that parents wage to prohibit the sexual activity of the child . . . causes the male to see in the mutilated female organ a reminder of inescapable punishment. When . . . fear and resentment of the opposite organ becomes insurmountable, the individual may escape into homosexuality. The male patterns are reassured by the presence in both of them of the male organ. Homosexuality is a deficient adaptation evolved by the organism in response to its own emergency overreaction and dyscontrol." (pp. 212–213)

Later Psychoanalytic Theories

Unlike Freud and Rado, several psychoanalytic authors completed special studies of homosexuality. This section reviews two approaches that view homosexuality as pathological and two that view it as a normal sexual variant. The latter view has represented a distinct minority opinion within the written opus of psychoanalysis, while the former view has been extensively held. It is beyond the scope of this chapter to review all psychoanalytic theories about male homosexuality, but interested readers should consult *The Psychoanalytic Theory of Male Homosexuality* (Lewes 1988).

Bieber et al. (1962) applied controlled studies to psychoanalytic research. One hundred and six homosexual men and 100 male heterosexual control subjects, all in psychoanalytic treatment, were compared to identify family patterns responsible for homosexuality. The authors concluded that their research confirmed Rado's theory of homosexuality: a particular family constellation caused homosexuality, and constitutional factors were unimportant; therefore, parental psychopathology was the cause of homosexuality. According to Bieber et al. (1962), the fathers of homosexuals had abandoned their sons to mothers who were only interested in satisfying their own needs:

> The majority of H-parents [of homosexual patients] in our study had poor marital relationships. Almost half the H-mothers were dominant wives who minimized their husbands. The large majority of H-mothers had a close-binding intimate relationship with the H-son. In most cases, this son had been his mother's favorite. . . . Most H-mothers were explicitly seductive, and even where they were not, the closeness of the bond with the son appeared to be in itself sexually provocative. In about two-thirds of the cases, the mother openly preferred her H-son to her husband, and allied with son against the husband. In about half the cases, the patient was the mother's confidant. (p. 313)

Socarides (1968) contested Freud's view that homosexuality is a developmental arrest and redefined it as conflictual, or an "illness" in the psychoanalytic sense. According to Socarides, the instinct has

> undergone excessive transformation and disguise in order to be gratified in the perverse act. The perverted action, like the neurotic symptom, results from the conflict between the ego and the id and represents a compromise formation which at the same time must be acceptable to the demands of the superego . . . the instinctual gratification takes place in disguised form while its real content remains unconscious. (pp. 35–36)

This conflict model is used to dispute Freud's pessimism about treatment, suggesting instead that therapeutic interventions intended to bring unconscious conflicts into awareness to reduce symptoms should be the basis for a psychoanalytic approach to treatment of homosexuality.

Socarides linked his work to Mahler's (1975) developmental model of separation and individuation. He saw homosexuality as a "resolution of the separation from the mother by running away from all women" (1968, p. 60). This preoedipal staging places homosexuality at a level of development between the borderline and psychotic and links it with severe psychopathology. Like Rado and Bieber, Socarides holds the family environment responsible for the boy's inability to achieve hetero-sexuality: "The family of the homosexual is usually a female-dominated environment wherein the father was absent, weak, detached or sadistic. This furthers feminine identification. The father's inaccessibility to the boy contributed to the difficulty in making a masculine identification" (1968, p. 38).

Friedman (1988) focused on constitutional factors promoting homosexuality. His approach, but not his conclusions, is reminiscent of Rado in its attempt to link psychoanalytic theory to contemporary re-search outside psychoanalysis, in this case, to psychoneuroendocrinol-ogy. Friedman believed that some types of homosexuality are caused prenatally, rather than preoedipally. For example, he asserted that de-ficient androgen exposure in the womb causes a subsequent distur-bance in the development of a masculine gender identity in some young boys. Homosexuality results from this "feminine or unmasculine self-concept" independent of family constellations. Friedman (1988) stated that "A strong case can be made for the hypothesis that a femi-nine or unmasculine self-concept during childhood is not only associ-ated with the emergence of predominant or exclusive homosexuality in men, it is the single most important causal influence" (p. 74).

Friedman thought of homosexuality along several dimensions. He used the Kinsey scale (Kinsey et al. 1948), which defines a continuum of homosexual experience spanning exclusive heterosexuality (Kinsey score = 0) to exclusive homosexuality (Kinsey score = 6), to make a case for a variety of homosexualities based on their origins: "[a] direct biological disposition toward homosexuality, indirect biological effects, and predominately psychodynamic influences" (p. 25). Using Kern-berg's (1975) theory of character structure, Friedman saw the level of personality organization as independent from sexual orientation (or psychostructural level). Therefore, he refuted both Freud and So-carides, claiming that he found homosexuality at the highest (neurotic) level of character organization.

Isay (1989) saw homosexuality as a nonpathological variant of hu-man sexuality. He attributed its causes to unelaborated constitutional factors and described the dilemma of a normative homosexual adap-tation in a heterosexual world. He believed that psychoanalytic theories labeling homosexuality as pathological reflected social biases. He rein-terpreted earlier psychoanalytic findings. Rejecting the assumption that distant fathers caused homosexuality in their sons, he wrote, "Gay men distance themselves from their fathers in their memory in order to avoid recognition of [their] erotic attachment and of their sexual arousal in early childhood" (p. 33). He went on to explain: "Some of the fathers of homosexual boys either consciously or unconsciously recognize that their sons have both a special need for closeness and an erotic attachment to them. These fathers may withdraw because of anxiety occasioned by their own homoerotic desires, which are usually unknown to them" (p. 34). Isay saw attempts to change homosexuals into heterosexuals as harmful to patients, leading to depression, anxiety, and loss of self-esteem. Isay (1991) has the historical distinction of being the first psychoanalyst to write about these issues as an openly gay man.

Discussion

The theoretical controversy regarding homosexuality exemplifies a larger contemporary psychoanalytic debate about the nature of the field itself (Eagle 1984; Langs 1993; Schafer 1995; Spezzano 1993; Stern 1991): Is psychoanalysis a science or a hermeneutic discipline? Does it deal with retrievable historical facts, or does it concern itself with the understanding or deciphering of meanings?

Psychoanalytic theories rely on clinical inferences to substantiate their metapsychologies. The fragmentation in the field today reflects the varied ways in which psychoanalytic data may be interpreted. Freud's drive theory competes with ego psychology, Kleinian object relations theory, interpersonal theory, and self-psychology, just to name a few. Each theory makes assumptions about normal development that may contradict the others. Spence (1982) proposed that analysts and patients generate narratives in their work together that are constructions, rather than reconstructions, of historical data. In other words, an analyst and patient generate a story that is meaningful to the two of them rather than discovering an objective history based on recollections of actual events. Analysts influence the outcome of narratives by asking leading questions and by directing their attention to certain patient responses. Patients in turn are adept at learning the clinical theory, attitudes, and technical language of their therapists.

The Bieber et al. study (1962) contained a priori assumptions, consistent with Rado's theory, that it subsequently claimed to confirm. The following are examples of these assumptions:

We have selected the patient-mother-father unit for analysis. . . . We believe that personality for the most part is forged within the triangular system of the nuclear family. It follows then that personality maladaptation must also be primarily rooted here. (pp. 140–141)

We assume that heterosexuality is the biologic norm and that unless interfered with all individuals are heterosexual. (p. 319)

We consider homosexuality to be a pathologic biosocial, psychosexual adaptation consequent to pervasive fears surrounding the expression of heterosexual impulses. In our view, every homosexual is, in reality, a "latent" heterosexual. (p. 220)

American culture vigorously persecuted homosexuality from the 1940s through the 1960s, when the psychoanalytic views of Rado, Bieber, and Socarides prevailed. In those years, patients and analysts usually began treatment with a shared view that homosexuality was a problem requiring treatment. Patient and analyst were both motivated to answer the question of how the family got the patient off the track toward normal heterosexuality. Schafer (1995) noted,

It seems like a straightforward technical principle that in doing character analysis one must render what is ego-syntonic ego-alien, thereby making it possible to analyze pathological character traits. . . . one realizes how much space this technical principle leaves for the analyst's personal values to be imposed on the patient. Here we need think only of the ego-syntonic homosexual orientation in whatever way that is structured in character, and of how so many analysts tried to make these orientations ego-alien or else resignedly thought it was hopeless even to try. (p. 200)

It is no surprise that the Bieber et al. study (1962), grounded in the values of the 1950s, found "the best interparental relationships" where "father dominates but does not minimize mother" (p. 158). Schafer (1995) remarked,

Many moral judgments have been taken for granted as factual statements, while many other moral judgments have been presented as reasoned conclusions based on careful exercises of curiosity in the form of purportedly scientific investigation or, even more simply, uncontroversial reality testing. (p. 189)

Cultural values equally play a role in the analyst's narrative of homosexuality as a normal variant. When social attitudes toward sexuality became more tolerant in the late 1960s through the 1980s, non-pathological theoretical models emerged. In one model, analyst and patient assume that homosexuality is intrinsic to the patient and share a belief in its normality. The origins of homosexuality are attributed to factors beyond the patient's conscious or unconscious control. Even if the analyst and patient believe that homosexuality is constructed, they do not believe it is inferior to a heterosexual orientation. Analyst and patient spare themselves the task of deciding what prevented the patient's heterosexual development. The narrative that emerges flows from the question of how the patient deals with a world that is hostile to homosexuality, or it may explore a patient's difficulties in accepting his own sexuality.

In his study of homosexuality and American psychiatry, Bayer (1981) concluded that "The status of homosexuality is a political question, representing a historically rooted, socially determined choice regarding the ends of human sexuality" (p. 5). Within psychoanalysis, the subject of homosexuality's status resembles a political debate in which two opposing camps refute each other's credibility. Each side frames the debate so that the legitimacy of its own narrative is based on what it believes to be objective scientific neutrality. By the same token, the opponent's narrative is refuted by devaluing the basis for its scientific credibility. Both sides present narratives generated in their clinical practices as scientific validation or "proof" of their theories.

In fact, however, Rado (1969) did not refute Freud's theory of bisexuality on the basis of results of a reproducible experiment. Instead, he denounced the anatomical analogy underlying Freud's theory, a belief in embryonic hermaphroditism, as a relic of unproved 19th-century theories (pp. 215–216). Friedman (1988) argued from a position of contemporary social tolerance. He used sparse scientific evidence to make a stronger case for the biological origins of homosexuality than actually exists in order to convince analysts that they should be more accepting of homosexuality. Socarides (1968) posited that an intrapsychic conflict leads to homosexuality, as opposed to Freud's contention that a perversion is nonconflictual, thus creatively redefining Freud's metapsychological construct. Socarides attempted to buttress his own scientific legitimacy by treating Freud's structural model as if it were a proven scientific fact, the composition of which he had scrupulously studied. Coming from the other side, Isay (1989) claimed that patient memories of distant fathers are distortions. He evoked the perennial issue of true and false memories that has plagued psychoanalysis since its origins. Isay denied the legitimacy of Bieber and Socarides's analytic data-gathering methods and undermined their claims that a truly faulty father-son relationship causes homosexuality.

As in any political debate, the findings of studies can seemingly be applied or disregarded at will. The discussion of Hooker's (1957) landmark study illustrates this point. Hooker gave projective tests to 30 matched pairs of nonpatient homosexual men and male heterosexual control subjects. "Blind" judges scored test results, unaware of their subjects' sexual orientations. The homosexual group showed no evidence of greater psychopathology. Here is an easily reproducible scientific test; however, Bieber et al. (1962) dismissed the study: "Since the tests and adjustment ratings were performed by competent workers and the implications of the findings and conclusions are at marked variance with those of our own and other studies, we suspect that the tests themselves or the current methods of interpretation and evaluation are inadequate to the task of discriminating between homosexuals and heterosexuals" (pp. 305–306). Socarides (1968) did not mention Hooker's study at all. Friedman (1988), on the other side of the issue, called Hooker's study "elegant research" that "indicates that the psychodynamic conflicts of adult homosexual and heterosexual men may be strikingly similar" (p. 235).

The history of psychoanalytic attitudes toward homosexuality reinforces the impression that psychoanalytic theories cannot be divorced from the political, cultural, and personal contexts in which they are formulated. The psychoanalytic method cannot determine whether homosexuality is biological in origin, although it may reveal a few cases where it is not. If and when the scientific evidence from other disciplines does make a legitimate case for homosexuality's biological or genetic origins, it is likely that some patients and analysts will regard homosexuality as a normal genetic variant, whereas other therapists and their patients will treat homosexuality as a genetic disease.

Future psychoanalytic theories about homosexuality may again move away from a tolerant position if society becomes less tolerant of homosexuality. For example, Nicolosi's (1991) recent work illustrates how contemporary religious intolerance of homosexuality can fuse psychoanalytic theories that pathologize homosexuality with pastoral counseling for homosexuals. Psychoanalysts will not be the ones who decide whether the culture will more fully accept its lesbian and gay members. History has shown that analysts can take positions that either facilitate or obstruct tolerance and acceptance. It is important to emphasize that the manner in which psychoanalysts choose to speak, act, and write about these issues is based on their moral and ethical beliefs rather than on the basis of scientific facts.

References

Bayer R: Homosexuality and American Psychiatry: The Politics of Diagnosis. New York, Basic Books, 1981

Bieber I, Dain HJ, Dince PR, et al: Homosexuality: A Psychoanalytic Study. New York, Basic Books, 1962

Breuer J, Freud S: Studies on hysteria (1893–1895), in Standard Edition of the Complete Psychological Works of Sigmund Freud, Vol 2. Translated and edited by Strachey J. London, Hogarth Press, 1955, pp 1–319

Drescher J: Anti-homosexual bias in training, in Disorienting Sexuality. Edited by Domenici T, Lesser R. New York, Routledge, 1995, pp 227–241

Drescher J: Psychoanalytic attitudes toward homosexuality. Gender and Psychoanalysis (in press)

Eagle M: Recent Developments in Psychoanalysis: A Critical Evaluation. Cambridge, MA, Harvard University Press, 1984

Freud E (ed): The Letters of Sigmund Freud. New York, Basic Books, 1960

Freud S: The interpretation of dreams (1900), in Standard Edition of the Complete Psychological Works of Sigmund Freud, Vols 4 and 5. Translated and edited by Strachey J. London, Hogarth Press, 1953, pp 1–751

Freud S: Three essays on the theory of sexuality (1905), in The Standard Edition of the Complete Psychological Works of Sigmund Freud, Vol 7. Translated and edited by Strachey J. London, Hogarth Press, 1953, pp 123–243

Freud S: "Civilized" sexual morality and modern nervous illness (1908), in Standard Edition of the Complete Psychological Works of Sigmund Freud, Vol 9. Translated and edited by Strachey J. London, Hogarth Press, 1959, pp 177–204

Freud S: Leonardo da Vinci and a memory of his childhood (1910), in Standard Edition of the Complete Psychological Works of Sigmund Freud, Vol 11. Translated and edited by Strachey J. London, Hogarth Press, 1957, pp 59–138

Freud S: On narcissism: an introduction (1914), in Standard Edition of the Complete Psychological Works of Sigmund Freud, Vol 14. Translated and edited by Strachey J. London, Hogarth Press, 1957, pp 67–102

Freud S: The dissolution of the Oedipus complex (1924), in Standard Edition of the Complete Psychological Works of Sigmund Freud, Vol 19. Translated and edited by Strachey J. London, Hogarth Press, 1961, pp 173–179

Friedman RC: Male Homosexuality: A Contemporary Psychoanalytic Perspective. New Haven, CT, Yale University Press, 1988

Hooker E: The adjustment of the male overt homosexual. Journal of Projective Techniques 21:18–31, 1957

Isay R: Being Homosexual: Gay Men and Their Development. New York, Farrar, Straus and Giroux, 1989

Isay R: The homosexual analyst: clinical considerations. Psychoanal Study Child 46:199–216, 1991

Kernberg O: Borderline Conditions and Pathological Narcissism. New York, Jason Aronson, 1975

Kinsey AC, Pomeroy WB, Martin CE: Sexual Behavior in the Human Male. Philadelphia, PA, WB Saunders, 1948

Langs R: Psychoanalysis: narrative myth or narrative science? Contemporary Psychoanalysis 29:555–594, 1993

Lewes K: The Psychoanalytic Theory of Male Homosexuality. New York, Simon and Schuster, 1988

Mahler MS, Pine F, Bergman A: The Psychological Birth of the Human Infant. New York, Basic Books, 1975

Marmor J (ed): Homosexual Behavior: A Modern Reappraisal. New York, Basic Books, 1980

Mitchell S: The psychoanalytic treatment of homosexuality: some technical considerations. International Review of Psycho-analysis 8:63–80, 1981

Nicolosi J: Reparative Therapy of Male Homosexuality: A New Clinical Approach. Northvale, NJ, Jason Aronson, 1991

Rado S: Adaptational Psychodynamics: Motivation and Control. New York, Science House, 1969

Schafer R: The evolution of my views on nonnormative sexual practice, in Disorientating Sexuality. Edited by Domenici T, Lesser R. New York, Routledge, 1995, pp 187–202

Socarides C: The Overt Homosexual. New York, Grune and Stratton, 1968

Spence D: Narrative Truth and Historical Truth: Meaning and Interpretation in Psychoanalysis. New York, WW Norton, 1982

Spezzano C: A relational model of inquiry and truth: the place of psychoanalysis in human conversation. Psychoanalytic Dialogues 3: 177–208, 1993

Stanton M: Sandor Ferenczi: Reconsidering Active Intervention. London, Jason Aronson, 1991

Stern D: A philosophy for the embedded analyst: Gadamer's hermeneutics and the social paradigm of psychoanalysis. Contemporary Psychoanalysis 27:51–80, 1991

12

Psychoanalytic Views of Female Homosexuality

Maggie Magee, M.S.W.
Diana C. Miller, M.D.

Several related factors have shaped psychoanalytic theory of female homosexuality: its phallocentric bias; its reliance on polarized dichotomies; its search for distinguishing etiologies, developmental lines, or clinical characteristics in those who desire homosexual relationships; and the exclusion of gay men and lesbian women from analytic training. Psychoanalysis remains largely ignorant about the anxiety particular to lesbian identity, desire, and relationships, namely, the ever-present, never-ending interpersonal and intrapsychic challenge of living in a world in which such desires and relationships are believed to be evidence of sinful character, disturbed or arrested psychological develop-

An earlier version of the chapter appeared as "She Foreswore her Womanhood: Psychoanalytic Views of Female Homosexuality." *Clinical Social Work Journal* 20:67–87, 1992.

ment, socially disruptive behavior, and disordered femininity.

Kenneth Lewes (1988) argued that the history of psychoanalytic concepts about male homosexuality has much in common with the history of psychoanalytic concepts about female sexuality. Homosexual men have been seen as

> deeply flawed and defective because they shared certain psychic characteristics with women. . . . What distinguishes the psychoanalytic theory of femininity from that of homosexuality, however, is the fact that almost from the beginning the former theory was elaborated, challenged, and qualified by . . . women analysts. (p. 237)

Slowly, against considerable resistance and inertia, psychoanalytic assumptions about female psychological development are changing. But troublesome assumptions remain to bedevil the clinical discussion of women in lesbian relationships.

Polarized Categories

Roy Schafer (1974) pointed to the difficulties Freud had working "within a nineteenth-century biological-medical tradition" that emphasized "great natural polarities or dichotomies" (pp. 482–483). Seeing the world as composed of great natural polarities—male and female as "opposite" sexes, homosexuality as the "inversion" of heterosexuality—leads easily to the conclusion that traits or characteristics believed to belong to members of one sexual category (e.g., male or heterosexual) must appear in some opposite form, be found deficient, or be missing altogether in the other sexual category (e.g., female or homosexual).

Freud attempted to address the limitations of this kind of thinking through qualifying statements in "Three Essays on the Theory of Sexuality," through his revisions of this work from 1910 to 1924, and through his writings on female sexual development. In footnotes and disclaimers Freud tries to assure himself and his readers that he is not disparaging women, and to insist that "psycho-analytical research is most decidedly opposed to any attempt at separating off homosexuals from the rest of mankind as a group of special character" (Freud 1905/1953, footnote added 1915, p. 145). But psychoanalytic theory is founded on the assumption that those with same-sex desires or relationships have categorically different (and more damaging) early developmental histories and different, or compromised, psychic functioning than those with other-sexed relationships and desires.

The Search for Early Developmental Disturbance

"What," asked Ernest Jones (1927, p. 460), in one of the earliest analytic papers on female homosexuality, "differentiates the development of homosexual from that of heterosexual women?" As psychoanalytic theory expanded from drive theory through ego psychology and object relations models, various answers to Jones's question emerged. The specific disturbances of early development said to characterize women with homosexual feelings or lesbian relationships have included the following:

◆ A disorder of drive/object caused by penis envy at the oedipal stage, which leads to a repulsion toward heterosexual relations and a regression to a fixation to an earlier object (Fenichel 1945; Freud 1920/1955).

◆ A disordered identification with the father in which identification replaces object relationship (Freud 1920/1955; Jones 1927), or an identification with the father in order to prevent psychotic symbiosis with mother (McDougall 1970).

◆ Failed identifications with mother due to maternal envy (Freud 1920/1955) or maternal narcissism (Siegel 1988) or the masochistic debased life of mother (Romm 1965).

◆ A disturbance of early (mother/child) object relations characterized by masochism (Brierley 1932; Deutsch 1932/1948; Socarides 1978) or failed separation-individuation (Socarides 1968).

◆ A premature genital awareness (Khan 1964); a precocious turn-on of erotic desire which "occurs when the child has been excluded from 'good enough' or 'long enough' primary bliss and seeks inclusion by a sexual bond and sexual wooing" (Eisenbud 1982).

Marmor (1980) and Stoller (1985) took exception to attempts to find a common psychodynamic denominator in female homosexuality. They stressed the multidetermined nature of any psychic phenomenon and pointed to the prejudices embedded in psychological theories about female homosexuality. Their perspectives are not, however, representative of most analytic approaches to the subject of female homosexuality. Two phallocentric assumptions cut across various theoretical orientations and underlie many formulations.

■ Phallocentric Assumption I: A Woman Who Loves a Woman Must Be a Man, or Be Like a Man, or Must Wish to Be a Man

Freud disagreed with beliefs of homosexual activists such as Magnus Hirschfeld that homosexuals were a "third" or "intermediate" sex and that homosexuality was, like left-handedness, constitutional. He particularly disagreed with the view that a male homosexual was "a feminine brain in a male body." Freud wished to distinguish physical sexual characteristics from what he called "mental qualities." A primary motivation seems to have been to rescue homosexual men from being seen as having feminine mental qualities: "It is only in the inverted woman that character-inversion of this kind can be looked for with any regularity. In men the most complete mental masculinity can be combined with inversion" (Freud 1905/1962, p. 142).

In 1920 Freud described the case of "a beautiful and clever girl of 18, . . . [who] had aroused displeasure and concern in her parents by the devoted adoration with which she pursued a certain 'society lady'" (Freud 1920/1955, p. 147). He noted that the girl had "intellectual attributes [which] . . . could be connected with masculinity: . . . acuteness of comprehension and her lucid objectivity" (p. 154). Freud said that to call these qualities "masculine" is merely convention. However, he did not feel it was merely convention to characterize as masculine her behavior toward her loved one: namely, her "humility" and her "sublime overvaluation of the sexual object" (p. 154). In speaking of the girl's bitter disappointment on discovering that not she, but her mother, was to have a baby from the father, he claims "she forswore her womanhood and sought another goal for her libido. . . . She changed into a man and took her mother in place of her father as the object of her love" (pp. 157–158).

Freud's language here illustrates a major phallocentric assumption about female homosexuality: one who loves a woman must be like a man. Although Freud, at this time, found it difficult to see a man who loves a man as sexually or psychically "feminine," he easily attributed "masculinity" to a woman's love for a woman. In summarizing the various factors contributing to this girl's homosexuality, he included the girl's "masculinity complex." As evidence of her masculinity complex he described her as a

> spirited girl, always ready for romping and fighting, she was not at all prepared to be second to her slightly older brother. . . . She was in fact a feminist; she felt it to be unjust that girls should not enjoy the same freedom as boys, and rebelled against the lot of woman in general. (p. 169)

The *masculinity complex*—variously defined as times and theory changed as masculine physical characteristics, masculine mental qualities, masculine identifications, or failed feminine identifications—has haunted analytic views of female homosexuality. In 1932, Helene Deutsch, writing about her experience with 11 cases of female homosexuality, begins by stressing

> the fact that none of these eleven women presented physical signs which might indicate that there had been a constitutional deviation, physiologically, in the direction of masculinity. . . . [T]he patients showed no physical signs of masculinity. (pp. 208–209)

In 1964, Khan, writing about a young woman patient in a sexual relationship with a woman, whom he continues to assure the reader was not a "true pervert," felt he must point out that it

> would be a misrepresentation of the emotional experience of this patient to conclude in this context that she was behaving in a "masculine way," was being a man or that the behavior was unfeminine. That phallic identifications (with the analyst-father-brother) helped her to find her way to this "infantile state of bliss" is true. But the aim was certainly feminine, tender and passive. (p. 251)

To rescue her from the charge of masculinity, Khan asserts that she was properly—that is, *passively*—feminine in her sexual aims.

A major shift in psychoanalytic theory occurred when "masculine identification" changed from being a describer of supposed mental qualities—such as acuteness of comprehension or lucid objectivity—to a manifestation of "disturbed gender identity." Many analytic therapists today who would never think to apply the concept masculinity complex to their women patients unquestioningly believe that female homosexuality is synonymous with a disturbance in gender identity. Joyce McDougall (1989), for instance, discussed "sexual identity formation and its inversions" (p. 206). For McDougall homosexuality was an inversion of gender identity, which occurs because of the different oedipal crisis which she believed besets homosexuals. Although she argued for "a measure of abnormality" in everyone, and pointed out that "it is hardly justifiable to label the sexual deviant according to his or her sexual practice alone" (McDougall 1985, p. 246), McDougall repeatedly attempted to distinguish heterosexual persons from homosexual persons on developmental grounds. In her attempt to explain female homosexuality, McDougall (1985) said that for a homosexual woman,

> the father's penis no longer symbolizes the phallus and she herself embodies the phallic object. Through unconscious identification with the father, and by investing her whole body with the significance of the penis, she is now able in fantasy to fulfill a woman sexually. (p. 133)

McDougall's ideas are reminiscent of Freud's notions that the little girl is a little man who desires her mother, whom she also believes to have a penis. Little girls (and lesbian women) are unconsciously (or originally) male. McDougall placed homosexual persons in an "intermediate" group which she called "third structure people" (1980) or "neosexualities" (1985), neither psychotic nor neurotic and characterized by the overall frailty of their psychic functioning.

From a very different perspective, Kirkpatrick and Morgan (1980) avoided polarized notions of identity or object choice. Following Stoller (1976), they suggested that since core female gender identity may be a more stable formation than male gender identity, sexual object choice may need to be less firmly fixed:

> Intimacy with women on some level may be continuous as a natural part of a woman's emotional life. . . . In women, homosexuality and heterosexuality do not appear to be at opposite ends of a continuum as Kinsey . . . suggested they were. Rather, the two trends might be seen as running a parallel course, capable of intermingling and of changing positions of ascendancy in consciousness and behavior under certain circumstances. (Kirkpatrick and Morgan 1980, p. 360)

■ Phallocentric Assumption II: A Relationship Between Two Women Must Always Be Incomplete Compared to the Fullness Possible in a Heterosexual Relationship; Lesbian Sexuality Is Immature and Lacking

In early psychoanalytic theory of feminine development, the little girl was a little man and the clitoris was a little penis. Libido was masculine because it was an active force. Masturbation was a masculine activity, which normal girls gave up when they discovered the poverty of their sexual equipment. Challenges and revisions to the theory have asserted that female development can rest on something other than disappointment in not being male and that the female body has its own anatomical pleasures.

Increasingly, in both the analytic and more popular literature, sexuality is seen to serve some different functions and have different importance in the psychological lives of men and women (Person 1980).

If female sexuality has been a territory difficult for psychoanalysis to explore, sexuality *between* two women is an even darker continent—one often imagined to be a primitive, underdeveloped region. In much psychoanalytic thinking, sexuality between two women is assumed to reflect preoedipal (mother-child) relationships and to be "caused" by disturbances in those relationships. Emotional regression, often espoused as a goal of heterosexual orgasmic experience, is seen as pathological when it occurs in female same-sex relationships.

Perspectives on sexuality premised on the two sexes being opposite (and thus complementary) assume something must be lacking in the sexual experience of two women. "How is it possible," wondered McDougall (1980, p. 88), "to maintain the illusion of being the true sexual partner to another woman?" To McDougall, who believed that lesbian women unconsciously deny sexual difference, sex without a penis was an illusion. For Elaine Siegel (1988), what lesbian women lack was not the penis, but a mental representation of the vagina. Siegel, like McDougall, believed that a common family dynamic produces homosexuality in women and believed she could distinguish the families of lesbian women from those of other women. For Kleinian Jean-Michel Quinodoz (1989) "manifest" homosexuality in women was unconsciously both a disavowal of envy of the mother and an envious attack on the mother, as well as an unconscious attempt to possess her so she can't have a husband and children (p. 59).

How can one explain these perspectives on female homosexuality? As Marmor (1980) noted about some others describing lesbian patients, many theorists may have

> fallen into the trap of defining the psychopathology in these women in terms of their sexuality instead of seeing them as females who suffer from certain characterologic problems which are reflected in their patterns of sexuality also. Preoedipal characterologic disorders with narcissistic defects . . . are not limited to lesbians. They are seen with considerable frequency among heterosexual females also. (p. 399)

Growing Up In or Out of the Closet

In the authors' psychoanalytic work with a variety of patients, they have not discovered common family histories or common and distinguishing early developmental disturbances. The authors have not found clinical phenomena—such as transference presentations, countertransference dilemmas, and internal conflicts—that are particular to their lesbian patients and that differentiate them from other patients.

The one aspect of development that *is* unique to lesbian women has received little psychoanalytic attention. What are the possible effects on psychic development (ego, drive, superego, self and object identifications) of growing up aware of attraction to and interest in other women while simultaneously trying to banish or hide such feelings? How do lesbian adolescents integrate a feminine sexuality, given devalued definitions and images of female homosexuality? In *Hidden Selves* Khan (1983) suggested a secret is "potential space": "The secret carries the hope that one day the person will be able to emerge out of it, to be found and met, and thus become a whole person, sharing life with others" (p. 105). He also saw the dangers of having to keep aspects of ourselves hidden: "a secret stays out of reach for any sort of further elaboration" (p. 106). For many women, feelings powerful and significant enough for Freud to call them "instinct" must be hidden from themselves and others, unable to be elaborated and organized through engagement with others.

Coming Out

When a woman says to herself and to others that she wants, or has, a primary relationship with another woman, she is faced with the immediate acquisition and management of a new, devalued social and psychological identity. Coming out is, therefore, always accompanied by anxiety and by wishes and impulses both to hide and to reveal. Although gay and lesbian therapists have addressed the psychological dimensions, developmental tasks, and stages of gay or lesbian identity (see Chapter 14 by Cass in this volume; Coleman 1982; de Monteflores 1986; Garnets and Kimmel 1993; Gartrell 1984; Hanley-Hackenbruck 1988; Stein and Cohen 1984), few psychoanalysts (Friedman 1988; Isay 1989; Magee and Miller 1994; Morgenthaler 1988) have discussed this developmental task. Instead, psychoanalysts have seen the revealing of a same-sex desire or relationship as either an impulsive acting-out of internal conflicts or deficits or as a resistance to working out these conflicts or deficits in the transference (Siegel 1988; Socarides 1978).

In myriad daily casual conversations, keeping silent is more than remaining private for a woman with a lesbian identity or relationship. At least, keeping silent means keeping a secret; often, it involves telling a lie. But the consequences of revealing lesbian identity or relationship may include disrupted or destroyed family and friendship relationships or loss of child custody, employment, professional advancement, and group membership. The accompanying anxieties about such consequences—not any special quality, quantity, or variety of preoedipal disturbance, narcissistic developmental arrest, oedipal anxieties, or self-disorder (all of which, of course, may also be present in any woman)—serve to distinguish lesbian patients from heterosexual female patients. A woman's abilities to develop a positive female self-image, to find and maintain a stable relationship, to disclose her lesbian identity and introduce her lesbian partner, and to manage the social consequences of such disclosures are all capacities which in other circumstances psychoanalysts might call ego strengths.

Lesbian Relationships

With a few notable exceptions (Deutsch 1932/1948; Eisenbud 1982; Lachmann 1975; Sanville 1991), published psychoanalytic case descriptions do not show that lesbian relationships were established or improved due to analytic treatment. Psychoanalysis has few conceptual tools for imagining psychologically mature, healthy, primary love between two persons of the same sex. Without such theoretical support, the anxieties and defenses in the patient that prevent the establishment of sound lesbian relationships may go unexamined. Instead, the analyst assumes that when the narcissistic deficits, separation anxiety, or oedipal conflicts are better resolved, the patient will be freer to have relationships with men, rather than assuming that when such issues are better resolved, the patient will become psychically freer to follow her attraction and find more satisfying relationships, which may continue to be with women. Deutsch (1932/1948) described such a patient:

> She knew that her erotic potentialities and fantasies were directed toward members of her own sex. . . . The women were not in any instance of a masculine type, and she herself was blond and feminine. She felt no hostility toward men . . . and had married a man of outspoken masculine appearance, and had several children by him. . . . (p. 209)

The patient had been aware of her attraction toward women since puberty. She came to treatment for her depressions, which had led to a number of serious suicide attempts, and for her timidity toward her women servants. The analysis focused on the patient's "aggressive, murderous hate against the mother" (p. 211). After a period of successful treatment, Deutsch referred her patient to a "fatherly male analyst," hoping that "the patient's libidinal future would shape up more satisfactorily with a revival of the father relationship" (p. 213). By accident about a year later she met her patient on the street and discovered

> she had become a vivid, radiant person. She told me that her depressions had entirely disappeared. The wish to die which had been continuously present . . . had apparently receded completely. At last she had found happiness in a particularly congenial and uninhibited sexual relationship with a woman. (p. 214)

Deutsch noted that "the result of the analysis was evident. Everything that had come to the surface so clearly in the analytic transference was now detached from the person of the analyst and transferred to other women" (p. 214). When the disturbance in internal early object relationships was relieved, the patient was freed to seek new relationships. To the surprise of her analyst, the patient left her husband and established a relationship with a woman.

Psychoanalytic Closets

A second reason for the lack of descriptions of improved or satisfying lesbian relationships in analytic literature is that analytic therapists of patients who do have such relationships often keep silent about their work and do not present or publish such cases. The authors believe that a closet has existed for some analysts who treat lesbian women. Such analysts are in the same position as their lesbian patients—ambivalent about whether to reveal or to hide and fearing that if they do come out, their work will at best not be appreciated and at worst be attacked by their analytic colleagues.

Psychoanalysts were active on both sides of the 1973 American Psychiatric Association (APA) debate over removing homosexuality as a pathological condition from the *Diagnostic and Statistical Manual of Mental Disorders* (Bayer 1981). It took 15 more years before the American Psychoanalytic Association endorsed the APA's resolution ("American Psychoanalytic Opposes Discrimination Against Homosexuals," 1991). Although institutional psychoanalysis has denied the existence of any barriers to analytic training for homosexual persons, openly gay or lesbian candidates were not admitted to American Psychoanalytic Institutes, and until very recently no openly gay or lesbian candidates trained at any psychoanalytic institutes. In 1988 Lewes, writing on male homosexuality and psychoanalysis, could still state: "There has not been in the history I have sketched a single analytic writer who could identify himself as homosexual" (p. 238). In the last 5 years, the voices of gay and lesbian analysts have begun to enter psychoanalytic discourse and to add their individual and varied perspectives to theory and practice (Blechner 1993; Domenici and Lesser 1995; Drescher 1993, 1994; Isay 1989; Lesser 1993; Magee and Miller 1994; Schwartz 1993).

New Analogies

Freud saw homosexuality in various ways: as an "aberration" of the sexual drive, an "inversion" of sexual object relations, a "perversion" of the drive's aim, and "one variety of the genital organization." Clara

Thompson (1947), objecting to Freud's drive theory, suggested that the term "homosexuality" had become a "wastebasket into which are dumped all forms of relationships with one's own sex" (p. 183). Then, she threw in some of her ideas. She called homosexuality a symptom, like "a headache [which] may be the result of brain tumor, a sinus, a beginning infectious disease, a migraine attack, an emotional disturbance, or a blow on the head. When the underlying disease is treated successfully, the headache disappears" (p. 187). Stephen Mitchell (1978) pointed out,

> The choice of analogies, again even among those questioning existing theory, tends to suggest pathology by offering conceptual frameworks for viewing the development of homosexuality that are derived from an understanding of ulcers (Friedman) or masochism (Lachmann). The problem is that even if one addresses secondarily adaptive or growth-enhancing aspects of the behavior, one is still employing a paradigm derived from a condition understood to be originally and most basically pathological. (p. 260)

The authors offer the analogies provided by two women patients. One woman's sexual attraction was to men; her sexual fantasies were about heterosexual relationships. She saw herself as a heterosexual woman with various blocks to achieving satisfying relationships with men. Therapy had helped, but in her late 30s, before entering analysis, she had suddenly and with very little difficulty formed a deeply satisfying lesbian relationship. Although she explored from many directions in her analysis the possible causes for this surprising development, finally it remained more than the sum of any explanations she could muster. One day she used a football analogy. "It's like a lateral pass," she said. "The intended receiver is not open. In order to continue forward motion one cannot throw down field. So one passes off laterally. Play is not interrupted and can go forward." Although amused by her own football metaphor, she felt it conveyed the motivation behind her "change of object." It allowed movement to continue. The metaphor also expressed her deep satisfaction at having her moves responded to by an "open" receiver and the excitement of that moment of connection.

Another woman offered a different metaphor based on her experiences. She had had a lesbian relationship in college and another in graduate school, had married, and after her divorce had begun a fulfilling relationship with a woman. "It's like 'Double Dutch' in jump rope," she explained. "You just keep jumping. One partner may move out of the rope and another may move in. But you keep jumping. It's the motion of the rope, the movement of your partner and how you relate to that person that enables you to stay in the game."

These analogies offer images of complicated interaction. In the first, life is seen as a football field where forward motion toward the goal of a satisfying relationship can be impeded. A change of object allows for the possibility of further adaptive movement, as well as possible conflict. One may miss one's intended lateral receiver, or that receiver may drop the ball, or defensive tackles may descend on both passer and receiver. In the second analogy, life is also likened to a game, this time a series of rope moves. Whether we master each series of moves is determined by the turns of the rope of chance and by our own abilities to match our rhythms with those with whom we share fate's revolutions.

Conclusion

The psychoanalytic search for distinguishing etiology and distinguishing clinical characteristics of gay men and lesbian women has to date met with no more success than the similar search undertaken by sexologists or biological investigators, and the authors suspect for similar reasons. The words *homosexual* and *heterosexual* identify socially determined categories of persons, not categories reflecting essential biological or clinical differences or distinguishing early developmental histories (see Chapter 6 by Stein and Chapter 9 by Byne in this book).

Of the various psychoanalytic formulations of the developmental disturbances said to characterize female homosexuality, none is specific to women who have homosexual feelings or relationships. To know that a woman patient is in a primary relationship with a woman or identifies herself as lesbian is to know nothing about her early developmental issues, the nature of her sexual experience, or the quality of her external or internal object relations. To understand these issues in a lesbian patient, one must, as with any patient, do the work of treatment.

References

American Psychoanalytic Association opposes discrimination against homosexuals. Psychiatric News, August 2, 1991, p 2

Bayer R: Homosexuality and American Psychiatry: The Politics of Diagnosis. New York, Basic Books, 1981

Blechner M: Homophobia in psychoanalytic writing and practice: commentary of Trop and Stolorow's "Defense Analysis in Self Psychology: A Developmental View" and Hanna's "False-Self Sensitivity to Countertransference: Anatomy of a Single Session." Psychoanal Dial 3:627–637, 1993

Brierley M: Some problems of integration in women. Int J Psychoanal 13:433–448, 1932

Coleman E: Developmental stages of the coming out process, in Homosexuality and Psychotherapy: A Practitioner's Handbook of Affirmative Models. Edited by Gonsiorek J. New York, Haworth, 1982, pp 31–45

de Monteflores C: Notes on the management of difference, in Contemporary Perspectives on Psychotherapy with Lesbians and Gay Men. Edited by Stein T, Cohen C. New York, Plenum, 1986, pp 73–101

Deutsch H: On female homosexuality (1932), in The Psychoanalytic Reader. Edited by Fleiss R. Madison, CT, International Universities Press, 1948, pp 208–230

Domenici T, Lesser R (ed): Disorienting Sexuality: Psychoanalytic Reappraisals of Sexual Identities. New York, Routledge, 1995

Drescher J: Psychoanalytic attitudes toward homosexuality. Paper presented at the annual meeting of the American Academy of Psychoanalysis, New York, December 1993

Drescher J: Contemporary psychoanalytic therapy with gay men. Paper presented at the annual meeting of the American Psychiatric Association, Philadelphia, PA, May 1994

Eisenbud R-J: Early and later determinants of lesbian choice. Psychoanal Rev 69:85–109, 1982

Fenichel O: The Psychoanalytic Theory of Neurosis. New York, WW Norton, 1945

Freud S: Three essays on the theory of sexuality (1905), in Standard Edition of the Complete Psychological Works of Sigmund Freud, Vol 7. Translated and edited by Strachey J. London, Hogarth Press, 1953, pp 123–245

Freud S: The psychogenesis of a case of homosexuality in a woman (1920), in Standard Edition of the Complete Psychological Works of Sigmund Freud, Vol 18. Translated and edited by Strachey J. London, Hogarth Press, 1955, pp 145–172

Friedman RC: Male Homosexuality: A Contemporary Psychoanalytic Perspective. New Haven, CT, Yale University Press, 1988

Garnets L, Kimmel D: Lesbian and gay male dimensions in the psychological study of human diversity, in Psychological Perspectives on Lesbian and Gay Male Experiences. Edited by Garnets, L, Kimmel D. New York, Columbia University Press, 1993, pp 1–51

Gartrell N: Issues in Psychotherapy with Lesbian Women. Wellesley, MA, The Stone Center Work in Progress Series, 1984

Hanley-Hackenbruck P: Psychotherapy and the "coming out" process. Journal of Gay and Lesbian Psychotherapy 1:21–39, 1988

Isay RA: Being Homosexual: Gay Men and Their Development. New York, Avon, 1989

Jones E: The early development of female sexuality. Int J Psychoanal 8:459–472, 1927

Khan M: The role of infantile sexuality and early object-relations in female homosexuality, in The Pathology and Treatment of Sexual Deviation: A Methodological Approach. Edited by Rosen I. New York, Oxford University Press, 1964, pp 221–292

Khan M: Hidden Selves. New York, International Universities Press, 1983

Kirkpatrick M, Morgan C: Psychodynamic psychotherapy of female homosexuality, in Homosexual Behavior. Edited by Marmor J. New York, Basic Books, 1980

Lachmann F: Homosexuality: some diagnostic perspectives and dynamic considerations. Am J Psychother 29:254–260, 1975

Lesser R: A reconsideration of homosexual themes: commentary on Trop and Stolorow's "Analysis in Self Psychology." Psychoanal Dial 3:639–641, 1993

Lewes K: The Psychoanalytic Theory of Male Homosexuality. New York, Simon and Schuster, 1988

Magee M, Miller D: Psychoanalysis and women's experiences of "coming-out": the necessity of becoming a "bee charmer." Journal of the American Academy of Psychoanalysis 22:481–504, 1994

Marmor J: Overview: the multiple roots of homosexual behavior, and Epilogue: homosexuality and the issue of mental illness, in Homosexual Behavior: A Modern Reappraisal. Edited by Marmor J. New York, Basic Books, 1980, pp 3–22, 391–401

McDougall J: Homosexuality in women, in Female Sexuality. Edited by Chasseguet-Smirgel J. Ann Arbor, MI, Michigan University Press, 1970, pp 171–213

McDougall J: Plea for a Measure of Abnormality. New York, International Universities Press, 1980

McDougall J: Theaters of the Mind. New York, Basic Books, 1985

McDougall J: The dead father: on early psychic trauma and its relation to disturbance in sexual identity and in creative activity. Int J Psychoanal 70:205–219, 1989

Mitchell S: Psychodynamics, homosexuality, and the question of pathology. Psychiatry 41:254–263, 1978

Morganthaler F: Homosexuality, Heterosexuality, Perversion. Hillsdale, NJ, Analytic Press, 1988

Person E: Sexuality as the mainstay of identity: psychoanalytic perspectives. Signs: Journal of Women in Culture and Society 5:605–630, 1980

Quinodoz J-M: Female homosexual patients in psychoanalysis. Int J Psychoanal 70:55–63, 1989

Romm M: Sexuality and homosexuality in women, in Sexual Inversion: the Multiple Roots of Homosexuality. Edited by Marmor J. New York, Basic Books, 1965, pp 282–301

Sanville J: The Playground of Psychoanalytic Therapy. Hillsdale, NJ, Analytic Press, 1991

Schafer R: Problems in Freud's psychology of women. J Am Psychoanal Assoc 22:459–485, 1974

Schwartz D: Heterophilia—the love that dare not speak its aim: commentary of Trop and Stolorow's "Defense Analysis in Self Psychology: A Developmental View." Psychoanal Dial 3:643–652, 1993

Siegel E: Female Homosexuality: Choice Without Volition. Hillsdale, NJ, Analytic Press, 1988

Socarides C: The Overt Homosexual. New York, Grune and Stratton, 1968

Socarides C: Homosexuality. New York, Aronson, 1978

Stein T, Cohen J: Psychotherapy with gay men and lesbians: an examination of homophobia, coming out and identity, in Innovations in Psychotherapy with Homosexuals. Edited by Hetrick E, Stein T. Washington, DC, American Psychiatric Press, 1984, pp 60–73

Stoller R: Primary femininity. J Am Psychoanal Assoc 24(5):59–78, 1976

Stoller R: Observing the Erotic Imagination. New Haven, CT, Yale University Press, 1985

Thompson C: Changing concepts of homosexuality in psychoanalysis. Psychiatry 10:183–189, 1947

13

Self Psychology and Homosexuality

Sexual Orientation and Maintenance of Personal Integrity

Bertram J. Cohler, Ph.D.
Robert Galatzer-Levy, M.D.

Changes in psychoanalysis over the past several decades have led to additional understanding of both the course of psychological development from earliest childhood to oldest age and the foundation of a more effective means of intervention to assist persons experiencing distress. However, these changes in both psychoanalytical developmental theory and technique have not been

Many of the ideas in this chapter had their origin in a group of therapists who met to discuss psychodynamic psychotherapy and sexuality. We are particularly indebted to Floyd Irvin, the late Bill Parker, Dennis Shelby, Jeff Slutsky, and Ed Tuder. This chapter particularly benefited from the support and guidance provided by Andrew Boxer, whose commitment as director of the Evelyn Hooker Center for Gay and Lesbian Mental Health inspires all of us who work in the area of sexuality and mental health. Comments by Colin Davis, David de Boer, and Dino Kostas regarding an earlier draft of this chapter are very much appreciated.

well recognized in much of the discussion of sexuality and mental health, which still focuses on problems of more traditional psychoanalytical perspectives emphasizing drive or instinctual elements. Contemporary contributions to self psychology recognize that sexual orientation and mental health must be understood as independent dimensions; there is little evidence that sexual orientation is related in any way to adjustment except as a consequence of stigma (Herdt and Boxer 1992; Hooker 1957).

Changes in our understanding of the significance of gay, lesbian, and bisexual lifestyles require reconsideration of both clinical theory and technique (Isay 1989). The experience of being gay, lesbian, or bisexual within recent generations or cohorts of young people is quite different from that of generations growing up prior to the Stonewall riots of 1969. As Herdt and Boxer's (1992) report of the study of a group of gay and lesbian adolescents has shown, young people who feel sufficiently safe not to hide or be ashamed of their sexual orientation are able to adjust in the same way as their nonhomosexual counterparts.

The case presented in this chapter was chosen to illustrate an approach to psychotherapeutic intervention with gay men, lesbians, and bisexual men and women in which choice of sexual orientation itself is not an issue; intervention seeks to foster enhanced personal integrity and vitality. It is important that discussion of psychotherapy and sexual orientation move beyond conflicts regarding conversion-affirmation of sexual orientation (Nicolosi 1991; Socarides 1978; Socarides and Volkan 1991) to focus on problems interfering in the patient's realizing an enhanced sense of well-being and a more effective attainment of personal goals. Statements such as those reported by Nicolosi (1991) that gay men are unable to maintain long-term monogamous partnerships and are particularly sexually promiscuous are both inaccurate generalizations regarding gay lifestyles and misrepresentations of the adjustment of gay men and lesbians.

More troubled men and women, regardless of sexual orientation, may use sexuality as a means of protecting themselves against feelings of personal depletion and fragmentation. Rather than sexual orientation, the primary focus of concern should be distress, together with reliance on sexualization in an effort to maintain a sense of vitality and coherence (Goldberg 1993). Too often, expression of sexuality among homosexual men and women is labeled *sexualization,* when comparable expression of sexuality among nonhomosexual counterparts is not seen as a "breakdown product." For example, homosexual cruising among gay men has often been portrayed as a classic instance of sexualization (Bollas 1992). However, the search may be for another person who will provide affirmation and companionship. A number of trial encounters may be necessary to define characteristics of this comforting partner. It is important to recognize that although the mode of expression may be different, such difference does not necessarily reflect greater psychopathology. The important issue is the meaning for persons of particular modes of sexual expression.

The meaning of *cruising* can be understood only in terms of the collaborative work of psychotherapy and the meaning that the patient and therapist make of this experience. The significance of sexual orientation must be understood in terms of the patient's cohort or generation and present social circumstances, as well as the life history as a whole (Boxer and Cohler 1989; Boxer et al. 1993). Changing norms within the gay, lesbian, and bisexual community play an important part in defining generational expectations of gay men and lesbians regarding both expression of sexuality and aspects of relationships. For example, among younger gay men and lesbians, the bar represents an important opportunity for affirming one's identity, being together with others like oneself, meeting friends, and enjoying music and dancing. Groups of young people arrive together and may or may not go home together afterward. The important factor in understanding the significance of sexuality for personal adjustment is less concerned, for example, with the fact of an evening spent in a dance bar than with the patient's experience during that evening.

Psychoanalysis and the Issue of Stigma

Other than as a means of providing better understanding of the determinants and expression of instinctual force, Freud (1905/1953, 1920/1955) had no views regarding the morality of any mode of sexual expression or the choice of a sexual partner. This is nowhere more clearly stated than in Freud's (1935/1951) letter to an American mother of a homosexual man in which he observed that "homosexuality is assuredly no advantage but it is nothing to be ashamed of. . . . It cannot be classified as an illness; we consider it to be a variation of the sexual function" (p. 787). Much of what has been assumed to be a psychoanalytical approach to understanding variation in choice of partner has come from a misreading of Freud's work. Freud made it quite clear in this letter that the goal of psychoanalytical intervention for homosexual men and women should be to facilitate adjustment, not to convert them to a heterosexual orientation.

It is particularly ironic that psychoanalysis has sometimes been identified with a particular position regarding the gender of a sexual partner. One major goal of clinical psychoanalytical intervention is that the analysand should become acquainted with the variety of wishes and the means of protection against recognition of these wishes. The analysand's discovery of the range of sexual wishes and the complex nature of sexuality should increase appreciation of the varieties of sexuality at the same time that the changing meaning of sexual expression throughout the course of life becomes a focus of analytic study. Awareness of the variety and complexity of wishes realized through personal psychoanalysis should lead to increased capacity for empathy; such stereotyping as represented by homophobia is inimical to psychoanalysis. As a consequence of enhanced self-understanding realized through self-exploration by means of analysis of the transference (Freud 1914/1958; Schafer 1982), psychoanalysis provides a means for overcoming prejudices such as homophobia that reflect projective identifications or attribution of one's own wishes to others, which are then experienced as a malignant attack on the self.

The analyst's concern should be to assist the analysand to enhance the capacity for self-inquiry, self-soothing, and solace, thereby fostering personal integrity. Some gay, lesbian, or bisexual patients may have problems in realizing effective personal integration because of both overt and covert homophobia and the stigma pervasive in society. All too often, patients and even openly gay, lesbian, or bisexual therapists exhibit homophobia (Malyon 1985). At the least, some gay, lesbian, or bisexual therapists share with their patients the belief that if they had not been gay, lesbian, or bisexual, they would not have had to experience stigma and thus would have had a less difficult life. Clearly, regardless of sexual orientation, it is essential that the therapist have considerable capacity for self-inquiry (Gardner 1983)—fostered by the therapist's personal analysis—and relative comfort with sexual orientation and varieties of lifestyles.

Furthermore, exploration of stigma experienced by lesbian, gay, or bisexual patients and their therapists provides an important opportunity for understanding the manner in which stereotyping adversely affects self-image and other aspects of adjustment (Allport 1954; de Monteflores 1986; Goffman 1963; Nash 1993). Homophobia is so endemic in our society, even among those who are openly gay, lesbian, or bisexual, that it may become an intrinsic element determining enactments of both the analyst and the analysand. The experience of stigma is likely to foster problems both in the analyst's capacity to maintain an empathic response to experiences reported by the analysand and in the analysand's particular intense search for mirror transferences. To an even greater extent than in the general population, lifelong experience of more or less subtle discrimination may lead the gay, lesbian, or bisexual analysand to be particularly sensitive to even nuances regarding the analyst's continuing concern and support for life choices and personal attainments within a "mirroring transference" (de Monteflores 1986; Kohut 1977, 1979, 1984).

Perspectives on Homosexuality From Self Psychology

Persons who are gay, lesbian, or bisexual may have conflicts stemming from the effort to resolve problems associated with the family romance accompanying the transition from early to middle childhood; in addition, they may encounter lifelong problems in experiencing a sense of personal coherence or integrity. Although Freud recognized the significance of concern with self-coherence, as a consequence of self-analysis in the aftermath of his father's death, he turned his attention to the impact of his discovery of the son's conflict between feelings of love and rivalry toward his father during the preschool years. This conflict leads to the nuclear constellation in which the boy or girl encounters feelings not only of love, but also of rivalry, fear of retaliation and consequent anxiety, and to both the appearance and resolution of the infantile neurosis, which is metaphorically akin to the phobia of the adult psychoneurosis (A. Freud 1965, 1971; Nagera 1966). Isay (1989) has suggested that a "negative," or "inverted," form of the nuclear neurosis generally accompanying early efforts to resolve the nuclear neurosis may be highlighted in boys who will become gay men. However, another version of the struggle of the young boy or girl to maintain personal integrity (including comfort with sexual orientation) focuses on concern with maintenance of coherence.

The long-term impact of the consequences of psychological conflict first experienced during the preschool years was initially described by Freud (1900/1958, 1915/1957) in terms of three systems of consciousness—unconsciousness, preconsciousness, and consciousness. Later, in the revised structural theory (S. Freud 1923/1961), this topographical perspective was reformulated in terms of a structural theory of the mind focusing on the macrostructures of id, ego, and superego. The effort to construct a model of the mind complemented Freud's initial concern with person and self, as reflected in the clinical essays of "Studies in Hysteria" (Breuer and Freud 1893–1895/1955). Changes in the model of the mind led, over time, first to a shift in focus from lifting repression to modifying a harsh and punitive superego modeled on the more benign superego of the analyst, and then to a developmental model based on restoration of personal functioning believed to have been distorted during the first years of life (Friedman 1988; Strachey 1934).

Regardless of whether this focus is portrayed as object relations theory (Guntrip 1971; Summers 1994; Winnicott 1953, 1960), relational psychology (Greenberg and Mitchell 1989), or self psychology (Kohut 1971, 1977, 1984), contemporary focus is on those factors that interfere with the patient realizing enhanced integrity or congruence through the collaborative construction by analyst and analysand of a revised life story. This "rewritten" life story should provide a more effective and comfortable integration of wish and experience throughout the present course of life than that described by the patient at the outset of psychotherapy (Freud 1909/1953; Schafer 1980, 1981). Following Kohut's (1977) initial discussion of homosexuality from the perspective of self psychology, additional reports by Shapiro (1985), de Monteflores (1986), Cornett (1993), and Magid (1993) have shown the contributions of self psychological psychoanalytical perspectives with lesbians and gay men who recognized an intense need for affirmation in response to lifelong stigma, leading to a sense of self-disparagement.

As contrasted with more traditional views within psychoanalysis, self psychological perspectives assume that we continue to use others psychologically across the course of self as a source of sustenance and support. Central to self psychological perspectives, as first portrayed by Fairbairn (1952), Winnicott (1953/1958, 1960, 1965), and Kohut (1959/1978, 1971, 1977, 1984), is increased recognition of the importance of experiencing integrity and congruence for continued mental health throughout life. Problems arise only when persons are unable to take advantage of available support or when this support is not sustaining or fulfilling. Self psychological perspectives suggest that initially the care provided by others is experienced by the child as care provided for oneself (Cohler 1980). To the extent that this initial care is, in Winnicott's (1960a) terms, "not good enough" for the child, it fails to provide solace and comfort; the consequence is the lifelong inability to modulate tension. This deficit in personality development may lead to a lasting deficit in the capacity for self-regulation. The deficit interferes with the ability to use others as a source of support and solace.

Over the past decade, the term "self psychology" has become identified with a particular approach to psychoanalytical intervention, and it has been associated with a formulation of origins and course of personality development, as reflected in the writing of Kohut, and most recently as elaborated by Elson (1986) and Wolf (1988). Although the work of Kohut and his associates is clearly an integral aspect of self perspectives within psychoanalysis, it is also a part of a much larger concern with person, context, psychological development, and mental health, as reflected by such psychoanalytical theorists as Winnicott (1953/1958, 1960, 1965), Guntrip (1971), Klein (1976), and Schafer (1980, 1981)—all of whom focus on circumstances that provide an enhanced sense of congruity and personal integration throughout life.

The self psychological perspective reflects an additional aspect of personality that is less specifically addressed within topographic or structural perspectives of psychoanalysis and that has specific relevance for the study of intervention with men and women who are characterized by variation in sexual orientation. Largely as a consequence of their lifelong experience of stigma, many gay men and lesbians have an experience of self that lacks coherence. Therefore, conflict with family members, such as that which may occur when "coming out," for example, may further challenge their experience of personal integrity. This struggle leads to increased vulnerability of self-esteem and requires the therapist's particular focus on the manner in which this vulnerability is expressed (de Monteflores 1986).

One such transference-like enactment (Kohut 1971), expressed through particular concern with the analyst's admiration, affirmation, and approval, has been portrayed by Kohut (1977, 1984) as a mirroring transference. However, particularly among lesbians and gay men in treatment with openly gay or lesbian therapists who have successfully negotiated coming out and are comfortable with their sexual orienta-

tion, the analysand may be more likely to develop an idealizing transference. These patients look up to their therapists as a model and find
renewed strength from basking in their glow. A third type of transference, twinship (alter-ego) transference (Kohut 1984), may be expressed
in the desire to spend time with the analyst or to be as much like the
therapist as possible. (Although issues of tact and timing are critical in
making interventions, a successful outcome of psychoanalysis or psychotherapy requires that the meaning of these enactments be made
explicit within the relationship of therapist and patient and resolved
in a manner similar to the more familiar "oedipal" transference associated with the nuclear neurosis).

Search for Self-Affirmation: Psychotherapy With Mr. A

Mr. A, a 26-year-old man working as a doctoral-level scientist in a major
laboratory, sought psychotherapy in connection with frustration in his
career and in his relationship with Mr. B, a partner of about 3 years.
Growing up in a small Midwestern community, the son of a prominent
Protestant minister, Mr. A had felt particular pressure almost since beginning school to be an exemplary member of the community. Both
Mr. A and his sister, who was 3 year older, had been asked by their
parents to be particularly aware of the family's position in the community. Mr. A described his parents as decent people who were very narrow
in their social outlook. His father struggled with his ministry and the
continuing conflicts within the congregation, leaving him little time for
his family. His mother was a somewhat depressed woman who had lost
her mother to cancer when she was in elementary school and had never
recovered from this loss. Mr. A had spent much time with his sister, who
had preceded him in going to college in another state and had later
become a physician.

Mr. A noted with a chuckle the sense of mourning so often expressed in contemporary society for the intimacy of the small town.
Aware since early adolescence of his homosexuality, Mr. A's first homosexual experience had been in high school while staying overnight with
a particularly close friend. Mr. A emphasized that although sex was
enjoyable, it was his friend's sharing of his experiences and feelings
and the similarity of interests and concerns that made the boys almost

inseparable over the succeeding months. Mr. A realized that he had never been able to mourn the loss of this friend, with whom he lost contact over time. He observed at one point that he and his mother shared the problem of not having been able to get over earlier losses.

Mr. A reported having felt "funny" in high school. He was sure that others knew of the significance of his relationship with his friend. He determined to go to college far from home and was accepted at an Ivy League university. He said that he felt liberated upon arriving at college in a large community in the mid-1970s, a time when the social turmoil of the preceding years had led to increased tolerance of both ethnic and sexual minorities. Relationships that Mr. A tried to develop during his college years led to disappointment when the prospective partner was unable to commit emotionally to a relationship. Mr. A said he was quite sure that he wanted an intimate relationship in which sexuality was an important part but in which there were also mutual understanding and caring.

Accepted into a doctoral program, Mr. A continued to show the outstanding intellectual attainments that had won him honors upon college graduation. Recently, however, he had become stuck on his dissertation project and had found it difficult to work with his emotionally distant and harried major adviser. Mr. A felt defeated by his lack of progress in completing his dissertation research and had become depressed in the absence of the affirmation he sought.

This feeling of futility had affected his relationship with his partner, who commented that the patient "moped about" and seemed to be unable to get himself motivated. Their relationship had become less intimate and satisfying as a result of Mr. A's problems. The two men had met at a gay bar in the city's predominately homosexual neighborhood and had "struck it off" from the outset. His partner was about 5 years older, a self-employed graphics designer who was reasonably successful in his work and more closely connected with the gay community than Mr. A, whose few homosexual experiences in graduate school had been with other students whom he had met through a local gay and lesbian organization. The two men had agreed to live together with the plan of becoming domestic partners, but they had become involved in conflict. Mr. B was more financially successful, and money issues had become a problem. Mr. A also resented his partner's community commitments, a reaction that he realized was similar to the way he had felt about his father's absence from the family.

Psychoanalytical psychotherapy lasted nearly 3 years and was concluded when Mr. A finished his doctoral degree and moved with his partner to another city for a postdoctoral fellowship. Mr. A was psychologically minded and concerned with understanding his present dilemma and his contribution to the problems with his partner. Referral for couples therapy was of assistance in helping the two men to work out details of their relationship, to come to a better understanding of such issues as family budget, and to resolve issues of sexual compatibility. Individual psychotherapy focused on Mr. A's search for affirmation, as reflected in a merger transference in which he sought assurance of his therapist's interest in him regardless of progress on his dissertation. This concern was also demonstrated in Mr. A's disappointment with his dissertation adviser's lack of support for his attainments in a manner similar to his father's response to him.

Much of the early work in therapy focused on Mr. A's concern that his therapist did not appreciate the significance of his achievements. Mr. A showed particular sensitivity to his therapist's acknowledgment of him. On one occasion, preoccupied with personal concerns far removed from treatment, his therapist invited Mr. A into the office but failed to say hello. The patient seemed to melt on the spot, looked crestfallen, and slumped into the chair in a way that was quite different from his usual, alert manner. When the therapist noted this change to himself and recalled the first moments of their meeting that day, he recognized his failure to greet Mr. A and explained that he was momentarily preoccupied with issues not related to treatment. This explanation led Mr. A to recall his continuing disappointment with his father's lack of affirmation for his achievements and the numerous times when his father had promised to spend time with him and then had let him down.

Continued effort to understand Mr. A's search for affirmation from his therapist and for praise for his honest struggle for enhanced self-understanding ultimately led to Mr. A's awareness of his resentment of his mother, who felt depleted and unable to respond to her children. Both he and his sister had encouraged their mother to seek psychiatric assistance for her pervasive depression, which had intensified over the past few years; Mr. A noted that his parents just weren't psychologically minded. His mother had been around during his childhood, helping his father with the church and assisting in the community, but she seemed to be happiest when away from home.

His concern that his mother didn't want to be with him or at home was repeated anew with his partner, also involved in the community, who seemed at times disinterested in him. This worry led to concern about whether his therapist wished to see him. Discussion of a lower fee raised the questions of why the therapist would want to see him and whether his therapist would stick by him as he struggled with his disappointments. Much effort was devoted to Mr. A's concern with his therapist's commitment to working with him. Over time, Mr. A was able to recognize the extent to which he was afraid that his mother's apparent indifference to him would be repeated with both his partner and his therapist. Mr. A struggled particularly with the issue of recognizing the difference between his partner and his mother and his need to support his partner's community involvement if their relationship was to grow. He began to join with his partner in work on community AIDS awareness and became an effective peer counselor. His partner appreciated Mr. A's increasing interest in this project, which led to increased intimacy and mutual satisfaction in the relationship. This enhanced mutuality, in turn, led Mr. A to recall times when he and his sister had helped their parents with the ministry.

In exploring his disappointments as reflected in the wish for his therapist's admiration, Mr. A was better able to understand his search for mirroring experiences, including those with his major adviser, his therapist, and his partner. Mr. A was able to connect his disappointment in his adviser with the longing he had felt for increased admiration and affirmation from his father. Consistent with Isay's (1989) formulation, it is possible that Mr. A's intense early childhood longing for a sexual relationship with his father had led his father to be wary of this bid for affection, leading to tension and subsequent problems in their relationship. Isay believes that the tension regarding the son's sexual wishes is a foundation of the father's effort to increase the emotional distance between them. From the perspective of self psychology, the son's experience of his father's increased distance, as a reaction to the father's discomfort with his son's bid for intimacy, is that of his father's failure to respond empathically to his son and an increased inability to obtain solace from relationships with others.

Although there is little evidence in the patient's mirroring transference to speak against this interpretation, the patient's recollection of his father was of his father's efforts on behalf of church and community, which left him too tired to be able to respond empathically to Mr. A's requests for affection. Mr. A came gradually to recognize that his adviser's cool manner was a part of his own upbringing and present manner of relating to both students and colleagues. In fact, his adviser had helped him with technical aspects of the project and had given freely of his time; however, there was little of the affection and admiration that Mr. A had sought.

Recognition of the connection between the empathic failure of both his father and his academic adviser and helplessness he had experienced as a reaction to this repeated empathic failure led Mr. A to be able to seek the help of a postdoctoral student in the laboratory who greatly admired Mr. A's nascent scientific attainments and his potential as a scientist; this recognition also led Mr. A to use his adviser in a more effective manner to conclude his experiment. The effort to understand the search for affirmation for his scientific work, frustrated by his rather austere supervisor, also led to enhanced concern with the mirror transference within psychotherapy reflected in his wish for his therapist to admire his scientific attainments.

Over time, Mr. A began to understand the events of his childhood somewhat differently and was able to recall times when he had felt affirmed by his father. For example, he recalled the evenings when he was in junior high school and the family cooperated to get the bulletin ready for Sunday service. Mr. A subsequently discovered that his father was nationally recognized for his reform efforts within his own denomination and began to see his parents in a different manner. At the same time, Mr. A did not yet feel comfortable disclosing his homosexuality and his partnership to them. The goals of this psychotherapy of helping the patient complete his doctoral studies and strengthen his relationship with his partner were realized. The patient wrote some time later that he had accepted a university position in another city and that his partner had been able to find work there as well.

Conclusion

Focus on issues of self and personal integrity both complements and extends more traditional psychoanalytical perspectives. In the case of Mr. A, it would be all too easy to assume that his work inhibition was a consequence of conflict regarding the possibility of surpassing his father's accomplishments and the presumed consequences. Issues of disappointment and of failure to realize effective tension management when confronted with such disappointment were explored through similar feelings evoked anew within the therapeutic relationship. Disappointments expressed toward the therapist and the patient's interest in exploring the source of these disappointments contributed to realization of the goals jointly agreed on when he had begun psychotherapy.

Psychotherapy was less successful in resolving the search for affirmation from Mr. A's father, reflected in the patient's concern that telling his father about his homosexuality would only further diminish the opportunity for realizing his father's admiration. It should be noted that the patient was successful in finding an environment likely to be supportive of his sexual orientation. Although he had experienced stigma in high school, this patient was fortunate in attending a liberal college in which students and faculty alike were supportive of diversity and alternative lifestyles and in selecting graduate study at an equally accepting university in which the primary concern was with intellectual attainment. Furthermore, the patient's commitment to maintaining a satisfying and intimate relationship reflected his relative personal strengths despite growing up in a family in which both parents were preoccupied and not entirely able to attend to the needs of their children. As Kohut (1987) has observed, the central issue is the person's capacity to tolerate moderate disappointments and to find appropriate persons with whom to seek satisfying merger experiences as "essential others" (Galatzer-Levy and Cohler 1993).

Focus on the manner in which patients experience the therapist, attention to concerns with idealization and affirmation, and the search for enhanced personal integrity all reflect enduring issues not always explicitly attended to in psychotherapy. This perspective has particular significance in psychotherapy with lesbians, gay men, and bisexual men and women, in which the combination of family and community stigma further compromises the effort to achieve appreciation, which is essential for a continued sense of well-being. Psychotherapy with these men and women, when it fosters grieving and reconciliation with this loss, can facilitate change, leading to increased capacity for self-soothing and for the more effective use of others to realize more complete development of personal integrity.

References

Allport GW: The Nature of Prejudice. Cambridge, MA, Addison-Wesley, 1954

Bollas C: Being a Character: Psychoanalysis and Self-Experience. New York, Hill and Wang, 1992

Boxer A, Cohler B: The life course of gay and lesbian youth: an immodest proposal for the study of lives. J Homosex 17:315–355, 1989

Boxer A, Cohler B, Herdt G, et al: The study of gay and lesbian teenagers: life-course, "coming out" and well being, in Handbook of Clinical Research and Practice With Adolescents. Edited by Tolan P, Cohler B. New York, Wiley-Interscience, 1993, pp 249–280

Breuer J, Freud S: Studies in hysteria (1893–1895), in The Standard Edition of the Complete Psychological Works of Sigmund Freud, Vol 3. Translated and edited by Strachey J. London, Hogarth Press, 1955, pp 1–305

Cohler B: Developmental perspectives on the psychology of self in early childhood, in Advances in Self Psychology. Edited by Goldberg A. New York, International Universities Press, 1980, pp 69–115

Cornett C: Dynamic psychotherapy of gay men: a view from self psychology, in Affirmative Dynamic Psychotherapy With Gay Men. Edited by Cornett C. Northvale, NJ, Jason Aronson, 1993, pp 45–76

de Monteflores C: Notes on the management of difference, in Contemporary Perspectives on Psychotherapy With Lesbians and Gay Men. Edited by Stein T, Cohen C. New York, Plenum, 1986, pp 73–138

Elson M: Self-Psychology in Clinical Social Work. New York, Norton, 1986

Fairbairn WRD: An Object-Relations Theory of the Personality. New York, Basic Books, 1952

Freud A: Normality and Psychopathology in Childhood: Assessments of Development. New York, International Universities Press, 1965

Freud A: The infantile neurosis: genetic and dynamic considerations. Psychoanal Study Child 26:79–90, 1971

Freud S: The interpretation of dreams (1900), in Standard Edition of the Complete Psychological Works of Sigmund Freud, Vol 4–5. Translated and edited by Strachey J. London, Hogarth Press, 1958

Freud S: Three essays on the theory of sexuality (1905), in Standard Edition of the Complete Psychological Works of Sigmund Freud, Vol 7. Translated and edited by Strachey J. London, Hogarth Press, 1953

Freud S: Notes upon a case of obsessional neurosis (1909), in Standard Edition of the Complete Psychological Works of Sigmund Freud, Vol 10. Translated and edited by Strachey J. London, Hogarth Press, 1953, pp 158–250

Freud S: Remembering, repeating and working through: further recommendations on the technique of psychoanalysis (1914), in Standard Edition of the Complete Psychological Works of Sigmund Freud, Vol 12. Translated and edited by Strachey J. London, Hogarth Press, 1958, pp 146–156

Freud S: The unconscious (1915), in Standard Edition of the Complete Psychological Works of Sigmund Freud, Vol 14. Translated and edited by Strachey J. London, Hogarth Press, 1957, pp 159–216

Freud S: The psychogenesis of a case of homosexuality in a woman (1920), in Standard Edition of the Complete Psychological Works of Sigmund Freud, Vol 17. Translated and edited by Strachey J. London, Hogarth Press, 1955, pp 147–172

Freud S: The ego and the id (1923), in Standard Edition of the Complete Psychological Works of Sigmund Freud, Vol 19. Translated and edited by Strachey J. London, Hogarth Press, 1961, pp 12–59

Freud S: A letter from Freud (1935). Am J Psychiatry 107:786, 1951

Friedman L: The Anatomy of Psychotherapy. Hillsdale, NJ, Analytic Press, 1988

Galatzer-Levy R, Cohler B: The Essential Other. New York, Basic Books, 1993

Gardner R: Self-Inquiry. Boston, MA, Little, Brown, 1983

Goffman I: Stigma: Notes on the Management of Spoiled Identity. Englewood Cliffs, NJ, Prentice-Hall, 1963

Goldberg A: Sexualization and desexualization. Psychoanal Q 62:383–399, 1993

Greenberg J, Mitchell S: Object Relations in Psychoanalytic Theory. Cambridge, MA, Harvard University Press, 1983

Guntrip H: Psychoanalytic Theory, Therapy, and the Self. New York, Basic Books, 1971

Herdt G, Boxer A: Children of Horizons. Boston, MA, Beacon Press, 1993

Hooker E: The adjustment of the male overt homosexual. Journal of Projective Techniques 21:18–31, 1957

Isay R: Being Homosexual: Gay Men and Their Development. New York, Farrar, Strauss and Giroux, 1989

Klein G: Psychoanalytic Theory: An Exploration of Essentials. New York, International Universities Press, 1976

Kohut H: The Analysis of the Self. Madison, CT, International Universities Press, 1971

Kohut H: The Restoration of the Self. Madison, CT, International Universities Press, 1977

Kohut H: Introspection, empathy, and psychoanalysis: an examination of the relationship between mode of observation and theory (1959), in The Search for the Self, Vol 1. Edited by Ornstein P, Madison, CT, International Universities Press, 1978, pp 205–232

Kohut H: The two analyses of Mr Z. Int J Psychoanal 60:3–27, 1979

Kohut H: How Does Psychoanalysis Cure? Chicago, IL, University of Chicago Press, 1984

Kohut H: The Kohut Seminars: On Self-Psychology and Psychotherapy With Adolescents and Young Adults. Edited by Elson M. New York, Norton, 1987

Magid B: The homosexual identity of a nameless woman, in Freud's Case Studies: Self-Psychological Perspectives. Edited by Magid B. Hillsdale, NJ, Analytic Press, 1993, pp 189–200

Malyon A: Psychotherapeutic implications of internalized homophobia, in A Guide to Psychotherapy With Gay Men and Lesbian Clients. Edited by Gonsiorek J. New York, Harrington Park, 1985, pp 59–69

Nagera H: Early Childhood Disturbances, the Infantile Neurosis, and the Adulthood Disturbances: Problems of a Developmental Psychoanalytical Psychology (Monograph 2, Monograph Series of Psychoanal Study Child). Madison, CT, International Universities Press, 1966

Nash J: The heterosexual analyst and the gay man, in Affirmative Dynamic Psychotherapy With Gay Men. Edited by Cornett C. Northvale, NJ, Jason Aronson, 1993, pp 199–228

Nicolosi J: Reparative Therapy of Male Homosexuality: A New Clinical Approach. Northvale, NJ, Jason Aronson, 1991

Schafer R: Narration in the psychoanalytic dialogue. Critical Inquiry 7:29–53, 1980

Schafer R: Narrative Actions in Psychoanalysis. Worcester, MA, Clark University Press, 1981

Schafer R: The relevance of the "here and now" transference interpretation to the reconstruction of early development. Int J Psychoanal 63:77–82, 1982

Shapiro S: Archaic selfobject transferences in the analysis of a case of male homosexuality, in Progress in Self Psychology, Vol 1. Edited by Goldberg A. Northvale, NJ, Jason Aronson, 1985, 164–174

Socarides C: Homosexuality. New York, Jason Aronson, 1978

Socarides C, Volkan V (eds): The Homosexualities and the Therapeutic Process. Madison, CT, International Universities Press, 1991

Strachey J: The nature of the therapeutic action of psychoanalysis. Int J Psychoanal 15:127–159, 1934

Summers F: Object Relations and Clinical Practice. Hillsdale, NJ, Analytic Press, 1994

Winnicott DW: Transitional objects and transitional phenomena (1953), in Collected Papers: Through Pediatrics to Psychoanalysis. Edited by Winnicott DW. New York, Basic Books, 1958, pp 229–242

Winnicott DW: The theory of the parent-infant relationship. Int J Psychoanal 41:585–595, 1960

Winnicott DW: Ego distortion in terms of the true and false self, in The Maturational Process and the Facilitating Environment. Edited by Winnicott DW. Madison, CT, International Universities Press, 1965, pp 140–152

Wolf E: Treating the Self: Elements of Clinical Self-Psychology. New York, Guilford, 1988

SECTION III

Homosexual and Bisexual Development Throughout the Life Cycle

From Childhood to Old Age

Sexual Orientation Identity Formation

A Western Phenomenon

Vivienne Cass, Ph.D.

In the past 25 years concepts such as "lesbian identity," "gay identity," "bisexual identity," and "coming out" have become an established part of the Western mental health practitioner's vocabulary. Without question we now assume that being lesbian, gay, bisexual, or heterosexual is a real event or experience, that being heterosexual is the default identity, and that homosexual and bisexual identities emerge after a unique process of psychological development.

These assumptions have been reinforced by a now considerable body of literature that has focused on the process by which individuals acquire a lesbian or gay identity (Ponse 1978; Raphael 1974; Schafer 1976, drawing on a sociological career-path approach; Plummer 1975; Troiden 1979; Weinberg 1983, drawing on symbolic interactionism; Cass 1979, 1984, 1985, 1990; Coleman 1981–2; Malyon 1982; Minton

227

and McDonald 1983–4; Schippers 1989, taking a psychological perspective). Some of these models of homosexual identity formation have been adopted by mental health professionals as a useful tool in helping clients "find themselves," "feel better about being lesbian, gay, or bisexual," "come to terms with a lesbian or gay sexual orientation," "find their true selves," and so on.

However, many mental health professionals (as well as theorists and researchers, unfortunately) have taken an ethnocentric viewpoint, making the incorrect assumption that all these concepts and processes are universal "truths" or "facts" that may be found in the psychology of all people, regardless of culture and social background. This viewpoint has been called the "essentialist approach" (see Chapter 6 by Stein; E. Stein 1992).

As a result of anthropological and historical evidence published in the last decade, we now know that many non-Western cultures take quite different viewpoints. Concepts such as sexual preference and orientation, sexual identity, coming out, homosexual identity formation, and bisexual identity, as well as some of the behaviors that (from a Western perspective) express these notions, do not exist in many of the world's sociocultural contexts. We also know that these concepts have not always existed in Western settings. From this it must be concluded that our ideas on sexual orientation and identity are specific to Western cultures at this particular period in our history (or to cultures that have been influenced by modern Western cultures). Such conclusions represent the social constructionist approach.

It is important for Western mental health practitioners to understand this broad context as they work with clients on issues of homosexual and bisexual identity formation. Several important implications arise from the constructionist understanding, such as the need to be aware of imposing our cultural norms on people from different sociocultural contexts and the need to recognize that ideas of sexual orientation, identity, and identity development may alter over time and hence may lead to changes in behavior.

Nevertheless, we cannot ignore the fact that practitioners regularly encounter clients who exhibit essentialist attitudes and behaviors—believing, for example, that their sexual attractions are a fixed part of their inner psychology and believing that the development of a lesbian, gay, or bisexual identity is a logical extension of this orientation. Hence, Western mental health professionals are required to work within a framework that accommodates the essentialist thinking of their clients, while recognizing the constructed nature of the issues on which their work is based.

The author's theory of lesbian and gay identity formation, described in this chapter, lies within such a framework. Known as *social constructionist psychology* (Bond 1988; Gergen 1985; Semin and Gergen 1990; Shotter 1991; Shweder and LeVine 1992; Stigler et al. 1992), this perspective seems most able to integrate these seemingly contradictory perspectives.

Social Constructionist Psychology and Sexual Orientation Identity Formation

Constructionist psychology, although neither antiuniversalist nor antirelativist, has identified broad-based support for its basic premise that *much of psychological functioning and human behavior is specific to the sociocultural environment in which people live, rather than the result of inner psychological mechanisms that can be found universally in all human beings.* (The latter view epitomizes the traditional psychology perspective in which most mental health practitioners have been trained.)

Within each sociocultural environment, setting, or world there exists an *indigenous psychology* (Heelas and Lock 1981), a system of psychological knowledge that forms part of the culture in which it resides. This system contains everything each world holds as the truth about human psychology (why human beings act the way they do) and is so integrated within the culture as to be taken for granted, that is, simply accepted as "the way things are." The indigenous psychology includes information about what constitutes a psychological concept; the kinds of psychological processes that occur; the behaviors that define these concepts and processes; and even the psychological problems, explanations, and solutions that exist in that culture. Indigenous psychologies direct and constrain the way individuals act, feel, think, and talk about themselves and others. In other words, each indigenous psychology defines a specific psychological reality for its people, a reality that is intricately linked with the ideological, moral, and historical foundations of the sociocultural setting.

Part of Western indigenous psychology is a system of "sexual" knowledge that informs us of the existence of sexual orientations and of sexual orientation identities, identifying behaviors, processes, and explanations that allow us to hold an understanding of what these concepts mean. We are acculturated with this knowledge, taking for granted a psychological reality that is assumed to have sexual orientations and related types or identities. Expressed in the language of essentialism, we perceive that lesbian, gay, bisexual, and heterosexual types of people exist and experience themselves as such; that development of a lesbian, gay, bisexual, or heterosexual identity occurs in a fairly predictable way; and so on. Hence some individuals are led by their Western indigenous psychology to experience *being* homosexual, bisexual, or heterosexual.

According to social constructionist psychology, *behavior (including actions, thoughts, and feelings) arises out of the relationship between individuals (both their biological and psychological capacities) and their sociocultural environments (including the indigenous psychology)*—a relationship that may be characterized as a process of *reciprocal interaction,* in which human beings simultaneously influence and are influenced by their environments during continual interchanges. Although biological and psychological capacities may include human processes that are universal as well as specific, the constructionist perspective recognizes that these factors can never be taken on their own as causes of behavior but must be seen as part of a larger process of reciprocal interaction.

According to this proposal, *lesbian, gay, or bisexual identity formation* is not a process of simply "finding an inner sense of self," as it has been traditionally formulated. Rather, *it is one in which people translate the everyday understanding of lesbian, gay, or bisexual identity provided by the Western indigenous psychologies into knowledge, behaviors, beliefs, and experiences about themselves via the process of reciprocal interaction.*

This understanding of identity formation calls for a shift in the thinking of mental health practitioners who have previously adopted the traditional psychological approach that a lesbian, gay, or bisexual identity is the result of inner developmental processes. Rather than a focus solely on inner psychological processes, it is the relationship between individual and environment, represented often in patterns of interaction between people, that now requires our attention.

Constructionist psychology directs us to ask quite different questions: What are the processes by which people come to move from a third-person approach to homosexuality or bisexuality ("*Some* people are lesbian, gay, or bisexual") to a first-person perspective ("I am a lesbian, gay, or bisexual")? How is it that Western individuals come to translate societal knowledge about sexual orientation into self-knowledge, making sense of and accounting for themselves by claiming the identity of lesbian, gay, or bisexual?

Lesbian, gay, or bisexual identity, in this sense, is a relatively constant understanding (perception, feeling, and experience) of self as "a lesbian," "a gay man," or "a bisexual" that arises (is constructed) out of constant and stable elements and processes within the interactional relationship between individuals and their environment.

However, against this understanding of the constructed nature of homosexual or bisexual identity formation, mental health practitioners must also recognize their clients' perceptions of what is happening. Derived from the indigenous psychology, the psychological reality for our clients is that they are "searching for identity," "finding myself," "needing to be a whole person." Their understanding draws on significant Western indigenous concepts such as personal growth, maturity, identity integration, and self-development to direct their needs and personal desires. We must give weight to these experiences. Hence practitioners, on the one hand, must acknowledge the formation of a lesbian, gay, or bisexual identity as a Western phenomenon that is guided by the directive of Western indigenous psychologies and constructed out of the reciprocal interaction process, and on the other hand, must simply accept their clients' psychological realities as real and significant experiences for them.

Stages in Lesbian and Gay Identity Formation

Within the lesbian and gay communities, the coming-out story is a widely held fact or truth. For the mental health practitioner, however, the question arises as to how this narrative becomes translated into feelings of identity. The following model describes this process, focusing on the evolving understanding of self as a lesbian or gay man that emerges as individuals confront and internalize notions of homosexuality and coming out that exist within their social environment.

Identity formation begins when someone first considers the possibility that the Western indigenous concept of homosexuality may be relevant to self ("There is something about my behavior that could be called homosexual, gay, or lesbian"). This awareness enters into the interactional relationship that exists between the individual concerned and his or her sociocultural setting. The ensuing sequences of interchange that result are never random but are constrained by the Western indigenous psychology as well as by the biological and psychological capacities of human beings.

As a result of these constraints, it is possible in Western cultures to identify patterns of interaction that give rise to differing degrees of cognitive awareness, self-understanding, and sense of identity in relation to the concept of homosexual sexual orientation and the impact these levels of self-knowledge have on the management of social interchanges.

The author has described these patterns as the six stages of identity formation (Cass 1979). The markers for each stage are provided by different levels of self-understanding that indicate an increasingly first-person account of self as lesbian or gay. These stages of identity formation are titled as follows: Stage 1—Identity Confusion, Stage 2—Identity Comparison, Stage 3—Identity Tolerance, Stage 4—Identity Acceptance, Stage 5—Identity Pride, Stage 6—Identity Synthesis.

Within each stage several pathways of interaction have been outlined, although these can be mentioned only briefly in this chapter. Although not detailed here, the process of reciprocal interaction leading to identity formation is complex and multivariable as individual factors (such as needs, desires, and learned behaviors) interact with biological factors (such as level of sexual desire) and environmental variables (such as social class, race, and location).

Each stage brings with it the following changes: 1) increasing use of the concept of homosexual, lesbian, or gay to account for and understand self; 2) use of terms "lesbian" or "gay" as an explanation of self within an increasingly wider number of interpersonal interchanges; 3) development of increasingly positive feelings about *being* a lesbian or gay man; 4) increasing belief that one belongs to the lesbian or gay social group and strengthening social ties with other lesbians or gay men; 5) gradual acceptance of positive values about homosexuals as a social group; 6) increasing independence from heterosexual values; and 7) a gradual shift in use of the concept of homosexual, lesbian, or gay from a means of labeling self to description of an inner belief in self.

Several factors (also defined by Western indigenous psychology) motivate people to adopt an understanding of self that is viewed negatively by (some) others: the need to maintain consistency in who we are; the need to increase and maintain positive feelings about ourselves or enhance self-esteem; adherence to the implicit cultural theory that if we experience sexual or emotional attraction to someone of the same sex we must *be* a lesbian or gay man; belief in other cultural "truths" about the importance of finding one's identity and being true to self; the imperative in some Western languages to describe persistent behavior by reference to a noun, for example, "I am a tennis player."

Because human beings are intentional creatures who have the capacity to act on as well as be acted on by their sociocultural context, some individuals will dynamically engage with their environment so as to prevent the acquisition of a lesbian or gay self-understanding. This process is termed "foreclosure."

In addition to individuals directing their actions toward foreclosure, the occurrence of homosexual identity formation processes will be restricted where there is an absence of those psychological capacities necessary to engage in the process of reciprocal interaction; for example, the ability to be self-aware; to learn and use language and meaning; to recognize actions for which one is held responsible; to be acculturated within the indigenous psychology; and to identify physical sensations, emotions, and cognitions as linked to homosexuality. Where such capacities are lacking—as may be seen in very young, developmentally disabled, mentally ill, and cognitively impaired individuals—identity formation and the maintenance of identity will not take place.

Although the following description applies to the development of lesbian and gay self-understanding, the psychological process of confronting personal information that relates to membership in a stigmatized social category is considered a generic one. Informal adaptations of the model have already been made to bisexual and cross-dressing individuals.

Prestage 1

Before the concept of homosexual, lesbian, or gay has acquired any personal relevance, Western individuals have already developed an understanding of themselves from previous engagement with the sociocultural setting: They assume their sexual orientation identity is that of "not lesbian/gay" or "not lesbian" or "not gay" and "heterosexual" or *supposed* to be heterosexual; they consider themselves more or less part of the majority group (heterosexuals) or recognize that they should be; and they understand that heterosexuality is desirable and acceptable and homosexuality is stigmatized and has minority status.

However, each individual also brings a uniqueness to the identity formation process. Differences exist in relation to personal and sociocultural factors such as the degree of negativity or positivity with which homosexuality and heterosexuality are perceived, the specific personal needs of individuals, levels and types of social support, personal styles in conflict management and communication patterns, and gender- and race-related experiences.

Stage 1—Identity Confusion

Stage 1 is marked by the first attempt to translate the concept of homosexual, lesbian, or gay from a third-person to a first-person perspective. Individuals observe, "There is something about my behavior (acts, thoughts, and feelings) that could be called homosexual, lesbian, or gay." When the observation has strong impact or when the homosexual interpretation of behavior persists, there is a questioning of self: "Does this mean I may be a lesbian/gay man?" "Am I really heterosexual?" "Who am I?" These are powerful questions to ask in a society such as ours and result in emotional reactions ranging from curiosity, bewilderment, and confusion to extreme turmoil.

The primary focus at Stage 1 is to cope with the confusion about who one is, to resolve the inconsistency brought about by attaching homosexual meaning to one's own behavior, and to reduce the discomfort that arises if this meaning is seen as undesirable; in other words, to deal with the impact on personal interchanges of labeling one's own behavior as "lesbian" or "gay."

Three patterns or pathways of interaction can be described at this stage (Figure 14–1), leading to two alternative end points: *either* the claim, "I may be a lesbian or gay man; I may not be heterosexual" *or* the rejection of any homosexual meaning as being relevant to one's own behavior (foreclosure). *Pathway 1* occurs for those individuals who accept the meaning of homosexual, lesbian, or gay to be an accurate and desirable account of their behavior. Using strategies to neutralize society's negativity toward homosexuality, they are led to consider, "I may be a lesbian/gay man; I may not be heterosexual" and to view this self-image positively.

Pathway 2 takes place when individuals accept the correctness of the homosexual meaning they place on their behavior but find this meaning undesirable. They then engage in actions to stop all relevant behaviors and so remove this undesirable element. If successful, they can return to an account of their behavior as nonhomosexual (foreclosure). If unsuccessful, the possibility of being lesbian or gay is acknowledged, although from a negative perspective.

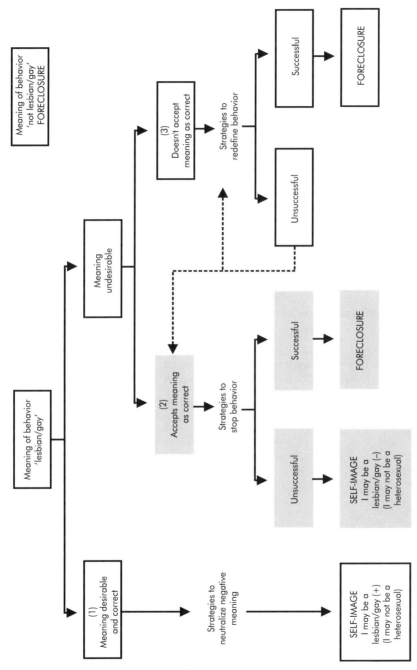

Figure 14–1. Stage 1 pathways of lesbian/gay identity formation.

Pathway 3 occurs when the meaning of one's behavior is considered neither correct nor desirable. The focus then becomes one of redefining this behavior to mean nonhomosexual. This redefinition can be done by changing either the meaning of the actions engaged in ("It was just the kiss of loving friends") or the meaning of the situation in which the behavior occurred, so that a stance of personal innocence can be adopted ("I was taken advantage of "). If successfully done, the original meaning of "heterosexual" is regained (foreclosure). Individuals unable to redefine their behavior are forced to accept that the meaning of lesbian or gay is applicable, and so they continue along Pathway 2.

■ Stage 2—Identity Comparison

Emerging from Stage 1 are two groups of individuals expressing the first tentative shift toward a homosexual, lesbian, or gay account of themselves: those positively disposed toward the self-image of "may be homosexual and may not be heterosexual" and those feeling negatively. Both groups now begin to consider the implications of this potential identity. Given Western approaches to lesbians and gay men, concerns surface about being different, ostracized, part of a minority, and at odds with society. The weight of possible membership in a negatively valued minority group is strongly felt. Feelings of alienation and estrangement are experienced. Furthermore, because the previously assumed heterosexual identity is now questioned, there is growing recognition that all plans and expectations linked with the heterosexual sexual orientation—for example, having children—may no longer apply. The continuity among past, present, and future is gone, leaving a sense of loss. Responses vary from intense feelings of rejection and grief to a sense of comfort as previous feelings of being different from others become clarified by the new self-understanding.

Individuals at Stage 2 engage in behaviors aimed at coping with the loss of direction, managing feelings of alienation and difference, and dealing with the incongruency provided by these events ("My behavior is lesbian/gay; I may be lesbian/gay but others see me as heterosexual"). Most pertinent to the way social interchanges are now handled is the degree to which individuals see the holding of a lesbian or gay self-image as bringing more positive consequences for them than negative ones (that is, more rewards than costs).

Four pathways of social interchange can now be described taken by those with 1) positive evaluation of self-image and perceived high rewards relative to costs; 2) positive evaluation and perceived low rewards; 3) negative evaluation and perceived high rewards; and 4) negative evaluation and perceived low rewards (Figure 14–2). The end point of these processes, when foreclosure does not occur, is the acceptance of the self-image: "I probably am a lesbian/gay man" (accompanied by positive or negative affect).

In *Pathway 1* the positive outlook and perceptions allow individuals to begin to recognize the personal value of lesbians and gay men and homosexuality, and correspondingly, the lack of personal relevance of heterosexuality. This leads to the understanding of self as "I probably am a lesbian/gay [positive evaluation]/probably am not heterosexual." However, those people with positive feelings toward themselves who anticipate costly results from holding a lesbian or gay account of self *(Pathway 2)* attempt to inhibit those overt and covert behaviors considered lesbian or gay in order to be able to reject the self-image of "may be a lesbian" or "may be a gay man." When this is difficult to do, the help of mental health practitioners may be enlisted. If successful, foreclosure will occur. If unsuccessful, the individual will conclude, "I probably am a lesbian/gay man [some degree of negative evaluation]" and adopt strategies to discount or lessen personal responsibility for his or her actions.

In *Pathway 3* attempts are made to deal with this personal conflict by finding ways of making the lesbian or gay account of themselves more palatable. This is done by placing the self-image of "may be a lesbian" or "may be a gay man" into frameworks that allow for an assessment of self as *potentially* heterosexual. There are four such frameworks: *special case* ("If not for this special person whom I love, I would be heterosexual"); *bisexual* ("I can also enjoy relationships with members of the opposite sex if I meet someone I really like"); *temporary* ("I'm just thinking or acting this way [homosexual] for now"); and *personal innocence* ("It's not my fault I've been made this way; with help I could be heterosexual"). *Bisexual* is used in this context as a strategy for reducing the sense of alienation and is distinct from the process of bisexual identity formation. If any of these strategies are successfully carried out, individuals make a partial commitment to the self-image: "I probably am *(partly)* a homosexual/probably not *(entirely)* heterosexual," and they feel less negative about the lesbian or gay account of themselves. If unsuccessfully applied, individuals are forced to move toward acceptance of the self-understanding, "probably a homosexual/probably not heterosexual," with accompanying negative affect.

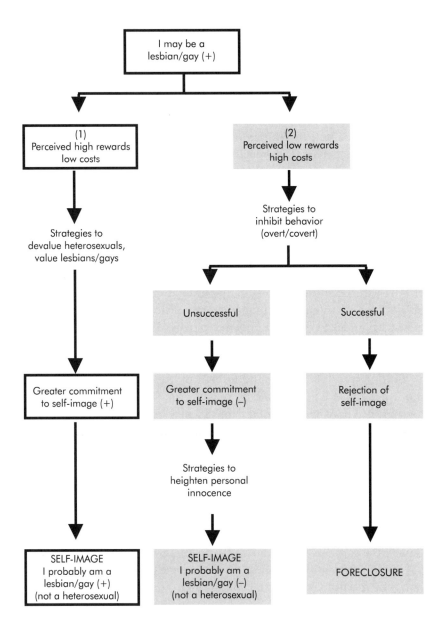

Figure 14–2.   Stage 2 pathways of lesbian/gay identity formation.

In *Pathway 4* there is a move to inhibit all behaviors leading to the understanding of self as "maybe lesbian" or "maybe gay," and these actions are reinforced by devaluing homosexuality and evaluating heterosexuality positively. If successful, the account of self is rejected (foreclosure). If unsuccessful, individuals are forced to accept the self-image of "probably lesbian" or "probably gay" (with increased negative evaluation of self), typically holding extreme levels of self-hatred that may lead to suicide or self-mutilation.

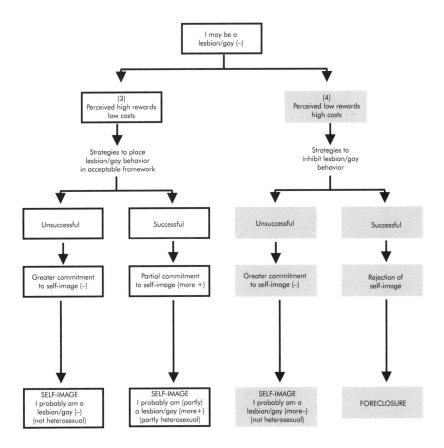

Figure 14–2.   Stage 2 pathways of lesbian/gay identity formation. *(continued)*

■ Stage 3—Identity Tolerance

At Stage 3, three groups of people acknowledge, "I probably am a lesbian/gay man": those who perceive this account as desirable, those who consider it undesirable, and those who feel fairly positive about themselves by adopting the "probably (partly) a lesbian" or "probably (partly) a gay man" account.

Freed from the previous search for an explanation of themselves, individuals at Stage 3 become more focused on social, sexual, and emotional needs that arise from seeing self as probably homosexual. This leads to considered disclosure of their self-image to some others in an attempt to have these needs fulfilled. All actions are guided, however, by awareness of the difference between self as a likely member of a group that is given negative minority status in society and members of the (valued) heterosexual majority with whom they interact. This sense of the heterosexual Goliath residing powerfully over the homosexual David/Dianne leads to an account of self that is couched in a context of *tolerance* of self. Needing to increase self-esteem and to reduce the intensity of alienation feelings, individuals begin to focus on making contact with other lesbians and gay men.

As attempts are made to juggle personal needs within this framework of tolerance, shifts begin to occur in the way individuals perceive themselves. For those who do not foreclose at Stage 3, the self-account "I *am* a homosexual/gay/lesbian" emerges. The quality of social contacts made with others is a vital factor in the development of this understanding. *Positive* social interchanges provide further evidence of the benefits of accounting for self as lesbian or gay, while *negative* ones are indicative of the high costs that may accompany such an identity. However, even negative contacts with others can have some benefits—for example, hearing positive attitudes about a homosexual sexual orientation—and with time there is increased likelihood of having positive experiences.

Six pathways are available to those who hold 1) a positive account of self as probably lesbian or gay and experience positive contacts, 2) a positive account and negative contacts, 3) a negative account of self and positive contacts, 4) a negative account and negative contacts, 5) a positive account of self as partly lesbian or gay and positive contacts, and 6) a positive account as partly lesbian or gay and negative contacts (Figures 14–3A and 14–3B). Although *Pathway 1* leads to increasing acceptance of the self-image, "I am a gay man/lesbian," *Pathway 2* highlights the personal costs of adopting an understanding of self as lesbian

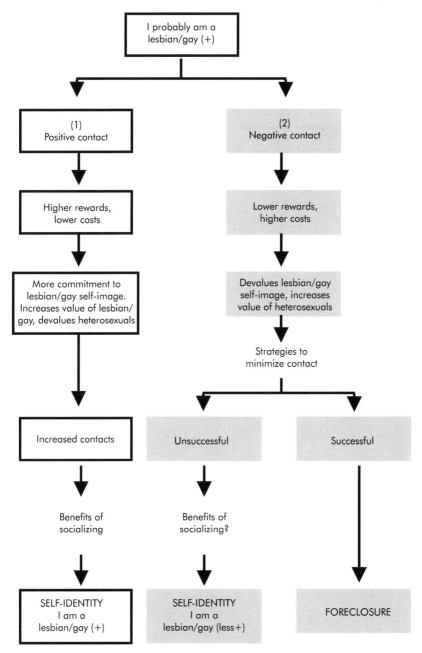

Figure 14–3A.   Stage 3 pathways (1–4) of lesbian or gay identity formation.

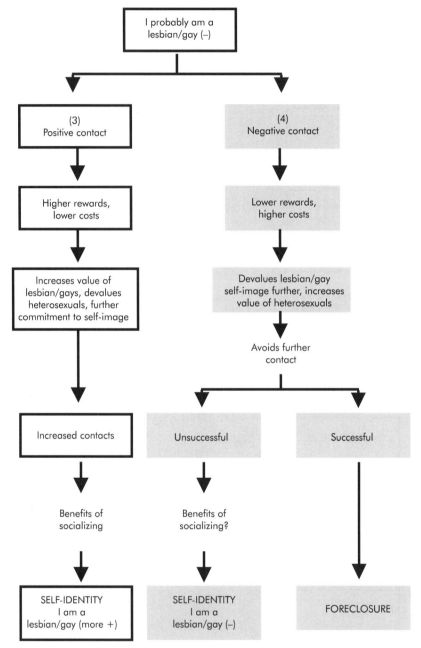

Figure 14–3A. Stage 3 pathways (1–4) of lesbian or gay identity formation. *(continued)*

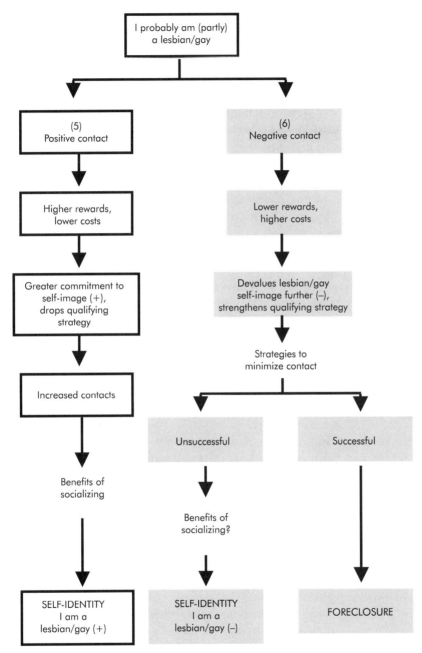

Figure 14–3B.   Stage 3 pathways (5 and 6) of lesbian or gay identity formation.

or gay. Strategies are adopted to minimize contact and devalue homosexuality so as to disengage from this account of self. If successful, foreclosure occurs. If unsuccessful, an understanding of self as lesbian or
gay emerges that is evaluated less positively than previously.

Similarly, in *Pathway 3* the negativity of the "probably lesbian"
or "probably gay" self-understanding is lessened by positive contacts
with others, leading to an acceptance that "I am lesbian/gay [more
positive evaluation]." On the other hand, the layering of negative
experiences on an already negative view of self, as seen in *Pathway 4,*
leads to strategies to avoid further contacts and, if successful, leads
to foreclosure. If not, a negative understanding of self as lesbian or
gay emerges that may be modified if positive contacts with others
are experienced.

For those individuals who had previously adopted the strategy of
partly lesbian or gay, positive contacts *(Pathway 5)* lead to a greater
commitment to self as a lesbian or gay man without use of the qualifier.
However, negative contacts will lead to a devaluation of homosexuality
(Pathway 6) and renewed efforts to maintain the existing account of self
as partly lesbian or gay. If these strategies are successful, foreclosure
occurs. If not, a somewhat negative account of self as lesbian or gay is
adopted.

■ Stage 4—Identity Acceptance

At the beginning of Stage 4 we see individuals who have come to
understand themselves as lesbian or gay and hold varying degrees
of acceptance in regard to this self-account. However, although the
perception of self is clearly formed, the *inner sense of self as lesbian or
gay* is still tenuous. Given that individuals at this point are en-
trenched in the societal belief that heterosexuality is where power
and acceptability lie, it is not surprising that little internalization of
this experience of self has occurred. During the processes that make
up the remaining stages, this inner sense of self as a lesbian or gay
person emerges.

With increasing and continued contact with other lesbians and gay
men, more and more people come to identify the individual as lesbian
or gay, and this encourages a stronger sense of being that kind of person. There is also increased disclosure to selected nonhomosexuals,
and this broadens the network of people who reinforce the lesbian or
gay understanding of self. These processes allow homosexuality and

homosexuals to be valued more positively, leading to a belief that "gays are just as good as straights." The power of heterosexuality is diffused at a personal level by the individual seeing homosexuality to be equally valid. The sense of oppression that comes from seeing oneself as a member of an "out group" is offset by these shifts, and the *tolerance* of Stage 3 is changed to *acceptance.*

For many people this stage is characterized by a sense of peace and fulfillment. Provided there is a continuation in the patterns of interaction that support the lesbian or gay understanding of self and that allow individuals to fit in with their sociocultural environment, a settled and stable account of self results. When negative reactions toward homosexuality are anticipated, the status quo is maintained by the use of strategies of deliberate passing as heterosexual, selective disclosure (carefully choosing to disclose one's identity to those likely to be supportive and prepared to uphold the individual's desire for secrecy in certain situations), and limited contact (keeping contact with unsupportive people to a minimum).

Where carried out successfully *(Pathway 1)*, individuals become buffered from the negativity or oppression of society and are able to account for themselves—"I am a lesbian/gay man and happily accept this; I can live with the minority status that goes with this identity"—a stance that is reinforced by a belief that being a lesbian or gay man is a private matter. However, when individuals cannot or will not maintain these strategies *(Pathway 2)*, their minority status is fully experienced ("I accept myself as homosexual, but when others don't I feel awful"). The need to resolve this inconsistency between self and others and to protect one's self-esteem from the heightened sense of alienation leads to the interactional processes found at Stage 5.

■ Stage 5—Identity Pride

At Stage 5 individuals enter interactions with others aware of the difference between their own total acceptance of themselves and the rejection of this self by the sociocultural environment in which they live. They recognize that the desire to fully express a lesbian or gay identity is made extremely difficult because of the dominant focus on heterosexuality.

A "them and us" attitude results in which the scales are tilted away from the position of Stage 4, in which homosexuality and heterosexuality were rated equal. Heterosexuality is markedly devalued, and homosexuality is given preferred status. The world is now divided into credible or significant lesbians and gays and discredited or devalued heterosexuals. Interactions with the latter are limited, heterosexuals are rejected as a legitimate reference group, and the perceived ideological base on which heterosexuality rests in Western society is attacked. A lesbian or gay account of self is the *preferred* identity. Individuals immerse themselves in the gay and lesbian subculture and experience a strong sense of group identification, expressed in feelings of pride, loyalty, and companionship.

The combination of pride and anger is empowering and leads to the abandonment of strategies to deliberately pass as heterosexual, although nonconcealment may be used as a compromise strategy. However, when thwarted in the drive toward validation as a lesbian or gay man, confrontation results. Lesbian or gay identity has now become a public pronouncement that is at odds with the ideological and moral framework of the sociocultural world in which it emerged. Two pathways are available as individuals process the reactions to their confrontational interactions with others. Those who receive consistently negative reactions take this as predictable evidence that the "them and us" understanding of the world is correct *(Pathway 1)*. Feelings of oppression and anger are increased, and heterosexuality is further devalued. The status quo is maintained and foreclosure occurs. For those who receive positive reactions to their confrontational actions *(Pathway 2)*, the clear division between them and us cannot be easily upheld. If such reactions are consistent or significant, these bring an incongruent element into the picture, and this element is processed in Stage 6.

◼ Stage 6—Identity Synthesis

When personal and ideological understanding of homosexuality is accepted by at least some heterosexuals, the simplistic belief that divided the world into "good" lesbians and gay men and "bad" heterosexuals is rejected (although opposition to heterosexuality as an ideology may still be upheld). Supportive heterosexuals are reevaluated positively and nonsupportive ones further devalued. This has the effect of increasing the network of others with whom the individual interacts positively as a lesbian or gay man. The level of anger, alienation, and frustration is lessened as the "enemy" is reduced in number at a personal level. Issues of oppression are now addressed in a less defensive manner and the level of identification with the lesbian or gay group seen in Stage 5 is reduced.

Interacting with others as openly lesbian or gay at an increasingly public level deepens and strengthens the inner psychological experience of identity. There is a sense of belonging to the world at large and of being "more than just a lesbian or gay man." Accounting for self as lesbian or gay is now an integrated part of the whole self and reinforces self-esteem and position in the world. This stance will be maintained as the individual's life continues in this way from day to day, unless something occurs to bring the focus back toward an image of the self as a member of the lesbian or gay group. Strategies will then be adopted to restore the individual's sense of being an independent, functioning person who is capable of being in control of his or her life.

The end points of "wholeness" and "personhood" achieved in Stage 6 are directed by the current Western indigenous psychology, driven by notions of individuality, self-actualization, personal maturity, development, and other concepts that form the cornerstone of our thinking.

Implications for Counseling and Psychotherapy

The model described above provides mental health practitioners with a number of counseling guidelines. First, care must be taken when talking with clients to use terms that are appropriate to the stage of identity formation into which they appear to fit. Describing someone as *being* gay, lesbian, or bisexual, for example, is quite inappropriate when the client is actually saying, "I'm confused about what I'm *doing*" (Stage 1) or "I might be . . ." (beginning of Stage 2).

Second, clients should be accepted as being in the stage they describe themselves to be, not where the counselor wants them to be. An 18-year-old woman, for example, who happily claims, "I'm a lesbian," (end of Stage 3 and onward) should not be told, "You're too young to know," because identity formation is already in progress.

Third, the theory indicates that there is a huge difference between behaving in a homosexual way and feeling oneself to be a lesbian or gay man. Behavior does not indicate the existence of identity, for example, as seen in prison situations. On the other hand, lack of apparent homosexual behavior does not indicate a lack of identity. People may proceed through the early stages of identity formation without ever having any sexual or emotional contact with another person (covert behaviors such as fantasies and bodily responses often provide the impetus to entering Stage 1).

Fourth, people who describe themselves via reference to lesbian or gay behaviors or identity should not be treated as identical on the basis of these characteristics. Both within and between stages, considerable differences may be apparent. The theory accommodates distinctions such as may be found between men and women and among different ethnic and religious groups. Practitioners need to take time to explore where clients may be in the process of identity formation, rather than to assume the label "homosexual/lesbian/gay" provides all the information they need.

Fifth, the theory indicates the importance of appropriate contacts with other lesbians and gay men. Mental health practitioners need to work with personal, social, and cultural issues that may prevent clients from making such contact successfully or at the appropriate time.

Sixth, identifying the stage at which clients are currently functioning allows the mental health professional to focus on the particular issues of that stage, rather than addressing homosexuality in general. For example, talking about the ideological aspects of lesbian and gay oppression is inappropriate when someone feels he or she has no future (Stage 2) or wants to meet other homosexuals (Stage 3).

Seventh, counselors should not judge any stage as better than other stages, or any individual as better than any other because his or her feelings and behaviors correspond with any particular stage. Our ideas about identity formation are guided by Western indigenous concepts such as maturity and self-actualization, and the practitioner must be alert to imposing clinical and personal judgment on clients who are in the early stages.

Finally, it is important to remember that homosexual identity formation does not occur in isolation from other processes and issues taking place. Coping with illness, aging, career changes, marriage, issues of ethnic difference, family dynamics, psychological dysfunction, and moving to another country are all examples of personal, social, and cultural factors that may interact with the development of an understanding of self as gay, lesbian, or bisexual. For example, a client in psychotherapy had great difficulty coping with the thought that she might be a lesbian because a childhood history of being teased for having large ears had left her sensitized to being alienated and isolated. Her identity formation experiences had raised to the surface all the pain of those early experiences so that past and present had become indistinguishable. Another client, who was 19 years old, had just left home for the first time, and was beginning to separate emotionally from an overprotective family. As part of this process, he had told his parents he was gay and was attempting to cope with their rejection of his homosexuality. The client then became HIV positive, which quickly progressed to AIDS. Working with him required an understanding of the intricate intertwining of homosexual identity formation, developing adulthood, and adjustment to illness and death.

The mental health practitioner should be mindful of the existence of complexities such as these and be aware that experienced therapeutic intervention is required.

Conclusion

The theory of homosexual identity formation can be a useful tool for understanding and helping individuals in Western cultures who confront the concept of gay, lesbian, or bisexual in a personal way. However, we should not forget that what is being addressed is a *process* of interaction, not a set of stagnant categories. Reference to stages is useful inasmuch as it allows us to recognize significant shifts occurring in individual cognitions and interactional relationships.

Nor should we forget the constructed nature of lesbian or gay identity formation. Because the indigenous psychologies directing our notion of identity formation can vary over time, we need to be alert to future shifts and changes that may occur in our Western sexual realities.

We must also be sensitive to cultural differences—for example, recognizing when discussion of sexual orientation identity is inappropriate with people from other cultures and being sensitive to the complexity of mixed-culture couples. Care must be taken to avoid presenting the concept of gay, lesbian, or bisexual identity as a universal norm, or the concept sexual orientation as necessarily being fixed. It is curious how often examples of behaviors that do not fit Western beliefs about sexual orientation will present themselves to the attentive mental health worker.

Nevertheless, while keeping in mind the larger cultural picture, we must also be able to accept that our clients often wish to hold on tightly to their essentialist beliefs. This need to balance the essentialist and constructed qualities of sexual orientation can create dilemmas for the mental health practitioner. Do we, as caring professionals, empathize with our clients' essentialist experiences of being lesbian, gay, or bisexual as the truth they hold about themselves (but contribute to maintenance of the ideological status quo); encourage them to abandon or change their beliefs related to the fixed nature of sexual orientation and sexual orientation identities (but deny the reinforcing qualities of sexual response and risk rejecting our clients' experiences); or try some kind of balancing trick between the two?

Unfortunately, there are no easy solutions to this dilemma, which itself has become a new element of our psychological reality. Indeed, the mental health professional must avoid grabbing at quick answers. We live in dynamic times. The theoretical grounds on which we work are being questioned, and our indigenous psychology, which continues to evolve, demands our attention. It would seem more important that we remain open to these changes and the discussion they generate, rather than become too quickly embroiled in the need to find simple solutions.

References

Bond M (Ed): The Cross-Cultural Challenge to Social Psychology. Newbury Park, CA, Sage, 1988

Cass V: Homosexual identity formation: a theoretical model. J Homosex 4:219–235, 1979

Cass V: Homosexual identity formation: testing a theoretical model. J Sex Res 20:143–167, 1984

Cass V: Homosexual identity formation: the presentation and testing of a socio-cognitive model. Unpublished doctoral dissertation, Murdoch University, Perth, Western Australia, 1985

Cass V: The implications of homosexual identity formation for the Kinsey model and scale of sexual preference, in Homosexuality/Heterosexuality: Concepts of Sexual Orientation. Edited by McWhirter D, Sanders S, Reinisch R. New York, Oxford University Press, 1990, pp 239–266

Coleman E: Developmental stages of the coming out process. J Homosex 7:31–43, 1981–2

Gergen K: The social constructionist movement in modern psychology. American Psychologist 40:266–275, 1985

Heelas P, Lock A (eds): Indigenous Psychologies: The Anthropology of the Self. London, Academic Press, 1981

Malyon A: Biphasic aspects of homosexual identity formation. Psychotherapy Theory, Research and Practice 19:335–340, 1982

Minton H, McDonald G: Homosexual identity formation as a developmental process. J Homosex 9:91–104, 1983–4

Plummer K: Sexual Stigma: An Interactionist Account. London, Routledge and Kegan Paul, 1975

Ponse B: Identities in the Lesbian World: The Social Construction of the Self. London, Greenwood Press, 1978

Raphael S: "Coming out": the emergence of the movement lesbian. Unpublished doctoral dissertation, Case Western Reserve University, Cleveland, Ohio, 1974

Schafer S: Sexual and social problems of lesbians. J Sex Res 12:50–69, 1976

Schippers J: Homosexual identity, essentialism and constructionism, in Homosexuality, Which Homosexuality? Edited by Altman D, et al. London, GMP Publishers, 1989, pp 139–148

Semin G, Gergen K (eds): Everyday Understanding: Social and Scientific Implications. London, Sage, 1990

Shotter J: The rhetorical-responsive nature of mind: a social constructionist account, in Against Cognitivism: Alternative Foundations for Cognitive Psychology. Edited by Still A, Costall A. New York, Harvester Wheatsheaf, 1991, pp 55–79

Shweder R, LeVine R (eds): Culture Theory: Essays on Mind, Self and Emotion. Cambridge, MA, Cambridge University Press, 1992

Stein E (ed): Forms of Desire: Sexual Orientation and the Social Constructionist Controversy. London, Routledge, 1992

Stigler J, Shweder R, Herdt G (eds): Cultural Psychology: Essays on Comparative Human Development. Cambridge, MA, Cambridge University Press, 1992

Troiden R: Becoming homosexual: a model of gay identity acquisition. Psychiatry 42:362–373, 1979

Weinberg T: Gay Men, Gay Selves: The Social Construction of Homosexual Identities. New York, Irvington Publishers, 1983

15

Latency Development in Prehomosexual Boys

Graeme Hanson, M.D.
Lawrence Hartmann, M.D.

T his chapter focuses on certain aspects of the early childhood development of boys who may be or will later become bisexual or homosexual. It is a cautionary chapter. Not much is known, yet many professionals and lay people assume that much is known. The scientific inquiry into the early childhood development of homosexual individuals is still in its infancy. Moreover, much of the literature in the mid-20th century was based on retrospective reconstructions derived from memories of adult patients in psychotherapy or analysis—a highly interesting, complex, and potentially triply biased sample. Also much of the data were collected and reported by clinicians who defined homosexuality as a disorder or a developmental arrest, and they gathered data through that filter, introducing a fourth and different kind of bias.

Some scientific studies of the developmental aspects of homosexuality have been done in the past 10 years, but they have been primarily studies of males. There is an even greater lack of information on the early development of lesbians. Rather than viewing female development, openly or implicitly, as a mere variant of or reaction to male development (which was unfortunately common until relatively recently [Gilligan 1982, Chehrazi 1984]), in this chapter the authors focus frankly on the development of boys who may be or will later become homosexual or bisexual, and there is no attempt to extrapolate to the childhood development of lesbians—about which one can hope there will soon be more data and theory.

A Developmental Perspective

The authors believe that nature and nurture are vital elements in the development of all humans; that maintaining a developmental perspective is crucial when therapists arrive at a formulation of any individual's current adaptation and functioning; and that an understanding of a person's development will inform any treatment plan for that person, no matter what the person's age or sexual orientation.

Beyond the interest of general knowledge of the variety of all major areas of human development, there are at least two practical reasons for trying to understand the early development of prehomosexual boys:

1. Having a clear picture of such early development will provide a better understanding for all therapists when patients explore or report memories of childhood; such reports are not necessarily accurate and may be heavily subject to cultural biases and individual defenses and distortions in patients, therapists, and nonclinical populations. It will help the therapist to know what areas to attend to in obtaining a developmental history and to be more acutely aware of dynamically determined omissions and distortions in the life stories that patients tell.

2. Perhaps of more importance, an understanding of the psychology of boys who may or will become homosexual will help parents and others who care for these children to be more sensitive to their individual strengths, plights, and needs. As the authors describe in this chapter, the life of many (no one knows even roughly how many) prehomosexual boys is fraught with conflict, self-doubt, and problems with self-esteem. These children at various developmental stages encounter subtle and unsubtle forms of rejection

and misunderstanding from their social environment and frequently from their families.

Although it is not at all possible to predict adult homosexual outcome and adaptation for most children, there are certain interests and behaviors in latency that, especially in extreme form, are associated with future homosexual adaptation. However, a significant proportion of future gay men do not exhibit these behaviors and interests as children, whereas a significant proportion of future heterosexuals do exhibit them (Baily and Zucker 1995; Bell et al. 1981; Green 1987; Harry 1982).

Human beings are best understood biopsychosocially (Engel 1977, 1979, 1980; Hartmann 1992). This is true of all people, patients and nonpatients, and it may be particularly usefully true in some areas such as homosexuality, in which it serves as a reminder that one should at present be modest about overvaluing single aspects of an interactive biopsychosocial picture. Reductionism is a danger.

Every 3- or 4- or 5-year-old boy arrives at that age with a good bit of biopsychosocial history. Psychoanalysis has tended to slight the biological and the social; current biological psychiatry tends to slight the psychological and the social. Although clinicians are now reassessing and discounting some of the extrapolations and false certainties of much mid-20th century psychoanalytical thinking about homosexual development (Friedman 1988; Lewes 1988), many psychoanalytical theories of oedipal and latency development likely apply to both prehomosexual and preheterosexual boys. So does the somewhat more behavioral and measurable transactional model of development (Sameroff and Chandler 1975), in which what infants or children bring to their environment (parents, siblings, extended family, school personnel, and so on) affects and changes that environment and produces particular responses. What children bring to their environment, in the case of prehomosexual boys, must on the basis of recent research be considered to include a significant amount of biological loading—genetic and prenatal hormonal—of relevance to sexuality. Environmental responses in turn affect and change the child, so that the child's next interaction with the environment will be different, and so on. The child is not passive but repeatedly influences and provokes responses from the environment and has a determining role in environmental responses. Back and forth, the child and parent, the child and the environment, contribute to continuing, evolving, interactive cycles of mutual influence. Behavior is the most measurable part of this cycle; however, feelings and fantasies are equally if not more important.

As an example, relatively simple and not at all rare, consider a father who was particularly invested in having a rough-and-tumble athletic son, but instead has a son who, for whatever complex biological, temperamental, and developmental reasons, is relatively passive and little interested in aggressive play or is relatively delicate or pretty; that father will probably be consciously or unconsciously disappointed in the son. The father may show his disappointment by, for example, being critical or by distancing himself from the son; this in turn affects the son's sense of himself and his relationship with his father, which then affects his subsequent attempts to interact with his father. Such transactions can lead to a troublesome cycle of increasing negativity and distancing, which may have many further consequences (many of them familiar from the clinical literature on children). The important point here is that both sides of the dyad repeatedly contribute to the interaction, transforming each other in the process.

Similarly, although a bit more complexly than two-sided interactions, oedipal development (at ages 3–5) of boys who may or will be homosexual or bisexual, like that of all boys, is in lively ways triangularly interactive with mother and father (or mother figures and father figures). It is extremely unlikely that there is one characteristic path and resolution for all prehomosexual or prebisexual boys; there are probably many. The overextrapolations of Bieber (1988), with their untenable implications of universality, have created clutter in a field in which their data regarding, for example, close-binding mothers and distant fathers might, if modestly treated, have clear usefulness in the understanding of some aspects of development in some gay men. In a similar vein, but probably even worse, the energetic pseudocertainties of Socarides (1989) about pre-oedipal and oedipal development have probably created flawed data and misinformation from which it will take scientific objectivity some time to reemerge. (See Friedman [1988] and Lewes [1988] for critical discussions of psychoanalytical theories of homosexuality.)

As mentioned above, it would be useful for many reasons to have a comprehensive understanding of the early development of boys who seem to be, or later may or will become, homosexual or bisexual. Although such study is difficult and time-consuming to undertake, there have been several important, pioneering attempts, in particular those of Bell et al. (1981), Green (1987), Harry (1982), and Isay (1989).

Except for the work of Green (1987), most of these attempts have been based on retrospective reconstructions derived from adult memories. This is a common and useful—but limited—approach, vulnerable to major inaccuracy, exaggeration, and overextrapolation. As research on memory has recently demonstrated, both childhood memories and adult memories of childhood (and suggestive memory fragments and derivatives embedded in psychoanalysis and psychotherapy) are inconsistently reliable (Loftus 1993), even in healthy people. Sometimes memories of factual events, times, and places can be validated by other sources, but such validation is often difficult to obtain. Child and adolescent psychotherapists and analysts have long learned to adapt to workable and clinically useful reconstructions and memory derivatives, including transference, without insisting on the pure truth and testability of memories. Memories of fantasies, feelings, attitudes, and other internal experiences are remarkably subject to the influences of repression, distortion, blending, contamination, wishes, fears, shame, and affective states at the time of encoding and at the time the recollection takes place; such memories are also subject to modification over time through the vicissitudes of development. Psychoanalytical case histories and theories of development have had to contend with these limitations, although in recent decades direct observations of children, testing, and building on and revising psychoanalytical ideas have added much useful data, if less in the area of childhood sexuality than in several other major areas.

Friedman (1988), in his work on male homosexuality, gave an excellent example of the ubiquitous difficulty of sifting meanings and importance in memory. He described twin men, one of whom became homosexual and the other became heterosexual. The two had strikingly different memories of their father. The heterosexual son remembered the father as being away on business a great deal; this was understood to be part of his father's work and was not taken as a personal rejection. The gay son remembered the father's absences and involvement with business as a pointed and hurtful rejection.

Long-term, wide-net prospective studies of boys and their future sexuality are needed. The one well-known, pertinent prospective study was done by Green (1987), who followed a somewhat small and relatively extreme sample of effeminate boys. Green's important research tends to confirm some of the retrospective studies that reported some correlation between particularly feminine behavior, attitudes, and identifications in early childhood and latency and the future development of homosexual adaptation. It is important to point out, as Green acknowledged, that a large but not yet clearly defined proportion of gay men do not recall, or have others who recall, feminine behavior or identification in their childhoods (Bell 1981; Isay 1989; Green 1987). Furthermore, even among boys who do exhibit such behavior and attitudes, a significant but still unknown percentage become heterosexual. The partial association of relatively extreme feminine behavior in boyhood and later homosexuality requires much more study. What other factors and mix of factors in boys influence, favor, tend to steer away from, or predict adult homosexuality are still unknown. This partial association is neither one-to-one nor a simple cause-and-effect relationship.

Prospective studies are complicated, long, and difficult to do. Yet some possible markers, such as the extreme feminine behavior and identifications that Green has usefully identified, can pragmatically identify some subgroups of boys for prospective study. Friedman (1988) suggests that a lack of traditional *masculine* interests or an aversion to rough-and-tumble play and physical conflict may be another characteristic in some boys that correlates highly with later homosexuality. This group of boys does not necessarily exhibit effeminate behaviors and could be another group for prospective study. It is likely, however, that a large portion of children who will become gay men who do not exhibit either of these two markers; it would be useful to conduct a more general prospective study to evaluate more widely what factors, and with what power, may be correlated positively or negatively with future homosexuality.

It is likely that the relatively average-looking population—in this case the heterosexual-looking or gender-conforming boys who go on to become heterosexual, gay, or bisexual—will be understudied in such research designs. Subsector research may clarify some correlated, causal, and adaptive factors but distort and underappreciate others, including some healthy and adaptive factors of sexuality and gender. Particularly likely to be ignored or understudied will be young children's sexual interests, feelings, and fantasies, as opposed to behavior, although these are important areas for study. Sexuality and presexuality are not just behavior.

There has been in the past century considerable theorizing and observation about childhood sexuality, much of it associated with psychoanalytical theory and derived from adult patients. However, especially in the realm of homosexuality, with recent data from several fields suggesting clear genetic and prenatal hormonal influence and considerable cultural and temporal influence, it is probably essential and timely to reassess with some skepticism and care psychoanalytical data and theories regarding homosexuality (Lewes 1988).

Few investigators have attempted systematic studies of the sexual lives and fantasies of young children (Friedrich et al. 1991). This seems a feasible and promising but difficult area for research, which may use and modify some psychoanalytical approaches and data. If the psychoanalytical and retrospective approach has major limitations and difficulties, the direct observation approach has its own significant problems. Children are taught, in this culture as in many cultures, both overtly and covertly, not to be sexual or not to show or act on their sexual feelings. Freud modified that climate, but there is still considerable denial and deprecation. It is clear from working with children in therapy that some will show or discuss some of their sexual thoughts and feelings with their peers and sometimes even act on them. Most show this area to their parents from time to time. However, to reveal this area to a relatively objective adult is difficult and rare for many or most children. Even trustworthy, playful, well-educated, and trained adult interviewers encounter significant denial, resistance, or flat lying about sex in otherwise largely open and honest youngsters. Moreover, many parents and clinicians think that a good bit of privacy and even denial about childhood sexuality are probably a good thing. Clearly, there are and will be many obstacles to gathering the data that would lead to a comprehensive understanding of the sexual fantasies and behavior of healthy as well as troubled children; yet such knowledge is vital to understanding the developmental patterns of childhood sexuality and the correlation between earlier fantasies and behaviors and later sexual orientation.

Latency Development

When the psychology of latency children who may or will become homosexual or bisexual is discussed, it is potentially useful to review certain developmental tasks of the latency period that are potentially helpful or problematic for these children. By age 2 to 3, almost all children have developed a clear, stable core gender identity: they know and feel they are male or female. Note that this is *gender identity* ("I am male or female") and is not the same as, although often confused with, *gender of object choice* ("I am attracted to the same or the other gender or to both genders"), which arrives and solidifies more slowly. Whereas gender and some gender roles are a stable reality for nearly all 3- or 5- or 8-year-olds, gender of sexual object choice for a child that age is probably to a large extent still in the realm of pale, variable, future-oriented, and only partly integrated fantasies, with varying levels of consciousness, certainty, and comfort.

An important change that takes place in early latency is a gradual but important shift in interest from the immediate sphere of the family to the world outside and to school and an increasing interest in the society of children. Children of elementary school age routinely begin to value or take into account the evaluation of themselves by their peers. Self concept is increasingly influenced by peer interaction and opinion. A child is no longer above all the 4-year-old in a family but now is one of many similar children in a group. Latency children also begin to elaborate their self concepts in a more complex way, now including social markers such as "I am a second-grader," or "I live in this or that neighborhood," or "I am of this or that group or ethnic/religious/cultural background." With peer comparisons, individual physical and mental characteristics also take on important meanings in evolving self concepts. For example, "I am short or tall, thin or fat," "I have red hair, freckles," "I am left-handed," and "I am good at kickball or arithmetic," can be important identifiers of the child by the social group as well as by the child. Of these social markers, the gender role as viewed by the child's particular society becomes a very important part of the developing child's sense of himself or herself.

In spite of sometimes valiant attempts in some subcultures to minimize the many nonessential differences between the sexes, in almost all cultures elementary school age boys and girls tend to separate into monosexual groupings for many play and social activities. Some adult and peer expectations of each gender's behavior and attitudes—gender role—are clear to the child and reinforced by the play group. In many settings, those boys who are relatively feminine in their behavior and attitudes (Green 1987) or who are less masculine but not necessarily effeminate (Friedman 1988) will be different from the norm. Some but not all gender-atypical children will at this point gravitate to opposite-sex playmates. Elementary school children are keenly aware of where they and their peers fit in the continuum of expectable and acceptable behavior, which may, at different levels of precision and importance in different groups, include gender role and gender-role–

labeled behavior. For the effeminate or less than traditionally masculine boy, this can be a time of anxiety or anguish because he is self-aware enough to know or feel he is in some ways different and not, or not quite, "one of the boys." There are many other reasons to feel not quite one of the boys, but sense of one's gender role seems to be one of the large, simple, final-seeming common paths for such ideas and feelings that one is a bit, or more than a bit, different.

Some children will reassure themselves that being different is not a bad thing or will develop a view that they are somehow special. Some may develop special talents, including musical, artistic, leadership, or theatrical, which become evident in latency and are often powerful forces in the developing child's social life as well as his or her internal sense of self. Also, given the continuing changes of childhood, the degree to which a difference is fixed usually takes a long time to determine and to be reasonably sure of. Adjustment to repeated particular situations depends on the child's prior and continuing development of self-esteem and on the parents' ability to provide reassurance and support, consciously or unconsciously, for this child. Because parents' social expectations of their latency child have both unique and societally determined features, one parent or both will often see the child as different from the norm, may interpret different as worse or wrong or as a precursor of badness, and may be worried, disappointed, critical, or rejecting.

The ego-ideal system has particular importance in latency. This is a time in life when children idealize certain heroes and heroines and elaborate more sophisticated fantasies of what they want to become when they grow up. Not uncommonly there is some group consensus and mutual sharing of these heroes and ego-ideal representations. If the prehomosexual boy has an ego-ideal figure different from the group consensus—such as a less aggressive, less conventionally masculine, or evenly overtly feminine one, or in some circles an artistic or scientific ideal rather than a sports hero—he may be subject to misunderstanding and sometimes disapproval, ridicule, and ostracism. Here parent availability, understanding, support, and encouragement can be most important. Some parents may usefully obtain professional help in working through their own conflicts regarding their child's "difference" or uniqueness.

To ego-ideal problems may be added problems in identifying with parents. It is likely to seem clear to many late latency and early adolescent children who are struggling not just with nontraditional or

non-gender-conforming ego ideals but with more explicitly sexual issues that their parents are in most cases not homosexual and that they
(the children) are therefore perhaps different in a profound and lasting
way from their parents. (Caution is in order again at this point because
many preheterosexual boys in adolescence have ideas from time to time
that they are or may be bisexual or homosexual.)

Early Experience and Feeling Different

Many gay men acknowledge that they felt different from a very early
age. Some claim that it began as far back as they can remember—age
2, 3, or 4; others far later; and still others that the feelings of being
different began early but that being "sexually different" came much
later. Sometimes the feeling of differentness was difficult to define (Bell
et al. 1981; Green 1987; Isay 1989). It may often be that the awareness
of fewer culturally defined masculine interests or identifications, or
more culturally defined feminine interests or identifications, is central.
In many cases a sexual differentness may not matter most, but in some
cases a sense of unusually strong sexual interest in other men accounts
for some of this early sense of differentness. Some adult gay men clearly
remember being strongly attracted to men as very young boys, with a
special erotic and excited interest in other male bodies. How many gay
men experience that, or for that matter, how many heterosexual men
do, is not known; later conscious and unconscious denial and distortion
make this difficult to study. A feeling that "somehow I am different" is
probably a significant factor for many prehomosexual and prebisexual
latency boys. Yet most boys at that age would be unlikely to be sophisticated enough (and so focused on sexual object choice as a stable or
central factor in themselves) that they would label themselves clearly
as gay or bisexual.

Certainly the most extremely effeminate boys, or even the not quite
traditionally masculine group, are often teased and derided by peers
and adults. The word "sissy" is an emotionally powerful, well-known
term of derision for these boys. It probably gains some of its strength
by confusion with "childish," "weak," "younger than your age," and this
confusion is generally less prominent with girls who show non-gender-
conforming behavior in latency than with boys who do so. Boys called
"sissies" often have few ways to express their distress about being different and about being teased. Some respond to social pressure by

increasing gender-conforming behavior, with or without consciously conflicted feelings. Others respond with some lowering of self-esteem, depression, and lowered ability to interact with, enjoy, and learn from peers.

Not infrequently the people to whom such boys would turn for adult support and comfort—their parents—may also be uncomfortable with, and lack understanding of, the child's being different. This can result in cumulative unfortunate and difficult circumstances. Parents often feel justified in demanding that such children "shape up." (That is a position justified by the earlier 20th-century assumption that homosexuality was not biological and was relatively easily changeable; however, it is a position called into serious question, if not yet fully invalidated, by the late–20th-century view that much of homosexuality is relatively fixed probably early on.) In addition, these boys are victims of misunderstanding and prejudice, but unlike other child victims of prejudice, many of them are not able to turn to their families for reassurance, support, and group identification.

Additionally, in latency, religious beliefs and commitments sometimes become important, and a boy whose religion flatly opposes homosexuality will have an additional powerful factor contributing to his struggle. All these factors result in a greater sense of isolation and a sense of not being understood or validated as a human being. Some of these boys will keep their thoughts and feelings quite secret on the basis of guilt, shame, or fear of ridicule. Having to, or feeling one has to, keep a secret from peers and family members results in a certain interference with trust of oneself, the development of a "social self," and growth and development in general. These effects can be carried forward into adulthood as a lifelong view of interpersonal relationships consisting of a kind of transference wariness or distrust of self and others that the young man will bring to future relationships.

Some prehomosexual boys, in trying to be accepted, make extraordinary efforts to conceal what they sense to be forbidden interests and wishes. This is not simply a conscious deception, but part and parcel of the average latency-age child's struggle to grow and mature, to master the requisite developmental steps, and to do what parents, peers, school, and culture expect. Some of these children, as they grow into later latency, become so successful at suppressing, denying, and disavowing aspects of their internal experience—especially in the realms of non-gender-conforming wishes and sexualized fantasies, including fantasies of other men—that they convince themselves they are indeed changing into more gender-conforming, or heterosexual, people. How frequent and real such changes are would be important to learn. Deep change seems, in the authors' experience, extremely rare and perhaps nonexistent, but more research would be central to determining how to help such children and their families to be as happy and effective as they can be.

Suppressing or disavowing parts of the self often results in a mental splitting-off of a part of the self, and in some boys this functions so firmly that it becomes part of the overall character. They go through life with the assumption that an important part of themselves has to be kept separate and not integrated into their self concept or the view others have of them. Such an assumption of unintegrability may be particularly prevalent among prehomosexual boys and homosexual men who, often from latency on, make attempts to develop a heterosexual adaptation and more or less fail. A good many such men marry and have families and not uncommonly in midlife come to a decision, consciously or unconsciously, to heal the split and integrate their homosexuality into the rest of their lives.

This sense of being different, the feeling of not being capable of being understood, the internal isolation that some of these children feel during an important developmental period may contribute to the rather assertive stance that some gay men take as adults in current American society (and differently in other cultures and eras) in announcing themselves. Their call for recognition and acceptance is in many cases not just an adult social and political statement, but at least partly it is an attempt to gain the recognition and personal validation that had been denied them in childhood.

One should point out that for some or many prehomosexual children, parents are supportive, encouraging, and proud of their child's accomplishments and ways of being in most areas, and the child's overall sense of self and self-esteem may be solid or not unduly damaged. It is not unlikely, however, that the parts of the self involved with sexual attraction and future love relationships remain at risk and affected.

The social and cultural environment for gay men in the United States in the late 20th century has been evolving, in some areas probably parallel to and sometimes following a decrease in sexism in general. In some communities it is now possible for young adolescents who are becoming increasingly aware of their possible or probable homosexuality or bisexuality to find opportunities for open discussion of these issues and to find role models among gay men—all of which can be very helpful in the elaboration of an integrated adult identity. Some, but for many reasons less, of this flexible acceptance and support of variety, including gayness, is probably trickling down to latency boys. The "love that dare not speak its name" can now be spoken of in a good many places with adolescents, and sometimes even with children. (The caption of a recent popular cartoon depicting a child at bedtime prayer read something like, "And God bless Mommy and Daddy and Uncle Bill and his roommate, Jack, who we're not supposed to talk about.") Increasingly, there is more education, understanding, and honesty among adults regarding homosexuality, which is likely to facilitate the more successful development and identity-consolidation for prehomosexual, prebisexual, and preheterosexual boys. Education, use of scapegoats, and tolerance for variety vary greatly among subcultures of society, however, and according to several recent polls, most Americans still disapprove of homosexuality so much that they do not want it to be considered as an acceptable "lifestyle."

Conclusion

In sum, one of the few areas that seems clear about prehomosexual boys is that one of the most important aspects of latency development for many of them is the psychology of feeling or being different—different in a way that is often inexplicable both to the child and to the environment, and perhaps different in a way that sets one apart from one's parents.

The typical latency-age child increasingly develops a sense of being both a public and a private individual. Usually even the private or mental life is to a considerable extent consistent with a socially acceptable model. For the boy who is aware of being different, his unacceptable part usually has to be split off, adaptively sometimes but also with potential interferences with integration and development. Coping with difference is a major stressful task for many or most prehomosexual latency boys.

References

Baily JM, Zucker KJ: Childhood sex-typed behavior and sexual orientation: a conceptual analysis. Developmental Psychology 31:43–55, 1995

Bell AP, Weinberg MS, Hammersmith SL: Sexual Preference: Its Development in Men and Women. Bloomington, IN, Indiana University, 1981

Bieber I: Homosexuality: A Psychoanalytic Study. Northvale, NJ, Jason Aronson, 1988

Chehrazi S: Female psychology: a review. J Am Psychoanal Assoc 34:141–162, 1984

Engel GL: The need for a new model: a challenge for biomedicine. Science 196:129–136, 1977

Engel GL: The biopsychosocial model and the education of health professions. Gen Hosp Psychiatry 1:156–165, 1979

Engel GL: The clinical application of the biopsychosocial model. Am J Psychiatry 137:535–543, 1980

Friedman RC: Male Homosexuality: A Contemporary Psychoanalytic Perspective. New Haven, CT, Yale University Press, 1988

Friedrich WN, Grambsch P, Broughton D, et al: Normative sexual behavior in children. Pediatrics 88:456–464, 1991

Gilligan C: A Different Voice. Cambridge, MA, Harvard University Press, 1982

Green R: The "Sissy Boy Syndrome" and the Development of Homosexuality. New Haven, CT, Yale University Press, 1987

Harry J: Gay Children Grown Up: Gender, Culture and Gender Deviance. New York, Praeger, 1982

Hartmann L: Presidential address: reflections on humane values and biopsychosocial integration. Am J Psychiatry 149:1135–1141, 1992

Isay BA: Being Homosexual: Gay Men and Their Development. New York, Farrar, Strauss and Giroux, 1989

Lewes K: The Psychoanalytic Theory of Male Homosexuality. New York, Simon and Schuster, 1988

Loftus E: The reality of repressed memories. Am Psychol 48:518–537, 1993

Sameroff AJ, Chandler MJ: Reproductive risk and the continuum of caretaking casualty, in Review of Child Development Research, Vol 4. Edited by Horowitz FD, et al. Chicago, IL, University of Chicago Press, 1975, pp 231–237

Socarides CW: Homosexuality: Psychoanalytic Therapy. Northvale, NJ, Jason Aronson, 1989

16

Lesbian, Gay, and Bisexual Development During Adolescence and Young Adulthood

Anthony R. D'Augelli, Ph.D.

Estimating the number of adolescents and young adults who are lesbian, gay, or bisexual is difficult because of the multidimensional aspects of sexual identity and its complex developmental progression. Several large-scale studies have investigated same-sex interests among adults, and their results have implications for prevalence among youth. For instance, one recent international study found that between 8.6% and 11.1% of females and 7.9% and 8.7% of males report same-sex attraction after age 15 (Sell et al. 1995). These researchers estimate that as many as 18% of females and 21% of males in the United States experience either same-sex attraction or behavior after age 15. With the use of results from a large probability sample of American adults, Laumann et al. (1994) found lower figures, with 7.7% of males and 7.5% of females indicating homoerotic interest or attraction after puberty. Many of the participants in these projects surely experienced homoerotic feelings before puberty or young adult-

267

hood. Unfortunately, data about homoeroticism before puberty are not available. In addition, obtaining reports about sexual orientation even from high school-age youths is problematic. On the basis of a large (over 36,000) study of junior and senior high school students in Minnesota, Remafedi et al. (1992) found that 11% were "unsure" of their sexual orientation; only about 1% labeled themselves lesbian, gay, or bisexual. However, 4.5% of the entire sample and 6.4% of the 18-year-old individuals in the sample reported same-sex attraction. Another study, of university men seeking routine medical care at a campus clinic, found that 11% identified themselves as bisexual (4%) or gay (7%) (Wiesmeier et al. 1986). Because the information in this study was not obtained anonymously, it is reasonable to assume that others in the study also were gay but would not acknowledge it.

The results from these studies suggest that as many as 15% of youth may experience nonheterosexual emotional and sexual attractions. Fewer engage in same-sex sexual activity, and far fewer identify themselves publicly as lesbian, gay, or bisexual. The tremendous stigma associated with homoerotic desire, action, and identity is even more pronounced among adolescents than among adults. A recent study of harassment in American high schools found that the type of harassment considered most upsetting was to be called gay (American Association of University Women 1993). A national survey of male teenagers aged 15–19 found that 89% thought the idea of homosexual sexual activity to be "disgusting," and only 12% were certain they could befriend an openly gay male (Marsiglio 1993). In addition, the stigma associated with same-sex sexual behavior may be greater now than previously as a result of the increased social visibility of lesbians and gay men and the association of same-sex orientation with AIDS. Finally, the barriers to obtaining accurate information about sexual practices among adults are daunting; gathering such information from junior and senior high school students is nearly impossible.

Because of the difficulty in estimating the population with same-sex orientations and the strong stigma associated with any manifestation of homoeroticism, especially during adolescence and within peer culture and within school settings, the recognition that many youth experience homoerotic desire and engage in homosexual activity and that some realize that they are not heterosexual has drawn the attention of mental health professionals and researchers (Boxer and Cohler 1989; Gonsiorek 1988; Herdt 1989; Remafedi 1987a, 1987b; Ross-Reynolds and Hardy 1985; Savin-Williams 1990, 1995; Schneider 1988;

Slater 1988). Much of the recent concern centers on adjustment, health, and mental health problems of youth that result from stresses associated with the emergence and management of sexual orientation. The most troublesome concern is the possibility that many youth suicides may be related to issues of sexual orientation and that many young lesbians and gay males contemplate suicide before integrating their sexual orientation into their lives (see Chapter 49 by Hartstein in this volume; Gibson 1989).

At a similar level of urgency is a concern about HIV infection among gay and bisexual male youth (Hunter and Schaecher 1994). Rotheran-Borus et al. (1994) identified six behavioral patterns that put gay male youths at risk: many sexual partners, early age of initiation of sexual activity, receptive anal intercourse, bartering of sex for money or drugs, inconsistent condom use, and frequent use of drugs or alcohol during sex.

In addition to these exceedingly serious problems, there are common—yet profoundly stressful—circumstances faced by nearly all youth who disclose their sexual orientation to peers, siblings, parents, and others in their lives. Those who refrain from disclosure or who are uncertain about their feelings also may run risks of jeopardizing their development (Malyon 1981). Regardless of their openness about their sexual orientation to others, all lesbian, gay, bisexual, and transgendered youth are exposed to frequent homophobic comments. Youth who are open about their sexuality or those who are assumed to be lesbian or gay become the direct targets of these comments. Victimization can be more serious than verbal abuse or threats, and many youth are the victims of the rising number of assaults and other hate crimes (Comstock 1991; D'Augelli and Dark 1995; Herek 1989). This chapter reviews the developmental challenges faced by adolescents and young adults who label themselves as lesbian, gay, or bisexual as well as youth who struggle with such a self-identification at different levels of awareness.

Developmental Milestones

The origin of sexual orientation remains a contested theoretical and empirical issue (see chapters in Section II of this volume), with increasing evidence pointing to a complex interaction of biological, psychological, familial, and cultural factors. Before the late 1980s, same-sex sexual orientation was conceptualized primarily as a characteristic of adulthood, and little attention was paid to homoeroticism during early adolescence and the teenage years. Many reasons exist for this adulto-centric point of view, including the practical issues that few lesbian or gay youth sought out psychiatric or psychological services and the difficulty of involving young females and males in research on same-sex sexual orientation. Thus, the clinical experience and the research base in this area are limited. This has led to the near invisibility of lesbian, gay, and bisexual youth in the professional literature, with a few early exceptions (Kramer and Rifkin 1969; Malyon 1981; Roesler and Deisher 1972).

Contemporary studies suggest that most adults who identify themselves as lesbian or gay realize their orientation during early adolescence. The largest of these studies are by D'Augelli and Hershberger (1993; includes 194 youths), Herdt and Boxer (1993; includes 202 youths), and by Savin-Williams (1990; includes 314 youth). Participants in these projects ranged in age from 14 to 23, far younger than participants whose lives are summarized in the heretofore available information about sexual orientation. For example, lesbian or gay participants in the Kinsey Institute report *Sexual Preference* (Bell et al. 1981) ranged from 27 to 37 years of age. The more accurate information obtained in the more recent research on the early emergence of sexual orientation occurs at the same time that lesbian, gay, and bisexual youth are increasingly open in our society. This greater openness allows researchers the opportunity to study increasingly young samples. Because these reports are relatively recent, these conclusions should be viewed as tentative, and subject to revision as our database increases.

A developmental approach to sexual orientation takes into account the developmental status of the individual. This means that same-sex eroticism will be experienced, thought about, and expressed not only in different ways at different ages but also in ways that reflect the physical, cognitive, emotional, and social development of the individual at a particular point in his or her life. Although no research based on representative samples has explicitly focused on sexual orientation before puberty, the conclusion of the most recent studies is that personal awareness of same-sex erotic feelings generally predates puberty and becomes increasingly crystallized at puberty. Sometime thereafter—and tremendous individual variability exists on this event—the person labels her or his feelings as homoerotic. The processes of self-awareness and self-identification occur simultaneously with the development of complex cognitive abilities, as well as the development of an increasingly autonomous social life less reliant on family and peers. Individual sexual behaviors—both solitary (fantasy, masturbation) and social (petting, mutual masturbation, oral sex, vaginal sex, and anal sex)—impact on the rate at which the solidification of a homoerotic orientation occurs. Interpersonal sexual activity is not a requirement for awareness of orientation, however, although the lack of such activity may delay self-labeling. In sum, as many developmental pathways exist to a same-sex sexual orientation as there are to a heterosexual or a bisexual orientation.

The biological processes of puberty accelerate the expression of same-sex orientation while the social pressures of adolescence in our current culture provide powerful barriers to its expression. This dynamic makes early adolescence, the teenage years, and early adulthood (from age 10 to 20) the most important developmental period for lesbians, gay males, and bisexuals. The paradox is intense during these years: both the repression and the expression of homoerotic desire strongly conflict. By the end of this period, the template of the life of the individual has been forged; a later revision is possible, but increasingly difficult, as more and more commitments to a particular orientation accumulate.

Although the articulation of these developmental complexities is beyond the scope of this chapter, the sequence of developmental milestones can be well set. The ages at which some of the critical milestones have been reported in the more recent research appear in Table 16–1.

These milestones take into account the distinctive quality of lesbian, gay, or bisexual development; it involves exiting from heterosexual socialization as well as creating a complex new "self" in the face of widespread cultural stigma and discrimination (D'Augelli 1994a, 1994b). Males report knowing about their orientation at or around puberty, at which point they label long-standing and often ambiguous feelings of "being different" as reflecting a gay sexual orientation (Malyon 1981; Troiden 1989). Females who label themselves lesbian do so several years after their male counterparts (Garnets and Kimmel 1991). Self-acknowledgment represents the beginning of the process of identity exploration and consolidation; this is called "coming out to oneself." Such personal acknowledgment precedes disclosure to someone else. Ordinarily telling another person for the first time is experienced as an extremely difficult act as it involves risk of rejection without the benefits of experience or helping resources. This first disclosure is the first of a lifelong series of coming-out processes. The first disclosure to another may not follow self-awareness and self-labeling for many years.

Multiple, overlapping processes are involved in the core lesbian-gay-bisexual developmental task of coming out (e.g., telling family, friends ranging from casual acquaintances to close friends, and many others in an individual's social network such as co-workers, religious leaders, and teachers). These disclosure processes facilitate an exiting from heterosexual identity and its social expectations. The more people who know the individual's sexual orientation, the more complete is the repositioning of the individual within a lesbian, gay, or bisexual identity. However, this exit from heterosexuality is stressful both for individuals, who have been socialized within a heterosexual model, and for their social networks, whose expectations have been violated.

Coming out also sets up new problems. Coming to terms with one's sexual orientation and the many personal and social dilemmas involved in coming out are considerably different for an individual age 14 compared with and individual age 25. Adolescents are still developing in many ways; more important, they are under the close scrutiny of parents, siblings, and peers and pressured to conform to heterosexual expectations. Lesbian, gay, and bisexual adolescents have few opportunities to explore their developing identities without severe risk. The

Table 16–1. Means and standard deviations of age of developmental milestones for lesbian, gay, and bisexual youth

| Milestone | D'Augelli & Hershberger (1993) | | Herdt & Boxer (1993) | |
	Females ($n = 52$)	Males ($n = 142$)	Females ($n = 55$)	Males ($n = 147$)
First same-sex attraction	11 ± 4	10 ± 4	10 ± 4	10 ± 4
First same-sex fantasy	n/a	n/a	12 ± 3	11 ± 3
First same-sex self-label	15 ± 3	15 ± 3	n/a	n/a
First same-sex sexual activity	15 ± 4	15 ± 3	15 ± 3	13 ± 4
First opposite-sex sexual activity	15 ± 4	12 ± 4	14 ± 4	14 ± 4
First disclosure to someone else	16 ± 2	17 ± 2	16 ± 2	16 ± 2

Note. Values are mean ± standard deviation.

lack of exploratory socialization options leads to many problems, as do the consequences of efforts at self-assertion.

Major Stressors in the Lives of Lesbian, Gay, and Bisexual Youth

◼ General Issues of Identity Development

Current studies find many serious dilemmas faced by lesbian, gay, and bisexual youth. Some stresses are related to concealment of sexual orientation; other stresses are related to openness about orientation. All lesbian, gay, and bisexual youth have learned the need to hide, and this long-standing manner of coping exacts its costs in terms of psychological well-being (Martin 1982). Herdt (1989) identified four characteristics of lesbian, gay, and bisexual youth that have consequences for their mental health: 1) their invisibility, 2) the assumptions of peers and family that they are defective, 3) the stigmatization that follows the assumption of deviance, and 4) the assumption by others that all lesbians and gay males are alike. Plummer (1989) added other factors that compromise development among young lesbians, gay males, and bisexuals, including the absence of positive role models, and the development of a "negative self" that results from the relentless heterosexism and homophobia of adolescent peer culture.

Given the stressors associated with lesbian, gay, or bisexual identity formation in contemporary society, it is not surprising that the most common experience of being a young lesbian, gay, or bisexual individual is a profound sense of difference. This sense of "otherness" results from isolation from those with similar feelings and from messages that homoerotic desire and identity are legitimate targets for rejection and hate. A cyclical pattern emerges; because youths feel different (and are often not able to understand the feeling), they may withdraw from others, may distort their life, or may try to act straight with varying degrees of success. This widens the gap between core identity and public identity. The process also intensifies social vigilance, lest others figure out the individual's "true" identity. As a result, anxiety and depression may increase, especially if the individual understands the nature of his or her difference. During this process, almost no sources of social support exist to offset the dynamic of withdrawal. Indeed, the avoidance of addressing sexual orientation concerns becomes highly reinforcing. This accounts for the large numbers of people who do not disclose their sexual feelings until later in life, often in circumstances free from the scrutiny of parents and friends.

During the initial period of recognition and labeling of homoerotic feelings, lesbian, gay, and bisexual youth have few, if any, helping resources to aid them in understanding their concerns. Lesbian- or gay-affirming materials may be inaccessible, or youths may feel embarrassed to buy them locally; casual discussions with family and friends are risky; and talking with counseling personnel in schools is hampered by fear of disclosure by counselors to others and by fear of judgment (Rofes 1989; Ross-Reynolds and Hardy 1985). In some urban areas, lesbian, gay, and bisexual youth can seek services from agencies devoted to their distinct concerns (Martin and Hetrick, 1988; Schneider, 1988). In other urban areas, youth can access telephone help or counseling systems anonymously, if they are aware of these systems and can overcome their fears. In many areas, particularly rural areas, however, such resources do not exist and the sense of isolation and lack of support can be profound. Sadly, even when there are helping resources available, only a slight percentage of lesbian and gay youth overcome hesitancies and seek help. Those who do not remain closeted tend to develop a small support system, divulging aspects of their emotional life to well-chosen family members and friends from whom they can predict support and confidentiality. Lesbian, gay, and bisexual youth are dependent on these small networks of knowing friends; disruptions in these friendships can be exceedingly stressful, because they often offer the only predictable validation the individual may have. Having a small network of friends who know, while hiding one's sexuality from most others (including parents and siblings) reinforces the sense of being different or deviant. Without the opportunity to discuss this feeling and have it proven to be wrong, lesbian, gay, and bisexual youth internalize the negative views of society further.

◼ Problems Resulting From Disclosure of Sexual Orientation to Family and Friends

Research on parental reactions to disclosure of sexual orientation finds considerable upset among parents, many of whom respond negatively at first to the disclosure and then recover slowly (Strommen 1989).

Remafedi (1987b) found that 43% of a sample of gay male adolescents reported strong negative reactions from parents about their sexual orientation; 41% reported negative reactions from friends. Cramer and Roach (1988), studying adult gay male subjects, found that 55% of their mothers and 42% of their fathers had an initially negative response. Robinson et al. (1989) surveyed parents of lesbian and gay adults through a national support group for parents and found that most reported initial sadness (74%), regret (58%), depression (49%), and fear for their child's well-being (74%). Boxer et al. (1991) studied youth aged 21 and younger as well as a sample of the parents of these youths. More youth had disclosed to their mothers than fathers. Of the lesbian youth, 63% had disclosed to mothers and 37% to fathers; of the males, 54% to mothers and 28% to fathers. Parents reported considerable family disruption after disclosure. Herdt and Boxer (1993) found that most youth first disclose their orientation to friends, with more males finding this difficult than females. More lesbian youth than gay male youth had disclosed their sexual orientation to their parents. Only a small group of youth perceived the response of their families to be supportive. D'Augelli and Hershberger (1993) found that only 11% of a sample of lesbian, gay, and bisexual youth received a positive response from parents on disclosure. Of parents aware of the orientation of their children, 20% of mothers and 28% of fathers were either intolerant or rejecting.

■ Victimization and Its Consequences

Research suggests that young lesbians and gay males are often the victims of assaults (D'Augelli and Dark 1995; Dean et al. 1992). Gross et al. (1988) found that 50% of a sample of gay men reported victimization in junior high school and 59% in high school; of lesbians sampled, 12% were victimized in junior high school and 21% in high school. In a study of New York City lesbian, gay, and bisexual youth, 41% had suffered from physical attacks; nearly half of these attacks were specifically provoked by the sexual orientation of the youths (Hunter 1990).

    Evidence exists of family victimization of lesbian and gay adolescents. Lesbians and gay males are more likely survivors of childhood physical or sexual abuse than heterosexual youth. In national surveys of victimization, 19%–41% of adult lesbians and gay males reported family verbal abuse, and 4%–7% reported family physical abuse (Berrill 1990). Pilkington and D'Augelli (1995) found that over 33% of their lesbian, gay, and bisexual youth sample had been verbally insulted by a family member, and 10% were physically assaulted by a family member because of their sexual orientation. Bradford et al. (1994) reported that 24% of 1,925 lesbians in their study had been harshly beaten or physically abused while growing up, 21% reported rape or sexual molestation in childhood, and 19% reported childhood incest. Of 1,001 adult gay and bisexual males attending sexually transmitted disease clinics, Doll et al. (1992) found that 37% said they had been encouraged or forced to have sexual contact (mostly with older men) before age 19. With the use of the same subjects, Barthalow et al. (1994) reported a significant association between earlier sexual abuse and current depression, thoughts of suicide, risky sexual behavior, and HIV-positive status. Harry (1989a) found that gay males were more likely to be physically abused during adolescence than heterosexual males, especially if they had a history of childhood femininity and poor relationships with their fathers. In comparison to the rates of victimization found in lesbian or gay subjects, prevalence estimates in general survey findings are much lower. For example, based on several national surveys, Finkelhor and Dziuba-Leatherman (1994) estimated the prevalence of physical abuse and rape directed to youth under 17 to occur at rates of 2% and 12%, respectively.

In addition to parental conflicts and violence, lesbian, gay, and bisexual youth who are open about their sexual orientation face verbal harassment and physical attacks at school and in their local communities. Between 33% and 49% of those responding to community surveys report being victimized in school (Berrill 1990), presumably in high school. The gay male youths in Remafedi's (1987a) report were similar, with 55% reporting peer verbal abuse and nearly 30% reporting physical assaults. Nearly 40% of the male youths in the study of Remafedi et al. (1991) said they experienced physical violence. In the study of Bradford et al. (1994), 52% of subjects said they had been verbally attacked and 6% said they had been physically attacked.

Pilkington and D'Augelli (1995) found that 80% of the lesbian, gay, and bisexual youth in their study reported verbal abuse specifically based on sexual orientation; 48% reported such abuse occurred more than twice. Gay male youth reported significantly more verbal abuse. Of the total group, 44% had been threatened with physical violence (19% more than twice), 23% had personal property damaged, 33% had objects thrown at them, 30% had been chased (16% more than once), and 13% had been spat on. As to more serious attacks, 17% had been assaulted (punched, kicked, or beaten), 10% had been assaulted with a weapon, and 22% reported sexual assault. Many youth in the Pilkington and D'Angelli (1995) study reported fear of verbal (22%) or physical (7%) abuse at home; more reported fear of verbal (31%) or physical (26%) abuse at school.

Widespread harassment and violence directed at open lesbian and gay male students on college and university campuses have been documented as well. In a review of studies of different universities, Comstock (1991) summarized the percentage of campus respondents victimized because of their sexual orientation. He found that 22% of lesbian or gay young adults had been chased or followed; 15% had objects thrown at them; 4% had been punched, hit, kicked, or beaten; 11% were the victims of vandalism or arson; 3% were spit at; and 1% were assaulted with a weapon. Comstock concluded that lesbian, gay, and bisexual students are victimized at a far higher rate than others on campuses, perhaps four times more often than the general student population. Managing sexual orientation involves active avoidance of threatening situations and people, even on college campuses, places typically seen as safe havens for free expression (Evans and D'Augelli 1995; Rhodes 1994).

Psychological and Psychiatric Problems

■ Critical Mental Health Issues

Lesbian, gay, and bisexual youth are at high risk for mental health problems (D'Augelli and Hershberger 1993; Gonsiorek 1988; Kourany 1987; Remafedi 1987a, 1987b; Savin-Williams 1994). As increasing numbers of young lesbians and gay males disclose their identities to others, researchers have been better able to study the psychological and psychosocial stressors in their lives (Gonsiorek 1988; Hetrick and Martin 1987). Table 16–2 shows the critical mental health issues of this population.

The most recent studies reveal considerable stress in the lives of these young people. A comprehensive analysis of a survey of mental health problems among lesbians was completed by the National Lesbian and Gay Health Foundation in 1987 and was later reported by Bradford et al. (1994). Of the more than 1,900 lesbians who were surveyed on their life concerns, 167 were aged 17 to 24. Mental health problems were common. When asked how often they were so worried that they "couldn't do necessary things," 13% of the females in this age bracket said they often felt this way, 29% sometimes felt this way, and 43% said rarely. Only 15% of these young lesbians responded that they never felt overwhelmed. Nearly two-thirds (62%) of those aged 17–24 had received counseling. The most frequently occurring problems taken to counselors were family problems (46%), depression (40%), problems in relationships (29%), and anxiety (26%).

Remafedi (1987a, 1987b) found that nearly 75% of the adolescent gay males in his study had received mental health services for emotional problems. A study of young gay males in college (D'Augelli 1991) revealed many personal and emotional problems; the most frequent concerns were dealing with parents about sexual orientation (93% reported it to be a concern), relationship problems (93%), worry about AIDS (92%), anxiety (77%), and depression (63%).

In D'Augelli and Hershberger's (1993) report, 63% of the youth said they were so worried or nervous in the last year that they could not function, 61% reported feeling nervous and tense at the time of the study (21% very much so), and 73% said they were depressed (38% very much so). In addition, 33% reported excessive alcohol use, and 23% reported illegal drug use. Yet, youths' reported symptoms in this research did not differ from other adolescents' symptoms (Hershberger and D'Augelli 1995). Although none of these studies had representative samples of young lesbians, gay males, or bisexuals (no representative sample of lesbians, gay males, or bisexuals have ever been obtained), the accumulated evidence supports the idea that stresses that jeopardize mental health are common in lesbian, gay, and bisexual youth and young adults. Such an idea is consistent with the unusual life

---

Table 16–2.   Critical mental health issues for lesbian, gay, and bisexual youth

---

◆   Stress associated with management of lesbian/gay/bisexual identity
◆   Disruptions in peer relationships
◆   Conflicts about disclosure to family and consequences of disclosure
◆   Emotional reactions to close relationship development
◆   Isolation from lesbian/gay/bisexual-affirming contexts
◆   Distress caused by discrimination, harassment, and violence based on sexual orientation
◆   Anxieties related to sexual health, especially HIV infection

---

stresses these young people face in addition to the stresses related to adolescent development and young adulthood in general.

■ Suicidality

The available evidence also suggests a disproportionately high incidence of suicide attempts among lesbian, gay, and bisexual youth. An early study of gay male youths aged 16–22 found that 31% had made a suicide attempt (Roesler and Deisher 1972). The first Kinsey report devoted exclusively to homosexuality (Bell and Weinberg 1978) found that 20% of the gay men studied reported a suicide attempt before age 20. A decade later, Martin and Hetrick (1988) found that 21% of their clients at a social service agency for troubled youth had made a suicide attempt. On the basis of his conclusions on earlier studies and on reports from community agencies, Gibson (1989) speculated that most suicide attempts by lesbians and gay males occurred in their youth; that lesbian, gay, and bisexual youth are two to three times more likely to commit suicide than their heterosexual peers; and that suicides of lesbians, gay males, and bisexuals may constitute up to 30% of all completed youth suicides. Gibson concluded that 20%–35% of lesbian, gay, and bisexual youth have made suicide attempts. Harry (1989b) concluded that lesbians and gay men were more likely to make suicide attempts at times of conflicts about sexual orientation, especially in adolescence. Unfortunately, Gibson's and Harry's conclusions were based on limited empirical data; nevertheless, these figures are considerably higher than current estimates of high school suicide attempts, which range from 6% to 13% (Garland and Zigler 1993).

Recent empirical studies have come to similar conclusions about a high risk for suicide among lesbian, gay, and bisexual youth. Remafedi (1987a, 1987b) found that 34% of his gay male adolescent subjects had attempted suicide. In a later study with a larger number of study subjects, Remafedi et al. (1991) found that 30% had made a suicide attempt. Those who had attempted suicide were younger, had more feminine gender role concepts, and were more likely to report drug and alcohol abuse. Another study of gay male youth found that 23% had attempted suicide at least once and that 59% evidenced serious suicidal thinking (Schneider et al. 1989). Of the young women in the National Lesbian Health Foundation survey (Bradford et al. 1994), 2% said they considered suicide often, 25% said sometimes, and 32% said rarely (59% of subjects at risk). Only 41% said they had never contemplated suicide. About 25% had made an attempt at suicide. D'Augelli and Hershberger (1993) found that 42% of a sample of lesbian, gay, and bisexual youth drawn from 14 metropolitan areas had made a suicide attempt. Only 40% of the youth in the study had never considered suicide. Herdt and Boxer (1993) found that 29% of lesbian, gay, and bisexual youth in a Chicago youth support group program had made a suicide attempt; 53% of the lesbian youth reported suicide attempts, compared with 20% of the gay male youths.

Unfortunately, linkages between personal, family, and social problems and suicide attempts, suicidal ideation, or other serious mental health problems have not been systematically studied. Until this is accomplished, we cannot distinguish suicidality unique to lesbian, gay, and bisexual youths from patterns found among youths in general. Possibly, factors associated with adolescent suicide attempts (e.g., a history of past attempts, depression, low self-esteem, and suicide attempts by friends) predict future attempts (Lewinsohn et al. 1994). On the other hand, unique stressors in the lives of lesbian, gay, and bisexual youths have been found to be associated with suicidality. For instance, Remafedi et al. (1991) found that 44% of their gay male youth subjects reported that their suicide attempts were precipitated by "family problems"; certainly family problems related to sexual orientation are unique to lesbian, gay, and bisexual youths. Schneider et al. (1989) found that suicide attempters had not yet established a stable sexual identity; attempts occurred most often before they acknowledged or disclosed their sexual identities to others. They also found that family background of paternal alcoholism and abuse, reliance on social support from people who rejected them because of their sexual orientation, and being aware of their sexual orientation at a earlier age were all associated with suicide attempts. D'Augelli and Hershberger (1993) found that suicide attempters were more open with others about their sexual orientation than youth who made no attempts, and had lost more friends because of their sexual orientation.

Probably, a complex interplay of sexual identity-related factors and other factors such as a history of victimization work together to produce suicide attempts (Hershberger and D'Augelli 1995). We know little about how variability in such crucial factors as prior victimization experience, psychiatric history, gender nonconformity, past suicide history, and sexual identity development status might influence how victimization results in mental health dysfunction. Until we have research on such questions, it is important to consider lesbian, gay, and bisexual youth at risk for mental health problems and suicide. Suicide is more likely in youth with serious mental health and adjustment problems, some of which may be related to sexual identity development. Suicide among lesbian, gay, and bisexual youth is more likely if there is a history of self-destructive behavior. Loss of important support from family and friends may be yet another important predictor of a suicide attempt, especially if the loss follows the disclosure of sexual orientation. Extreme negative reactions to conflicts within same-sex relationships (especially relationship termination) might precipitate suicide attempts, especially among youths who have few experiences in same-sex relationships. Finally, suicide potential may exist for youth who have been subject to persistent and long-lasting forms of victimization, especially sexual abuse.

Identity Consolidation Among Lesbian, Gay, and Bisexual Youths

The late adolescent and early adulthood years are the most important years for identity exploration for lesbian, gay, and bisexual youth. The normative expectations of identity exploration (e.g., career or relationships) are more complex for these youth as they must simultaneously confront the processes of lesbian or gay identity development. The many conflicts and confusions of these years are intensified as young lesbians, gay males, and bisexuals resist heterosexual imperatives, "re-create" themselves, and construct a new life trajectory. Although most lesbian and gay adults acknowledge their sexual orientation to themselves during their teenage years, most have not come out, except to a handful of others, by the time they leave high school. Only a small minority of lesbian, gay, and bisexual youth disclose in junior or senior high school, and these youth face the most difficult challenges. Probably, more youths will be disclosing their sexual orientation during these years, and professionals must be prepared to offer them protection and support. All indicators suggest that the earlier a youth comes out to others, the more external negative reactions the individual will endure.

In addition to the stresses associated with heterosexual expectations, and the problems created directly or indirectly by heterosexism, homophobia, and discrimination, lesbian, gay, and bisexual youths must build a personal identity within a gay or lesbian context (D'Augelli and Garnets 1995). Lesbians, gay males, and bisexuals must relate to other lesbian, gay, or bisexual individuals; socialize in lesbian, gay, or bisexual settings or communities; and integrate their sexual orientation into all domains of personal life. Many of these processes involve stressful experiences, because they bring additional risks, including ventures into new situations and the creation of relationships with people in different social circles. For most youths, being seen in lesbian, gay, or bisexual settings or associating with others who are lesbian, gay, or bisexual exposes them to added stress.

On the basis of the research literature, some general predictions are possible about the needs of lesbian, gay, and bisexual youths. More youths will be "coming out" at earlier ages. As youth label themselves at earlier ages, they will experience greater stress and will be at higher risk unless given support (Remafedi et al. 1991). The increased cultural visibility of lesbians, gay males, and bisexuals will escalate negative reactions, causing greater conflicts among lesbian and gay youth. As more and more conflict is experienced, more will seek mental health services. Some will seek help as a result of the psychological consequences of persistent harassment, and some will need help to deal with reactions to incidents of violence. More youths will self-identify as lesbian, gay, or bisexual during their college years (Evans and D'Augelli 1995; Rhodes 1994). These youths who disclose their sexuality will meet the challenges of developing into well-functioning lesbians, gay men, and bisexual individuals if given access to helping resources such as peer support and affirming professional helping resources. This cohort of lesbian, gay, and bisexual youths has benefited from the accomplishments of earlier generations, which have led to a greater sense of collective self-esteem. For lesbian, gay, and bisexual youth in the 1990s, sexual orientation issues are psychologically salient. The issues have been in their awareness for longer periods than for earlier cohorts (Herdt 1989). Greater social acceptance makes denial increasingly difficult to sustain.

The problems lesbian, gay, and bisexual youths will present to mental health professionals are predictable (D'Augelli 1993). Probably, they will seek help mostly under crisis conditions, having exhausted the usefulness of lesbian, gay, and bisexual peer support. The most predictable crises will concern disclosure of sexual orientation to others (especially family) and concerns about developing relationships. Crises may be exacerbated by experiences with neglectful, troubled, or abusive families, as well as becoming enmeshed in abusive or exploitive close relationships. Less routine crises related to victimization also will occur, as will concerns related to HIV status for gay and bisexual males. The accumulated experience of coping with years of societal, peer, and familial ambivalence will manifest as depression or anxiety. The new assertiveness of this generation of lesbian, gay, and bisexual youth is a double-edged sword: it is hard for these young people to look back on the hurts of the past because they are too busy hoping to move ahead. The seeking of professional help is generally not acceptable, yet most young lesbian, gay, and bisexual youth are in need of more support and nurturance than they receive. Young lesbian, gay, and bisexual people are the most poorly served group in public schools and on college campuses as far as health and mental health services are concerned. Fearing the consequences of allowing themselves to be vulnerable, they do not make their needs known and prefer to obtain help from peers. Many psychosocial and personal issues may remain unaddressed as a result.

Conclusion

Mental health professionals must take the lead in the development of affirmative services and the creation of supportive settings for lesbian, gay, and bisexual youth. We must not victimize these youth again by colluding with social and political forces that render them invisible in public schools, on college and university campuses, and in community settings. Nor can we ignore the pervasive heterosexism, homophobia, and discrimination that occur in the social contexts in which they spend a crucial decade of their preparation for adulthood. Increased professional attention must be directed toward helping lesbian, gay, and bisexual young people deal with the distinct dilemmas of becoming a lesbian, gay male, or bisexual adult. The need for interventions directed toward this population is intense and urgent.

References

American Association of University Women: Hostile Hallways: The AAUW Survey on Sexual Harassment in America's Schools. Washington, DC, American Association of University Women, 1993

Barthalow BN, Doll LS, Joy D, et al: Emotional, behavioral, and HIV risks associated with sexual abuse among homosexual and bisexual men. Child Abuse Negl 18:753–767, 1994

Bell AP, Weinberg MS: Homosexualities: A Study of Diversity Among Men and Women. New York, Simon and Schuster, 1978

Bell AP, Weinberg MS, Hammersmith SK: Sexual Preference: Its Development in Men and Women. Bloomington, IN, Indiana University Press, 1981

Berrill KT: Anti-gay violence and victimization in the United States: an overview. Journal of Interpersonal Violence 5:274–294, 1990

Boxer AM, Cohler BJ: The life course of gay and lesbian youth: an immodest proposal for the study of lives. J Homosex 17:315–355, 1989

Boxer AM, Cook JA, Herdt G: Double jeopardy: identity transitions and parent-child relations among gay and lesbian youth, in Parent-Child Relations Throughout Life. Edited by Pillemer K, McCartney K. Hillsdale, NJ, Erlbaum, 1991, pp 59–92

Bradford J, Ryan C, Rothblum ED: National Lesbian Health Care Survey: implications for mental health care. J Consult Clin Psychol 62:228–242, 1994

Comstock GD: Violence Against Lesbians and Gay Men. New York, Columbia University Press, 1991

Cramer DW, Roach AJ: Coming out to mom and dad: a study of gay males and their relationships with their parents. J Homosex 15:79–92, 1988

D'Augelli AR: Gay men in college: identity processes and adaptations. Journal of College Student Development 32:140–146, 1991

D'Augelli AR: Preventing mental health problems among lesbian and gay college students. Journal of Primary Prevention 13 (suppl 4):1–17, 1993

D'Augelli AR: Identity development and sexual orientation: toward a model of lesbian, gay, and bisexual development, in Human Diversity: Perspectives on People in Context. Edited by Trickett EJ. San Francisco, CA, Jossey-Bass, 1994a, pp 312–333

D'Augelli AR: Lesbian and gay male development: steps toward an analysis of lesbians' and gay men's lives, in Lesbian and Gay Psychology: Theory, Research, and Clinical Applications. Edited by Greene B, Herek GM. Newbury Park, CA, Sage, 1994b, pp 118–132

D'Augelli AR, Dark LJ: Vulnerable populations: lesbian, gay, and bisexual youth, in Reason to Hope: A Psychosocial Perspective on Violence and Youth. Edited by Erong LD, Gentry JH, Schlegel P. Washington, DC, American Psychological Association, 1995, pp 177–196

D'Augelli AR, Garnets LD: Lesbian, gay, and bisexual communities, in Lesbian, Gay, and Bisexual Identities Over the Lifespan: Psychological Perspectives. Edited by D'Augelli AR, Patterson CJ. New York, Oxford University Press, 1995, pp 293–320

D'Augelli AR, Hershberger SL: Lesbian, gay, and bisexual youth in community settings: personal challenges and mental health problems. Am J Community Psychol 21:421–448, 1993

Dean L, Wu S, Martin JL: Trends in violence and discrimination against gay men in New York City: 1984 to 1990, in Hate Crimes: Confronting Violence Against Lesbians and Gay Men. Edited by Herek GM, Berrill KT. Newbury Park, CA, Sage, 1992

Doll LS, Joy D, Bartholow BN, et al: Self-reported childhood and adolescent sexual abuse among adult homosexual and bisexual men. Child Abuse Negl 16:855–864, 1992

Evans NJ, D'Augelli AR: Lesbians, gay men, and bisexual people in college, in The Lives of Lesbians, Gays, and Bisexuals. Edited by Savin-Williams RC, Cohn KM. New York, Harcourt Brace, 1995, pp 201–226

Finkelhor D, Dziuba-Leatherman J: Victimization of children. Am Psychol 49:173–183, 1994

Garland AF, Zigler E: Adolescent suicide prevention: current research and social policy implications. Am Psychol 48:169–182, 1993

Garnets L, Kimmel D: Lesbian and gay male dimensions in the psychological study of human diversity, in Psychological Perspectives on Human Diversity in America. Edited by Goodchilds J. Washington, DC, American Psychological Association, 1991, pp 143–192

Gibson P: Gay male and lesbian youth suicide, in ADAMHA, Report of the Secretary's Task Force on Youth Suicide, Vol 3 (DHHS Publ No ADM-89-1623). Washington, DC, U.S. Government Printing Office, 1989, pp 110–142

Gonsiorek JC: Mental health issues of gay and lesbian adolescents. J Adolesc Health Care 9:114–122, 1988

Gross L, Aurand S, Adessa R: Violence and Discrimination Against Lesbian and Gay People in Philadelphia and the Commonwealth of Pennsylvania. Philadelphia, PA, Philadelphia Lesbian and Gay Task Force, 1988

Harry J: Parental physical abuse and sexual orientation. Arch Sex Behav 18:251–261, 1989a

Harry J: Sexual identity issues, in ADAMHA, Report of the Secretary's Task Force on Youth Suicide, Vol 2. (DHHS Publ No ADM-89-1622). Washington, DC, U.S. Government Printing Office, 1989b, pp 131–142

Herdt G: Gay and lesbian youth: emergent identities and cultural scenes at home and abroad. J Homosex 17:1–42, 1989

Herdt GH, Boxer AM: Children of Horizons: How Gay and Lesbian Teens are Leading a New Way Out of the Closet. Boston, MA, Beacon Press, 1993

Herek, GM: Hate crimes against lesbian and gay men: issues for research and social policy. Am Psychol 44:948–955, 1989

Hershberger SL, D'Augelli AR: The consequences of victimization on the mental health and suicidality of lesbian, gay, and bisexual youth. Developmental Psychology 31:65–74, 1995

Hetrick ES, Martin AD: Developmental issues and their resolution for gay and lesbian adolescents. J Homosex 14:25–43, 1987

Hunter J: Violence against lesbian and gay male youths. Journal of Interpersonal Violence 5:295–300, 1990

Hunter J, Schaecher R: AIDS prevention for lesbian, gay, and bisexual adolescents. Families in Society 75 (suppl 6):346–354, 1994

Kramer MW, Rifkin AH: The early development of homosexuality: A study of adolescent lesbians. Am J Psychiatry 126:129–134, 1969

Kourany RFC: Suicide among homosexual adolescents. J Homosex 13 (suppl 4):111–117, 1987

Laumann EO, Gagnon JH, Michael RT, et al: The Social Organization of Sexuality: Sexual Practices in the United States. Chicago, IL, University of Chicago Press, 1994

Lewinsohn PM, Rodhe P, Seeley JR: Psychosocial risk factors for future adolescent suicide attempts. J Consult Clin Psychol 62:297–305, 1994

Malyon AK: The homosexual adolescent: development issues and social bias. Child Welfare 60:321–330, 1981

Marsiglio W: Attitudes toward homosexual activity and gays as friends: a national survey of heterosexual 15- to 19-year-old males. J Sex Res 30:12–17, 1993

Martin AD: Learning to hide: socialization of the gay adolescent. Adolesc Psychiatry 10:52–65, 1982

Martin AD, Hetrick ES: The stigmatization of the gay and lesbian adolescent. J Homosex 15:163–184, 1988

Pilkington NW, D'Augelli AR: Victimization of lesbian, gay, and bisexual youth in community settings. J Community Psychol 23: 33–56, 1995

Plummer K: Lesbian and gay youth in England. J Homosex 17:195–223, 1989

Remafedi G: Adolescent homosexuality: psychosocial and medical implications. Pediatrics 79:331–337, 1987a

Remafedi G: Male homosexuality: the adolescent's perspective. Pediatrics 79:326–330, 1987b

Remafedi G, Garrow JA, Deisher RW. Risk factors for attempted suicide in gay and bisexual youth. Pediatrics 87:869–875, 1991

Remafedi G, Resnick M, Blum R, et al: Demography of sexual orientation in adolescents. Pediatrics 89:714–721, 1992

Rhodes RA. Coming Out in College: The Struggle for a Queer Identity. Westport, CT, Bergin and Garvey, 1994

Robinson BE, Walters LH, Skeen P: Response of parents to learning that their child is homosexual and concern over AIDS: a national survey. J Homosex 18 (suppl 1/2):59–80, 1989

Roesler T, Deisher R: Youthful male homosexuality. JAMA 219:1018–1023, 1972

Rofes E: Opening up the classroom closet: responding to the educational needs of gay and lesbian youth. Harvard Education Review 59:444–453, 1989

Ross-Reynolds G, Hardy BS: Crisis counseling for disparate adolescent sexual dilemmas: pregnancy and homosexuality. School Psychology Review 14:300–312, 1985

Rotheran-Borus MJ, Rosario M, Meyer-Bahlburg HFL, et al: Sexual and substance use acts of gay and bisexual male adolescents in New York City. J Sex Res 31 (suppl 1):47–57, 1994

Savin-Williams RC: Gay and Lesbian Youth: Expressions of Identity. New York, Hemisphere, 1990

Savin-Williams RC: Verbal and physical abuse as stressors in the lives of lesbian, gay male and bisexual youths: associations with school problems, running away, substance abuse, prostitution and suicide. J Consult Clin Psychol 62:261–269, 1994

Savin-Williams RC: Lesbian, gay male, and bisexual adolescents, in Lesbian, Gay, and Bisexual Identities Over the Lifespan: Psychological Perspectives. Edited by D'Augelli AR, Patterson CJ. New York, Oxford University Press, 1995, pp 265–189

Schneider MS: Often Invisible: Counseling Gay and Lesbian Youth. Toronto, ON, Central Toronto Youth Services, 1988

Schneider SG, Farberow NL, Kruks GN: Suicidal behavior in adolescent and young adult gay men. Suicide Life Threat Behav 19:381–394, 1989

Sell RL, Wells JA, Wypij D: The prevalence of homosexual behavior and attraction in the United States, the United Kingdom, and France: results of national population-based samples. Arch Sex Behav 24:235–248, 1995

Slater BR: Essential issues in working with lesbian and gay male youths. Professional Psychology: Research and Practice 19:226–235, 1988

Strommen EF: Hidden branches and growing pains: homosexuality and the family tree. Marriage and Family Review 14:9–34, 1989

Troiden RR: The formation of homosexual identities. J Homosex 17:43–74, 1989

Wiesmeier E, Forsythe AB, Sundstrom MJ, et al: Sexual concerns and counseling needs of normal men attending a university student health service. J Am Coll Health 35:29–35, 1986

17

Midlife Gay Men and Lesbians

Adult Development and Mental Health

Robert M. Kertzner, M.D.
Margery Sved, M.D.

G ay men and lesbians, like their heterosexual counterparts, are likely to experience important changes
in self-identity and social roles as they enter their midlife years. This
is a largely uncharted time of life for gay men and lesbians, despite
recent advances in knowledge of homosexuality and refinements in
understanding of midlife. A generation of gay men and lesbians who
"came of age" during the inception of the modern gay rights movement may be creating a unique developmental trail through the middle years of life.

This work was supported, in part, by center grant P50-MH43520 from the National Institute of Mental Health, Anke A. Ehrhardt, Ph.D., Principal Investigator.
The chapter was presented as a poster at the Sixth International AIDS Conference, San Francisco, CA, June 1990, SD 906, Vol 3, p 316.

In delineating such a trail, this chapter discusses the mental health of gay men and lesbians in midlife with consideration of traditional perspectives of midlife development, homosexual identity development, the life experiences and expectations of current gay men and lesbians in midlife, and the impact of the human immunodeficiency virus (HIV) epidemic on gay adult development. Two preconceptions are at hand: 1) it is useful to describe psychological adaptations in gay men and lesbians with a longitudinal perspective (Stein 1993); and 2) normative descriptions of age-related concerns provide an essential backdrop for evaluating clinical problems (Nemiroff and Calorusso 1990).

General Midlife Issues

Midlife psychology for any population is strongly influenced by contemporary culture and history; this may be particularly true for the generation of gay men and lesbians in their 40s and early 50s, men and women who were in their teens and 20s during the era of social change leading up to Stonewall. This generation also experienced many of the first casualties of the HIV epidemic and has arguably sustained the greatest cumulative mortality rates attributable to AIDS. In discussing the current generation of gay men and lesbians in midlife, this chapter adopts a restricted definition of midlife as the span between ages 40 and 55 years. Given the heterogeneity that characterizes gay and lesbian midlife, the selection of a narrower age range may help to limit historic age-cohort effects that significantly affect adult development.

The chronological borders of midlife are ambiguous, with some research reports using age ranges of 40–69 and even 30–74 to study midlife (Bumpass and Aquilino 1995). Gay men and lesbians consider the chronological range of middle age to be similar to the general population; in a study of age-category labeling by gay men ranging in age between 28 and 68, for example, Minnigerode (1976) found that the mean chronological ages given for the onset of middle and old age were 41 and 65 years, respectively.

With these chronological caveats in mind, the current generation of gay men and women in midlife is arguably different, or will be different, from past and future cohorts of midlife gay men and lesbians. Moreover, there is a large diversity of life experience among current middle-aged gay men and lesbians; clearly, many factors other than midlife membership influence psychological adjustment and mental health. Race and economic status create additional developmental histories that must be considered in describing adult development in gay men and lesbians (Kimmel 1978). Many other factors contribute to the diversity that characterizes gay men and lesbians in midlife, such as the presence or absence of children, family life, community of residence (e.g., urban versus rural), and general health. The chronological age and developmental stage at which gay men and women "come out" also affect the course of midlife development.

Although this chapter discusses gay and lesbian lives, gender is associated with important developmental differences for homosexual as well as heterosexual midlife. Earlier theories of adult development were primarily based on observations of relatively affluent and presumably heterosexual white men; only recently have life-cycle descriptions considered the unique adult developmental issues of racial minorities and of women (Baruch and Brooks-Gunn 1984; Gilbert 1993).

In this chapter, the authors limit discussion of adult development to self-identified gay men and lesbians; bisexual men and women, whose identities and life experiences introduce an element of additional complexity to an already heterogeneous populace, are beyond the scope of this review (see Chapter 10 by Fox). Bisexuality may signify a transitional phase from heterosexuality to homosexuality (or vice versa), nonoverlapping serial phases of homosexual and heterosexual activity, a single departure from exclusive heterosexual or homosexual behavior, or substantial overlapping of heterosexual and homosexual activities (Boulton 1993). As such, adult development may vary widely among bisexual individuals and share features of both homosexual and heterosexual midlife.

Few descriptions exist of midlife adaptation in gay men and lesbians (Cornett and Hudson 1987; Kimmel and Sang 1995; Sang 1991), particularly in relation to their developmental histories in adolescence and early adulthood. Little has been written about life after coming out in terms of individual change and the effects of life events on homosexual identity across the life course (Herdt and Boxer 1992); moreover, little is known about how gay men and women change their perceptions of homosexual identity as "central, desirable, significant, or permanent" during life (Troiden 1984). Although homosexual identity formation in youth or young adulthood has been described (see Chapter 14 by Cass; Coleman 1981) and psychological adjustment in older gay men and women has been studied (see Chapter 18 by Berger and Kelley in this volume), few reports have focused on adaptations to midlife.

During the midlife years, many gay men and lesbians experience an increasing awareness of being older and interpret the passage of time within the context of both the dominant heterosexual culture and gay subculture. This awareness may entail redefining self-identity as no longer being young, despite prevailing norms that greatly value youthfulness, or more specifically confronting negative stereotypes about older gay men and lesbians. Psychological adaptation to midlife also may be shaped by gay identity development and self-acceptance, proximity to the HIV epidemic, and more traditional predictors of individual mental health, such as psychiatric status, physical health, social support, life events, and ego strengths.

Given these variables, what age-related concerns might be common to gay men and lesbians in midlife and how are they similar or dissimilar to the concerns of middle-aged heterosexual men and women? Certain key tenets of midlife developmental theory seem relevant to gay and lesbian lives as well as heterosexual lives. Middle age has been described as a time for men when personal limitations are realized and possibilities reassessed (Levenson 1978), and when an outer directedness, concerned with establishing social identity, is replaced by an inner reflectiveness, attuned to the finiteness of life and the passage of youth (Jung 1933; Neugarten 1968). In addition, the adult in midlife becomes increasingly concerned with the gains of others, particularly those of another generation; Erikson describes this period as one of generativity, referring principally to procreation and parenting but also to productivity and creativity (Erikson 1959).

Midlife responsibilities in the general population are primarily related to work and family, with changing roles in caring for young children and aging parents (Bumpass and Aquilino 1995). Because many lesbians and a significant minority of gay men are parents, the maturation or emancipation of children is an important factor influencing the midlife development of significant numbers of gay men and women. Presumably many gay men and women, as do many heterosexual men and women, enter midlife with two living parents and experience parental illness and mortality as normative events during middle adulthood. The statistical probability of these events may not differ by sexual orientation, but the meaning and developmental implications of these milestones may be different for gay men and women.

Other aspects of traditional perspectives on adult development seem less applicable to gay men and lesbians in midlife, although, as stated earlier, this is a greatly diverse group. First, many theories of adult development suggest that middle-aged men and women experience significant challenges to their social identity for the first time in their adult lives (Vaillant 1977); for example, a middle-aged businessman may realize that he is no longer competitive with younger colleagues and thus feels threatened by the change in his social status. Gay men and lesbians, however, are likely to experience a profound social crisis much earlier in life when they disclose their sexual orientation to families. Kimmel (1978) describes a "crisis competence" forged by the coming out process and argues that this may buffer gay men and women from crises in later life. Gay men and lesbians prepare for self-reliance during later years by developing self-created friendship networks and social supports.

Second, life-cycle models such as the eight stages of psychosocial development discussed by Erikson (1959) presume an optimal sequence in which maturational tasks are resolved. Erikson believed that achieving the capacity for intimate relationships, which is attained by most individuals during the stage of "intimacy versus isolation," precedes and enhances the ontogenic stage of "generativity versus stagnation," during which individuals maximize self-realization through work, creativity, or the provision of care to others.

Given the unique issues of homosexual identity formation, such as the frequently delayed consolidation of sexual identity, the sequence of developmental tasks for a large number of lesbian and gay adults may differ from that of heterosexual adults. Some gay men and lesbians, for example, have resolved issues of generativity more fully than those of intimacy, despite the sequence of maturation postulated above (R. M. Kertzner, unpublished observations, 1994).

In addition, whereas greater integration of masculine and feminine qualities is described as a key midlife transition by Levenson (1978) and Jung (1933), many gay men and lesbians experience a wider range of gender roles throughout their lives (Robinson et al. 1982). In comparison to middle-aged heterosexual women, lesbians in midlife may have already cultivated both career and intimate relationships in their lives; the challenge of midlife for lesbians may be to achieve a balance of commitments rather than the task of developing new capacities (Sang 1991).

As discussed below, the HIV epidemic has made the presumption of good health in midlife no longer possible for many gay men.

Significant numbers of gay men in several major urban centers in this country are HIV-infected; even larger numbers of gay men and many lesbians have experienced multiple AIDS bereavements and the premature loss of friends, partners, and colleagues.

Finally, optimal midlife development occurs in lives unhampered by discrimination (Erikson 1959), a condition that is not applicable to many gay men and lesbians. Indeed, the experience of stigmatization and discrimination may overlay the spectrum of adult development for gay men and lesbians (Cohen and Stein 1986). Whether one is able to participate openly in gay community life, teach younger generations, or adopt children is subject to the vagaries of law and social tolerance.

Midlife Development and Mental Health Issues for Lesbians

▮ Multiple Roles and Diverse Lives

Lesbians in midlife are a heterogeneous group whose diverse experiences are shaped by factors such as prior heterosexual life, including marriage; the presence and timing of children; role in the work force; the impact of sexism; and involvement in the feminist movement—variables that pertain to adult development in heterosexual women as well.

Lesbians in midlife, as do their heterosexual counterparts, may find themselves adapting to their children's increasing independence, to menopause and other physical changes, and to ongoing and competing demands of career and personal life. In these respects, the midlife development of lesbians may more closely resemble the adult development of women in general, rather than the life cycle of gay men.

Unlike their heterosexual counterparts, however, lesbians may need to place a greater emphasis on work in midlife than in younger years because of the importance of economic self-sufficiency. Moreover, most lesbians have never had an expected path of midlife development and, with few role models to follow, many have developed a highly individualized balance of personal commitments. This heterogeneity is reflected in the divergent age at which lesbians and bisexual women become aware of their sexual orientation; not uncommonly, this may occur toward the end of early adulthood or during midlife (Sang 1991).

■ Health

The most significant health issues for lesbians and bisexual women in midlife (as with younger and older lesbians) result from invisibility, ignorance of medical professionals about lesbian health concerns, and lack of access to health care. Little is known about lesbian health in midlife. The National Lesbian Health Care Survey completed in 1985 provided a description of the demographics and health status of 2,000 lesbians. In an analysis of survey respondents between ages 40 and 60, Bradford and Ryan (1991) found that "lesbians appear similar to all women of the same age, both in general health and the prevalence of typical problems" (p. 162). Lesbians in midlife, however, experienced significant financial problems, despite high levels of education and professional experience, and many were not receiving adequate health care because of financial reasons or past negative experiences related to their lesbianism.

Significant questions concerning the health of midlife lesbians, including whether lesbian and heterosexual women differ in the onset or experience of menopause and the relative risk of lesbians developing breast cancer, remain unanswered. Little is known about HIV transmission between women, as data on this route of transmission are not routinely collected. Beyond questions of HIV infection, many lesbians play significant roles as caregivers, members of AIDS service organizations, and family members and friends of HIV-infected individuals. Many have experienced multiple bereavements as a result of AIDS.

■ Work

Those heterosexual women who experience midlife most successfully are described as having a professional identity—a sense of self not just as wife or mother—in addition to economic independence and intellectual commitment. These characteristics are applicable to most lesbians, who have often known since adolescence that they would not be living in traditional heterosexual marriages and would most likely be self-supporting.

Bradford and Ryan (1991) report that lesbians in midlife are four times as likely to be employed in professional or technical roles, considerably more likely to work as managers or administrators, and less likely to occupy clerical positions, when compared to all working women in midlife. However, their incomes do not reflect occupational status, with few lesbians reporting annual incomes of over $40,000 in 1985. Lesbians in the workplace are subject to the same difficulties as all women, such as sexual harassment, lower wages, and "glass ceilings," in addition to discrimination because of sexual orientation.

■ Family and Relationships

Like other women, most lesbians strongly value relationships (see Chapter 20 by Klinger and Chapter 44 by Herbert). Many identify friendship networks as their greatest source of support, whereas heterosexual women are more likely to rely on extended families for support. In addition to friendship networks, most lesbians are involved in a primary relationship with another woman (Bradford et al. 1994). The lack of legal recognition of these relationships, however, may create additional stress throughout adulthood. For example, midlife or younger lesbians may be engaged in custody battles that require concealment of their sexuality or relationships.

Parenting raises many issues for many lesbians (see Chapter 21 by Kirkpatrick). These issues include the decision whether or not to undertake parenting and, if undertaken, caring for young children and adolescents; balancing career demands; and creating or finding support within the lesbian community to help manage the multiple roles associated with parenthood, partnership, and work identity. For lesbians who do not have children, generativity may be expressed in relationships with other women, community involvement, or contact with older or younger lesbians.

Midlife Development and Mental Health Issues for Gay Men

■ Perceptions of Aging

The awareness in midlife of no longer being young can be a potent realization and may lead to increased psychological distress, personal growth, or both. Earlier reports of adjustment in middle-age gay men emphasized concerns about decreasing physical attractiveness (Levy

1981). Some middle-age gay men continue to be strongly affected by social norms equating sexual and personal desirability with youthfulness; these men may experience heightened concerns about growing older (Harry 1982). Nevertheless, the expanding range of self-definition and life choices available to many gay men in midlife provide an opportunity for ongoing personal growth during adulthood. Thus, gay men in their 40s and 50s may find themselves raising children or assuming important roles in an array of political, social, or community organizations.

◼ Generativity

Gay men in midlife may be at the height of their need to be generative (Cornett and Hudson 1987). In an ongoing study of adaptation to midlife in gay men between 40 and 55, one of the authors (R. M. Kertzner, unpublished observations, 1994) found that many participants cite the quality of friendships they cultivate and provide to others as a major source of pride and personal meaning in their lives. Intergenerational commitments also may be developed during this time. In a study of middle-age gay men without children, Farrell (1992) found that many of his subjects had strong feelings of loss concerning their childlessness and in response had strengthened kinship ties, established "fictive kin" relationships, served as mentors or "big brothers," or pursued foster or adoptive parenthood. Gay men in midlife also may be fathers, through previous marriage, adoption, or biological coparenting (see Chapter 22 by Patterson and Chan). Gay fathers, as with lesbian mothers, are likely to experience additional developmental tasks, such as those arising from parenting older children or adolescents and incorporating children into new family life, often with a male coparent. Gay men, along with lesbians, are creating novel configurations of family with significant implications for self-identity and personal growth in midlife.

◼ Work Identity

Career consolidation—a clear, specialized career identification as measured by occupational satisfaction, commitment, and skill—is thought to be a normative process for men in young adulthood (Vaillant 1980).

This consolidation may be applicable to homosexual as well as heterosexual men, with some gay men in professional or managerial positions describing their 30s and 40s as a time when jobs evolve into careers that become important means of self-realization, creativity, and generativity (R. M. Kertzner, unpublished observations, 1994).

Some gay men working in institutional or business settings may resist greater identities as "company men" as they ascend work hierarchies. Gay men with advanced degrees from colleges and universities may not promote themselves at work or may hold themselves back from advancement, fearing an exposure of their homosexuality. As such, a "lavender ceiling" may be just as much self-imposed as it is a reality of discrimination in the workplace (Horn 1994).

In one of the authors' (R.K.) experience, some gay men in their 30s may sense that they are no longer the "golden, fair-haired boy," or that prized relationships with older mentors cannot be indefinitely maintained. If these real or pending terminations evoke feelings of paternal rejection initially experienced during childhood (Isay 1989), work transitions in midlife may rekindle feelings of early loss with resultant decreased self-esteem and depression.

■ The HIV Epidemic

In the "nexus of disease, culture, sexuality, stigma, death and survival which is the HIV epidemic" (Gorman 1991), it is difficult to discern issues specific to midlife and aging. HIV infection has profoundly touched the lives of many gay men and women, particularly those residing in large metropolitan areas, and has had myriad effects on gay male development and mental health (see Chapter 51 by Ostrow). Two factors emerge, however, that may be particularly relevant for a discussion of midlife issues.

First, HIV serological status affects perceptions of time remaining in life, a hallmark of midlife reconceptualization of the self (Neugarten 1968). Hopcke (1992) describes an "AIDS-induced midlife" for some gay men in which a confrontation with mortality provides an opening to a classic midlife psychological transformation. The HIV epidemic may have moved a generation of gay men concerned with consolidating personal identity into a period of heightened generativity as reflected in widespread care-partnering and increased community involvement. If so, this may represent a seismic coincidence of individual and social change.

Second, the experience of AIDS-related bereavement is a key determinant of mental health in gay men (Martin and Dean 1993) and also may strongly influence perceptions of midlife. Although all ages of gay men have been affected by HIV, those in midlife have perhaps experienced the greatest number of cumulative AIDS deaths. With the decimation of friendship networks, many gay men feel a diminished sense of family and a heightened apprehension about loneliness in the future. Clinical and research reports describe problems of anxiety, depression, and "survival guilt" in some HIV-negative gay men, particularly those with higher numbers of past partners who have died (Odets 1992; Wayment et al. 1990). Many HIV-negative gay men report that the HIV epidemic has altered their sense of growing older; some gay men no longer take for granted a normal life expectancy or feel "lucky and grateful about getting this far in life" (Kertzner et al. 1994).

Conclusion

Midlife is a time of maximal opportunities for gay men and lesbians, and in this sense, homosexual adult development may depart from more classic descriptions of midlife in heterosexuals. Without the developmental "headstart" of a conventional sexual orientation or the social facilitation of a gay identity, the developmental task of young adulthood may be to consolidate homosexual identity and to explore individual sexuality. By midlife, the urgency of these tasks may yield to a readiness to undertake more expansive pursuits, such as making a mark on the world, creating a legacy, or sharing life experiences, tasks that may be achieved by establishing families or nurturing friendships, or through creative work. Paradoxically, for gay men and lesbians most affected by the HIV epidemic, midlife also requires adjusting to the closeness of death and accepting the evanescence of life, which are developmental tasks usually associated with old age.

The overriding developmental task of homosexual adulthood may be that of striking a balance between maintaining positive self-identity as a gay or lesbian individual and undergoing the more universal self-transformations associated with middle age (assuming the individual has good health). All gay men and lesbians must maintain certain aspects of a positive gay self-identity in what Brooks (1992) has called "an assumptive world that negates their existence, and which directly or indirectly rewards their invisibility and punishes healthy disclosure" (p. 211). In addition, midlife gay men and lesbians may need to reintegrate their homosexual self-identity into a larger, changing self-identity based on an awareness of aging and the discovery or heightened realization in adulthood of "what and whom you can take care of " (Erikson 1973, p. 124).

Within these broad themes, important gender differences may characterize the adult development of gay men and lesbians. Specific issues associated with the developmental tasks of adulthood (e.g., intimacy or generativity) may vary by gender in homosexual as well as heterosexual midlife (Kimmel and Sang 1995). Psychological well-being in midlife also may be associated with gender differences, in gay men and lesbians as well as in the general population (Ryff 1989).

The relationship between adult development, psychological well-being, and the maintenance of gay identity is complex and to date poorly delineated. As more gay men and lesbians establish healthy sexual identities in young adulthood, a greater need exists to extend descriptions of normative homosexual life into middle adulthood. Medical advances against HIV and the continuing evolution of social tolerance and legal rights, as recognized by the recognition of domestic partnerships, parenting rights, and homosexual marriage, and the adoption of antidiscrimination measures will undoubtedly help to shape the future course of midlife development for gay men and lesbians. In a world of greater possibility, homosexual midlife would become a way station en route to a full realization of human potential.

References

Baruch G, Brooks-Gunn J: Women in Midlife. New York, Plenum, 1984

Boulton M: Research on bisexual men: sociodemographic or social context? AIDS 7:1267–1268, 1993

Bradford J, Ryan C: Who we are: health concerns of middle-aged lesbians, in Lesbians at Mid-life: the Creative Transition. Edited by Sang B, Warshow J, Smith AJ. San Francisco, CA, Spinster Books, 1991, pp 147–163

Bradford J, Ryan C, Rothblum ED: National lesbian health care survey: implications for mental health care. J Consult Clin Psychol 6:228–242, 1994

Brooks WK: Research and the gay minority: problems and possibilities, in Lesbian and Gay Lifestyles. Edited by Woodman NJ. New York, Irvington Publishers, 1992, pp 201–215

Bumpass LL, Aquilino WS: A Social Map of Midlife: Family and Work Over the Middle Life Course. Vero Beach, FL, MacArthur Foundation Research Network on Successful Midlife Development, 1995

Cohen CJ, Stein TS: Reconceptualizing individual psychotherapy with gay men and lesbians, in Contemporary Perspectives on Psychotherapy with Gay Men and Lesbians. Edited by Stein TS, Cohen CJ. New York, Plenum, 1986, pp 27–53

Coleman E: Developmental stage of the coming out process. J Homosex 7:31–43, 1981–1982

Cornett CW, Hudson RA: Middle adulthood and the theories of Erikson, Gould, and Vaillant: where does the gay man fit in? Journal of Gerontological Social Work 10(3/4):61–73, 1987

Erikson EH: Identity and the life cycle. Psychological Issues 1(1):50–100, 1959

Erikson EH: Dimensions of a New Identity: Jefferson Lectures. New York, WW Norton, 1973

Farrell K: The Psychosocial Adaptations of Middle-Aged Gay Men to Being Childless. Master's thesis, California State University, Long Beach, CA, December 1992

Gilbert LA: Women at midlife: current theoretical perspectives and research. Women and Therapy 14:105–115, 1993

Gorman EM: Anthropological reflections on the HIV epidemic among gay men. J Sex Res 28:263–273, 1991

Harry J: Gay Children Grown Up. New York, Prager, 1982

Herdt G, Boxer A: Introduction: culture, history, and life course of gay men, in Gay Culture in America: Essays From the Field. Edited by Herdt G. Boston, MA, Beacon Press, 1992, pp 1–28

Hopcke RH: Midlife, gay men, and the AIDS epidemic. Quadrant 35(1):101–109, 1992

Horn M: Making your life your life's work. Metrosource, Autumn/Winter, 1994, p 52

Isay RA: Being Homosexual: Gay Men and Their Development. New York, Farrar, Straus, Giroux, 1989

Jung CG: Modern Man in Search of a Soul. New York, Harcourt, Brace and World, 1933

Kertzner RM, Todak G, Goetz R, et al: Living in a sero-possible world: adaptations of HIV-negative gay men. Poster presented at the Second Annual Biopsychosocial Conference on AIDS, Brighton, UK, 1994

Kimmel DC: Adult development and aging: a gay perspective. Journal of Social Issues 34(3):113–130, 1978

Kimmel DC, Sang BE: Lesbians and gay men in midlife, in Lesbian, Gay, and Bisexual Identities Over the Lifespan: Psychological Perspectives. Edited by D'Augelli AR, Patterson CJ. New York, Oxford University Press, 1995

Levenson DJ: The Seasons of a Man's Life. New York, Alfred A Knopf, 1978

Levy N: The middle-aged male and female homosexual, in Modern Perspectives in the Psychiatry of Middle Age. Edited by Howells JG. New York, Brunner Mazel, 1981, pp 116–113

Martin JL, Dean L: Effects of AIDS-related bereavement and HIV-related illness on psychological distress among gay men: a seven year longitudinal study. J Consult Clin Psychol 61:94–103, 1993

Minnigerode FA: Age-status labeling in homosexual men. J Homosex 1:273–276, 1976

Nemiroff RA, Calorusso CA: Frontiers of adult development in theory and practice, in New Dimensions in Adult Development. Edited by Nemiroff RA, Calorusso CA. New York, Basic Books, 1990, pp 97–124

Neugarten BL: The awareness of middle age, in Middle Age and Aging. Edited by Neugarten BL. Chicago, IL, University of Chicago Press, 1968, pp 93–98

Odets W: Unconscious motivations for the practice of unsafe sex among gay men in the United States. Poster presented at the Eighth International AIDS Conference, Amsterdam, July 1992, PoD 511, p D418

Robinson BE, Skeen P, Flake-Hobson C: Sex role endorsement among homosexual men across the life span. Arch Sex Behav 11:355–359, 1982

Ryff CD: Happiness is everything, or is it? Explorations on the meaning of psychological well-being. J Pers Soc Psychol 57:1069–1081, 1989

Sang B: Moving toward balance and integration, in Lesbians at Midlife: The Creative Transition. Edited by Sang B, Warshow J, Smith AJ. San Francisco, CA, Spinster Books, 1991, pp 206–214

Stein TS: Overview of new developments in understanding homosexuality, in American Psychiatric Press Review of Psychiatry, Vol 12. Edited by Oldham JM, Riba MB, Tasman A. Washington, DC, American Psychiatric Press, 1993, pp 9–40

Troiden RR: Self, self-concept, identity, and homosexual identity: constructs in need of definition and differentiation. J Homosex 10:97–109, 1984

Vaillant GE: Adaptation to Life. Boston, MA, Little, Brown, 1977

Vaillant GE, Milofsky E: Natural history of male psychological health: IX. Empirical evidence for Erikson's model of the life cycle. Am J Psychiatry 137(11):1348–1359, 1980

Wayment HA, Kemeny ME, Silver RC: Survivor syndrome in the gay community. Poster presented at the Sixth International AIDS Conference, San Francisco, CA, June 1990, SD 906, Vol 3, p 316

Gay Men and Lesbians
Grown Older

Raymond M. Berger, Ph.D.
James J. Kelly, Ph.D.

B ecause the professional literature on aging rarely mentions older gay men and lesbians, the reader may believe that homosexuality does not exist among elderly people. However, the authors' knowledge of the Kinsey data, which shows that gay men and lesbians exist in substantial numbers across the age span (Kinsey and Gebhard 1953; Kinsey et al. 1948), as well as their impressions gained from conversations with older gay men, suggest otherwise.

If we assume that 8% of the adult population is same-sex oriented (Berger 1982), then gay men and lesbians ages 65 and older number over 1.75 million in the United States alone. Older gay men and lesbians have been ignored by both gerontological researchers and mental health providers. Their special needs have nearly always gone unidentified and unmet, and they have withstood the effects of societal hate and discrimination to an extent at which many younger gay men and lesbians might marvel. This is changing.

In this chapter, the authors review recent research that has debunked much of the mythology of gay male and lesbian aging, and highlight some ways in which being gay or lesbian can actually make it easier to grow old. Although most psychosocial needs of older gay men and lesbians are the same as those of other older people, several special needs are reviewed, and the authors discuss how clinicians can be helpful to this group.

Fiction and Fact

No gay person can ignore the extreme stereotypes of gay male aging that are popular in our culture. Plays, novels, and even (until recently) scholarly presentations have painted a bleak future for young gay men and lesbians. The older gay man is said to become increasingly isolated and effeminate as he ages. Lacking family and friends, he is portrayed as desperately lonely. He must settle for no sex life at all, or he must prey upon young boys to satisfy his lust.

The older lesbian, where she is said to exist at all, is purported to be a cruel witch. Cold, unemotional, and heartless, she despises men. Devoted solely to masculine interests and career pursuits, she has no friends and is repeatedly frustrated by the rejections of younger women whose attention she solicits.

These stereotypes have had a devastating effect on both young and old gay men and lesbians. Many sociologists believe that our self-concepts are determined by our beliefs regarding evaluations of us by others (Weinberg and Williams 1975). Negative stereotypes, then, are the most important weapon in the arsenal of low self-esteem messages that society wields against unpopular groups, and they have helped to ensure that gay men and lesbians remain unpopular.

Fortunately, the authors have enough research evidence (less for women, unfortunately) to say with confidence that only a small minority of older gay men and lesbians fit the negative stereotypes. For example, in a questionnaire study of 1,117 gay men of all ages, Weinberg and Williams (1975) found older respondents to be as well adjusted as younger ones and in some ways more so. Compared with younger gay men, older gay men worried less about disclosure or discovery of their homosexuality, were less likely to desire psychiatric treatment, and had more stable self-concepts. Minnigerode (1976) found that gay men do not perceive themselves as aging sooner than heterosexual men. In a study of 43 gay men aged 32–76, Friend (1980) found high levels of personal adjustment, particularly among men who were open about their homosexuality. Rather than being isolated, these men had support systems composed of both family and friends. Kelly (1977) reported that although older gay men visited gay bars less frequently than their younger counterparts, no evidence existed that they had disengaged from others. About one-third of these men reported feelings of loneliness, but more than one-half had a lover, and the majority were satisfied with their sex lives. Most older gay men had many gay friends. Older respondents had more positive views of other older gay men than did younger gay men.

To date, the most comprehensive study of older gay men is Berger's (1984) survey of 112 gay men aged 41–77. None of the men in this study fits the stereotype of extreme social isolation. Rather than preying on younger men, these older men preferred to socialize with age peers, particularly other gay men. Only about one-third lived alone, and almost one-half lived with a lover. About one-third had been heterosexually married. Almost three-fourths described themselves as "well accepted" or "popular" among other gay men. However, their participation in gay community institutions such as bars, social clubs, and organizations was low.

Berger (1984) also measured older gay men's self-acceptance, depression, and psychosomatic symptoms. On average, his respondents scored well within the healthy range. Eighty-four percent of Berger's respondents said they were "very happy" or "pretty happy," and only a few reported that the knowledge that they were homosexual "weighed on their mind." About one-half worried at least sometimes about growing older, but few ever worried about dying. Only a small number desired counseling for their homosexuality or for any other personal issues. The two strongest predictors of good psychological adjustment were commitment to homosexuality and integration into the gay community. With minor exceptions, age was not associated with measures of psychological adjustment, suggesting that aging is not associated with poor adjustment among older gay men.

Berger's findings failed to support the stereotype that older gay men always conceal their homosexuality and are uptight about being known as gay. More than one-third of these men agreed that they did not care who knew about their homosexuality. About one-third were "out" to all or most of their heterosexual acquaintances, relatives, and work associates.

Although older lesbians have been less studied, available findings also debunk the myths about this group. In an early study, Saghir and Robins (1973) reported that about half their sample of 31 younger lesbians believed they would grow old gracefully and would remain involved and interested in life. Wolf (1980) suggested that older lesbians use "fictive kin"; that is, they use friends as substitutes for the family relationships that are more prevalent among straight women. This idea was confirmed by Raphael and Robinson (1980) on the basis of 20 interviews with lesbians who were age 50 and older. All except one (a woman who relied solely on her lover) had friendship networks, and none of the respondents fit the stereotype of the desperately lonely lesbian. Middle-aged and older lesbians preferred other older women as intimate partners and were often able to find them.

A questionnaire study (C. Almvig, unpublished master's thesis, 1984) of 74 lesbians age 50 and older depicted similar patterns. Almost three-quarters described their mental health as good or excellent and said their lesbianism had been a source of great joy and satisfaction to them. A few more than half had a current lover, and only half lived alone. Although Bell and Weinberg (1978) found that older lesbians were less sexually active than younger lesbians, the majority were still sexually active, primarily with age-peer partners.

These research findings paint a new picture. Most older gay men and lesbians are reasonably well adjusted. They are generally well integrated into social networks and relate primarily with age peers.

Lessons To Be Learned

Studies of older gay men and lesbians are beginning to show ways in which the unique adaptations of this group provide healthy pathways for a good adjustment to aging. In some ways, being gay can be an advantage for the aging individual.

Francher and Henkin (1973) suggested that early life experiences of older gay men led them to develop skills and attitudes that helped them adapt to growing older. For example, one of the tragedies of growing older in our culture is that old people are stigmatized: they are treated as useless and incompetent. However, many gay men and lesbians learned how to cope with a stigmatized identity early in life and are able to insulate themselves from the worst effects of societal stigma by developing self-affirming attitudes and by seeking support from others. These skills and attitudes also are useful in adapting to the stigmatized status of being an older person.

A closely related idea is that gay people also experience a "crisis of independence" in early adulthood. Because they cannot take family and other social supports for granted, they learn self-reliance skills that become crucial in old age as friends and lovers die and as social roles become constricted. One of these skills is role flexibility. The sex role divisions that are the norm in heterosexual relationships are less common among same-sex couples, where both partners generally learn to do "male" and "female" tasks.

There is another factor related to sex roles that may play an important part in the adjustment of older gay men and lesbians to aging. One of the most difficult parts of growing older for all of us is learning to accept the physical changes of aging. They are rarely welcome. From the point of view of traditional heterosexual sex roles, the changes that come with age often make men less masculine and women less feminine. For example, many older men have trouble adjusting to diminished physical capacities and older women are perceived to be less feminine. Again, earlier life experiences may serve older gay men and lesbians well in meeting this challenge. They are likely to have less personal investment in following traditional notions of virility and masculinity or sexiness and femininity, respectively. The physical changes that accompany old age, then, may not seem like insurmountable hurdles.

When Things Go Wrong

Not all is rosy for older gay men and lesbians. Being old is not easy in a society that treats elderly people badly. The problems faced by older gay men and lesbians are, for the most part, the problems faced by all older people. The two most important concerns are: "Will I have good health?" and "Will I have enough money to live comfortably?"

On top of these concerns are several issues unique to older gay men and lesbians. Social service agencies and helping professionals often fail to recognize the needs of their older gay and lesbian clients. The reluctance of most gay men and lesbians (older and younger) to reveal their sexual orientation perpetuates the problem, but their reluctance did not create it. When seeking services, gay men and lesbians are not likely to come out because they have assessed, often accurately, that this will cause difficulty or result in poor service.

In some situations, the sexual orientation of the older person will not be relevant. But what if a same-sex partner dies? How many social service agencies are able to provide sensitive and well-informed bereavement counseling for a gay male or lesbian surviving partner? Where will a sexually dysfunctional same-sex couple seek help? Will an older gay man have to hide his orientation from a homemaker or home health aide on whom he depends heavily? What about the older lesbian who needs help in handling life's difficulties: can she really open up to a counselor who may not accept her homosexuality?

Little information, other than anecdotal data, is available about the treatment of older gay men and lesbians by helping professionals. The authors often hear comments from their colleagues about the lack of responsiveness of mainstream social service agencies to the needs of the gay and lesbian communities and about the ways in which helping professionals have added to oppression by misdiagnosing, stigmatizing, and "treating" such clients. The authors suspect these problems are even more severe for elderly gay and lesbian people, although no hard data exist to support this suspicion.

When elderly people come to the attention of a helping professional, they are likely to be dependent and vulnerable. This is true, for example, of elderly nursing home residents and frail older individuals who need in-home services. That these people might be gay or lesbian is never considered. Inasmuch as most helping professionals in gerontological services believe that all elderly individuals are heterosexual, they are unequipped to provide adequate service to their gay and lesbian clients.

Several years ago a social worker brought to the authors' attention a survey of human service agencies that was conducted in 1984 in a medium-sized midwestern city (J. J. Gerhardstein, personal communication, 1984). Each human service agency in the community was asked whether it provided any resources specific to gay men and lesbians, if it did outreach to them, if it had any philosophy about such services, and if it had any staff with particular expertise or sensitivity in this area. The survey results were most notable for the consistency with which most agencies answered "No" to all these questions.

Of all the agencies in this city, there were 13 that provided services specifically to elderly people. All medical centers were included because older adults are heavy consumers of health care. None of the

13 agencies provided any outreach to gay or lesbian elderly people nor did they have a specialized resource or staff person. Five of the agencies stated that their philosophy included nondiscrimination, but the remaining agencies either made no comment about services to gay men and lesbians or were hostile to the researcher.

Of the six nursing homes in the community, only two completed the questionnaire, and both of these responded they were unaware of how homosexuality related to their services. One response was that a philosophy about services to this group was "not needed." The response of another home, which refused to complete the questionnaire, was all too typical: "As a skilled nursing facility providing medical care to the elderly, we feel this questionnaire is inappropriate/irrelevant to our services." Consider that a nursing home with a patient census of 200 residents is likely to have 16 to 20 elderly gay men and lesbians. Also consider what sort of treatment these people would be likely to receive in such a home if their sexual orientation were to become known.

Institutional policies present some of the most difficult problems for older gay men and lesbians because of the vulnerability of patients. Disclosure of the homosexuality of a patient may result in ostracism or abuse by other patients. The quality of life of nursing home patients is most affected by their treatment at the hands of nonprofessional staff, who provide assistance for activities of daily living. Regardless of the patient's sexual orientation, concerns often exist about the care of institutionalized patients. Attendants are poorly paid and receive little or no training in basic care skills and almost no training in personal or interactional skills. In many urban areas, staff may not speak the same language as patients, further complicating personal interactions with them. Although training about the full range of human sexuality among older persons would alleviate this problem, such training is rarely available to institutional staff.

Few nursing homes allow conjugal visits or sexual expression of their heterosexual residents. They are even less likely to allow an older lesbian or gay man to have an intimate visit with a lover.

Formal policies may create problems for the older gay man or lesbian. Most intensive care units allow visits by blood relatives and spouses only, excluding lifelong same-sex partners. When the older person is incompetent or otherwise unable to make decisions, the patient's lover must often stand by helplessly while relatives (who may be distant or hostile to the patient's homosexuality) make life-and-death decisions.

The legal system can also create severe problems for the older gay man or lesbian. Most often these are problems of omission rather than commission, that is, the problem is not created by laws that prohibit sexual conduct but rather by the fact that gay men and lesbians are not afforded benefits or protection that apply to heterosexuals. For example, an older gay man or lesbian may experience discrimination in renting or buying a home, securing employment, and purchasing insurance. In most areas, such discrimination is legal.

Finally, same-sex partners are rarely able to share job-related benefits, such as health insurance, that are routinely made available to heterosexual spouses. Until recently this was true everywhere. Today, however, more than two dozen local jurisdictions and a number of corporations have instituted domestic partner laws and policies that extend these benefits to both opposite-sex and same-sex unmarried partners (Berger and Kelly 1994).

Clinical Implications

Clinicians who treat younger homosexuals often assume (incorrectly) that the client's sexual orientation is the "problem." For the older gay male or lesbian client who comes to the clinic with a lifelong adaptation to homosexuality, it is even less appropriate to assume that the client's sexual orientation is the problem. The client may simply need help adapting to the challenges that face all older persons. Therefore, clinicians who treat older gay men and lesbians must be familiar with the mental health challenges that face older persons in general.

Depression is the most common mental health problem of older persons. This mood disorder may be the result of many factors: the older person's perception that his or her life goals were not achieved, the death of a spouse or of one's friends and family, declining health and loss of physical abilities, and financial limitations. Clinical intervention may involve supportive counseling, cognitive therapy, restructuring of social support systems and daily activities, financial counseling, evaluation of medical problems, and use of antidepressant medication. These interventions are applicable regardless of the older client's sexual orientation.

Despite these considerations it is hard to imagine how the treatment of an older gay male or lesbian client can be effective unless the clinician is knowledgeable about gay and lesbian people, their communities, and the resources available to them. Because the clinician's warmth, genuineness, and empathy are the most critical ingredients of a successful intervention, the clinician must feel comfortable and confident about working with older gay men and lesbians. In addition, that comfort must extend to discussion of intimate issues such as the loss of a same-sex partner and concerns about sexual issues. Clinicians can become more comfortable in working with older gay male and lesbian clients by having older gay and lesbian friends or direct contact with older gay and lesbian persons, learning about the local community, attending training workshops designed to counter homophobia, and confronting their own fear and discomfort about homosexuality.

One of the thorniest issues in treating the concerns of older gay men and lesbians is the issue of client self-disclosure. Is it essential for the clinician to know the client's sexual orientation? Should the clinician ask? In general, asking older clients directly about their sexual orientation is not the best approach. Most older persons in our culture—homosexual and heterosexual—tend to be reticent about all forms of personal self-disclosure. The clinician who respects this reticence is most likely to establish the kind of trusting therapeutic relationship that is critical to success.

It is often important, however, for the clinician to be aware that the client is gay or lesbian. Experienced clinicians know that they are most effective when their clients feel free to self-disclose. For example, in bereavement counseling it is essential for the older client to be able to reminisce freely about his or her life partner, without fear of censure. To facilitate the open sharing of information between the clinician and an older gay male or lesbian client, the authors advocate an indirect but multifaceted approach. The goal is to establish a therapeutic environment in which the client can feel free to self-disclose. This can be accomplished at every stage of the client's involvement with the clinic.

In its public information and agency brochures, announcements of specialized programs, and media presentations a clinic can include older gay men, lesbians, and bisexual people. This information must establish that gay men and lesbians are welcomed, just as are other groups. The clinic should avoid any implication that its programs intend to "change" gay, lesbian, or bisexual individuals into heterosexuals.

On a clinic's intake form and in its intake interview, clients can be asked to respond to an optional question about their sexual orientation. Clinicians should not assume that all older clients are heterosexual, even if the clients are heterosexually married. In addition, the assessment process should recognize that older adults may have varied sexual histories, with heterosexual and homosexual interests dominating at different times in their lives. For older gay male or lesbian clients who are comfortable discussing their sexuality, this will facilitate their self-disclosure and will expedite establishment of an open therapeutic relationship. For clients who are referred to other agencies, the clinic's referral list of services should include local agencies that serve or publicly support gay male and lesbian clients. Even in rural areas where these agencies do not exist, the clinic's referral list can include contact information for national groups that the client can contact by mail or phone.

Clients who come to the clinic should see literature supporting gay men and lesbians in the waiting room and on the bookshelves of its treatment rooms. Gay bookstores, which are located in most large cities, can provide a list of appropriate magazines and books.[1] When clinicians administer paper-and-pencil assessment instruments, such as marital or relationship inventories, assessment items can be reworded so they apply to both opposite-sex and same-sex situations.

It is sometimes useful for clinicians to let clients know that they are supportive of gay men and lesbians and that they are experienced in dealing with issues of concern to older gay men and lesbians. Openly gay male or lesbian clinicians can self-disclose their own sexual orientation. Agencies can sponsor workshops to educate staff about sexual orientation. When colleagues and clients participate directly in providing this training, it has particular impact on staff attitudes and feelings toward gay men and lesbians.

Clinicians can also put their older gay and lesbian clients at ease by reviewing the clinic's policy governing confidentiality of client information. This is particularly true in rural areas or small towns where the consequences of being publicly labeled are greatest. Older gay men and lesbians who are employed may be legitimately concerned about

---

[1] The Gay and Lesbian Task Force of the American Library Association provides up-to-date reading lists of gay and lesbian fiction and nonfiction, lists of gay and lesbian bookstores, professional associations, and other materials. Readers may obtain an order form by writing to: GLTF Clearinghouse, ALA Office for Outreach Services, 50 East Huron Street, Chicago, IL 60611.

passing as heterosexual in their workplaces, but those who are retired may have few concerns. The degree of anxiety about disclosure may also be related to the older client's lifelong pattern of "passing" and to the nature of his or her support network. These considerations are more important than chronological age in determining the client's attitude about disclosure. Clinicians do best when they ask their gay male and lesbian clients how they feel about this matter, rather than make the assumption that all older gay men and lesbians want to pass at all times.

A final clinical issue concerns the availability of referral resources that are gay- and lesbian-positive. In many areas, gerontological services are characterized by homophobia or by the heterosexist belief that gay men and lesbians do not exist among older persons.

When making a mental health referral for an older gay or lesbian client—especially one who is openly gay—clinicians should consider whether that resource is likely to be gay-positive. For example, a clinician may need to request a psychiatric hospitalization for an older gay male client. Although a specialized gay unit is not likely to exist, staff at the local gay and lesbian services center may know about psychiatric units that are staffed by gay-sensitive personnel. Clinicians should also be familiar with local gay and lesbian resources such as support groups, information and referral services, and social clubs.

Because of dramatic social and health changes in the past two decades, there may be differences among future cohorts of older gay men and lesbians. For example, the cohort of gay men who are today in their 40s and 50s may be smaller than past or future cohorts, because AIDS has claimed many lives in this group. Although today's older gay men and lesbians have often adapted to societal oppression, the more activist cohort of current "twenty-something" gays and lesbians may bring greater levels of political activism to tomorrow's older homosexual population. Whatever the future brings, gay men and lesbians will continue to be an important part of the elderly population.

References

Bell AP, Weinberg MS: Homosexualities: A Study of Diversity Among Men and Women. New York, Simon and Schuster, 1978

Berger RM: The unseen minority: older gays and lesbians. Soc Work 27:236–242, 1982

Berger RM: Gay and Gray: The Older Homosexual Man. Boston, MA, Alyson Press, 1984

Berger RM, Kelly JJ: Gay men: overview, in Encyclopedia of Social Work, Vol 2, 19th Edition. Edited by Edwards. Washington, DC, National Association of Social Workers, 1995, pp 1064–1075

Francher JS, Henkin J: The menopausal queen: adjustment to aging and the male homosexual. Am J Orthopsychiatry 43(4):670–674, 1973

Friend RA: GAYging: adjustment and the older gay male. Alternative Lifestyles 3(2):231–248, 1980

Kelly JJ: The aging male homosexual: myth and reality. Gerontologist 17(4):328–332, 1977

Kinsey AC, Gebhard PH: Sexual Behavior in the Human Female. Philadelphia, PA, WB Saunders, 1953

Kinsey AC, Pomeroy WB, Martin CE: Sexual Behavior in the Human Male. Philadelphia, PA, WB Saunders, 1948

Minnigerode FA: Age-status labeling in homosexual men. J Homosex 1:273–275, 1976

Raphael SM, Robinson MK: The older lesbian: love relationships and friendship patterns. Alternative Lifestyles 3(2):207–229, 1980

Saghir MT, Robins E: Male and Female Homosexuality: A Comprehensive Investigation. Baltimore, MD, Williams and Wilkins, 1973

Weinberg MS, Williams CJ: Male Homosexuals: Their Problems and Adaptations. New York, Penguin, 1975

Wolf DG: Life cycle change of older lesbians and gay men. Paper presented at the Annual Meeting of the Gerontological Society, San Diego, CA, 1980

SECTION IV

Creating Relationships

Gay and Lesbian Couples, Children, and Families

Male Couples

David P. McWhirter, M.D.
Andrew M. Mattison, M.S.W., Ph.D.

Male couples are a new social construct. A product of the second half of the 20th century, this construct arises from the visibility of the contemporary gay movement and the subsequent identification and establishment of social structures and organizational support systems. Although gay men have been living as couples for centuries, their social identification in their relationships had not been recognized. In the past 30 years, recognition of relationships of gay men and lesbian women has gone from nonexistent to the current legal establishment of same-sex marriages in Denmark and Sweden and legal domestic partnerships in some United States cities. There is a continuing clamor for federal and state legislatures to provide universal legalization of domestic relationships, whatever the partner's sex. The movement toward legalization and

Partial support for the writing of this chapter was provided by the HIV Neurobehavioral Research Center, NIMH Center Grant 5 P50 MH45294.

acceptance has continued to encounter severe and vitriolic opposition, arising mainly from religious conservatives.

As gay couples became more visible, they began seeking establishments catering to their needs as couples. Gay entrepreneurs began to respond with an array of professional, social, and business services marketed to these couples. Scientific researchers also became interested in this newly visible phenomenon and began describing and defining it more clearly.

Definitions

■ Male Couple

For the purpose of this chapter, a male couple is defined as two men, usually self-identified as gay, who are in a primary relationship with each other, similar to cohabiting or married heterosexual couples.

■ Varieties of Relationships

Most commonly, gay men in primary relationships choose to live together some time after a courtship period. However, because of their minority status and because they lack traditional norms and expectations, gay men have experimented with a variety of other relationship styles. The following are four such examples:

Two men living apart who describe themselves as a couple.   Such individuals may spend most of their free time together. They may sleep together in one partner's home, or sometimes each stays in his own. Reasons for this arrangement include considerations such as the occupation of each man, concern for family sensibilities, and the need for mutual independence.

Two men who describe themselves as a couple, living in different cities or continents.   Sometimes these couples live as they do because of their jobs, or perhaps because one is attending school in a distant city. They see each other on a regular basis, as often as every weekend or as infrequently as three or four times a year. Others live in this fashion because they describe their separation as one important ingredient that helps them to enjoy the relationship. These couples exchange letters, phone calls, faxes, and E-mail and may have sexual and affectionate relationships with others, while considering their lover as the primary partner.

A male couple, one member of which is in a heterosexual marriage. One partner maintains his own home, while the married partner lives with his wife and children. Sometimes the wife is fully aware of the gay relationship and accepts it; in other instances, the relationship is clandestine. Some couples consist of two heterosexually married men. It is no longer uncommon for a gay man to be married to a lesbian woman for convenience, cover, and children while continuing a primary relationship with a same-sex partner. Heterosexually married men involved in love relationships with other men appear to be more numerous than previously believed (Weinberg et al. 1994).

Brief relationships lasting less than 1 year. Brief relationships occur with the greatest frequency. For some people, moving from one brief relationship to the next becomes a way of life. For many, there is a series of brief relationships used for learning—as stepping stones leading to a more enduring partnership. For others, longer relationships may be interspersed with one or more brief ones.

Ethnic Diversity

Gay people can be found among all racial and ethnic groups. In the past 20 years ethnic minorities have formed their own openly gay and lesbian organizations. The visibility of male couples in all these groups has increased the general awareness of the universality of homosexuality. Many cross-cultural and mixed racial couples exist; some have national organizations like Black and White Men Together. Hispanic-Anglo relationships are very common, as are Asian-Pacific Islanders and Anglos. Despite considerable cultural boundaries, the visibility of male couples within ethnic groups is increasing, although there is no definitive research on this issue.

Incidence of Male Couples

There is serious controversy over the incidence of both male and female homosexuality in the United States and, for that matter, in the world community. Without entering into that controversy, suffice it to say that the original extrapolations from the Kinsey data and subsequent communications between Gebhardt and Voeller establishing 10% as the figure for homosexuality among U.S. males has not been substantiated by other research (McWhirter and Mattison 1984; see Chapter 4 by Michaels in this volume).

It is difficult to obtain a large enough random sample of the population to establish reliable data. For this chapter, the authors have elected to use Diamond's conclusion (1993) from his meta-analysis of all the important data studies that a mean of 5.5% of males have engaged in same-sex behaviors for some significant period in their lives. Further, by conservative extrapolation from other studies (Bell and Weinberg 1978; Jay and Young 1977; Spada 1979), the authors estimate that there are over one million male couples living in the United States. These couples live throughout the country, in large cities, in middle-American suburbs, on farms, in small towns, and among the very wealthy, the middle class, and the very poor.

Literature on Male Couples

The illness theory of homosexuality dominated the research about gay people until well after the 1973 decision by the American Psychiatric Association to delete homosexuality per se as a mental disorder. Before 1973 most research on homosexuality involved patients in therapy or men in prison (Berger 1990). Even after that, as more extensive studies of homosexuality were published, the focus was on individuals, not couples (Bell and Weinberg 1978; Saghir and Robins 1973). If couples were discussed, the focus was usually on sexuality with no attention to other qualities in relationships. For example, in the Saghir and Robins (1973) research, all the relationships between gay men were treated as affairs, with the assumption that they were short-lived.

Bell and Weinberg (1978) were the first researchers to offer a typology of gay relationships. The wrote about "closed-coupleds" and "open-coupleds," but they only included couples living together. Closed-coupleds were described as "happy" and similar to married men in levels of psychological adjustment. They described a close emotional bond between partners. They had few sexual problems and were sexually exclusive and accepting of their homosexuality. Open-coupleds lived with a primary partner but experienced a limited level of commitment. They admitted to limited satisfaction with their relationships and therefore sought outside sexual experiences. This group was less accepting of their homosexuality. In contrast, Kurdek and Schmitt (1987) found no difference between the psychological adjustment of closed-coupleds and open-coupleds but did find improved relationship quality in closed-coupleds.

Blumstein and Schwartz (1983) published a landmark comparative study including heterosexual married and cohabiting couples along with gay and lesbian couples. They identified major relationship issues including sex, finances, career, and work. Financial issues played an important part in determining satisfaction and partner autonomy in all couples, but male couples had the most difficult time resolving money issues. In the study done by McWhirter and Mattison (1984), pooling of money and the complete blending of finances were the most important evidence of commitment the couples made; it usually did not happen completely until after the couples had been together 10 years or more.

Silverstein (1981), Mendola (1980), Harry and DeVall (1978), and Harry (1984) all wrote books on male couples based on surveys and interviews with couples. These descriptive and survey research data provided unbiased and nonprejudiced phenomenological information about the day-to-day lives and issues of gay couples. For example, Harry's study (1984) of male couples focused attention on characteristics of male couples to see how they differ from heterosexual ones, which are traditionally structured around sex roles.

A special issue of the *Journal of Homosexuality*, edited by Peplau and Jones (1982), was devoted entirely to a symposium on couples. A series of articles examined not only love and sex in gay and lesbian couples, but also investigated other components of coupling, such as partners' attitudes about closeness, distance, loyalty, power, decision making, age differences, and sex roles.

The Male Couple (McWhirter and Mattison 1984) was the first systematic, longitudinal study of male couples, and it gained the attention of both nongay and gay readers. The in-depth study of 156 male couples undermined many long-held myths about gay men. The work demonstrated that gay male relationships characterized by longevity, satisfaction, and lifetime dedication do exist. A theory of relationship stages emerged from this work, discussed later in the chapter.

A recent review article on lesbian and gay couples (Kurdek 1995) is a very comprehensive overview of the research work that has been done over the last 20 years, with highlights of Kurdek's and Kurdek and Schmitt's multiple contributions on comparisons, relationship satisfaction, stability, and predictors of relationship functioning (Kurdek 1994; Kurdek and Schmitt 1987). Kurdek's work demonstrated, as he said, the need to develop conceptual frameworks that integrate current findings and generate testable predictions.

Permanent Partners (Berzon 1988) represents a genre of works about lesbian and gay couples written for gay and lesbian couples themselves. The appearance of such books showed the interest of same-sex couples in building and nurturing relationships that last. *The Male Couple's Guide* (Marcus 1992), *Love Between Men* (Isensee 1990), and *Intimacy Between Men* (Driggs and Finn 1991) are but a few of these popular books for male couples.

Models of Relationships

There are three historical models for male-male relationships as described by Harry (1984): the Latin-American model, patterned after traditional sex roles; the Greek model, involving a mature adult male and a younger male; and the more modern form between males of approximately the same ages that predominates today.

Studying how these relationships are established and develop has been the work of a number of researchers (Blumstein and Schwartz 1983; Harry 1984; Kurdek and Schmitt 1987; Larson 1982; McWhirter and Mattison 1984; Peplau and Jones 1982). The theory McWhirter and Mattison (1984) proposed uses a model of developmental stages, which has gained significance in the past decade. This theory was derived from the analysis of interviews with 156 male couples who were together from 1 to 37 years. Some findings of that study showed that gay men can and do establish long-term, committed relationships, which are characterized by stability, mutual caring, generosity, creativity, intimacy, love, support, and nurturing.

Before this research, only anecdotal reports provided evidence for the existence of these relationships. Some findings from the research are particularly cogent. For example, it was telling that gay males needed to find alternate ways to maintain intimacy and longevity in their relationships. Gay men have lacked models for their relationships other than the traditional heterosexual ones, and yet many values and practices that are cornerstones of heterosexual relationships are absent in male couples. In fact, some qualities identified with stability and intimacy between men and women can be detrimental for lesbian and gay male relationships. As an example, although most gay couples begin their relationships with implicit or explicit commitment to sexual exclusivity, few of the couples in the authors' original group reported that they had been consistently sexually monogamous through the years of their relationship. Sexual exclusivity is not an ongoing expectation among many male couples.

Another important finding was the assumption of equality between two men in a relationship, which is difficult for heterosexual partners. In most heterosexual relationships, the woman has been expected to be dependent on the man whether because of biology, tradition, religion, or oppression. Traditionally, the man has been expected to make more money and support her. He has greater earning power. Only a small percentage of heterosexual couples have succeeded in establishing relationships of complete equality, despite modern feminism calling attention to this inequity. Lacking the difference in sex, there is a tendency toward greater equality between gay partners, as expressed in attitudes toward each other and exemplified in their maintenance of financial separateness during the early years of their relationship.

Some theoretical constructs began to develop as the data from the McWhirter and Mattison study (1984) were analyzed. Different answers and an emerging pattern developed when men responded to questions about family, friends, social lives, sexuality, and how problems developed and were resolved in the relationship. The length of the relationship tended to predict the nature of the responses. The responses of couples who had been together for only a few years were similar to one another, as were the responses of couples who had been together 10 years and those of couples who had been together 20 years. It became clear that factors keeping couples together in the first years are very different from factors that keep them together in the 5th, 10th, or 20th year. Although every relationship is unique, male couples, in general, move through a characteristic series of stages in their relationship, which are mainly related to the length of time together.

Six stages, each with a time frame and a name that describes what happens in that stage, were identified. The four characteristics that are associated with each stage describe the major components of that stage (see Table 19–1). Each relationship stage has many more characteristics than the four listed, but those reported here are the ones reported most frequently by the study participants. There are no good or bad characteristics, and often those from one stage become the building blocks for those in other stages. The stages are not necessarily linear or flat but spiral-shaped and multidimensional. Characteristics from one stage also may be present in other stages, and they sometimes overlap.

Not all male couples fit this model. However, after over 12 years of using and reevaluating it and having others use these findings in other research, the authors believe that the model has acquired greater validation. The authors have always seen this model as a beginning to understanding the complex phenomenon of male couples.

Stages of Relationships

Stage One: Blending (Year 1)

Blending is experienced as the intensity of togetherness gay men feel early in their relationships. Their similarities bind them; their differ-

Table 19–1. Developmental stages and their characteristics of the male couple

Stage 1: blending (year 1)	Stage 4: building (years 6–10)
Merging	Collaborating
Limerence	Increasing productivity
Equalizing of partnership	Establishing independence
High sexual activity	Dependability of partners
Stage 2: nesting (years 2 and 3)	**Stage 5: releasing (years 11–20)**
Homemaking	Trusting
Finding compatibility	Merging of money and possessions
Decline of limerence	Constricting
Ambivalence	Taking each other for granted
Stage 3: maintaining (years 4 and 5)	**Stage 6: renewing (beyond 20 years)**
Reappearance of the individual	Achieving security
Risk taking	Shifting perspectives
Dealing with conflict	Restoring the partnership
Establishing traditions	Remembering

Source. Adapted from McWhirter and Mattison 1984.

ences are mutually overlooked. They tend to do everything together, almost to the exclusion of others. Limerence is intense and most often reciprocal, although there are variations here. Equality is usually manifested in shared financial responsibility and equal distribution of the chores of daily living, but most importantly as a shared attitude. Sexual activity varies but usually includes several encounters weekly and de facto sexual exclusivity.

■ Stage Two: Nesting (Years 2 and 3)

During the first year together, men appear to have limited concerns about their living environment. By the second year, however, attention to their surroundings takes the form of homemaking activities, decorating a new home, or rearranging an old one. Couples in this stage also tend to see each other's shortcomings and discover or create complementarities that enhance compatibility. The partners' decline in limerence is usually not simultaneous and is often a cause for worry and concern. The search for compatibility and the decline in limerence set the stage for the mixture of positive and negative feelings about the value of the relationship, termed "ambivalence."

■ Stage Three: Maintaining (Years 4 and 5)

Maintaining the relationship depends on establishing balances between individualization and togetherness, conflict and its resolution, autonomy and dependence, and confusion and understanding. The intense blending of stage one clears the path for the reemergence of individual differences, identified here as individualization. As this process begins, individualization is accompanied by some necessary risk taking, whether in outside sexual liaisons, more time apart, greater self-disclosure, or new, separate friendships. These risks often result in conflicts, including jealousy and differences of opinion, interests, or tastes that are dealt with either by confrontation and resolution or by avoidance.

The fourth characteristic of stage three (establishing traditions) may well be the ingredient that counters the other three characteristics and thus helps sustain the relationship. After 3 or 4 years together, two gay men tend to look on their relationship as if it were a third person possessing certain dependable qualities, such as steadfastness, comfort, and familiarity, which sustain the momentum of their partnership. It should be noted here that recognition and support of the relationship by family and friends often begin only after a couple has been together 3 years.

Stage Four: Building (Years 6–10)

Besides the usual meaning of *cooperation,* collaboration also implies giving aid to an occupying enemy. Couples in stage four can unwillingly collaborate in this sense and aid the development of boredom and feelings of entrapment. After 5 years together, couples experience a new sense of security and a decreasing need to process their interactions. On the one hand, this decline in communication frequently gives rise to making unverified assumptions about each other. On the other hand, their collaborative adjustments often lead to effective complementarity. This complementarity, combined with the coping mechanisms for dealing with conflict and boredom, yields new energy for enriching their horizons beyond the relationship. This energy leads to mutual as well as individual productivity of a visible nature, such as business partnerships, financial dealings, estate building, or achieving personal gains in professional or academic worlds. The individualization of stage three can progress to the establishment of independence, sustained by the steady, dependable availability of a partner for support, guidance, and affirmation.

Stage Five: Releasing (Years 11–20)

Trust develops gradually for most people. As the years pass and as they gain experience, gay couples trust each other with greater conviction. The trust of stage five includes a mutual lack of possessiveness and a strong positive regard for each other. The slow merger of money and possessions may be a manifestation of this trust. Among men in the latter half of stage five, the authors also found a gradual isolation from the self as manifested by lack of feelings and inattention to personal needs, isolation from the partner because of withdrawal and lack of communication, and sometimes isolation from friends for the same reasons. The authors identified this characteristic as a type of constriction; it may be a result of the men's ages. The attitude of taking the relationship for granted develops as a result of the other characteristics of this stage.

Stage Six: Renewing (Beyond 20 Years)

The 20th anniversary appears to be a special milestone for gay male couples. The authors found a surprising number of couples reporting a renewal of their relationship after being together for 20 years or more. Most men's goals include financial security; the men in the sample had usually attained this goal after 20 years. Other goals included business, professional, and academic success. These couples also assumed that they would be together until separated by death. Most men expressed a series of personal concerns, such as for health and security, fear of loneliness, and death of partners or themselves. Most were struck by the passage of time and would reminisce about their years together.

Stage-Related Problems

Each of the stages has a unique set of problems. What follows is not intended to be a complete list of such problems, but rather some examples of common stage-related difficulties.

Couples in stage one tend to believe that the love and togetherness of blending and high limerence are the critical indicators of their relationship; they see the least rupture in this togetherness as heralding the end of the relationship. When each partner begins to feel less intense, or when there is a mutual diminution of feelings, men withdraw from each other. This is the most common cause of gay men ending their relationships before the end of the first year. An accompanying problem is the fear of intimacy generated by the intensity of the blending. This fear, which can be as difficult as the loss of feelings of limerence, may also be manifested in the individual's resistance to the process of blending.

The most common problems in stage two arise from differences between the partners, in contrast to the problems caused by similarities in stage one. High passion declines and no longer shields partners from the annoyances with each other. Familiarity brings the diversity of their values and tastes to the surface and sets the stage for disagreement. The partners begin to notice each other's failures and shortcomings. This stage also sees the onset of outside sexual interests and a resulting increase in jealous possessiveness.

The problems in stage three are provoked by the beginning of individualization and the consequent fears of loss. Misunderstandings arise from the partners' newly felt needs to be separate—specifically, their increasing desire for sex with others. The risk taking involved at this stage tends to generate new anger and anxiety.

As a consequence of the activity taking place outside the relationship, stage four is a time of considerable distancing from each other. This distancing generates fears of loss, but it is also partially responsible for cementing the dyad. Despite the distancing, there is a consolidation in the couple's efforts together outside of the relationship.

In addition to problems related to the length of time in the relationship (10–20 years), couples in stage five have the burden of concerns accompanying the process of aging. Routine and monotony can become the enemies in stage five. The tendency to become more fixed or rigid in personality characteristics while struggling to change each other can also plague men who have been together over 10 years.

Couples in stage six often continue to have the problems seen in stage five, but with the increase in age and the attainment of goals there is restlessness, sometimes withdrawal, and feelings of aimlessness. Most men currently in this stage grew up as gay men in a more repressive era; their beliefs and feelings may reflect antihomosexual attitudes. Although at the present time these problems appear to be stage related, they may not be found to the same extent among gay men in the future.

Stage Discrepancy

More often than not, partners in a couple do not progress through the stages simultaneously. If there is a wide difference, problems arise that the authors have identified as "stage discrepancies." It is very common to find couples together 3–5 years with one partner in an individualized, comfortable position (stage three) and the other still dependent and clinging (stage one). Regardless of their presenting problems, the authors find that over half the couples seen in their clinical practice have some degree of stage discrepancy (Mattison and McWhirter 1987). Couples experience considerable relief when this concept is explained to them, just as the man with chest pain is relieved when the physician tells him it is only muscle strain and not a heart attack.

When couples understand the concept of stage discrepancy, they realize that their problems are not flaws in themselves or their partnerships but correctable, developmental differences in the growth of their relationships. Although all discrepancies may not lend themselves to rapid adjustment, the understanding derived from the cognitive framework of stage discrepancy makes the affective problems easier to handle and to treat. After all, when a man with chest pain knows the exercise will not injure him, running need no longer be anxiety provoking.

Problems in Relationships

Male couples experience the same wide range of interpersonal problems that are found in all relationships (see Chapter 28 by Cabaj and Klinger in this volume). However, some problems may be unique to gay men. Establishing intimacy is generally a goal in all relationships. Depending on developmental conditions, gay men, as a rule, have less trouble with this than their straight brothers and fathers, perhaps due to the relative "demasculinization" of their childhood development. It has been suggested that most gay men have histories of some cross-gender childhood behaviors and attitudes that prepare them to become more nurturing and available to each other in relationships (McWhirter and Mattison 1984). Nonetheless, many gay men also suffer from the predominantly masculine condition of being out of touch with their feelings, or lacking the ability to express or share them.

One of the more common problems for male couples, often unrecognized by the couples themselves, is differences between their value systems. Religious differences and a tendency to make heterosexual assumptions about their relationship are often responsible. For example, holding different values about sexual exclusivity and emotional fidelity can be very problematic and induce jealousy.

◼ Background Differences

One of the more interesting problems male couples face is differences in their backgrounds, which often are not recognized. (Fortunately, this problem sometimes is one of the most easily solved.) Couples coming from different socioeconomic, religious, ethnic, or family backgrounds often have difficulty finding compatibility in their relationship simply because they were reared with different expectations, values, and ways of behaving. Understanding the differences in backgrounds and how they affect relationships can be one of the most effective means of resolving problems in some relationships.

Differences in leadership and dominance in male relationships can be destructive. The use of power and the establishment of equality or balance are real necessities early in the relationship if it is to survive.

Sexual exclusivity is a general expectation in most new relationships. Many studies investigated questions about exclusivity and openness in male couples (Bell and Weinberg 1978; Blasband and Peplau 1985; Blumstein and Schwartz 1983; Deenen et al. 1994; Harry 1984; Harry and DeVall 1978; Kurdek and Schmitt 1986; McWhirter and Mattison 1984; Peplau and Cochran 1981). Almost all these studies showed that gay men seem to have a more permissive attitude over time about sexual fidelity than do heterosexuals and lesbians (Peplau and Cochran 1990). This very permissiveness can lead to complicated rules established by the couple to deal with jealousies and injured feelings that often threaten the existence of the relationships. Others have worked out compromises with respect to permissiveness that complement their lives together and that some report as being responsible for relationship survival.

Another problem that may affect gay relationships is difficulty maintaining feelings of closeness. The pervasiveness of antihomosexual attitudes touches every person but affects gay people profoundly. These responses include ignorance, prejudice, oppression, and homophobia. In addition, problems can arise from chemical dependency or excess drug and alcohol use, physical illness, or any psychiatric problems including depression and anxiety.

■ HIV and Couples

Human immunodeficiency virus (HIV) infection or the presence of the acquired immunodeficiency syndrome (AIDS) in one or both partners brings with it an array of issues. Mattison and McWhirter (1990) offered an analysis of 27 male couples with AIDS, demonstrating some common problems and issues encountered by them all. For example, one of the early responses to an AIDS diagnosis in many male couples is for the individuals to draw closer together. Threats, such as facing a life-threatening illness, seem to lead to early consolidation of the relationship. Most couples also seek to reconcile with families of origin if there has been an estrangement. If intact, the family bonding becomes more intense.

Couples facing AIDS, whatever the length of their relationship, seem to act like stage six couples, leaping over the earlier stages to deal with shifting perspectives and the threat of illness and death. These couples have a great deal in common with much older couples who have been together many years and are facing death from natural causes. One partner or the other sometimes deals irrationally with mourning and loss, almost like an approach-avoidance situation. One individual said, "If I don't get too close to him, the loss won't be as bad."

Based on clinical work with numerous couples in which one partner is HIV negative and the other is HIV positive, the authors defined approaches to the psychotherapeutic assessment of and intervention with male couples who are serodiscordant for HIV. These couples report an increase in the expectation of sexual exclusivity in their relationships (Mattison and McWhirter 1994).

Regardless of the HIV status of the individuals, more male couples report that they have agreements of sexual exclusivity because of the threat of HIV infection. Thus, there does seem to be a change in the sexually permissive attitudes seen earlier. In the age of AIDS, there also seems to be an increase in the value placed on relationship longevity. Finding a partner and settling down is more common than in the past.

AIDS has introduced a tragic element into the lives of male couples. In the early years of the epidemic, partners were becoming sick and dying not after a long life together but during the beginning years of their relationships. Illnesses were sudden and hospitalizations frequent; painful physical deterioration was the norm; and death was the outcome. More recently, due to the advances in antiviral and other therapies, lives are being extended for many persons with HIV-related diseases. However, there is hardly a male couple—young or old, "newlyweds" or "long-timers"—whose lives have not been directly affected in some way by the AIDS epidemic.

■ Other Important Issues for Male Couples

There are many additional issues for male couples. Families and children are covered in this book (see Chapter 29 by Stein and Chapter 22 by Patterson and Chan). The development of extended families should, likewise, be seen as a creative and vital part of male couples' lives.

Benefits and Joys

The old notion that aging gay men are disgruntled, lonely, or misanthropic is belied by the growth and strength of organizations like Seniors Active in a Gay Environment (SAGE). The robust participation in the full panoply of the gay lifestyle by men of all ages may be a new phenomenon (see Chapter 18 by Berger and Kelly in this volume). In the 25 years since Stonewall, numbers of men originally involved in the liberation of the community have reached the senior citizen category (Adleman et al. 1993). Contrary to previous expectations, aging gay men are generally welcomed by younger men and interact with them on a day-to-day basis socially and through a variety of gay organizations. Friend (1990) postulated that gay men who accept their homosexuality and actively participate in the community accept aging with grace and dignity.

The authors' more recent interviews with male couples who have been together for more than 20 years revealed men in coupled relationships for 50 years and more. Just as men in the first few years of a relationship must establish compatibility, so it is with the older gay couples. They continue to focus on compatibility and companionship as crucial ingredients of their ongoing commitment.

Conclusion

Although the concept of male couples may be a construct of the 20th century, the work of John Boswell, *Same-Sex Unions in Premodern Europe* (1994), highlights the existence of male-male love relationships for many hundreds of years. The character, structure, and visibility of these relationships have changed, developed, and evolved over the centuries and even more so in the past 30 years of open gay awareness. Research with these couples is beginning to tell society how they are similar to and different from other types of couples. The presence of a life-threatening disease has molded these gay men's lives in different directions.

The important point stated here is that these relationships do exist. They are real and viable pairings that enrich and expand the lives of the participants. They are as committed and long term as any relationship. These couples believe in human family values carried over from their own backgrounds. They believe that their relationships and families contribute significantly to the well-being, health, and stability of their lives as individuals and couples. They deserve not only to be recognized but also to be celebrated and nurtured.

References

Adleman J, Berger R, Boyd M, et al: Lambda Gray. North Hollywood, CA, Newcastle Publishing, 1993

Bell AP, Weinberg MS: Homosexualities: A Study of Diversity Among Men and Women. New York, Simon and Shuster, 1978

Berger RM: Men together: understanding the gay couple. J Homosex 19:31–50, 1990

Berzon B: Permanent Partners: Building Gay and Lesbian Relationships That Last. New York, Dutton, 1988

Blasband D, Peplau LA: Sexual exclusivity versus openness in gay male couples. Arch Sex Behav 14:395–412, 1985

Blumstein P, Schwartz P: American Couples: Money, Work, Sex. New York, William Morrow, 1983

Boswell J: Same-Sex Unions in Premodern Europe. New York, Villard, 1994

Deenen AA, Gijs L, van Naerssen AX: Intimacy and sexuality in gay male couples. Arch Sex Behav 23:405–420, 1994

Diamond M: Homosexuality and bisexuality in different populations. Arch Sex Behav 33:291–310, 1993

Driggs J, Finn S: Intimacy Between Men: How to Find and Keep Gay Love Relationships. New York, Plume, 1991

Friend R: Older lesbian and gay people: a theory of successful aging. J Homosex 12:3–4, 1990

Harry J: Gay Couples. New York, Praeger, 1984

Harry J, DeVall W: The Social Organization of Gay Males. New York, Praeger, 1978

Isensee R: Love Between Men: Enhancing Intimacy and Keeping Your Relationship Alive. New York, Prentice Hall, 1990

Jay K, Young A: The Gay Report: Lesbians and Gay Men Speak Out About Sexual Experiences and Lifestyles. New York, Summit, 1977

Kurdek LA: The nature and correlates of relationship quality in gay, lesbian, and heterosexual cohabiting couples: a test of the contextual, investment, and discrepancy models, in Lesbian and Gay Psychology: Theory, Research, and Clinical Applications. Edited by Greene B, Herek GM. Thousand Oaks, CA, Sage, 1994, pp 133–155

Kurdek LA: Lesbian and gay couples, in Lesbian, Gay, and Bisexual Identities Over the Lifespan: Psychological Perspectives. Edited by D'Augelli AR, Patterson CJ. New York, Oxford University Press, 1995, pp 243–261

Kurdek LA, Schmitt JP: Relationship quality of partners in heterosexual married, heterosexual cohabitating, and gay and lesbian relationships. Journal of Personal and Social Psychology 51:711–720, 1986

Kurdek LA, Schmitt JP: Partner homogamy in married, heterosexual cohabitating, gay, and lesbian couples. J Sex Research 23:212–232, 1987

Larson P: Gay male relationships, in Homosexuality as a Social Issue. Edited by Paul W, Weinrich JDF, Gonsiorek JC, et al. Beverly Hills, CA, Sage, 1982

Marcus E: The Male Couple's Guide: Finding a Man, Making a Home, Building a Life. New York, HarperCollins, 1992

Mattison AM, McWhirter DP: Stage discrepancy in male couples. J Homosex 14:89–99, 1987

Mattison AM, McWhirter DP: Emotional impact of AIDS: male couples and their families, in AIDS and Sex: An Integrated Biomedical and Biobehavioral Approach. Edited by Voeller B, Reinisch JM, Gottlieb M. New York, Oxford University Press, 1990

Mattison AM, McWhirter DP: Serodiscordant male couples. Journal of Gay and Lesbian Social Services 1:83–99, 1994

McWhirter DP, Mattison AM: The Male Couple: How Relationships Develop. New York, Prentice Hall, 1984

Mendola M: The Mendola Report: A New Look at Gay Couples in America. New York, Crown, 1980

Peplau LA, Cochran S: Value orientations in the intimate relationships of gay men. J Homosex 6:1–19, 1981

Peplau LA, Cochran S: A relationship perspective on homosexuality, in Homosexuality/Heterosexuality: Concepts of Sexual Orientation. Edited by McWhirter DP, Sanders SA, Reinisch JM. New York, Oxford University Press, 1990, pp 321–349

Peplau LA, Jones R (eds): Symposium on Couples. J Homosex 8:1–89, 1982

Pillard RC, Weinrich JD: Evidence of familial nature of male homosexuality. Arch Gen Psychiatry 43:808–812, 1986

Saghir MT, Robins E: Male and Female Homosexuality: A Comprehensive Investigation. Baltimore, MD, Williams and Wilkins, 1973

Silverstein C: Man to Man: Gay Couples in America. New York, William Morrow and Company, 1981

Spada J: The Spada Report: The Newest Survey of Gay Male Sexuality. New York, Signet, 1979

Weinberg MS, Williams CJ, Pryor DW: Dual Attraction: Understanding Bisexuality. New York, Oxford University Press, 1994

Lesbian Couples

Rochelle L. Klinger, M.D.

Lesbians form relationships for the same reasons as heterosexual women do: to satisfy basic needs for love, companionship, creativity, and sexuality. In the more than two decades since homosexuality has not been viewed as a mental illness, there has been an increasing focus on lesbians in couples. However, as with research on women in general, lesbians have been neglected in terms of careful study of their relationships, compared with those of gay men (McWhirter and Mattison 1984).

Studies of lesbian couples reviewed in this chapter share several basic shortcomings. First, it is impossible to obtain a representative sample of lesbians and gay men because of homophobia and fear of disclosure. Accordingly, most lesbians studied have been relatively active in the lesbian community and tend to be well educated, white, and middle class; lesbians of color, those from lower socioeconomic classes, and those who are less "out" are unlikely to be identical to the

The author wishes to thank Barbara Dill, R.N., M.S.N., and Mary T. Walker, M.S.W., for their help in preparation of this chapter.

groups actually studied. Second, most existing studies are primarily based on self-report methods, such as surveys or interviews, rather than on behavioral measures. Overall, however, the increase in interest in lesbian couples is heartening and will hopefully lead to more inclusive and comprehensive studies in the future.

This chapter summarizes research findings about psychologically healthy lesbian couples. The specific topic of couples therapy with lesbians and gay men is covered in Chapter 28 by Cabaj and Klinger in this volume. Among the important questions about lesbian couples are the following:

1. What do we know about lesbian couples, and what are the areas where data are missing?
2. What are the similarities and differences between lesbian, gay male, and heterosexual couples?
3. What are possible explanations for these differences?

Descriptive characteristics of lesbian couples are summarized in Table 20–1 and discussed in the text, and important internal and external influences on lesbian couples are presented. Finally, a model for the life cycle of healthy lesbian couples is described.

Descriptive Characteristics of Lesbian Relationships

Table 20–1 summarizes 11 studies of 50 or more lesbian couples each (Bell and Weinberg 1978; Blumstein and Schwartz 1983; Bradford and Ryan 1988; Caldwell and Peplau 1984; Kurdek 1988, 1989; Loulan 1988; Peplau and Gordon 1982; Peplau et al. 1982; Weinberg and Williams 1974; Zacks et al. 1988). Multiple studies of the same group of subjects are considered together.

■ Rate and Longevity of Coupling

Overall, 60%–80% of individual lesbians studied were coupled, the majority in committed relationships. When reported, the relationships had a fairly short mean longevity of 2–5 years, although they ranged

Table 20–1. Studies of lesbian couples

Study	Number of subjects	Percentage coupled	Equality	Longevity	Relatedness	Sexuality
Bell and Weinberg 1978 Weinberg and Williams 1974	278	82	High	—	High	—
Blumstein and Schwartz 1983	90 couples	100	High	Median 2.2 years Less than hetero-sexual couples Pooled finances correlated with longevity	High	Lower frequency than heterosexual or gay male couples Frequency < once/month after 1 year together High rate of inhibited sexual desire High rate of extra-marital affairs
Bradford and Ryan 1988	1,925	60	—	—	—	—
Kurdek 1988, 1989	47 couples	100	High	Mean 4.5 years Less than gay male couples in study	High (compared with gay male couples)	93% sexually exclusive

Table 20–1. Studies of lesbian couples *(continued)*

Study	Number of subjects	Percentage coupled	Equality	Longevity	Relatedness	Sexuality
Loulan 1988	1,566	61% coupled; 12% casually coupled	—	—	—	55% had sex 2–10 times/month Frequency decreased with time together; but satisfaction remained stable
Peplau et al. 1978 Caldwell and Peplau 1984 Peplau and Gordon 1982	127	60	97% endorsed equal power; 61% had it on objective measures	Median 2.9 years Less longevity than heterosexual couples in study	High	—
Zacks et al. 1988	52 couples	100	High	Median 3.54 years Range 1–34 years Less than heterosexual couples in study	High	—

Note. Equality = degree of belief in equal status of partners; *relatedness* = degree of affiliation and dependency; *sexuality* = characteristics of sexual interaction.

from 1 to 34 years. Of note is that lesbian couples are less likely to stay together than gay male or heterosexual couples, contrary to the stereotype that lesbians form more solid relationships than gay men. Blumstein and Schwartz (1983) and Schneider (1986) noted that lesbian couples who were more interdependent financially were less likely to dissolve the relationship.

It is difficult to know for certain how many lesbian families include children. Bradford and Ryan (1988) noted that 29% of their sample of 1,925 lesbian women had been pregnant, and 16% were mothers at the time of the survey. An additional 30% wanted to be mothers.

■ Sexuality

Almost 100% of lesbian couples who have been studied state that they are sexually exclusive. Blumstein and Schwartz (1983) noted that when nonmonogamy occurred in their sample of lesbian couples, it was usually in the form of a romantic affair outside the relationship with extensive emotional involvement rather than outside contacts that were primarily sexual. In couples from this study in which romantic affairs occurred, they were usually divulged to the primary partner and led to the couple breaking up.

Lesbian couples show a lower frequency of sexual contact than heterosexual or gay male couples. All studies reported a decreased frequency of sexual interactions within lesbian relationships after 1 year together, for example, less than once per month in the Blumstein and Schwartz (1983) study. However, this decreased frequency was balanced by significant nongenital physical activity such as hugging and cuddling, shared in an egalitarian way. Loulan (1988) noted that despite decreased frequency of genital sexual contact, satisfaction with sex remained high in long-standing couples (see Chapter 44 by Herbert in this volume).

■ Relatedness and Equality

As might be expected based on the course of women's psychological development (Gilligan 1982; Miller 1976), a number of the studies showed that lesbian couples demonstrate a higher degree of cohesion and relatedness than gay male or heterosexual couples, as measured by objective and subjective measures. High relatedness is cited by lesbian couples in many studies as a positive attribute of their relationships.

Lesbian couples in general endorse a higher degree of equality in their relationships compared with gay male and heterosexual couples. However, Caldwell and Peplau (1984) noted that although nearly 100% of their couples wanted an equal balance of power, only 61% felt they had achieved it. Lower income and education and higher dependence on the partner predicted lower power for an individual in the relationship. Finally, these studies consistently reported a high degree of masculine/feminine role flexibility between lesbian partners and offered no evidence for butch and femme role-playing.

Influences on Lesbian Relationships

Influences on couples can be examined as internal, including intrapsychic and couples issues, and external, encompassing social and systemic issues.

■ Internal Influences

A growing body of literature describes differences in psychological development in women versus men (Chodorow 1978; Gilligan 1982; Jordan et al. 1991; Miller 1976). By virtue of socialization and object relations with the mother, boys are pushed toward autonomy, whereas girls tend toward relatedness. Therefore, a lesbian couple, consisting of two women, can be expected on the average to have a high tendency toward relatedness (Burch 1993), which may account for the high levels of cohesion, equality, and relatedness noted in the studies of lesbian couples.

The nature of women's psychological development also helps to explain the findings that lesbians tend to become aware of their same-sex attraction at a later age and to be more flexible in their sexual orientation than gay men (de Monteflores and Schultz 1978). Some authors (Burch 1993; Golden 1987) divided lesbian women into two categories: primary lesbians, defined as women who feel they have always been lesbian and will always remain so, and bisexual lesbians, who have had some degree of sexual and affective involvement with men but are more comfortable with women. Kirkpatrick and Morgan (1980) suggested that, rather than being on the opposite ends of a continuum as for men, heterosexuality and homosexuality for women "might be seen as running a parallel course, capable of intermingling and of changing positions of ascendancy in consciousness and behavior under certain circumstances" (p. 360).

The role of complementarity in lesbian relationships deserves careful consideration. Complementarity can be understood as the tendency for persons with different characteristics to be attracted to each other. In heterosexual relationships, an obvious difference is sex. Burch (1993) made a strong point that successful lesbian relationships also exhibit complementarity. She emphasized the construct of bisexual and primary lesbians being partners as a frequent source of complementarity in lesbian relationships. Other complementary variables that are observed in couples might include differences in age, religious background, and racial and ethnic background. Some clinicians believe that, given the absence of sex complementarity, these types of differences may be more common in gay male and lesbian couples than in heterosexual couples (R. P. Cabaj, personal communication, December 1992; Carl 1990).

Fusion, which some consider to be a maladaptive closeness, occurs when partners give up their individuality and interrupt the normal ebb and flow of intimacy. Fusion is common in lesbian couples and is encouraged by women's psychological development as well as by external stigma. It has been examined in the literature primarily as a source of psychopathology in lesbian couples (Burch 1986; Kaufman et al. 1984; Krestan and Bepko 1980). Slater and Mencher (1991) made a strong case that the perception of fusion as always problematic is biased because it equates fusion with pathology and is based on observations of a clinical sample (i.e., lesbian couples seeking therapy). They believed that a degree of fusion is necessary for the healthy functioning of a lesbian couple because of the need to counteract the effects of ongoing homophobia and invisibility. They saw fusion along a continuum, with too little being dangerous because of the risk of dissolution and too much carrying the risk of loss of individuality and intimacy. There appears to be a waxing and waning of fusion in the life cycle of couples, depending on the degree of external homophobia. Fusion should be assessed for a lesbian couple within a lesbian, rather than a heterosexual, community norm.

Each individual's progress in the coming-out process is also an important influence on the functioning of the lesbian couple (Klinger and

Cabaj 1993). Coming out is a process, not an end point, and involves self-acceptance of a same-sex orientation in the face of external obstacles. Disclosure to some degree is an integral part of the process and is a task that partners often have to negotiate.

Unexamined internalized homophobia can be a negative factor in lesbian relationships, leading to a sense that one or both partners lack confidence in the viability of the relationship. Because homophobia is ubiquitous, no individual can totally get over her internalized homophobia. Therefore, conscious awareness and active processing of internalized homophobia, rather than total elimination, are the goals for the couple.

Lesbians lack the internalized sex-based role models for their relationships that heterosexuals have. These are not obtained in the family of origin, and the media and popular culture provide few gay and lesbian role models, most of which are highly stereotypical and stigmatized. Loulan (1988) showed that lesbians in couples do not assume rigid sex-based roles, but resolve questions of who does what sex-stereotyped task in unique ways. For example, one partner may do the laundry, a traditionally female task, but may also do the home maintenance, a traditionally male task, while the other does auto maintenance and cooking.

The lack of rigidity may be an asset, allowing creativity and flexibility as lesbians, as a couple, negotiate tasks and roles. However, it can also cause anxiety, especially in new couples who are early in the coming-out process. Contacts and role-modeling within the lesbian community can be helpful for these couples (Slater and Mencher 1991).

Finally, the influence of each individual's personality and psychological traits should not be underestimated. For example, Kurdek (1988) noted that strong intrinsic motivation to be in the relationship is an excellent predictor of relationship quality in lesbian couples. Individual personality traits, as well as possible psychopathology, can be quite relevant to the quality, character, and longevity of lesbian relationships.

■ Case Example 1

Ms. A and Ms. B were 39 and 26 years old, respectively, and had been together for 9 months. Ms. A had previously been married. She was successful as an out lesbian in her career. Ms. B had recently finished graduate school and was looking for a job. After the intense sexuality and limerence of the first phase of the relationship wore off, they began to argue about how out to be, with Ms. A feeling that Ms. B was too closeted, and Ms. B feeling that Ms. A disclosed her (and their) sexual orientations indiscriminately. Each woman had to acknowledge and discuss her internalized homophobia to negotiate this impasse successfully.

▉ External Influences

Homophobia is a major external influence on lesbian couples. The impact of active homophobia is fairly easy to detect and includes the effects of prejudice in employment, expressed in ways such as discrimination against lesbian teachers or lesbians in the military. Discrimination also results from antisodomy laws and from denying lesbian mothers custody of their children.

The influence of homophobia can be much more subtle, however, as manifested by the invisibility and lack of legitimacy of lesbian couples. Legally, lesbian couples cannot marry anywhere in the United States and are denied the social, economic, and legal benefits of marriage. Unless they make specific arrangements, lesbian couples have no legal link to each other even if they have long-standing relationships. To protect each other in the event of serious illness or death, each member of a lesbian couple has to execute three documents: 1) a will or revocable trust; 2) a power of attorney for asset management if incapacitated; and 3) a durable power of attorney for health care, allowing one partner to make medical decisions for the other if she is unable to do so for herself. See Chapter 46 by Purcell and Hicks for more information regarding legal issues for gay men and lesbians.

Lesbian couples and families are also excluded from the rituals and from many forms of social support for their unions that heterosexual couples take for granted. Slater and Mencher (1991) decried the lack of ritual and legitimacy for lesbian couples, which extends into invisibility in the family therapy literature.

Lesbian couples fare poorly in the economic arena compared with gay male and heterosexual couples. This, of course, is due to the decreased earning power of women in general in our society. In Bradford and Ryan's study (1988), 70% of the women had advanced degrees and worked in full-time professional or managerial positions. Nevertheless, 64% earned less than $20,000 per year, and only 12% earned more than $30,000.

Family and community influences have significant impact on lesbian couples. Relationships with families of origin, ex-spouses and ex-lovers, religious and community organizations, and employers and co-workers can be influential.

Lesbian couples differ in the degree of disclosure of their sexual orientation to families of origin. Members of the family must go through their own coming-out process when they discover that their relative is lesbian. A major problem for the lesbian couple is the uncertain outcome of coming out to the family. If family members have sufficient psychological resources, they may go through a process of grief and readjustment and may eventually be a good support for the couple. If they lack the resources or are influenced by things such as fundamentalist religious beliefs, disclosure may cause rejection. In a couple, rejection by one or both families can reawaken internalized homophobia and feelings of lack of legitimacy (Brown 1989).

Bradford and Ryan (1988) confirmed the impression that few lesbians are out at their places of employment, finding that only 17% of their sample were completely out at work. Conflict can arise within a couple regarding the degree of outness when they have different degrees of perceived risk in their employment. Remaining closeted may be viewed as safer, but it deprives the couple of the social support for their relationship that people normally get from activities such as office parties and informal conversation at lunch.

Lesbian couples who have children are confronted with the need for another layer of community involvement. In many states, it is dangerous to be an openly lesbian mother, and community support for lesbian mothers is usually nonexistent. Networks of lesbians with children are growing as more lesbians choose to be parents.

■ Case Example 2

Ms. C and Ms. D were both in their mid-40s. Ms. C had been married and had a teenage child, and Ms. D was a primary lesbian. When they met, both were teachers, and neither was out to her family of origin. In the conservative state in which they lived and worked, they felt that any disclosure to the community at large would be dangerous in terms of employment and custody issues. To maximize other support for their relationship, they built a strong network of lesbian and gay male friends and a few trusted heterosexual friends with whom they could be out. This network helped them weather the inevitable stressors encountered as they moved from the early limerence stage of their relationship to dealing with the more mundane details of life together.

Life Cycle of Lesbian Couples

The concept of a life cycle, with expected progression through stages with predictable pitfalls, can be useful for understanding couples and families. Carter and McGoldrick (1980, 1989) extensively elaborated a life-cycle model for heterosexual families. McWhirter and Mattison (1984) developed a life-cycle model for gay male couples consisting of six stages: blending, nesting, maintaining, building, releasing, and renewing (see Chapter 19). There is no comparable model at present for lesbian couples, and given the differences between gay male and lesbian relationships, it is doubtful that the McWhirter and Mattison model would apply to lesbian couples. Some of the special issues that have been described for lesbian couples need to be considered in developing such a model for these couples.

Studies to date suggest that lesbians go through the same initial stage as gay male couples, consisting of merging, limerence, and intense sexual activity (Kurdek 1988, 1989). This stage lasts 6 months to 1 year for gay men; however, the degree of merging may not drop off as quickly for lesbian couples as it does for gay male couples. Although the tasks of nesting, building, and releasing need to occur for lesbians as well as for gay men, their sequence and timing may be very different. For example, merging of finances may occur earlier, and reemergence of the individual may occur later. It is important not to assume that the gay male model fits lesbian couples until empirical research comparable to McWhirter and Mattison's ground-breaking study of gay male couples is done with lesbian couples.

Conclusion

In returning to the questions posed at the beginning of the chapter, some answers emerge after a review of the major studies of lesbian couples. Despite recent increased interest in lesbian couples, far less is known about these couples than remains unknown. Several helpful survey studies were reported, but we are missing a prospective, longitudinal study of lesbian couples; studies of subgroups such as lesbian couples of color, those from lower socioeconomic groups, and less-out lesbian couples are also absent. A large-scale study with objective measures of couples' functioning would also be helpful. Difficulties with recruiting study participants make studies of lesbian couples difficult to do, as has been noted.

Existing studies reveal that there are both differences and similarities between lesbian, gay male, and heterosexual couples. The similarities are in the basic bonds of love and intimacy that are the same in all couples (Dailey 1979; Laner 1977). Differences are noted in terms of higher levels of sexual exclusivity, relatedness and fusion, and equality for lesbian couples than for gay male and heterosexual couples. Conversely, less frequent sexual contact, less rigidity of same-sex orientation, and shorter relationship longevity are seen in lesbian couples compared with gay male and heterosexual couples.

The basis for these differences can be traced to sources within as well as outside the couple. Internal sources include women's psychological development, which tends to lead to more relatedness, equality, and flexibility of sexual orientation; progress in negotiating the coming-out process and managing internalized homophobia; and individual personality factors. External factors include the effects of ubiquitous active and subtle homophobia and family and community influences. Lesbian couples should be encouraged to take all legal steps possible to protect themselves against the effects of external homophobia and discrimination.

We live in a time when interest in healthy lesbian couples is at an all-time high, but unfortunately homophobia remains widespread as well. Clinicians and researchers need to advocate for studies of lesbian couples now and in the future.

References

Bell AP, Weinberg MS: Homosexualities: A Study of Diversities Among Men and Women. New York, Simon and Schuster, 1978

Blumstein P, Schwartz P: American Couples: Money, Work and Sex. New York, William Morrow, 1983

Bradford J, Ryan C: The National Lesbian Health Care Survey. Washington, DC, National Lesbian and Gay Health Foundation, 1988

Brown LS: Lesbians, gay men and their families: common clinical concerns. Journal of Gay and Lesbian Psychotherapy 1:65–78, 1989

Burch B: Psychotherapy and the dynamics of merger in lesbian couples, in Contemporary Perspectives on Psychotherapy With Lesbians and Gay Men. Edited by Stein TS, Cohen CC. New York, Plenum, 1986, pp 57–72

Burch B: On Intimate Terms: The Psychology of Difference in Lesbian Relationships. Urbana, IL, University of Illinois Press, 1993

Caldwell MA, Peplau LA: The balance of power in lesbian relationships. Sex Roles 10:587–599, 1984

Carl D: Counseling Same-Sex Couples. New York, WW Norton, 1990

Carter B, McGoldrick M: The Family Life Cycle: A Framework for Family Therapy. New York, Gardner Press, 1980

Carter B, McGoldrick M: The Changing Family Life Cycle: A Framework for Family Therapy. Needham Heights, MA, Allyn & Bacon, 1989

Chodorow N: The Reproduction of Mothering: Psychoanalysis and the Sociology of Gender. Berkeley, CA, University of California Press, 1978

Dailey DM: Adjustment of heterosexual and homosexual couples in pairing relationships: an exploratory study. J Sex Res 15:143–157, 1979

de Monteflores C, Schultz SJ: Coming out: similarities and differences for lesbians and gay men. Journal of Social Issues 34:59–72, 1978

Gilligan C: In a Different Voice. Cambridge, MA, Harvard University Press, 1982

Golden C: Diversity and variability in women's sexual identities, in Lesbian Psychologies: Explorations and Challenges. Edited by Boston Lesbian Psychologies Collective. Urbana, IL, University of Illinois Press, 1987, pp 18–34

Jordan JV, Kaplan AG, Miller JB, et al: Women's Growth in Connection. New York, Guilford, 1991

Kaufman P, Harrison E, Hyde M: Distancing for intimacy in lesbian relationships. Am J Psychiatry 141:530–533, 1984

Kirkpatrick M, Morgan C: Clinical aspects of female homosexuality, in Homosexual Behavior: A Modern Reappraisal. Edited by Marmor J. New York, Basic Books, 1980, pp 357–375

Klinger RL, Cabaj RP: Characteristics of gay and lesbian relationships, in American Psychiatric Press Review of Psychiatry, Vol 12. Edited by Oldham JM, Riba MB, Tasman A. Washington, DC, American Psychiatric Press, 1993, pp 101–125

Krestan J, Bepko C: The problem of fusion in the lesbian relationship. Fam Process 19:272–289, 1980

Kurdek LA: Relationship quality of gay and lesbian cohabitating couples. J Homosex 15:93–118, 1988

Kurdek LA: Relationship quality in gay and lesbian cohabitating couples: a 1-year follow-up study. Journal of Social and Personal Relationships 6:39–59, 1989

Laner MR: Permanent partner priorities: gay and straight. J Homosex 3:21–39, 1977

Loulan J: Research on the sex practices of 1566 lesbians and the clinical applications. Women and Therapy 7:221–234, 1988

McWhirter DP, Mattison AM: The Male Couple: How Relationships Develop. Englewood Cliffs, NJ, Prentice Hall, 1984

Miller JB: Toward a New Psychology of Women. Boston, MA, Beacon, 1976

Peplau LA, Gordon SL: The intimate relationships of lesbians and gay men, in Changing Boundaries: Gender Roles and Sexual Behavior. Edited by Allgeier R, McCormick NB. Palo Alto, CA, Mayfield, 1982, pp 226–244

Peplau LA, Cohran S, Rook K, et al: Loving women: attachment and autonomy in lesbian relationships. Journal of Social Issues 34:7–27, 1978

Schneider MS: The relationships of cohabitating lesbian and heterosexual couples: a comparison. Psychology of Women Quarterly 10:234–239, 1986

Slater S, Mencher J: The lesbian family life cycle: a contextual approach. Am J Orthopsychiatry 61:372–382, 1991

Weinberg MS, Williams CJ: Male Homosexuals: Their Problems and Adaptions. New York, Oxford University Press, 1974

Zacks E, Green RJ, Marrow J: Comparing lesbian and heterosexual couples on the circumplex model: an initial investigation. Fam Process 27:471–484, 1988

21

Lesbians as Parents

Martha Kirkpatrick, M.D.

I n 1975, a Texas jury removed Mary Risher's 9-year-old son Richard from her custody and placed him with his father because of Ms. Risher's admitted lesbianism. In 1975 clinicians knew little more about lesbian mothers and their children than did that jury. The American Psychiatric Association had removed homosexuality from its list of mental disorders in 1973, but motherhood and lesbianism were still considered a contradiction in terms.

Lesbian mothers were not a new phenomenon—Sappho of Lesbos herself had a child; but fear of public condemnation and ostracism forced many lesbian mothers to live in secrecy, their lesbianism often hidden from their own children. Lesbians often mothered other people's children as nannies, governesses, nurses, and teachers, as single women were often preferred for these occupations. Furthermore, these ways for lesbians to mother "in disguise" were supported by the then commonly held assumption that lesbians were revolted by heterosexual activity and by quintessential feminine states such as motherhood.

Early Research

During the early 1970s, some lesbians took courage from the growing women's movement and the gay liberation movement to disclose their current lesbian relationship during custody proceedings rather than live in fear of being discovered. Although the consequences were often similar to Ms. Risher's, lesbian mothers started to become a visible segment of the nonclinical population. A few anecdotal reports began to appear suggesting, contrary to expectation, that lesbian mothers were ordinary mothers beset by worries and cherishing joys similar to those of heterosexual mothers (Bryant 1975; Goodman 1973). Pagelow (1980) compared 20 lesbian mothers with 43 children to 23 heterosexual divorced mothers with 51 children. The lesbian mothers had more custody problems but were more often self-employed and more likely to own their own home. The two groups of mothers were equally burdened by low wages, lack of adequate child-care arrangements, housing problems, and concern over the children's health. Mucklow and Phelan (1979) looked for statistical differences in the responses of 34 lesbian mothers compared with 47 "traditional" mothers to a series of slides of children's behaviors. They failed to find differences in the responses of the mothers. They concluded that parental behavior was a highly complex matter, a product of the mother's attitudes, values, and personality characteristics, not the consequence of sexual orientation. These early studies reflected the concern at the time that there were defects in the personal and social development of lesbians compared with heterosexual women that would negatively impact their mothering.

After in-depth interviews with 43 lesbian mothers and 37 divorced heterosexual mothers, Lewin and Lyon (1979) documented the similarities in the organization of family life in these two groups. Both sets of mothers placed strong emphasis on the maintenance of ties with kin, including ongoing connections with the children's fathers. Homosexual orientation, they stated, far from being a determinant of lifestyle, appeared to have no consistent effect on the organization of the mothers' lives or friendship patterns. The most salient feature of identification for both groups of women was motherhood.

Previously Married Lesbian Mothers

This lack of distinguishing differences between lesbian mothers and heterosexual divorced mothers has been confirmed in a variety of settings: observations of support groups for mothers (Goodman 1973), responses from questionnaires (Bryant 1975), home interviews

(C. Steirn, unpublished manuscript, 1973; St. Marie 1976), and by research studies comparing lesbian mothers with heterosexual mothers.

■ Studies With Control Groups

In 1980, four studies using control populations were presented at the
annual Orthopsychiatry meeting in Toronto. One (Lewin and Lyons
1980) dealt with the support system for single mothers as reported
above. The other three presentations (Hoeffer 1981; Hotvedt and
Mandel 1982; Kirkpatrick et al. 1981a) compared both mothers and
children in lesbian households with those in divorced heterosexual
households. The three studies supported each others' findings in several unexpected areas. Almost all mothers in both groups had been
married at the time of their children's conception. The researchers
found that in all samples the two groups of mothers, including those
with previous lesbian relationships, reported marrying at approximately the same age and for the same reasons—love of husband and
desire for marriage. In both groups almost all children had been conceived out of desire for a family. In both groups a small number of
women had married for other reasons (to escape from home or to give
the child a name) or had conceived accidentally.

Although these studies were completed in different areas of the country—in San Francisco and southern California and in the East and Southeast—the average length of marriage was the same, 7–8 years. Hotvedt
and Mandel (1982) found that 25% of the lesbian mothers stated they
would consider remarriage if it would benefit their children. This finding
suggests a lack of exclusivity in sexual partnering for a certain number of
women and helps explain the finding in some studies of nonclinical populations of lesbians that 25%–30% have been married (Bell and Weinberg
1978; Saghir and Robins 1973). These studies also suggest that there is
no reason to believe that lesbian desire arises primarily out of a revulsion
for men. Two studies (Golombok et al. 1983; Kirkpatrick et al. 1981a)
found relationships with men, especially fathers (Golombok et al. 1983),
to be much better in the lesbian households than the divorced heterosexual households. The author and colleagues (Kirkpatrick et al. 1981a)
found the lesbian mothers to be less angry at men, possibly because their
marriages had been less chaotic and violent. The lesbian mothers had
almost all initiated divorce because of a lack of intimacy in contrast to the
frequent reports from heterosexual mothers of violence, substance abuse,
or infidelity by ex-husbands.

In addition to interviewing the two groups of mothers, all three research teams reported the mothers' scores on the Bem Sex Role Inventory Scale (Bem 1974). Lesbian mothers were reported to be as high on the femininity scale as the heterosexual mothers, to have higher scores on the masculinity scale, and to be less likely to be classified as undifferentiated (Hoeffer 1981). Undifferentiation on the Sex Role Inventory Scale has been linked with problems of self-esteem, seemingly a greater risk for the heterosexual mothers in these samples.

Explorations of the pregnancy histories and infant parenting failed to reveal any evidence of underlying conflicts about maternal activities in the lesbian group compared with the heterosexual group. In a study of previously married lesbian mothers, Javaid (1993) found these mothers hoping to be grandmothers and preferring their children, especially their sons, to be heterosexual.

Children of Previously Married Lesbians

When acknowledged lesbian mothers began appearing in custody litigation, the judicial system was not alone in wanting to know whether lesbian mothers unintentionally caused unwanted consequences for their children. Many lesbian mothers also were deeply concerned with the burden their sexual orientation might place on their children. Many also feared their children would turn against them in later years. Clinicians and child specialists needed to know how to advise their clients. Courts indicated fears that the children would inevitably have gender disorders, sexual difficulties, or show disturbances of psychological or social development as a result of stigmatization.

It would be naive to assume that a child's development is simply the result of the mother's capacity to parent effectively. The genetic makeup; health, social, and economic status; and other family relationships and experiences all play a vital role in the development of a child. Nevertheless, the mother's role is certainly instrumental, and the child's psychological functioning provides some evidence of the adequacy of maternal functioning. Thus, studies of the children in lesbian families served many interests, including providing data on the capacity of lesbians to raise healthy children.

Green (1978) reported on 21 children who were raised in lesbian households and examined during custody litigation. The responses of children to the Draw-a-Person (Koppitz 1968), favored peer group, and favored toy fell well within conventional expectations, as did the sexual fantasies of the adolescent children.

The previously mentioned 1980 reports (Hoeffer 1981; Hotvedt and Mandel 1982; Kirkpatrick et al. 1981a) were the first studies of children of lesbian mothers that used control groups. These studies compared the social and sexual development of the children in lesbian mother families with that of children in heterosexual divorced mother families. Almost all of the children of lesbians had been born during marriages and thus experienced divorce as well. Most of the children studied were in the custody-sensitive age range of 5–14 years; a few were older. The studies regularly included in-depth interviews with the mother to obtain a history of the child's development and relationships. The children responded to projective tests, including the Draw-a-Person, as well as a semistructured playroom interview. High on the agenda was the collection of data related to the child's inchoate sexual identity. Judges had indicated their fear that such children would inevitably be homosexual as adults, suffer emotional disturbances, or be stigmatized by peers.

Despite the concern that the children in lesbian households would have difficulty with gender identity or sexual role development, no comparison study has found one group of children to differ from the other in this respect (Golombok et al. 1983; Green 1978; Hoeffer 1981; Hotvedt and Mandel 1982; Kirkpatrick et al. 1981a). Intellectual, social, and psychological development was comparable in the two groups in all studies.

In 149 children of lesbian mothers examined in five studies (Golombok et al. 1983, 37 children; Green 1978, 21 children; Hoeffer 1981, 20 children; Hotvedt and Mandel 1982, 51 children; Kirkpatrick et al. 1981a, 20 children) no childhood disorder or developmental problems were identified in relationship to the sexual orientation of the mother. The author and colleagues (Kirkpatrick et al. 1981a) concluded that 10% of the children had some degree of psychological difficulty, but this was true for children in the heterosexual group as well. Golombok et al. (1983) obtained information from teachers who described the children of lesbians in the sample as better adjusted and performing at a higher academic and social level than the children in the control group.

Golombok's group of children of lesbians also had more contact with fathers than did the children in the control group. The author and colleagues (Kirkpatrick et al. 1981a) found the cohort of lesbian mothers to be more concerned with providing male figures in their children's lives than were the heterosexual mothers. This was especially true of those lesbians who had a domestic partner. Although the study (Kirkpatrick et al. 1981a) did not evaluate this effect, the author was impressed with the benefit to children of households that contained more than one adult. Those households provided a richer, more diversified social life and had less distress over daily burdens as well as a higher income. Furthermore, the mothers in these households were more available to their children. These factors should be taken into consideration when courts recommend custody arrangements that restrict the presence of the partner of the lesbian mother. Almost all these children had experienced family discord and divorce, and they showed signs of the suffering these experiences imposed. If the lesbian relationship dissolved, they experienced the pain of loss again. Although the partner of the lesbian related in various ways with the children, most were experienced by the children as an aunt, adult friend, or big sister. None played the role of "father."

Hoeffer (1981) examined a sample of 20 lesbian mothers and 20 divorced heterosexual mothers and their only or oldest child between ages 6 and 9. The mothers did not differ in self-reports of encouraging sex role traits and behavior in their children. The children were asked to rate themselves on five male-valued traits ("outgoing," "adventuresome," "never cries," "strong," and "likes to be the leader") and five female-valued traits ("aware of others' feelings," "gentle," "behaves," "neat," and "quiet"). Boys in both groups rated themselves conventionally masculine. However, boys in the lesbian group rated themselves higher on "awareness of others' feelings" and "gentleness." Boys in both groups felt their peers were closer to their ideal than they were. Girls of the two groups rated themselves similarly on female-valued traits. In addition, the girls of lesbians rated themselves higher on "adventuresomeness" and "likes to be the leader." The girls of both groups, unlike the boys, felt themselves to be as close to their ideal as their peers. Hoeffer (1981) theorized that this finding was the result of the mothers in both groups providing a less effective role model for boys than for girls. This finding, if replicated, seems related to the absence of an effective male figure rather than the sexual orientation of the mother.

None of these studies found evidence of more disorders of gender identity, gender role, sexual orientation, or social or psychological functioning in one group of children compared with the other. The studies up to this time have given convincing evidence that lesbianism does not impair effective mothering. (For more detailed review of these studies see Kirkpatrick et al. 1981b and Patterson 1992.)

Support groups for children of lesbian mothers are available in large urban centers. Reports on these groups identify the concerns of young children with the problem of secrecy while adolescents present concerns about their own sexual futures (Hall 1978; Javaid 1983; Lewis 1980). Support groups are helpful in relieving these anxieties.

▮ Limitations of the Studies

All the studies were driven by a need to respond to the previous assumptions about differences between lesbians and heterosexual women, especially in regard to mothering capacity. These studies demonstrated that there is no specific effect to be predicted from the rearing of a child by a lesbian mother. However, no new information about the desire for motherhood or its sources and development in lesbians was identified. The studies revealed little about ways lesbians and children cope with a homophobic society.

A serious flaw in the design of all the above-mentioned studies was the use of "single mother" in the legal sense to characterize the cohorts. In most of the lesbian cohorts, many lesbian mothers had partners who either shared the household or lived nearby. Thus a more appropriate control group would have been reconstituted heterosexual families. The presence of another adult enriches the child's (and the mother's) life, and partnering may in itself reflect a higher level of psychological functioning (Bell and Weinberg 1978). If this is so, the studies restricted the heterosexual cohort, but not the lesbian cohort, in a way that maximized the number of persons with social or psychological dysfunction in the former group.

An additional limitation was the small number of adolescents represented in the studies. The evaluations of the sexual orientation of preadolescent children were only suggestive at best. Furthermore, no longitudinal or follow-up studies are in print. No study contained more than one or two women who had given birth to children in a committed lesbian relationship. Thus almost all the children had had fathers in the home during the first 1–2 years. New research with lesbian mothers raising children from birth is discussed below.

■ Older Children of Previously Married Lesbians

To correct one deficiency in the early reports, the children of the first wave of identified lesbian mothers were studied again when they became adolescents (Cushing 1983; Huggins 1989). Huggins (1989) evaluated the self-esteem of 18 adolescents aged 13–19 raised by lesbian mothers with the self-esteem of 18 age-matched adolescents in the households of divorced heterosexual mothers. No significant difference was noted in the two groups on the Coopersmith Self-Esteem Inventory (1969). In addition, the children whose mothers were involved in a stable ongoing relationship scored higher than those whose mothers were without partners. The daughters of fathers who were accepting of the lesbian relationship of the mother had higher self-esteem scores, possibly related to identification with a more clearly valued female figure.

Gottman (1990) compared 35 adult daughters of lesbian mothers with 35 adult daughters of divorced heterosexual mothers who had remarried during the daughters' childhood and 35 adult daughters of divorced heterosexual mothers who had remained single. The daughters' ages ranged from 18 to 44 with a mean age of 24. Using a variety of scales, Gottman measured gender identity, gender role, sexual orientation, and social adjustment of the daughters. No differences in these measures in the three groups of daughters were related to the sexual orientation of the mothers. Two interesting differences were found: 1) a trend for daughters with older brothers to score higher on masculine gender role and 2) daughters of lesbian mothers (all of whom had had lesbian partners at some time) and rematched heterosexual mothers scored higher on well-being than daughters whose mothers had remained single. Again the presence of a coparent, regardless of sex, seems valuable in enhancing a sense of well-being in children.

■ Discussion

Despite limitations, these early studies were of value to concerned parents and to the judicial system searching for grounds on which to determine the best interests of the child. From the clinical perspective, although most clinicians and researchers continue to believe that changes in family structure and parental behaviors always have an effect on children, these studies demonstrated that the sexual orientation of the mother, at least after the first 2 years of the child's life does not have a predictable effect on the child. Either the sexual orientation of the mother is a weak influence or is embedded in other more powerful influences unrelated to family structure and more likely related to family process. The greater effect on development seems to arise from the quality of the mother's relationship with her child, rather than from her sexual orientation.

New Lesbian Mothers

No easy way exists to accurately estimate the number of lesbians with children or the number of children in lesbian and gay households. Estimates of numbers of lesbian mothers range from 1 to 5 million (Gottman 1990; Hoeffer 1981), with the number of children ranging from 6 to 14 million (Editors of the Harvard Law Review 1990). Most of this group of parents conceived their children in heterosexual marriages. Recently, however, an increasing number of lesbians have conceived children and raised them from birth either as single parents or in committed lesbian relationships. These are the "new" lesbian mothers who are participating in the "lesbian baby boom" (Patterson 1994). In addition, adoption, foster care, and various forms of coparenting have made it possible for more lesbians to fulfill their desire to parent.

■ Planning Pregnancy

Lesbians rarely become pregnant by accident. However, contrary to traditional assumptions, many lesbians who wish to parent would like to become pregnant. If coupled, their situation has some similarity to infertile heterosexual couples. The struggle to achieve a mutual decision to adopt or to try alternate methods of conception is similar. Both must consider how best to achieve pregnancy, how to prepare for the procedures, pay the cost, and minimize health hazards. The similarity ends there. Lesbian couples must decide who is to become pregnant, although both may wish to eventually bear children. Many infertility services in the country accept heterosexual couples, but few accept single women, much less lesbians, for insemination procedures. One such clinic in Boston received a grant in 1993 from the Lesbian Health Fund to study alternate methods of insemination for lesbians to determine efficacy, cost, and safety. This study is comparing home-based insemination (known as the turkey baster method) with office-based procedures such as the pericervical cap, the low-technology intracervical procedure, and the high-technology intrauterine procedure.

No evidence exists that fertility problems are more common in lesbians than in heterosexual women. Endometriosis may be more common in lesbians because they are less likely to have used birth control pills, which protect against the condition.

To help with the many decisions to be made at this time, discussion groups are available in some urban areas for lesbians considering parenthood. Jennifer Firestone (personal communication, July 1994), who facilitates such groups in Boston, reports that lesbians tend to spend many months or years planning for pregnancy and childrearing. The complexity of the personal, medical, legal, and family issues requires deeper introspection and more careful exploration by lesbians than by heterosexuals.

■ Maternal Desire

The presumed dichotomy between motherhood and lesbianism was supported by the belief that lesbians were revolted by their own genitals and female reproductive functions and instead identified with males, male interests, and values. These interests are as variable among lesbians as among heterosexual women. The experience of loving and desiring a woman as a sexual partner may be all that lesbians have in common with men. On the other hand, a lesbian may have many stereotypically male values and interests without having lost interest in pregnancy and childrearing. Lewin (1993) points out that lesbian mothers and heterosexual mothers, like most women, "share in the system of meaning that envelops motherhood in our culture" (p. 182). Motherhood signals adulthood and mature functioning capacities, both physiologically and psychologically.

For lesbians, as for other women, motherhood is a profound foundation for adult identity (Lewin 1981). To some extent, lesbians may feel normalized by motherhood and thus more a part of the same life events and responsibilities that society expects of women in general. Motherhood links them to other mothers in maintaining the continuity of society as well as their own. Lesbians, perhaps more than other women, tend to prize intimacy, nurturance, feminine sensibilities, and "nest building." For lesbian couples, as for many heterosexual couples, loving deeply is a creative experience. Having a child is an announcement and a celebration of this love. However, unlike most heterosexual couples, lesbian couples must involve a third party.

■ Donors

Who should the donor be? If the donor is known, what will be his role and that of his family after the birth? In many states the semen of the donor must be given to the mother by a physician, otherwise the donor retains paternal rights.

In some communities, single lesbians or lesbian couples are creating parenting units with gay males or gay male couples. A thoughtful and detailed parenting contract in writing can define the rights and responsibilities of each member of the unit, including the rights and responsibilities should either couple separate (Martin 1993; Pies 1985; Schulenberg 1985). In this circumstance, the number of extended family members can become quite large.

Other lesbians prefer to find anonymous donors through friends, their physician, or a sperm bank. Under any circumstances it is essential to know the health of the donor. According to Johnson (1994), seven women to that date had been infected with the AIDS virus from fresh donor semen. The use of frozen semen or washed semen increases safety. Semen banks provide a catalogue giving race, physical characteristics, ethnic ancestry, occupation, and interests of each donor. These banks are inspected and accredited by national standardizing associations and state licensing departments. Coparents need to reach a consensus on the type of donor and the relationship anticipated. A decision also must be reached about the last name the child will carry.

■ Disclosure

How to respond to the child's questions about his or her father requires many hours of discussion. A plan that is satisfactory for a 3-year-old child may be unacceptable for an older child. Children may become preoccupied with a "ghost parent" father (Margolis 1989). Many lesbian mothers believe their child will benefit from knowing the real father in addition to acknowledging his function as semen donor. This has led to increased interest in parenting contracts with a known donor or the preference for a "yes" donor (i.e., one who agrees to be identified when the child reaches age 18). In addition, decisions must be made about informing the mother's and her partner's families. Some prospective grandparents may be delighted, others shocked or disapproving.

The nonpregnant partner, unlike a heterosexual mother's partner, has no recognized position in the child's future life. She may be unable to tell co-workers or various family members about this exciting change in her life. During the pregnancy she may begin to feel invisible or dismissed, unless both partners are attentive to this possibility. Despite a parenting contract, she has no accepted legal rights or duties even if she provides primary care. A number of legal cases regarding visitation rights of a separated coparent have come to litigation in the last 5 years with various outcomes according to the National Center for Lesbian Rights.

If, when, and how disclosure of the lesbian relationship will be made to the child also require careful thinking and a common approach between coparents. Mothers who were able to disclose their lesbian identity to bosses, ex-husbands, and children were found by Rand et al.(1982) to have a more positive sense of well-being than those who could not disclose. The increased sense of well-being may enhance effective mothering. Disclosure to children prior to adolescence appears to be less difficult than during adolescence (Cushing 1983; Huggins 1989). Children who could negotiate disclosure in a discriminating way also were found to have higher self-esteem (Gershon, in press). Lewis (1980) suggested from observations of such children in support groups that silence about their mother's orientation with schoolmates created feelings of isolation that were alleviated by discussion with other children in similar households.

■ Coparent

The social invisibility of the lesbian coparent during pregnancy and the lack of legal parental rights after delivery cause anxiety for the live-in coparent and place stress on the couple's relationship. The biological mother may feel vulnerable and fearful of increased dependency on her partner. Couples struggle to create and maintain a family unit for which there is no model. McCandlish (1987) found insignificant bonding differences between lesbian coparents during the pregnancy and in the first 2 postpartum years. The biological mother expected to bond to the infant, but the nonbiological mother was shocked by the unexpected feelings of immediate attachment. The intensity of this feeling, legally and socially discontextual, produced anxiety in the coparent about the child's bond to her for the first 2 years. Osterweil (1991) found lesbian couples to derive satisfaction from relational values and skills. These skills, especially effective communication and equality of involvement with the child, were the foundation for neutralizing the difficulties encountered in this new family form and for providing satisfaction.

■ Adoption and Foster Care

The above-mentioned problem of the legal invisibility of the nonbiological mother has been addressed by a variety of awkward maneuvers such as a draft by an attorney allowing the nonbiological parent to give consent for medical care or to be nominated as the child's guardian. In the past few years, a number of jurisdictions have allowed "second parent adoptions" in which the biological mother need not relinquish her relationship to her child to allow her partner to have equal parental rights.

A New York case in 1992 became the first such reported decision in the country (in re: Evan, 583 N.Y.S. 2nd 977, 1992). The supreme courts of several states, including Vermont and Massachusetts, have decided in favor of legal coparenting. The National Center for Lesbian Rights (1370 Mission Street, 4th Floor, San Francisco, CA 94103) provides current information on the rapidly changing legal scene as well as legal guide books.

Lesbians have been able to openly adopt as single parents in some states, although they are defined as presumptively unfit because of lesbianism in others. Since the mid-1980s, some states have permitted joint adoptions by lesbian couples. Similarly, Foster parenting has been variously treated. Terry de Crescenzo, who initiated the Gay/Lesbian Adolescent Social Services in Los Angeles in 1984, refers to a "motherlode of gay and lesbian couples longing to parent" who are available for providing foster care. She has initiated such a program and currently reports supervising 55 children under the age of 4 in homes, almost all of which are gay or lesbian. Children stay for periods of a few days up to 18 months. Some foster parents become legal guardians of children in their care, and a few are permitted to adopt.

In addition to the many decisions surrounding lesbian parenting already suggested is the necessity to think through the repercussions on social life and on participation in the larger lesbian community. Some lesbian mothers avoid lesbian mother groups because of pressure to raise children according to the perceived ideological demands of the group (Lewin 1993).

■ The Children

The Women's Action Coalition (1993) in San Francisco estimated that in the United States 10,000 children who were conceived by alternate insemination are being raised by single or coupled lesbians. A few studies on these children have been completed. The first study (Steckel 1987), compared the process of separation-individuation between 11 preschool children born by alternate insemination and raised by lesbian couples and 11 similarly aged children of heterosexual couples. The study included structured parent interviews, parent and teacher Q-Sort, and a projective Structured Doll Technique interview with each child. Evaluating independence, ego function, and object relations by this means did not reveal any differences between the two groups of children. However, suggestive differences were noted in the children's perceptions of themselves. Children of heterosexual parents saw themselves as more aggressive, as did their parents and teachers, whereas children of lesbians saw themselves as more lovable and were seen by their parents and teachers as more affectionate and protective of younger children. Steckel concluded that the presence of a female rather than a male coparent did not impair the separation-individuation process but did establish a qualitatively different experience.

Patterson (1994) examined 37 children born to or adopted by single or coupled lesbians. Coparents completed the Achenbach and Edelbrock Child Behavior Checklist to assess social competence and behavior. The Eder Children's Self-View Questionnaire was administered to the children through the use of hand puppets. Sex-role behavior was assessed by asking preferences for playmates, toys, games, and favorite characters.

The results were compared with norms for children of this age. As with earlier studies, no significant differences were found with one exception—the children of lesbian mothers reported both more stress and a greater sense of well-being. Although different from Steckel's finding of more affectionate natures in younger children born into lesbian households, this finding also suggests enhanced presence of emotional expressiveness, another female-valued trait.

Future Research

Early studies dispelled the notion that the children of lesbian mothers would show specific problems in the area of gender development and sexual orientation. As noted earlier, the sexual orientation of the mother appeared to be a weak influence and was not correlated with any identified characteristic in the children. These studies confirmed that lesbians are a heterogeneous group, a portion of whom desire pregnancy or the opportunity to parent. This group of mothers provides an opportunity to study the meaning and construction of motherhood separated from heterosexual orientation. We have yet to examine how racial and cultural differences impact on lesbians choosing motherhood and their children. Several early studies suggest the great value of the presence of more than one adult caregiver, regardless of gender or relationship, although this has not yet been studied as a separate variable.

Although greatly idealized in the 20th century, the nuclear family has had serious difficulties. A mother and her children form a small unit, often isolated and overly interdependent, even if in a heterosexual marriage. The 21st century will probably see an increase in a variety of new family forms, including lesbian mother families with various arrangements with fathers. The efforts made by these parenting units to form contracts specifically for the children's welfare (unlike the marriage contract, which is primarily to define the ownership and management of property) may instruct the larger community. The many forms of parenting units, the arrangements with fathers and donors, the management of disclosures, the role of the coparent, and the consequences of alterations in the parenting unit and support systems (or lack thereof) represent some of the diversities that intrigue current researchers. The management of stigma in the schools (Casper 1992), the effects of participation in the gay community on the development of tolerance, and the individual ways of coping with prejudice in the larger community all should be studied.

Longitudinal studies of lesbian families and children's development in these families are essential. Clearly, family process, rather than family structure, is the significant feature in a child's development. Hopefully, these studies will help illuminate the significant features of beneficial family process for all children.

References

Achenbach TM, Edelbrock C: Manual for the Child Behavior Checklist and Revised Child Behavior Profile. Burlington, University of Vermnont, Department of Psychiatry, 1983

Bell A, Weinberg M: Homosexuality: A Study of Diversity Among Men and Women. New York, Simon and Schuster, 1978

Bem SL: The measurement of psychological androgeny. J Consult Clin Psychol 42:155–162, 1974

Bryant B: Lesbian mothers. Unpublished master's thesis, California State University of Social Work, Sacramento, CA, 1975

Casper V, Schultz S, Wickens E: Breaking the silences: lesbian and gay parents and the schools. Teachers College Record 94(1):109–137, 1992

Coopersmith S: The Antecedents of Self-Esteem. San Francisco, CA, WH Freeman, 1967

Cushing B: Adolescent children of lesbian mothers: an exploratory study. Unpublished master's thesis, California State University, Fresno, CA, 1983

Eder RA: Uncovering young children's psychological selves: individual and developmental differences. Child Development 61:849–863, 1990

Editors of the Harvard Law Review: Sexual Orientation and the Law. Cambridge, MA, Harvard University Press, 1990

Gershon TD: Lesbian and gay parents, in Developmental and Behavioral Pediatrics: A Handbook for Primary Care. Edited by Parker S, Zuckerman B. New York, Little, Brown (in press)

Golombok S, Spencer A, Rutter M: Children in lesbian and single-parent households: psychosexual and psychiatric appraisal. J Child Psychol Psychiatry 24:551–572, 1983

Goodman B: The lesbian mother. Am J Orthopsychiatry 43:282–284, 1973

Gottman JS: Children of gay and lesbian parents, in Homosexuality and Family Relations. Edited by Bozett F, Sussman MB. New York, Harrington Park Press, 1990, pp 177–196

Green R: Sexual identity of 37 children raised by homosexual or transsexual parents. Am J Psychiatry 135:692–697, 1978

Hall M: Lesbian families: cultural and clinical issues. Soc Work 23:380–385, 1978

Hoeffer B: Children's acquisition of sex-role behavior in lesbian mothers' families. Am J Orthopsychiatry 51:536–643, 1981

Hotvedt M, Mandel J: Children of lesbian mothers, in Homosexuality: Social, Psychological and Biological Issues. Edited by Weinrich P, Gonsiorek J, Hotvedt M. Beverly Hills, CA, Sage, 1982, pp 275–285

Huggins S: A comparative study of self-esteem of adolescent children of divorced lesbian mothers and divorced heterosexual mothers. J Homosex 18:123–135, 1989

Javaid G: The children of homosexual and heterosexual single mothers. Child Psychiatry Hum Dev 23:235–248, 1993

Javaid G: The sexual development of the adolescent daughter of a homosexual mother. Journal of the American Academy of Child Psychiatry 22:196–201, 1983

Johnson SR: The health care needs of lesbian women. Presented at the annual meeting of the American Society of Psychosomatic Obstetrics and Gynecology, San Diego, CA, February 27, 1994

Kirkpatrick M, Smith K, Roy R: Lesbian mothers and their children: a comparative study. Am J Orthopsychiatry 51:545–551, 1981a

Kirkpatrick M, Smith K, Roy R: Studies of a new population: the lesbian mother, in Modern Perspectives in the Psychiatry of Middle Age. Edited by Howells J. New York, Brunner/Mazel, pp 132–143, 1981b

Koppitz EM: Psychological evaluation of children's human figure drawings. New York, Grune & Stratton, 1968

Lewin E: Lesbian Mothers: Accounts of Gender in American Culture. Ithaca, NY, Cornell University Press, 1993

Lewin E: Lesbianism and motherhood: implications for child custody. Hum Organ 40(1):6–14, 1981

Lewin E, Lyons T: Lesbian and heterosexual mothers: continuity and difference in family organization. Paper presented at the annual meeting of Orthopsychiatry, Toronto, April 1980

Lewis K: Children of lesbians: their point of view. Soc Work 25:198–203, 1980

Margolis Z: The new lesbian mothers: an exploratory study. Unpublished master's thesis, UCLA School of Social Welfare, Los Angeles, CA, 1989

Martin A: The Lesbian and Gay Parenting Handbook. New York, Harper Perennial, 1993

McCandlish BM: Against all odds: lesbian mother family dynamics, in Gay and Lesbian Parents. Edited by Bozett FW. New York, Praeger, 1987, pp 23–38

Mucklow B, Phelan G: Lesbian and traditional mothers' responses to adult response to child behavior and self concept. Psychology Reporter 44(3):880–882, 1979

Osterweil DA: Correlates of relationship satisfaction in lesbian couples who are parenting their first child together. Unpublished doctoral dissertation, California School of Professional Psychology, Berkely, CA, 1991

Pagelow M: Heterosexual and lesbian single mothers: a comparison of problems, coping, and solutions. J Homosex 5:189–204, 1980

Patterson C: Children of lesbian and gay parents. Child Dev 63:1025–1042, 1992

Patterson C: Children of the lesbian baby boom: behavioral adjustment, self-concepts and sex-role identity, in Lesbian and Gay Psychology: Theory, Research and Clinical Applications. Edited by Greene B, Herek G. Beverly Hills, CA, Sage, 1994

Pies C: Considering Parenthood: A Workbook for Lesbians. San Francisco, CA, Spinsters Ink, 1985

Rand C, Graham DLF, Rawlings EI: Psychological health and factors the court seeks to control in lesbian mother custody trials. J Homosex 8:27–39, 1982

Saghir M, Robins E: Male and Female Homosexuality: A Comprehensive Investigation. Baltimore, MD, Williams and Wilkins, 1973

Schulenberg J: Gay Parenting: A Complete Guide for Gay Men and Lesbians with Children. Garden City, NY, Anchor Books, 1985

St. Marie D: A descriptive study of lesbian mothers. Unpublished master's thesis, University of Hawaii School of Social Work, Honolulu, HI, 1976

Steckel A: Psychosocial development of children of lesbian mothers, in Gay and Lesbian Parents. Edited by Bozett FW. New York, Praeger, 1987, pp 75–85

Women's Action Coalition: The Facts About Women. New York, The New Press, 1993

22

Gay Fathers and Their Children

Charlotte J. Patterson, Ph.D.
Raymond W. Chan

The concepts of heterosexuality and parenthood are intertwined so deeply in cultural history and in contemporary thought that, at first glance, the idea of gay fatherhood can seem exotic or even impossible. Undeniably, however, some men identify themselves both as fathers and as gay. Most of these men have been able to avoid media attention, but others have become the subjects of intense public discussion and controversy (Campbell 1994; Ricks 1995). For instance, in 1993 when Ross and Luis Lopton, a gay couple living in Seattle, attempted to complete a legal adoption of their young foster son, the boy's biological mother, Megan Lucas, raised objections and attempted to halt the adoption process. Even though the Loptons

---

This chapter is an edited and condensed version of Patterson CJ, Chan RW: "Gay Fathers," in *The Role of the Father in Child Development*, 3rd Edition. Edited by Lamb ME. New York, Wiley, 1996. Copyright 1996 John Wiley and Sons, Inc. Reprinted by permission of John Wiley and Sons, Inc.

refused to discuss the case in public, considerable controversy never-theless ensued. Eventually, the men were allowed to complete the adoption (Ricks 1995). Although this was not the first adoption of its kind (Seligmann 1990) and the Loptons are not the first gay men to become fathers through adoption (Patterson, in press a), the publicity surrounding their case brought more attention to the issue of gay fatherhood than ever before.

In the wake of the Lopton matter, gay fatherhood has emerged into public awareness and brought questions. Who are gay fathers, and how do they become parents? What kind of parents do gay men make, and how do their children develop? What special challenges and stresses do gay fathers and their children face in daily life, and how do they cope with them? What can acquaintance with gay fathers and their children offer to the understanding of parenthood, child development, and family life? Although the research literatures bearing on such questions are quite new and relatively sparse, existing studies address some issues raised by the existence of gay fathers.

Who Are Gay Fathers and How Do They Become Parents?

Gay fathers are a varied group. In addition to diversity engendered by age, education, race, ethnicity, and other demographic factors, some of the issues specific to gay fathers also create important distinctions among them and among their families.

■ Diversity Among Gay Fathers

Probably the largest group of gay fathers are divorced (Bozett 1982, 1989; Green and Bozett 1991). These men generally entered into a heterosexual marriage and had children before declaring a public gay identity. After coming out, many say that they got married because they wanted to have children, because they loved their wives, because they wanted a domestic, married life, and because of social pressures. Some report that they married despite their knowledge of being attracted to other men, sometimes in the hope that marriage would dispel such desires. Others explain that they were not fully aware of their sexual desires for other men until well into their marriages. Although some men remain married after coming out, most separate from their wives and eventually divorce (Bozett 1982, 1989).

When couples divorce after a husband comes out as gay, custody of children is likely to be granted to the wife (Editors of the Harvard Law Review 1990; Rivera 1993). If the courts have biases about which parent should be given custody of minor children, they are likely to favor mothers over fathers and heterosexual over homosexual parents (Thompson 1983). Together, these two factors usually combine to ensure that primary physical custody of children goes to the mother in such cases. Thus, the largest group of divorced gay fathers are nonresidential parents (Strader 1993). Visitation arrangements may vary. One divorced gay father's children may visit with him every other weekend (Fadiman 1983), whereas another man's children may visit only rarely and be forbidden to stay in his home overnight (Campbell 1994). A newly divorced gay father without primary custody is likely to encounter issues related to grieving the loss of daily contact with his children while adjusting to his new life as a gay man.

A smaller group of divorced gay fathers has custody of their children and act as their primary caregivers. In some cases, extenuating circumstances may place one or more children in the father's custody. For instance, in one family, the mother felt that she could care for two of the couple's three children but believed that bearing responsibility as a single parent for the third (a 10-year-old child who had been diagnosed with Down's syndrome) would overwhelm her; this family agreed that the gay father would take custody of the 10-year-old child (Fadiman 1983). In another instance, a mother's serious illness precluded her taking custody of the couple's child during a period of chemotherapy (*Roe v. Roe* 1985). Divorced gay fathers with primary custody of their child or children may need time to adjust to being the primary caregiver for children (often as a single parent) while also striving to accommodate to their new identities as gay men.

Another group of gay fathers have become foster or adoptive parents after coming out as gay. Two states (Florida and New Hampshire) have laws forbidding the adoption of minor children by gay or lesbian adults, but foster placements with and adoptions by gay adults have taken place in many jurisdictions (Ricketts 1991; Ricketts and Achtenberg 1990). Foster or adoptive placements may involve children who are relatives of the adoptive father, or they may involve unrelated children (Patterson 1995c). Gay men also have legally adopted the children of their gay partners (Patterson 1995c; Seligmann 1990). Because of antigay prejudices in adoption and foster care circles and in the courts, gay men have often had to fight for the right to adopt or to become foster parents (Ricketts 1991), with cases sometimes remaining in the courts for years (Patterson 1995c); others who have been given the opportunity to become foster or adoptive parents have been offered only children who are considered difficult to place because of age, ethnicity, illness, or disability. Gay men also have completed interracial or international adoptions (Martin 1993). Foster and adoptive gay families are thus a diverse group.

Gay men also have become parents by fathering children with a surrogate mother (Martin 1993; McPherson 1993; Sbordone 1993). For instance, a gay couple might make a contract with a woman to bear a child or children conceived with the use of the sperm of one member of the couple. At the child's birth, the woman agrees to relinquish parental rights and responsibilities, and the father becomes the sole legal parent. The child is then reared by the two men (McPherson 1993; Sbordone 1993) and may eventually be adopted by the nonbiological father (for example, *In re W.S.D.* 1992).

Another route to parenthood taken by some gay men is to conceive and raise children jointly with a woman or women with whom the men are not sexually involved (Martin 1993; Van Gelder 1991). In one common scenario, a gay couple and a lesbian couple might undertake parenthood together, with sperm from one of the men being used to inseminate one of the women. In an arrangement sometimes called "quadra-parenting," the child or children might spend part of the time in one home and part of the time in the other home. Gay men can undertake such arrangements with women who are heterosexual or lesbian or who are single as well as in relationships with partners. The details of child custody and visitation also may vary considerably from family to family and over time. Thus considerable diversity exists among gay fathers and among their families (Patterson 1992).

■ Prevalence of Gay Fatherhood

Because gay parenthood is so diverse, providing accurate estimates of the numbers of gay fathers in the United States is difficult (see Chapter 4 by Michaels). In response to widespread prejudice and discrimination, many gay and lesbian individuals believe that they must conceal their sexual identities in many environments. This is especially true of gay fathers and lesbian mothers, who may fear that child custody or visitation will be curtailed or even terminated if their sexual identities become known (Campbell 1994). For these and other reasons, many gay fathers attempt to conceal their gay identities, sometimes even from their own children (Dunne 1987; Robinson and Barret 1986).

Despite difficulties, estimates of the number of gay parents in the United States have been made (Bozett 1987; Miller 1979). Some estimates begin with the assumption (from Kinsey et al. 1948) that 10% of the male population is predominantly gay. According to results of large-scale survey studies (Bell and Weinberg 1978; Bryant and Demian 1994; Saghir and Robins 1973), about 10% of gay men are parents. Calculations based on these figures suggest that there are between 1 million and 2 million gay fathers in the United States (Bozett 1987; Miller 1979); if each of these fathers has, on average, two children, then one might estimate that there are between 2 million and 4 million children of gay fathers.

Like any estimates, these are only as good as the figures on which they are based, and reasons exist to question these estimates. Recent research has suggested that the gay population may be smaller than previously estimated, perhaps in the range of 3%–5% (Gagnon et al. 1994). However, younger gay men may be increasingly likely to consider parenthood in the context of their established gay identities. In a recent survey of gay couples (Bryant and Demian 1994), one-third of respondents under age 35 years were either planning to have children or considering having children. Secular trends may thus influence both the prevalence of gay fatherhood and the characteristics of the population of gay fathers, making any numerical estimates unstable at best.

Gay Fathers as Parents

Despite the diversity of gay fatherhood, with few exceptions research has been conducted with relatively homogeneous groups of participants, and using a relatively narrow range of methodological approaches (Patterson 1992, 1994b, 1995a, 1995d). Samples of gay fathers have been mainly white, well educated, affluent, and living in major urban centers. Although recent evidence suggests that self-identified gay men are more likely to live in large cities than elsewhere (Gagnon et al. 1994), how well the samples of gay fathers studied to date represent the population of gay fathers is not known. The existing research falls into two categories: studies of divorced gay fathers and studies of gay men who became parents after establishing their gay identities (Bigner and Bozett 1990; Gottman 1990; Patterson 1995a, 1995d).

■ Divorced Gay Fathers

Research on gay fathers was initiated by two investigators, one in Canada (Miller 1979) and one in the United States (Bozett 1980, 1981a, 1981b, 1987), and focused on concerns about gay father identities and their transformations over time. Both Miller and Bozett sought to provide conceptualizations of the steps through which a man who considers himself to be a heterosexual father may begin to identify as a gay father in public as well as in private. On the basis of extensive interviews with gay fathers, these authors emphasized the centrality of identity disclosure and of the reactions to disclosure by significant people in a man's life in the process of identity acquisition. By disclosing his status as a gay man to those in the heterosexual world, by disclosing his status as a father to members of the gay community, and by receiving validating responses from significant others, Bozett argued that a gay father is gradually able to integrate these previously separate aspects of his identity.

Miller's (1979) model of the acquisition of gay father identities, based on his interviews with 50 gay fathers, involves four steps. At the outset, a married man who wants sexual contact with other men engages in "covert behavior," seeking secretive sexual encounters with men, often using excuses such as drunkenness to explain away his behavior (Ortiz and Scott 1994). A man engaging in covert behavior of this kind is likely, according to Miller, to see his children and family life as "duties" and not to see life as a gay man as a viable option.

In Miller's next step, a man may have "marginal involvement" in the gay community. Although the man continues to live with his wife and children, and generally presents himself in public as heterosexual, he may have occasional contact with gay men, either sexually or in gay community meeting places or organizations. At this point, a man is likely to feel guilty about his growing need to conceal important aspects of his identity from his wife and children and may begin to think about living separately from them.

In the third step of Miller's model, the "transformed participation" step, a man begins to assume a gay identity for the first time. Many individuals move away from their wives and children and begin to disclose their sexual orientation to people outside the family. At this stage, Miller argues, men begin to worry about possible interventions by the courts into their relationships with their children and about the possibility that the legal system may curtail or deny their visitation with their children. With the demise of pretense, however, many men feel better and experience heightened self-esteem and more favorable mental health.

The fourth step in Miller's model is called "open endorsement." At this point, individuals have solidified their identities as gay men and are often working professionally or in volunteer capacities for various gay causes. Miller describes their lives as organized around gay communities, often involving a gay partner. By this time, men have disclosed their gay identities to family members, and these relationships are now unencumbered by the psychological distance that was once involved in keeping secrets about their sexual orientation. Concerns mentioned by such men center on the difficulties of integrating identities as gay men and as fathers in a world that valorizes one identity but denigrates the other.

Some ideas about what propels a man through the steps of acknowledging an identity as a gay father to himself and to others have been proposed. Miller and Bozett concur that, although a number of factors such as occupational autonomy and amount of access to gay communities may affect how rapidly a man acquires a gay identity and discloses it to others, the most important of these is likely to be the experience of falling in love with another man. This experience more than any other, suggest Miller and Bozett, is likely to lead a man to integrate the otherwise compartmentalized parts of his identity as a gay father. This hypothesis is open to empirical evaluation, but to date such research has not been reported.

The contributions of Miller and Bozett to research on gay fathers have been substantial, and Miller's model is apparently an accurate compilation of the retrospective reports of men he interviewed. On the other hand, their models are not helpful in predicting which married men who engage in covert sexual relations with other men will eventually divorce and identify themselves as gay fathers. Furthermore, such models explain little about the behavior of gay fathers in parenting and other roles.

Research on the parenting attitudes of gay versus heterosexual divorced fathers has, however, been conducted (Barret and Robinson 1990, 1994). Bigner and Jacobsen (1989a, 1989b, 1992) compared 33 gay and 33 heterosexual divorced fathers, each of whom had at least two children. With one exception, results showed no differences between motives for parenthood among gay and heterosexual men. The single exception was the greater likelihood of gay than heterosexual fathers to cite the higher status accorded to parents compared with nonparents as a motivation for parenthood (Bigner and Jacobsen 1989a). The best interpretation of this finding is not clear. One possibility is that gay fathers were more candid and hence more likely to acknowledge that their desire for children might have been driven at least in part by self-serving motives. Another possibility is that, because of the stigma associated with gay identity, gay fathers were less likely to take for granted the respect accorded to parents. Additional research will be necessary to clarify these and other possibilities.

Bigner and Jacobsen (1989b) also asked gay and heterosexual fathers in their sample to report on their behavior with their children. Although no differences emerged in the fathers' reports of involvement or intimacy, gay fathers reported that their behavior was characterized by greater responsiveness, more reasoning, and more limit-setting than did heterosexual fathers. These reports by gay fathers of greater warmth and responsiveness, as well as greater control and limit-setting, are strongly reminiscent of findings from research with heterosexual families and would seem to raise the possibility that gay fathers are more likely than their heterosexual counterparts to exhibit authoritative patterns of parenting behavior such as those described by Baumrind (1967) and Baumrind and Black (1967). Caution must be exercised, however, in the interpretation of results such as these, which stem entirely from paternal reports about their own behavior.

Similar results were reported earlier (Scallen 1982 cited in Flaks 1994). Scallen collected self-report information from 30 gay and 30 heterosexual fathers, all of whom were divorced. In areas of problem solving, providing recreation for children, and encouraging the autonomy of children, no differences were reported as a function of sexual orientation. In concert with the findings of Bigner and Jacobsen (1989b), gay fathers placed greater emphasis than did heterosexual fathers on paternal nurturance. At the same time, gay fathers also placed less importance on their role as economic providers for children.

Although the study thus revealed many similarities in the responses of gay and heterosexual divorced fathers, the gay fathers seemed to be somewhat less traditional in their views of the paternal role.

In addition to research comparing gay and heterosexual fathers, a few studies have made other comparisons. Robinson and Skeen (1982) compared sex role orientations of gay fathers with those of gay men who were not fathers and found no differences. Skeen and Robinson (1985) found no evidence to suggest that retrospective reports from gay men about relationships with their parents varied as a function of whether they were parents themselves. Comparing gay fathers and lesbian mothers, Harris and Turner (1985/1986) reported that, although gay fathers had higher incomes and were more likely to report encouraging their children to play in conventionally sex-typed ways, lesbian mothers were more likely to believe that their children received positive benefits such as increased tolerance for diversity from growing up with lesbian or gay parents. Studies such as these begin to suggest a number of issues for research on gender, sexual orientation, and parenting behavior, and research in this area could take many valuable directions.

Crosbie-Burnett and Helmbrecht (1993) examined the sources of individual differences within families with gay fathers. These authors focused on a group of 48 gay stepfamilies (i.e., on families composed of a gay father, his lover or partner, and at least one child who either lives in or visits the gay father's household). In assessing aspects of the functioning of stepfamilies that were associated with family happiness, Crosbie-Burnett and Helmbrecht found that, both for gay fathers and for children, the best predictors of family happiness were concerned with the integration and inclusion of gay stepfathers. Interestingly, however, the integration of stepfathers did not predict their own ratings of family happiness. Gay fathers also reported greater openness about their sexual orientation than did their children; whereas only 4% of gay fathers reported that they were not open with heterosexual friends about being gay, 54% of adolescents reported that their heterosexual friends did not know about the father's sexual orientation. Thus, children were more circumspect than their gay fathers about their status as members of a gay family, and they reported receiving less support from nongay friends. Given negative societal attitudes toward same-sex sexual relationships, it is not surprising that some gay fathers and many of their children felt the need to monitor disclosures about the gay identities of their fathers (Baptiste 1987).

■ Gay Men Choosing to Become Parents

Although for many years, gay fathers were generally assumed to have become parents only in the context of previous heterosexual relationships, both men and women are increasingly believed to be undertaking parenthood in the context of already established lesbian and gay identities (Patterson 1994a, 1995b). The research literature describes the transition to parenthood among heterosexual couples (Cowan and Cowan 1992), but no research has addressed the transition to parenthood among gay men. Many issues that arise for heterosexual individuals are also faced by lesbians and gay men (e.g., worries about how children will affect couple relationships and economic concerns about supporting children). Gay men and lesbians, however, must also cope with additional issues because of their situation as members of stigmatized minorities.

Gay men who wish to become parents often face a number of related issues (Martin 1993; Patterson 1994a), and the logistics of becoming parents can seem daunting. Prospective gay parents need accurate, up-to-date information about how they could become fathers, how their children are likely to develop, and what supports are likely to be available in the community where they live. Another issue is whether to father children in a coparenting or surrogacy arrangement or to become foster or adoptive parents. Gay men who seek to father a child also are likely to encounter various health concerns (e.g., medical screening of the prospective birth parents and assistance with techniques for donor insemination). As matters progress, legal concerns about the rights and responsibilities of all parties are likely to emerge. Associated with all of these will be financial issues; the cost of medical and legal assistance, in addition to the support of a child, can be considerable. Finally, social and emotional concerns of various kinds are likely to be significant (Patterson 1994a).

As this overview suggests, numerous questions are posed by the emergence of prospective gay parents (Patterson 1994a). What are the factors that influence the inclinations of gay men to make parenthood a part of their lives? What impact does parenting have on gay men who undertake it, and how do the effects compare with the ones experienced by heterosexuals? How effectively do special services such as support groups serve the needs of gay fathers and prospective gay fathers? What are the elements of a social climate that is supportive for gay and lesbian parents and their children? As yet, little research has addressed such questions.

Only two studies of men who have become fathers after identifying themselves as gay have been reported. Sbordone (1993) studied 78 gay men who had become parents through adoption or through surrogacy arrangements and compared them with 83 gay men who were not fathers. No differences were noted between fathers and nonfathers on reports about relationships with the men's own parents. This result is consistent with the findings of Skeen and Robinson (1985) for divorced gay fathers. Gay fathers did, however, report higher self-esteem and fewer negative attitudes about homosexuality than did gay men who were not fathers (Sbordone 1993).

An interesting observation of Sbordone's (1993) study was that most gay men who were not fathers indicated that they would like to rear a child. Those who said that they wanted children were younger than those who said they did not, but the two groups did not differ on income, education, race, self-esteem, or attitudes about homosexuality. Given that fathers had higher self-esteem and fewer negative attitudes about homosexuality than either group of nonfathers, Sbordone speculated that the higher self-esteem of gay fathers might have been a result, not a cause or simple correlate of parenthood. Longitudinal research would be useful in evaluating this idea.

A study of gay couples choosing parenthood was conducted by McPherson (1993), who assessed division of labor, satisfaction with division of labor, and satisfaction with couple relationships among 28 gay and 27 heterosexual parenting couples. Consistent with evidence from lesbian parenting couples (Hand 1991; Osterweil 1991; Patterson 1995b), McPherson found that gay couples reported a more even division of responsibilities for household maintenance and child care than did heterosexual couples. Gay couples also reported greater satisfaction with their division of child care tasks than did heterosexual couples. Finally, gay couples also reported greater satisfaction with their couple relationships, especially in the areas of cohesion and expression of affection.

Research on Children of Gay Fathers

Gay fathers are by definition members of families; they have children and often have wives or ex-wives as well as gay partners. Of course, gay fathers most often have other family members as well, including parents, aunts, uncles, siblings, nieces, nephews, and cousins. Because research on other family members has scarcely began (for exceptions, see Buxton 1994; Hays and Samuels 1989), this section focuses on the children of gay fathers, including research on the sexual identity and aspects of personal and social development of children. The research to date has focused on children of divorced gay fathers (Patterson 1992, 1995d).

Sexual Orientation

Much research on the offspring of gay fathers has examined the development of sexual identity. In response to the popular stereotype that children of gay fathers may grow up to become gay themselves, a number of researchers have studied sexual orientation among the offspring of gay fathers. In contrast to common beliefs, research has revealed that most children of gay fathers grow up to become heterosexual adults.

The earliest findings about sexual orientation among children of gay fathers were reported by Miller (1979) and by Bozett (1980, 1982, 1987, 1989). In their research, fathers were asked to report on the sexual orientation of their adolescent and young adult children. In Miller's (1979) sample, 4 of 48 children were said by their fathers to be gay or lesbian. In the two samples of Bozett (1980, 1982, 1987, 1989), 0 of 25 and 2 of 19 children were described by their fathers as gay or lesbian. Small sample sizes and varied sampling procedures suggest that interpretations of these data should be made with care. If, however, the findings from these three studies are combined, the results reveal that 6 of 92 offspring (6.5%) were reported by their fathers to be gay or lesbian.

In the largest study of sexual orientation among the offspring of gay fathers to date, Bailey et al. (1995) studied 82 adult sons of 55 gay fathers. They obtained self-reports from most of the sons as well as reports about the sexual orientation of the sons from fathers, which allowed them to assess the reliability of reports in cases where both father and son had been interviewed. Bailey et al. reported that, in the 41 cases in which fathers said they were "virtually certain" or "entirely certain" of the sexual orientation of their sons and in which sons also provided information, fathers and sons agreed in all but one case; the lone disagreement occurred when a father described his son as heterosexual and the son described himself as bisexual. The reports of fathers were thus accurate overall, allowing the confident use of paternal reports when sons could not be contacted. Of sons whose sexual orientation could be rated with confidence, 68 of 75 were said by their fathers to be heterosexual, indicating that about 9% were reported to be gay or bisexual.

An interesting aspect of the Bailey et al. (1995) study was its assessment of environmental factors. If exposure to gay fathers increases the likelihood that their sons grow up to be gay men, then sons who have lived in the household of their gay father over longer periods might be expected to show greater likelihood of being gay. In contrast to such an expectation, Bailey et al. reported that the sexual orientation of sons was unrelated to the number of years spent living in the household of a gay father, to frequency of current contact with the gay father, or to the rated quality of current father-son relationships. For instance, gay sons had lived with their fathers an average of only about 6 years, whereas heterosexual sons had lived with their fathers, on average, for about 11 years. Although this difference was not statistically significant, clearly no evidence for environmental transmission of sexual orientation was provided by these data.

The available data thus suggest that, although most children of gay fathers grow up to be heterosexual, a minority (perhaps 5%–10%) are gay or bisexual. Appropriate interpretation of these results rests heavily on estimates of the population base rates for homosexuality, and—as noted above—these are the subject of considerable controversy (see Chapter 4 by Michaels). Estimates of male homosexuality range from 1% to 2% up to about 5% or more, depending on the details of sampling, assessment, and other aspects of methodology (Bailey 1995). Whatever the ultimate resolution of this issue, it is clear that most children of gay fathers grow up to be heterosexual adults.

■ Other Aspects of Personal and Social Development

Many aspects of the personal and social development of children of gay fathers have not been studied, but some evidence exists about relationships between parents and their children. Harris and Turner (1985/86) studied 10 gay fathers, 13 lesbian mothers, 2 heterosexual fathers, and 14 heterosexual mothers, most of whom had custody of their children. The respondents had 39 children, who ranged from age 5 to 31 years. Parents described relationships with their children in generally positive terms, and no differences were noted among gay, lesbian, and heterosexual parents in this regard. Most gay and lesbian parents did not report that their sexual identities had created special problems for their children. Heterosexual parents were more likely to report that their children's visits with the other parent presented problems.

One long-standing cultural stereotype about gay fathers suggests that they may be more likely than other parents to sexually abuse their children. In contrast to the stereotype, however, most sexual abuse can be characterized as heterosexual in nature, with an adult male abusing a young female (Jones and McFarlane 1980). Available evidence shows that gay men are no more likely than heterosexual men to commit child sexual abuse (Groth and Birnbaum 1978; Jenny et al. 1994; Sarafino 1979).

For example, Jenny et al. (1994) found that of all children seen for sexual abuse during 1 year at a large urban hospital, only 2 of 269 (1%) of adult offenders could be identified as gay or lesbian. Of the 219 sexually abused girls, one attack (0.4%) was attributed to a lesbian woman; of the 50 sexually abused boys, one attack (2%) was attributed to a gay man. In contrast, 77% of abuse against girls and 74% of abuse against boys were committed by the adult male heterosexual partner of a family member (e.g., a mother, foster mother, or grandmother). No evidence was noted for the belief that gay men are more likely than other men to perpetrate sexual abuse against children.

Bozett (1980, 1987, 1989) has provided much of what is known about the peer relations of the children of gay fathers. On the basis of interviews with adolescent and young adult offspring of gay fathers, Bozett concluded that, although children affirmed their fathers in parental roles and generally considered their relationships with gay fathers as positive ones, they nevertheless expressed some concerns. Primary among these was that, if their fathers' sexual identities were widely known, then the children too might be seen as nonheterosexual. For instance, one teenager said, "I don't tell anyone else because I'm afraid that they'll think I'm gay" (Bozett 1989, p. 227).

To avoid problems, children reported using various strategies. These include selective disclosure of the sexual identities of their father, nondisclosure, and what Bozett termed "boundary control," in which children attempted to limit the expressions of gay identity by their fathers. Some gay fathers were reported to have accommodated to the requests of children in this regard by putting away gay publications during the visits of children's friends or by avoiding expressions of affection for a gay partner when in the company of their adolescent or adult children. Bozett suggested that these kinds of negotiations were affected by the age of the child, by the nature of the father-child relationship, by the perceived visibility of the sexual orientation of the father, and by other factors. Systematic research on the ways in which children of gay fathers cope with the potentially stigmatizing nature of their fathers' orientation could make important contributions toward the understanding of children's coping with prejudice as well as toward the understanding of ways that sexual orientation affects family dynamics.

Overall, research on children of gay fathers, although still sparse, has produced some important information. Contrary to popular stereotypes, little evidence exists to suggest that children of gay fathers are any more likely to encounter difficulties in the development of their own sexual identities, to be the victims of sexual abuse, or to be placed at any significant disadvantage relative to otherwise similar children of heterosexual fathers. Although children of gay fathers do appear to encounter some special challenges (e.g., in learning how to cope with potentially stigmatizing information about the sexual orientations of their fathers), every indication is that most children surmount these without undue difficulty. Probably the most important finding in the literature on children of gay fathers is that, despite the undoubted prejudice and discrimination against their fathers, children nevertheless described relationships with their gay fathers as generally warm and supportive.

Directions for Additional Research

As the preceding discussion makes clear, most research on gay fathers and their families is of relatively recent vintage, and researchers have many important questions still to address. In considering the substantive issues for future research on gay fathers, it is useful to distinguish between normative questions and individual differences questions. Normative questions concern the central tendencies of a population, whereas individual differences questions concern differences among members of a population. In this context, these include questions about gay fathers as a group and also about diversity among gay fathers.

One important task for research is to provide normative information about parenting behaviors of gay fathers with infants, children, adolescents, and adult children. As contemporary research on heterosexual families attests (Lamb 1981, 1986), relationships with fathers are significant aspects of the family environment of the child, yet little is known about the qualities of relationships of children with their gay fathers or about how these may compare to the relationships of children with heterosexual fathers. Is there any correlation between the sexual orientation of their fathers and their involvement in parenting or style of parenting? And what effects might such differences, if any, have on children's development?

Another direction for research is to identify patterns of family organization and family climate that may be characteristic of families with gay fathers. Are there ways in which families with gay fathers differ from families with heterosexual or lesbian parents and, if so, what are they? In studies of lesbian, gay, and heterosexual couples without children, Kurdek (1995) has reported that many issues for couples depend more on the length of time that a couple has been together than on the gender or sexual orientation of partners. Similar research on couples with children has not, however, been reported. Recent studies have suggested that gay and lesbian couples are more likely than heterosexual couples to divide the labor involved in child care evenly between the partners (Hand 1991; McPherson 1993; Patterson 1995b); what impact, if any, does this egalitarian tendency have on the overall family climate in gay, lesbian, and heterosexual families?

A third direction for research involves exploration of interfaces between families with gay fathers and major educational, religious, and cultural institutions with which they have contact. What are the most common issues and concerns for families with gay fathers in their contacts with settings such as their children's school or the work environment of the parents, and how are they usually addressed? Are the family issues of gay fathers the same or different compared with those of families with lesbian mothers or of members of other stigmatized minorities such as ethnic or religious minorities?

Research also should examine in a normative spirit the issues of subgroups of gay fathers. For example, following the work of Bozett (1980, 1981a, 1981b) and Miller (1979), researchers could examine the normative life trajectories of nonresidential gay fathers after divorce, examining the challenges and stresses of such life transitions and of noncustodial parenting. In the same vein, one might examine the issues of gay stepfathers over time, comparing them with those of both heterosexual stepfathers and lesbian stepmothers.

From an individual difference perspective, a central concern is to identify and examine factors that add to or detract from the quality of life in families with gay fathers. For instance, with the use of different levels of analysis, family, community, and cultural factors could be examined for evidence of their impact on the well-being of individual gay fathers as well as that of their family members. Drawing on results of research with families with heterosexual parents (e.g., Lewis et al. 1981), one would expect psychologically healthy men, living in supportive families and communities in a favorable cultural milieu, to cope in more favorable ways with the challenges of life in families with gay fathers. The relative importance of various levels of analysis is, however, far from clear, and there is much research still to be done in this area.

In addition, issues of contemporary relevance to gay communities should be examined as these may influence the experience of life in families with gay fathers. Prejudice and discrimination against gay men and lesbians are important factors that must be considered. Another is the special health concerns faced by gay men, especially the long illnesses and premature deaths attributable to human immunodeficiency virus (HIV) disease (Paul et al. 1995). Families with gay fathers, more often than families with heterosexual parents, may be faced with caretaking responsibilities for family members and friends who are ill and with grieving the loss of loved ones to a stigmatized illness. How do these special challenges, and the environments in which they occur, affect the experiences of those who live in families with gay fathers?

Families with gay fathers and lesbian mothers also provide an opportunity to assess the long-assumed significance both of gender and of sexual orientation in parenting. Comparisons of the dynamics of gay father and lesbian mother families could prove as interesting as comparisons of gay and heterosexual parents. The results of such work should clarify the adequacy of fundamental assumptions about the significance of gender and sexual orientation in parenting that have long been taken for granted but rarely if ever subjected to rigorous test. The results of this process should provide a better understanding of gay father families and a better understanding of families and parenting in general.

From a methodological perspective, the authors also can offer suggestions for research. The first of these concerns sampling methods. Existing research has tended to involve small, unsystematic samples of unknown representativeness. Larger, more representative samples of individuals and families would be helpful. In addition, longitudinal research with observational and other varied assessment procedures would be valuable. Multisite studies that systematically assess the impact of environmental and personal and familial processes hold great promise. Except in the case of qualitative work, rigorous statistical procedures should be used. Methodological improvements of these kinds would increase the likelihood that future research has a major impact on knowledge in this area (Patterson 1995a).

Summary and Overview

Social science research on gay fathers is a relatively recent phenomenon. Because the research has arisen in the context of widespread prejudice against members of sexual minorities, much research has been concerned to evaluate negative stereotypes about families with gay fathers. Although a great deal in this regard remains to be done, the results of existing research fail to provide evidence for any of the prevailing stereotypes about gay fathers or about their children. On the basis of existing research, no reason exists for concern about the development of children living in the custody of gay fathers; on the contrary, there is every reason to believe that gay fathers are as likely as heterosexual fathers to provide home environments in which children grow and flourish. Additional research is, however, needed.

As researchers seek to expand the evidence relevant to traditional stereotypes, it will also be important to begin to examine individual differences among gay fathers and among their children. In this regard, it will be important for researchers to remember that, despite widespread prejudice, many gay fathers and many of their children are competent, well-functioning members of society. Now that research has begun to address negative assumptions embodied in psychological theory and popular opinion, researchers are in a position to examine personal, social, community, and cultural factors that affect the quality of life for gay father families. Much important work remains to be done in order to understand the structure and functioning of gay father families.

References

Bailey JM: Biological perspectives on sexual orientation, in Lesbian, Gay and Bisexual Identities Over the Lifespan: Psychological Perspectives. Edited by D'Augelli AR, Patterson CJ. New York, Oxford University Press, 1995

Bailey JM, Bobrow D, Wolfe M, et al: Sexual orientation of adult sons of gay fathers. Developmental Psychology 31:124–129, 1995

Baptiste DA: Psychotherapy with gay/lesbian couples and their children in "stepfamilies": a challenge for marriage and family therapists, in Integrated Identity for Gay Men and Lesbians: Psychotherapeutic Approaches for Emotional Well-Being. Edited by Coleman E. New York, Harrington Park Press, 1987, pp 223–238

Barret RL, Robinson BE: Gay fathers. Lexington, MA, Lexington Books, 1990

Barret RL, Robinson BE: Gay dads, in Redefining Families: Implications for Children's Development. Edited by Gottfried AE, Gottfried AW. New York, Plenum, 1994, pp 157–170

Baumrind D: Child care practices anteceding three patterns of preschool behavior. Genet Psychol Monogr 75:43–88, 1967

Baumrind D, Black AE: Socialization practices associated with dimensions of competence in preschool boys and girls. Child Dev 38:291–327, 1967

Bell AP, Weinberg MS: Homosexualities: A Study of Diversity Among Men and Women. New York, Simon and Schuster, 1978

Bigner JJ, Bozett FW: Parenting by gay fathers, in Homosexuality and Family Relations. Edited by Bozett FW, Sussman MB. New York, Harrington Park Press, 1990

Bigner JJ, Jacobsen RB: The value of children to gay and heterosexual fathers, in Homosexuality and the Family. Edited by Bozett FW. New York, Harrington Park Press, 1989a, pp 163–172

Bigner JJ, Jacobsen RB: Parenting behaviors of homosexual and heterosexual fathers, in Homosexuality and the Family. Edited by Bozett FW. New York, Harrington Park Press, 1989b, pp 173–186

Bigner JJ, Jacobsen RB: Adult responses to child behavior and attitudes toward fathering: gay and nongay fathers. J Homosex 23:99–112, 1992

Bozett FW: Gay fathers: How and why they disclose their homosexuality to their children. Family Relations 29:173–179, 1980

Bozett FW: Gay fathers: evolution of the gay father identity. Am J Orthopsychiatry 51:552–559, 1981a

Bozett FW: Gay fathers: identity conflict resolution through integrative sanctioning. Alternative Lifestyles 4:90–107, 1981b

Bozett FW: Heterogeneous couples in heterosexual marriages: gay men and straight women. Journal of Marital and Family Therapy 8:81–89, 1982

Bozett FW: Children of gay fathers, in Gay and Lesbian Parents. Edited by Bozett FW. New York, Praeger, 1987, pp 39–57

Bozett FW: Gay fathers: a review of the literature, in Homosexuality and the Family. Edited by Bozett FW. New York, Harrington Park Press, 1989, pp 137–162

Bryant AS, Demian: Relationship characteristics of American gay and lesbian couples: findings from a national survey, in Social Services for Gay and Lesbian Couples. Edited by Kurdek LA. New York, Haworth, 1994, pp 101–117

Buxton AP: The Other Side of the Closet: The Coming Out Crisis for Straight Spouses and Families, 2nd Edition. New York, Wiley, 1994

Campbell K: A Gay Father's Quiet Battle. Washington Blade, November 18, 1994, p 5

Cowan CP, Cowan PA: When Partners Become Parents: The Big Life Change for Couples. New York, Basic Books, 1992

Crosbie-Burnett M, Helmbrecht L: A descriptive empirical study of gay male stepfamilies. Family Relations 42:256–262, 1993

Dunne EJ: Helping gay fathers come out to their children. J Homosex 13:213–222, 1987

Editors of the Harvard Law Review: Sexual Orientation and the Law. Cambridge, MA, Harvard University Press, 1990

Fadiman A: The double closet: how two gay fathers deal with their children and ex-wives. Life May:76–78, 82–84, 86, 92, 96, 100, 1983

Flaks D: Gay and lesbian families: judicial assumptions, scientific realities. William and Mary Bill of Rights Journal 3:345–372, 1994

Gagnon JH, Laumann EO, Michael RT, et al: The Social Organization of Sexuality. Chicago, IL, University of Chicago Press, 1994

Gottman JS: Children of lesbian and gay parents, in Homosexuality and Family Relations. Edited by Bozett FW, Sussman MB. New York, Harrington Park Press, 1990

Green GD, Bozett FW: Lesbian mothers and gay fathers, in Homosexuality: Research Implications for Public Policy. Edited by Gonsiorek JC, Weinrich JD. Thousand Oaks, CA, Sage, 1991

Groth AN, Birnbaum HJ: Adult sexual orientation and attraction to underage persons. Arch Sex Behav 7:175–181, 1978

Hand SI: The lesbian parenting couple (unpublished doctoral dissertation). The Professional School of Psychology, San Francisco, CA, 1991

Harris MB, Turner PH: Gay and lesbian parents. J Homosex 12:101–113, 1985/86

Hays D, Samuels A: Heterosexual women's perceptions of their marriages to bisexual or homosexual men, in Homosexuality and the Family. Edited by Bozett FW. New York, Harrington Park Press, 1989, pp 81–100

In re W.S.D., No. A-308-90 (D.C. Superior Court Family Division, April 30, 1992)

Jenny C, Roesler TA, Poyer KL: Are children at risk for sexual abuse by homosexuals? Pediatrics 94:41–44, 1994

Jones BM, McFarlane K (eds): Sexual Abuse of Children: Selected Readings. Washington, DC, National Center on Child Abuse and Neglect, 1980

Kinsey AC, Pomeroy WB, Martin CE: Sexual Behavior in the Human Male. Philadelphia, PA, WB Saunders, 1948

Kurdek LA: Lesbian and gay couples, in Lesbian, Gay and Bisexual Identities Over the Lifespan: Psychological Perspectives. Edited by D'Augelli AR, Patterson, CJ. New York, Oxford University Press, 1995, pp 243–261

Lamb ME (ed): The Role of the Father in Child Development, 2nd Edition. New York, Wiley, 1981

Lamb ME (ed): The Father's Role: Cross-cultural Perspectives. Hillsdale, NJ, Lawrence Erlbaum Associates, 1986

Lewis M, Feiring C, Weinraub M: The father as a member of the child's social network, in The Role of the Father in Child Development, 2nd Edition. Edited by Lamb ME. New York, Wiley, 1981, pp 259–294

Martin A: The Lesbian and Gay Parenting Handbook. New York, HarperCollins, 1993

McPherson D: Gay parenting couples: parenting arrangements, arrangement satisfaction, and relationship satisfaction. Unpublished doctoral dissertation, Pacific Graduate School of Psychology, Palo Alto, CA, 1993

Miller B: Gay fathers and their children. Family Coordinator 28:544–552, 1979

Ortiz ET, Scott PS: Gay husbands and fathers: reasons for marriage among homosexual men. Journal of Gay and Lesbian Social Services 1:59–71, 1994

Osterweil DA: Correlates of relationship satisfaction in lesbian couples who are parenting their first child together (unpublished doctoral dissertation). California School of Professional Psychology, Berkeley/Alameda, 1991

Patterson CJ: Children of lesbian and gay parents. Child Dev 63:1025–1042, 1992

Patterson CJ: Lesbian and gay couples considering parenthood: an agenda for research, service, and advocacy. Journal of Gay and Lesbian Social Services 1:33–55, 1994a

Patterson CJ: Lesbian and gay families. Current Directions in Psychological Science 3:62–64, 1994b

Patterson CJ: Lesbian mothers, gay fathers, and their children, in Lesbian, Gay and Bisexual Identities Over the Lifespan: Psychological Perspectives. Edited by D'Augelli AR, Patterson CJ. New York, Oxford University Press, 1995a, pp 262–290

Patterson CJ: Families of the lesbian baby boom: parents' division of labor and children's adjustment. Developmental Psychology 31:115–123, 1995b

Patterson CJ: Adoption of minor children by lesbian and gay adults: a social science perspective. Duke Journal of Gender Law and Policy 2:191–205, 1995c

Patterson CJ: Lesbian and gay parenthood, in Handbook of Parenting, Vol 3: Status and Social Conditions of Parenting. Edited by Bornstein MH. Hillsdale, NJ, Lawrence Erlbaum Associates 1995d

Paul JP, Hays RB, Coates TJ: The impact of the HIV epidemic on U.S. gay male communities, in Lesbian, Gay and Bisexual Identities Over the Lifespan: Psychological Perspectives. Edited by D'Augelli AR, Patterson CJ. New York, Oxford University Press, 1995, pp 347–397

Ricketts W: Lesbians and Gay Men as Foster Parents. Portland, ME, National Child Welfare Resource Center, University of Southern Maine, 1991

Ricketts W, Achtenberg R: Adoption and foster parenting for lesbians and gay men: creating new traditions in family, in Homosexuality and Family Relations. Edited by Bozett FW, Sussman MB. New York, Harrington Park Press, 1990, pp 83–118

Ricks I: Fathers and son. Advocate 674:27–28, February 7, 1995

Rivera R: Sexual orientation and the law, in Homosexuality: Research Implications for Public Policy. Edited by Gonsiorek JC, Weinrich JD. Newbury Park, CA, Sage, 1993, pp 81–100

Robinson BE, Barret RL: Gay fathers, in The Developing Father: Emerging Roles in Contemporary Society. Edited by Robinson BE, Barret RL. New York, Guilford Press, 1986, pp 145–168

Robinson BE, Skeen P: Sex-role orientation of gay fathers versus gay nonfathers. Percept Mot Skills 55:1055–1059, 1982

Roe v. Roe, 324 S.E. 2d 691, 228 Va. 722 (1985)

Saghir MT, Robins E: Male and female homosexuality: a comprehensive investigation. Baltimore, MD, Williams and Wilkins, 1973

Sarafino EP: An estimate of nationwide incidence of sexual offenses against children. Child Welfare 58:127–134, 1979

Sbordone AJ: Gay Men Choosing Fatherhood (unpublished doctoral dissertation). Department of Psychology, City University of New York, 1993

Seligmann J: Variations on a theme: gay and lesbian couples. Newsweek (Special Issue on the 21st Century Family), 1990, pp 38–39

Skeen P, Robinson B: Gay fathers' and gay nonfathers' relationships with their parents. J Sex Res 21:86–91, 1985

Strader SC: Non-custodial gay fathers: considering the issues. Paper presented at the annual meeting of the American Psychological Association, Toronto, August 1993

Thompson RA: The father's case in child custody disputes: the contributions of psychological research, in Fatherhood and Family Policy. Edited by Lamb ME, Sagi A. Hillsdale, NJ, Lawrence Erlbaum Associates, 1983

Van Gelder L: A lesbian family revisited. Ms. March/April:44–47, 1991

SECTION V

Finding Support and Achieving Growth

Psychotherapy With Gay Men, Lesbians, and Bisexuals

23

Psychotherapy With Women Who Love Women

Kristine L. Falco, Psy.D.

W omen who love women make up such a diverse group that describing them is a most challenging task. This diversity also makes the formulation of a systematic psycho-therapeutic format difficult to develop. Women who have romantic or erotic love for another woman may or may not identify with this aspect of their existence. They may or may not call themselves lesbian or bisexual. They may or may not be aware of a lesbian subculture. They may or may not feel any need to let their love be known to others. They may be wealthy or poor, may be politically active or not, may be edu-cated or not, may have careers in any field, may have children or not, may have been married or not, may be able-bodied or disabled, may or may not have mental illnesses, and may be of any race and religion.

These diverse characteristics must be taken into consideration in any psychotherapeutic approach to the treatment of women who love women; such factors are woven into the fabric of each woman's charac-ter, style, capacities, and beliefs. In spite of these sundry traits, some useful generalities can be stated about women who romantically or erotically love a woman, regardless of how much they identify with this aspect of themselves, and about the manner in which a psychotherapist can view treatment with these women. Whether or not they define themselves as lesbian or bisexual, a large percentage of women who love women experience similar identifiable stressors that warrant attention in a psychotherapeutic setting. As a group, they may also possess certain assets that can be utilized as therapeutic strengths.

Furthermore, the manifestation of mental illnesses or other forms of distress that may bring a woman to the therapist's office may be influenced by her lesbian status, that is, by her ability to love women, and the degree to which her psychological identity is invested in this ability. Thus, diagnostic entities and other states resulting from psychological pain may present themselves in somewhat different forms in a lesbian or bisexual patient than in a patient who is heterosexual.

Because there is as yet no systematic formulation for providing psychotherapy to women who love women, therapists must instead rely on a broad knowledge of the interpersonal and intrapersonal dynamics that are implicit in being a woman who intimately loves another woman. This knowledge is then woven into the fabric of therapeutic assessment and treatment planning.

Some Generalities

A woman's identification with the fact that she is capable of loving another woman is quite variable in degree. Some women, for example, have no question that their feelings for other women are clearly recognizable as lesbian feelings, and such women can take on a strong, internalized, positive lesbian identity. Still other women see their love for a woman as simply a special exception, and do not consider themselves to be lesbian at all. For others, the idea of lesbianism has been inculcated with such cultural negativity that they either do not accept the label of lesbianism, or they may live their lives outwardly as heterosexual while having sexual affairs with women on the side, often accompanied by much confusion and shame. Numerous permutations of these varying degrees of lesbian identity exist. The term "women who love women" is meant to encompass this entire gamut.

Many times, there is no clear congruency between how a woman experiences her sexual behavior, her emotional drives, her affectional interests, and her internally defined identity. This state of incongruence is often a matter for therapeutic examination; such examination must focus on the effects and personal meanings of the inconsistencies, rather than working toward an expected goal of complete congruence. Some women do not find the congruence necessary, while others may consider it an important personal goal.

Thus, a most important part of psychotherapy with women who love women is the investigation of the degree to which the patient identifies with her ability to love women, and whether or not she considers herself a lesbian. Again, a specific goal is not as important as the process of understanding the personal meanings and effects of such matters as identity and labels. The therapeutic process will be tailored to fit the woman's identity, whether she calls herself a lesbian, a bisexual, asexual, or a heterosexual in a special relationship, or eschews labels altogether, which in turn will influence directions taken in treatment planning.

When lesbian issues are a part of the therapeutic venue, a more direct or educational approach is often called for than many therapists are used to providing. This more active role may be called for especially during inquiry about the meaning and effects of the patient's homosexuality and when ascertaining the degree to which homosexuality will be a *focus* for therapy versus the *context* of the therapy. Either way, homosexual feelings can never be ignored in the therapeutic process.

A significant number of lesbians will, consciously or unconsciously, minimize many of the difficulties of their lesbianism, reporting simply, "I'm used to it." If the therapist were to inquire no further after such a statement, important therapeutic material could be missed that might reveal patterns of psychological coping, interpersonal dynamics, the effects of the hiding of the self, and internalized homophobia. Of course, there is indeed such a thing as really being "used to it" that signals a true integration and a working through of the losses and choices involved in loving another woman, which the therapist can help ascertain. An active inquiry and investigation, then, can augment the assessment and treatment planning process, as well as assist in the evaluation process of the stressors and assets that are particular to each patient.

The knowledge required of the therapist in order to provide services to this population is substantial. Factors such as common stressors and assets, lesbians' use of mental health services, diagnostic manifestations, and treatment planning are discussed here. To provide sound psychotherapy to this population, the therapist must have in addition a thorough familiarity with the process of lesbian identity formation (see Chapter 14 by Cass in this volume). Also, familiarity with the literature on the psychology of women provides an important background for delivery of lesbian positive psychotherapy.

Common Stressors and Assets

Following is a description of some of the stressors and strengths that may be common to lesbians and bisexual women as a group. Each consideration may not apply to every individual, but warrants evaluation in treatment to determine applicability. These become important aspects of any in-depth treatment plan.

▓ Disclosure Choices Are Continual

The process of "coming out," or identifying oneself as lesbian or bisexual, does not happen just once; rather, it is a lifelong process (Stein and Cohen 1986). Additional decision points will continually present themselves throughout the patient's lifetime. Always there will be more decisions to make about how much to tell and to whom, as the people in the patient's life come and go over the years and as internal identity shifts. Every day can present new opportunities for serious rejection or reprisal in the lesbian's life.

Although the research literature suggests that greater disclosure is associated with better psychological health (Bell and Weinberg 1978; Gartrell 1984; Greene 1977), patients must make very individualized decisions about their disclosure level. Such choices are best made in light of considerations of personality style, needs for privacy or for openness, the personal costs of either hiding or disclosing, and the impact of potential responses from others. Character structures and defense mechanisms that relate to the patient's need for safety and the strength of her need for acceptance or approval are of importance here. The therapist can assist this continual decision process.

Nondisclosure Generalizes to Other Areas

Most women who love women make complex and inconsistent choices about revealing their lover's gender, and very few reveal this information to everyone; certain people in the patient's life are simply never informed, regardless of the reason. Whether or not these decisions are considered to be well made, the psychological phenomenon of nondisclosure generalizes to other psychological areas of the patient's life. The act of nondisclosure requires self-censoring, carefully chosen words, and vigilance. A rigidity can ensue that generalizes to many other areas of life, particularly in interpersonal relationships.

When the self is thus constricted, self-esteem often deteriorates, for the psyche tends to interpret *hidden aspects* of the self as *bad* aspects. Therapists can help evaluate the impact of this generalization and can encourage the patient to develop positive antidotes in her life to counter these negative effects.

Lack of Support

The absence of social support for a woman's ability to love another woman is deeply pervasive and has effects on both the conscious and subconscious mind; sometimes these effects are minor, other times they can be quite extreme. Negative cultural attitudes about lesbianism, as well as deeply ingrained, internalized negative attitudes about lesbianism, can cause profound psychological suffering. This invisibility and insinuated (and sometimes overt) degradation have kept countless women in denial of their own true self-expression and identity, have caused countless suicides and aborted relationships, have ravaged self-esteem, have kept many women in unhappy marriages, and have kept many women in pain and hiding, from the world and from themselves. The therapeutic atmosphere can help correct the negativity that a patient may have experienced throughout her lifetime.

If troubles arise in a lesbian partnership or in the process of lesbian identity formation, many women feel they have few people they can turn to who will understand the depth of their tumult. Indeed, many fear that their pain will be mocked by being told that they deserve their turmoil for having "chosen" such a lifestyle. This fear is especially likely to occur for women who do not possess a lesbian identity or who have little contact with a lesbian community. Further, women who love women are often thought by their friends and relatives to be in waiting for the "right man" to come along. This attitude devalues the reality of the patient's feelings toward women.

When evaluating these aspects of the patient's life, the therapist can encourage involvement in positive social alliances to counter any negative effects of otherwise poor social support. Therapeutic strengthening of the ability to withstand being different, especially being different in a way that is so scorned in most cultures, can also be provided.

■ Absence of Role Models and Cultural History

The need for symbols, imagery, myths, traditions, and other nonrational aspects of life is associated with a great void for women who love women. In schooling, in television, in history, in the arts, in printed sources, and in everyday culture, the absence of lesbian references is resounding, and quite consequential. Lesbian poets, writers, politicians, musicians, inventors, scientists, or artists are rarely mentioned, although there are many. Each lesbian therefore faces the task of finding her way through disbelief in her own feelings in the cultural context. Many women who love women experience this journey with great fright and self-doubt, particularly those women who are just coming out or who have not yet found a satisfactory resolution to their lesbian identity.

The therapist can assist the patient in finding lesbian culture, lesbian literature, and lesbian social events. Finding individual models is also very helpful, which may make a case for lesbian therapists to disclose their lesbianism in some cases to patients (see Chapter 30 by Cabaj in this volume).

■ Internalized Homophobia

Women who love women often operate under the negative messages transmitted from the social context to an internalized context, despite personal acceptance of their capacity to love women. Some lesbians and bisexual women believe that heterosexuality is superior to homosexuality. Many wish they did not love women, and go to great lengths to hide their love from themselves or from others, causing much psychological distortion. Some patients search for the "reason" they have homosexual feelings, usually looking for a negative event, as if homosexuality is a process of heterosexuality gone awry.

Still other expressions of internalized homophobia (Margolies et al. 1987) include a fear of telling others, feeling superior to heterosexuals (instead of inferior), discomfort in the company of other gay or bisexual people, belief that lesbians are no different from heterosexual women, uneasiness with the idea of children being raised in a lesbian home, having very short relationships, or restricting involvements to women who are unavailable. Recent data on gay men, which may be extrapolated to women who love women, indicate that internalized homophobia is a distinctive and measurable factor that can account for important intrapsychic and developmental events (Shidlo 1994). The data suggest that an internalized negativism toward homosexuality is associated with overall psychological distress, depression, somatic symptoms, low self-esteem, loneliness, and distrust. These expressions of internalized homophobia may not be obvious, so the therapist needs to be alert to subtle evidence of their presence.

■ Identity Development

The recognition of the ability to love women and the accomplishment of a lesbian identity are complex and often lengthy psychological processes. The process can be seen as a developmental progression through stages (see Chapter 14 by Cass in this volume; Cass 1979) or from the perspective of an interactionist model (Gramick 1984; Ponse 1978).

A stage model describes the psychological movement from an initial glimmer of recognition of attraction to women, through stages of doubt and concern, to eventually finding a positive stance to take within oneself, along with the development of a community of support and an intrapsychic system for managing emergent identity issues. Such models rarely apply exactly to an individual woman, and suggest an endpoint or goal to be reached for satisfactory completion of the developmental identity process, which may be a false notion. Nevertheless, it can be useful in both the assessment and treatment of a lesbian patient for a therapist to view identity formation as a series of stages through which the patient will navigate; the stage theory can also be used as a guide for mapping therapeutic interventions (Falco 1991).

Interactionist models, on the other hand, describe a nonlinear trajectory of events that can happen in any order, and that will lead to adoption of a congruent identity. Such events include recognizing one's feelings toward women, accepting the significance of these feelings, creating a sexual-emotional relationship, and creating a community.

Whichever system a therapist finds more useful to use as a template with which to conceptualize a patient's identity development, it is most important to appreciate that there may be no completely satisfactory way for a woman to integrate all the diverse aspects of her identity (Elliott 1985). Resolving identity to the mutual satisfaction of society and the individual is probably not possible, as long as lesbianism is rejected by the larger society. Seeking a "good enough" match may be a reasonable therapeutic goal.

Further, it is important to distinguish between lesbian *erotic interests*, lesbian *sexual behavior, emotional attachments* to women, and a lesbian *identity*. These four factors may not be in complete agreement with each other, which will create some inner dissonance. Again, identity formation is a developmental process that is highly individualized. All of these characteristics can also be fluid rather than fixed, with changes small or large happening over the life span. The therapist can help measure the varied aspects of this process, helping the patient to make choices that match her attributes of style, character structure, and needs, and to be able to live well with inevitable incongruences.

■ Androgyny and Ego Strength

Lesbians as a group show a greater tendency than do heterosexual women to possess both feminine and masculine traits (Riddle and Sang 1978; Vance and Green 1984). This is true in behavioral realms (doing both so-called masculine and feminine chores around the home) and in psychological realms (having masculine traits such as being agentic, active, and independent, and feminine traits such as being nurturing and interactive). Possession of both masculine and feminine traits is usually considered to be associated with better psychological health than is possession of a preponderance of one or the other (Falco 1991).

In order to recognize their love for women, lesbians and bisexual women have to take a psychological step outside of standard social and ego norms. The capacity to find a definition for oneself that is beyond any of the models presented by one's culture, and that is not associated with negative stereotypes, calls for a certain degree of ego strength to be present. Further, ego strength may be augmented in the process of this self-definition. Thus, lesbians as a group may have some psychological advantages over heterosexual women as a group. These gender role and ego strength aspects can be evaluated in therapy, and these strengths can be utilized and amplified.

■ Female Socialization and Its Impact on Relationships

Although all women differ in the degree to which they adopt prescribed female gender roles, and in the degree of female biological traits that are present, the manifestation of these roles and traits cannot help but have some influence on the interpersonal dynamics of a two-female relationship. For example, because of both biology and socialization, each of the women in a couple may be sexually unaggressive and may value feelings of love and affection over sex (Blumstein and Schwartz 1983; Loulan 1990). Also, both women may subscribe to an "ethic of care" and have more permeable psychological boundaries (Chodorow 1978; Gilligan 1982), which may affect the dynamics of merger and separation–individuation in the relationship (see Chapter 20 by Klinger in this volume).

These attributes can be either assets or liabilities in a relationship, suggesting the need for an evaluative process that the therapist can expedite. Probably, healthier relationships are those in which the members can move comfortably back and forth between psychological merger and psychological individuation (Elise 1986; Lindenbaum 1985), and this flexibility may be the therapeutic goal.

Use of Mental Health Services

In 1987, The National Institute of Mental Health (NIMH) published the results of a mental health survey of approximately 2,000 women who identified themselves as lesbian, perhaps the most extensive survey of its type to date. One of the striking features of the survey is that nearly three-fourths (73%) of the subjects had received some form of counseling or mental health services. Some of the reasons for seeking counseling were as follows (percentages overlap): sadness or depression, 50%; problems with lover, 44%; problems with family, 34%; anxiety or fears,

31%; personal growth, 30%; being gay, 21%; loneliness, 23%; alcohol or drug problems, 16%; problems at the job, 11% (NIMH 1987).

Among this sample, half of the subjects had been in counseling for less than 1 year, 18% for 1 to 2 years, 11% for 2 to 3 years, 7% for 3 to 4 years, and 14% for more than 4 years. This survey indicates that lesbians are very heavy users of mental health services. This fact would once have been seen as an indication of lesbians' poor mental health, but can now be seen as evidence of the toll taken by living in an unaccepting environment, and of many lesbians' commitment to optimizing their lives.

The lesbians in the survey reported symptoms that are similar to symptoms seen in other high-stress groups, such as physicians. Twenty-seven percent of the lesbians surveyed had considered suicide at some time, and 18% had tried to kill themselves. The suicide risk is the highest during adolescence. Many subjects reported experiencing discrimination, being verbally attacked, and losing jobs because of their lesbianism. It is clear that the stresses produced by the lack of acceptance of lesbianism in the world can contribute to mental health deterioration in some individuals.

Other factors were the same among this lesbian sample as among heterosexual women, such as the rates of physical abuse, rape, and childhood molestation. These results confirm that lesbianism is not associated with abusive experiences with men. Eating disorders and alcoholism were also reported with the same frequency as is seen in heterosexual women.

Diagnostics

Describing the effects of lesbianism on mental health diagnostics is a speculative endeavor, for very few studies have been done on this topic. Nevertheless, this is an important consideration, and one that the therapist may be faced with repeatedly during assessment and treatment planning.

It is useful to ask if the ability to love women is a central issue to the therapeutic goals, or provides instead just the backdrop for therapeutic investigation. It is important also to assess whether lesbianism or bisexuality could be exacerbating or attenuating the diagnostic signs presented. At a time when a woman is just coming to terms with the meaning and ramifications of her homosexuality, she is at most risk either for deterioration of her mental health or for misdiagnosis.

Beyond the lesbian mental health survey noted above, a few clinicians and researchers have provided description and theory about the demographics of mental health disorders among lesbians (Gonsiorek 1982; Rothblum 1989; Smith 1988). Among the disorders first evident in childhood and adolescence, it may be speculated that a young lesbian who is experiencing discomfort over her "differentness" may show signs of conduct disorder, avoidant disorder, anxiety, or attention deficit disorder. Also, various reactive states could occur during adolescence, arising from internalized homophobia and manifesting with symptoms such as tics, stuttering, and identity disorder (some young lesbians think that their ability to love women is evidence that they must want to be a man). Defenses such as denial and reaction formation may also be likely.

Frequently, psychological surveys, such as those mentioned above, have suggested that affective disorders are more common among lesbians than nonlesbians, but recent quantifiable research does not bear this out. Rothblum (1989) proposes that although the rates of depression are the same, the mitigating factors may be different for the two groups. For example, Rothblum notes that known risk factors for depression in heterosexual women include marriage, raising young children, and lack of employment outside the home. For most lesbians, the presence of these risk factors is less common. Nevertheless, lesbians may more often be exposed to the risk factors that are derived from lack of social support, self-concealment, and discrimination on the job and elsewhere.

Regarding bipolar disorders, again there is no difference in frequency between homosexual and heterosexual women (NIMH 1987; Rothblum 1989). However, misdiagnosis is occasionally possible in cases where a patient in a sexual identity crisis, or coming-out crisis, responds with mood swings, hyperactivity, and impulsive behaviors reminiscent of hypomania. Resolution of the sexual-affectional issue may alleviate symptoms and can help clarify the diagnosis.

The borderline and narcissistic disorders may be overdiagnosed among lesbian patients. This is partly due to traditional (Caprio 1954), now disproved, notions that lesbians are too self-involved and suffer from an unstable identity, two hallmarks of these personality disorders. A sexual identity crisis may precipitate a period of poorly made judgments about differentiations and boundaries. Further, the sense of invisibility and need for deception that many lesbians experience can produce incongruent body cues, trouble establishing intimacy, psychological rigidity, anxiety, and anger (Zevy and Cavallero 1987), which could be interpreted as signs of narcissistic or borderline disorders, but again the symptom picture and diagnosis will be clearer when the crisis has abated.

The social withdrawal that many lesbians use as a survival tool (especially early in the coming-out process) can be misdiagnosed as avoidant or schizoid personality disorder. Also, a brief period of acting-out behaviors that are unconsciously motivated to accomplish needed visibility can be misdiagnosed as passive-aggressive traits, conduct disorder, or oppositional disorder.

Temporarily deferring diagnosis for lesbian and bisexual women clients can increase accuracy of assessment and treatment planning. The need to hide and the internalized negative opinion of oneself are the forces behind many signs and symptoms. Only if the signs and symptoms persist after resolution of the identity crisis is the diagnosis clear.

Most other mental disorders are probably seen with the same frequency in lesbian and bisexual women as in heterosexual women. These include psychotic disorders, anxiety disorders, somatoform and dissociative disorders, sexual disorders, factitious and impulse control disorders, adjustment disorders, sleep disorders, personality disorders, and most substance abuse disorders. Recent studies (NIMH 1987) contradict the findings of previous research on the frequency of alcoholism; earlier studies sometimes showed an increased frequency of alcoholism among lesbians as compared to heterosexual women, but more recent studies show that this increased frequency is limited to lesbians who are over 55 years of age. Further, the NIMH study speculates that these findings do not represent a tendency for lesbians to drink more alcohol as they age, but the findings instead indicate a cohort phenomenon. Lesbians who are now over the age of 55 were often coming out during a time in history when taverns and bars were the only places available to them to meet other lesbians, which provided an atmosphere conducive to drinking.

Assessment and Treatment Planning

A lesbian-affirmative psychotherapy, regardless of the school of psychotherapeutic thought it is based on, should contain the following key themes in assessment and treatment (Garnets et al. 1991):

◆ The understanding that homosexuality is not a sign of developmental arrest or psychopathology, and that women who love women can live fulfilling lives.

◆ Appreciation of the multiple ways that societal prejudice and discrimination can create problems that lesbians may seek to address in therapy.

◆ Understanding that sexual orientation is just one of many important attributes that characterize the patient, and that an evaluation must be made as to whether the patient's sexual orientation forms a relevant backdrop to the therapy or whether it is integral to the foreground of the patient's therapeutic goals.

◆ Perception of the synergistic effects of multiple social statuses experienced by ethnic minority lesbians, lesbians with disabilities, and bisexual women.

◆ An ability to help patients overcome negative attitudes about homosexuality, both overt and covert.

The therapist's preferred style of psychotherapy probably makes little difference; effective lesbian-affirmative therapy can be based upon a dynamic, cognitive-behavioral, humanistic-existential, Jungian, Gestalt, systems theory, and perhaps any other approach. Each modality warrants its own modifications to incorporate the implications of lesbianism in both its theory and its application.

In developing a treatment plan, all of the stressors and strengths previously mentioned should be evaluated and interwoven with assessment of the intrapsychic and interpersonal deficits and strengths of the individual patient. This presents a most challenging therapeutic task.

Furthermore, a woman's navigation of the personal meanings that she places on her homosexuality will frequently result in some substantial strengths and resolutions, despite the difficulty that many women experience in accomplishing a positive lesbian identity. Many women who love women may remain in a somewhat foreclosed state of psychological growth as a result of extreme difficulties with differentiation from external pressures, or internalizing those pressures, but most of them instead move toward more integration, more ability to withstand cultural disapproval, more self-definition, and more comfort with the choices made about levels of disclosure and development of support systems. These goals are perhaps the heart of the treatment plan; they help establish which therapeutic interventions are to be provided to the patient, and in what developmental order.

A treatment plan from almost any therapeutic approach is likely to include appraisal of the following: the patient's style of expressiveness, degree of contact with inner life, relationship status and quality, expression of psychological boundaries, press for needs (conscious and unconscious), repertoire of coping mechanisms, flexibility, authenticity, a consistent set of values, and perception of self and the world. Additional factors often assessed may be particularly emphasized because of the way they can interface with lesbianism, including character style, "stage" of identity formation, signs and symptoms, degree and type of internalized homophobia, and generalization of constrictions. By covering all of these components the therapist can be assured of providing a fairly thorough assessment that will lead to development of an appropriate treatment plan.

In summary, to fully tailor the therapy to meet the needs of the lesbian or bisexual woman patient, the therapist initially can make the usual assessment of clinical syndromes, personality traits, and the patient's approach to the world. Then each of these features can be reviewed to examine how the effects of a culturally stigmatized identity might influence or exaggerate these signs.

An examination of the effects of internalized homophobia is also often called for. Therapist and patient may check for unresolved doubts the patient harbors about the healthiness of her homosexuality, what stresses she encounters because of her love, and what her beliefs are about lesbianism. This material may be very sensitive or even unrecognized by the patient, and requires careful approach.

A search for unconscious processes that may be affected by lesbianism is also warranted. This calls for evaluation of the degree of disclosure the patient embraces regarding her love for a woman, and the pros and cons of these choices. It also calls for analysis of ways in which nondisclosure and constriction may generalize to other aspects of the patient's life. Noting that there may be no perfect solution to these matters, the therapist can help the patient come to terms with the best choices for her own life.

Assessment may also include discovery of particular strengths the patient may have developed as part of her ability to love women. These could include self-definition skills, interdependence skills, stamina, a strong set of values, and ego strength.

Finally, whether or not the patient identifies as a lesbian, it may be useful to distinguish for her among lesbian erotic interests, lesbian sexual behavior, and love for women. These factors need not completely correlate, but awareness of them can contribute to stabilization of identity or increased comfort with a fluid identity. Also, these factors should be evaluated for the potential to interface with the patient's personality traits or her approach to her world.

References

Bell AP, Weinberg MS: Homosexualities: A Study of Diversity Among Men and Women. New York, Touchstone, 1978

Blumstein P, Schwartz P: American Couples. New York, William Morrow, 1983

Cass V: Homosexual identity formation: a theoretical model. J Homosex 4:219–235, 1979

Caprio F: Female Homosexuality: A Modern Study of Lesbianism. New York, Grove, 1954

Chodorow N: The Reproduction of Mothering. Berkeley, CA, University of California Press, 1978

Elise D: Lesbian couples: the implications of sex differences in separation–individuation. Psychotherapy 23:305–310, 1986

Elliott PE: Theory and research on lesbian identity formation. International Women's Studies 8:64–71, 1985

Falco KL: Psychotherapy with Lesbian Clients. New York, Brunner/Mazel, 1991

Garnets L, Hancock K, Cochran S, et al: Issues in psychotherapy with lesbians and gay men: a survey of psychologists. Am Psychol 46:964–972, 1991

Gartrell N: Combating homophobia in the psychotherapy of lesbians. Women and Therapy 3:13–29, 1984

Gilligan C: In a Different Voice. Cambridge, MA, Harvard University Press, 1982

Gonsiorek JC: The use of diagnostic concepts in working with gay and lesbian populations, in Homosexuality and Psychotherapy: A Practitioner's Handbook of Affirmative Models. Edited by Gonsiorek JC. New York, Haworth, 1982, pp 5–7

Gramick J: Developing a lesbian identity, in Women-Identified Women. Edited by Darty T, Potter S. Palo Alto, CA, Mayfield, 1984, pp 13–44

Greene DM: Women loving women: an exploration into feelings and life experiences. Dissertation Abstracts International 37:3608, 1977

Lindenbaum JP: The shattering of an illusion: the problem of competition in lesbian relationships. Feminist Studies 11:85–103, 1985

Loulan J: The Lesbian Erotic Dance. San Francisco, CA, Spinsters, 1990

Margolies L, Becker M, Jackson-Brewer K: Internalized homophobia: identifying and treating the oppressor within, in Lesbian Psychologies. Edited by Boston Lesbian Psychologies Collective. Urbana, IL, University of Illinois Press, 1987, pp 229–241

National Institute of Mental Health: National Lesbian Health Care Survey (Contract No. 86MO19832201D). Washington, DC, DHHS Publication, 1987

Ponse B: Identities in the Lesbian World. Westport, CT, Greenwood, 1978

Riddle DI, Sang B: Psychotherapy with lesbians. Social Issues 34:84–100, 1978

Rothblum ED: Depression Among Lesbians: An Invisible and Unresearched Phenomenon. Paper presented at the annual convention of the American Psychological Association, New Orleans, LA. August 1989

Shidlo A: Internalized homophobia: conceptual and empirical issues in measurement, in Lesbian and Gay Psychology. Edited by Greene B, Herek G. Thousand Oaks, CA, Sage, 1994, pp 176–205

Smith J: Psychopathology, homosexuality, and homophobia. J Homosex 15:9–73, 1988

Stein TS, Cohen CJ: Contemporary Perspectives in Psychotherapy with Gay Men and Lesbians. New York, Plenum, 1986

Vance BK, Green V: Lesbian identities: an examination of sexual behavior and sex role attribution as related to age of initial same-sex sexual encounter. Psychology of Women Quarterly 8:293–307, 1984

Zevy L, Cavallero SA: Invisibility, fantasy, and intimacy: Princess Charming is not a prince, in Lesbian Psychologies. Edited by Boston Lesbian Psychologies Collective. Urbana, IL, University of Illinois Press, 1987, pp 83–94

24

Psychotherapy With Gay Men

Terry S. Stein, M.D.
Robert P. Cabaj, M.D.

A large number of volumes on the topic of psychotherapy with gay men, as well as lesbians, became available in the 1980s and 1990s (Coleman 1987a; Cornett 1993; D'Augelli and Patterson 1995; Gonsiorek 1982; Hetrick and Stein 1984; Isay 1989; Ross 1988; Silverstein 1991; Stein and Cohen 1986). Recognizing that this literature represents the thinking of a maturing group of clinicians and researchers who present a growing sense of confidence in and knowledge about their subject, Charles Silverstein (1991) designated the 1980s as the historical period of "The Third Generation" of therapists who are gay.

Until the 1970s virtually all writing about psychotherapy with gay and bisexual men assumed that homosexuality was pathological and described attempts to change the sexual orientation of these men. In contrast, the literature cited above is written from the perspective of a gay-affirmative psychotherapy, described by Malyon (1982a) in the following manner:

> This theoretical disposition regards homosexuality as a nonpathological human potential. The goals of gay-affirmative psychotherapy are similar to those of most traditional approaches to psychological treatment and include both conflict resolution and self-actualization. (p. 62)

Most gay men enter psychotherapy with the same types of problems as the general population. In addition, sometimes they seek help with problems specifically related to their being gay. Regardless of the presenting problem, however, the gay man will most often discuss issues that in some way relate to his homosexuality. In some instances, concerns about being gay may be in the foreground; in others, a depiction of being gay provides background information, or part of the setting or context for the discussion of some other problem. For example, presentation with a specific mental disorder, like a mood or an anxiety disorder, or with an interpersonal problem in a relationship or at work may or may not involve concerns about being gay, but talking about these problems will generally include discussion of some aspects of being gay, such as availability of a gay community or support system, level of development and disclosure of one's gay identity, and presence or absence of a committed relationship. Therefore, when evaluating the meaning of a gay-related topic for a gay man in therapy, the therapist should neither define it as a problem simply because it has become a part of the content of therapy nor ignore the possibility that the patient has some concern about being gay of which he is unaware or which he is unable to raise directly.

Often gay men and lesbians are presented together in discussions about psychotherapy and homosexuality; bisexuals of both sexes are frequently ignored. In this chapter, the particular issues for gay men in psychotherapy are described. Chapter 23 by Falco in this volume offers an elaboration of the topic of psychotherapy with lesbians, and Chapter 25 by Matteson provides a discussion of psychotherapy with bisexuals. While these groups share similar sexual orientations and are subject to related types of oppression and discrimination, differences in their experiences are so profound that it is appropriate to describe approaches to psychotherapy with them in separate texts. This chapter is divided into the following sections: the effects of gender and development on psychotherapy with gay and bisexual men; the role of acceptance and acknowledgment in the conduct of psychotherapy; and special issues in psychotherapy with gay and bisexual men.

The Effects of Development on Gay Men

The biological sex and gender identity of gay men, like heterosexual men, are male; the gender role of some gay men is less stereotypically masculine than that of many heterosexual men; and the sexual orientation of gay men, unlike heterosexual men, generally involves a greater degree of attraction for other men than for women (Herron et al. 1993). Thus, the central differences in sexual identity development experienced by gay and bisexual men in contrast to heterosexual men derive from the effects of their sexual orientation and, for some, their gender, or social-sex, role.

Self-awareness of a homosexual sexual orientation, which does not generally occur until adolescence, may be preceded by a sense of difference in some pregay boys (Isay 1989; Troiden 1988). In a society that promotes and supports heterosexuality, the sense of difference in these boys, even if it is not yet labeled as homosexuality, may be alienating, leading to reactions such as social isolation and denial. For those boys who are also effeminate or less masculine, profound deficits in self-esteem and in other aspects of the personality may result from being shunned, humiliated, and derided by their peers (see Chapter 15 by Hanson and Hartmann in this volume).

Malyon (1982a) has eloquently described how pregay boys internalize "the mythology and opprobrium which characterize current social attitudes toward homosexuality" (p. 60), which results in an internalized homophobia that shapes the ego through both unconscious negative introjects and conscious derogatory attitudes and beliefs about homosexuality and the self. Malyon (1982b) further describes a biphasic development for gay men that results from the vicissitudes of such socialization, consisting of a first phase with incomplete identity formation and ego development due to the need to adapt to cultural expectations to be heterosexual during childhood and adolescence, and followed by a second phase in which identity formation can be completed in conjunction with "coming out" as a gay man. Chapter 14 by Cass in this volume describes various points at which identity formation foreclosure may occur.

For the pregay boy, the complex processes of physical, psychological, and social development during childhood and adolescence are thus further complicated by the countervailing forces of internalized homophobia, pressuring the boy to reject an essential and integrative aspect of his identity. If the effects of internalized homophobia are also compounded by incidents of overt discrimination or violence in response to the boy's differences, the personality may be severely damaged, leading to serious impairment in the capacity for psychological, social, and work adaptation.

Gay men's true sexual orientation can remain hidden, unclear, or unknown throughout childhood, and for some, until well into adulthood. Although there is a greater tendency for an adult gay sexual orientation in a boy with gender nonconforming behavior (Bell et al. 1981), sexual orientation itself may not be obvious or apparent during childhood. Given the heterosexist views of our society, the vast majority of parents raise their children either assuming they will be heterosexual, or not thinking about their sexual orientation at all. Such nonconfirming behavior and parental expectations may tend to enhance the feelings of difference, of standing apart, reported by many gay men in their childhood, and add to their confusion about their identity.

Although the pregay boy and his parents may not have words to describe their impressions and perceptions, they may react to the subtle differences that result from having affectional and sexual needs that are different. As Isay (1989) notes, the fathers of such boys may pull back or treat these boys differently; and mothers may react the same way, or, in some instances, may give their sons extra attention and concern, trying to make up for their fathers' distance. The latter pattern suggests an alternative explanation for the traditional psychoanalytic description of the distant father and close-binding mother (Bieber et al. 1962) in the development of the prehomosexual boy. Commonly, however, as observed in the authors' clinical experiences, gay men as children learn to disconnect and dissociate from their true selves and sexual orientation and adapt to parental expectations by creating and presenting a false self or behaviors that are not genuine reflections of the true self.

As is true for all children, pregay boys want the love and acceptance of their parents and other caregivers. If their parents cannot respond to or give support for what is unfamiliar or uncomfortable for them—the awareness of difference in their son in this case—they will either ignore those attributes of the child that suggest difference or try to change them. This process of ignoring may be quite subtle, a process of neglect similar to that described by the Swiss psychoanalyst Alice Miller in her early works (1981, 1984). Miller's description of parents who form, and deform, the emotional lives of their talented or different children may have strong parallels with the development of some gay children. Parental reactions help to shape and validate the expression of the needs and longings of their children, and parents more frequently reward what is familiar and acceptable to them and tend to discourage or deemphasize behavior and needs they do not value or understand.

Some boys who will grow up to be gay may require or desire a closer and more intimate relationship with their fathers, which is generally not encouraged in our society. As a result, these boys may hide their needs and longings, again putting on a false front and creating a false sense of self. Dissociation and denial may become major defenses in the personality structures of these children. Through this process, some gay men learn early that their feelings and needs are not acceptable and must be hidden and suppressed.

The psychological effects of being different and being discriminated against, and the adaptation necessary to live in a society that does not readily accept difference (de Monteflores 1986), profoundly shape the sexual identity development of many boys who will be gay when they emerge from childhood. When parents and others recognize and affirm a "false self" in these children, such children may massively suppress their more natural feelings. In addition, these children are unlikely to have clear and positive role models of gay adults available to them—for example, the sexual orientation and relationship status of gay and lesbian teachers are rarely revealed, and there is little positive media attention given to gay men and lesbians. In latency, children who recognize sexual attraction for other children or adults of the same sex, especially boys who may also be effeminate, usually begin to fear other children, to feel even more different, and to become socially isolated. In adolescence, their sexual feelings emerge with greater urgency, but there is rarely any context or permission for their expression. Adolescents in particular often reject and isolate those who are different and encourage conformity, which further supports denial and suppression of the emerging gay feelings. As a result, the adolescent who is gay may even further split off any awareness of affect and behavior related to his homosexuality (Martin 1982).

When adolescents who have disconnected themselves from any awareness of their homosexual feelings begin to recognize the source of their sense of difference, their sexual attraction to boys and men, they may work even harder to suppress these feelings by isolating themselves and avoiding situations that may stir up their longings. Some of these youth may devote extraordinary energy to academic or career success to cover up for their underlying shame and sense of being defective; others may become depressed, isolated, guarded, and lonely, expecting to be rejected and ignored if their true feelings are revealed (Hetrick and Martin 1987). Often they become ashamed not only of their sexual feelings, but also of their bodies, their social interactions, and other aspects of the self.

Although not all gay men have the same degree of difficulty traversing childhood and integrating a sexual identity that is generally stigmatized into a healthy personality structure, most of them will show some residual signs of this difficult developmental pathway. In addition to the developmental tasks required of all children as they go through childhood and adolescence, gay men have also had to deal with the effects of internalized homophobia, the coming-out process, and the impact of gender role socialization and sexual orientation on their capacity for intimacy with other men and with women. Some gay men will need to process the effects of direct victimization as children resulting from discrimination and physical violence. Most gay men must come to terms with a profound sense of difference. While a supportive family and social environment may mitigate the negative effects of these factors for some gay men, none of them will have escaped entirely the consequences of these stigmatizing forces and events.

Wide-ranging sociocultural factors will also significantly shape the experiences and expectations of gay men who seek psychotherapy. These factors include an increase in public awareness about homosexuality; the development of a visible gay culture during the past three decades; the growth in antigay and lesbian violence; the appearance of AIDS during the 1980s; and the generational effect of growing up today, in contrast to growing up before 1950, in the 1950s, the 1960s, the 1970s, or the 1980s. These differences between age cohorts of gay men must be considered in the mental health evaluation and treatment of gay men and are discussed further in this chapter.

Role of Acceptance and Acknowledgment

Because of the developmental patterns described above and the resulting internalized homophobia, the need for explicit acceptance and acknowledgment of their homosexuality can be expected to be a major factor in psychotherapy with many gay men—acceptance by the patient of his own sexual orientation and acceptance by others, including the therapist. Similarly, because of their need for acceptance and acknowledgment for themselves as they truly are, many gay men may also be extremely sensitive to signs of rejection or ridicule. The manner in which gay men who have achieved some degree of self-acceptance present themselves or express their sexual feelings to others may have been significantly shaped by an expectation of being ignored, rejected, or ridiculed. Such gay men will face the same fears about negative reactions when they seek help from medical or mental health providers, regardless of the sexual orientation of the provider (see Chapter 30 by Cabaj).

During the initial evaluation and treatment planning stage, the powerful impact on gay men of being straightforwardly acknowledged and accepted by the therapist cannot be overestimated, even when concerns about being gay are not part of the presenting problem. For example, directly asking a gay man if the adjustment to his sexual orientation was difficult will not suggest that the therapist sees homosexuality as pathological or problematic, but rather, that homosexuality is something that can be openly discussed. Such inquiry can create an empathetic frame that lets the patient know he is free to talk about his sexual orientation if he wishes to do so and suggests that the psychotherapist can, if necessary, help provide a corrective experience to past parental avoidance or rejection.

The acceptance and acknowledgment that a therapist provides must be genuine and nonintrusive, and presented in a manner that allows the patient to discuss his own feelings about being gay. Unreflective and premature reassurances that being gay is perfectly all right and not a problem will not be helpful (Cabaj 1988); by not allowing full awareness and discussion of self-doubts and uncertainties, this stance may replicate the rejection by the patient of his own feelings and fears. Allowing an open presentation and exploration of the patient's feelings about his sexual orientation, and how he came to those feelings, will set the stage for an understanding and an acceptance based on the actual experiences of the patient. The following case example illustrates such a situation:

■ Case Example 1

Mr. A is a 42-year-old white gay man who entered therapy because of difficulties in making contact with other gay men. He clearly recognized that he was gay, but was fearful of almost any contact with men and, in his rare sexual encounters, was always impotent. He reported an extremely stressful experience when he was in the military: a peer reported to a commanding officer that Mr. A was gay. Mr. A was subsequently hospitalized on a psychiatric unit, interrogated, forced to name others who might be gay, and dishonorably discharged. After leaving the service, he became socially isolated, living in a set of rooms in his family's house. After avoiding all contact with any gay men or gay situations for nearly 5 years, he began to desire the company of other gay men. He was only aware of bars as possible gay social outlets, and he went to them with great anxiety, and would often panic when he was in one.

Mr. A said he had come to believe, especially after reading some articles about homosexuality, that it was all right to be gay, and now he wanted help with his difficulty socializing. The therapist accepted the patient's self-evaluation, did not point out possible signs of internalized homophobia, and said he was willing to work with Mr. A as the openly gay man that he saw himself to be.

During therapy, Mr. A recalled how he was in awe of, fascinated by, and excited by looking at military men who would visit with his father during World War II. He recalled that when he was 5, his father caught him staring at one of these men and told him never to look at a man like that again. This recollection led to an acknowledgment of his internalized homophobia, including a belief that he was defective or bad just for being gay. Eventually, Mr. A was not only able to go to gay bars comfortably, but also found additional gay social outlets, and had some successful sexual encounters with other men.

This case demonstrates the importance of initial acceptance by the therapist of the gay patient and his feelings at the level of his experience and makes the point that the therapist should not prematurely interpret a gay male patient's negative feelings as internalized homophobia (Malyon 1982a). The treatment in this case was able to move quickly because the patient was reassured by the fact that the therapist expressed acceptance of him as a gay man and did not reject his feelings. The patient's awareness of his own self-doubts and self-loathing emerged later, as a result of the supportive therapeutic frame.

Negative feelings about being gay can arise at any point in therapy, but especially, perhaps, when exploring past relationships and personal interactions, including those with parents. The patient may regress or retreat to a psychological stage when he felt that it was not all right to be gay and that he had to hide or try to change himself in order to be acceptable or to be loved (Cohen and Stein 1986). Rejections in current relationships or job or health setbacks may serve to precipitate such a reaction. The therapist must appreciate the psychodynamic basis for these reactions and not move too quickly to counter the expressions of resurgent internalized homophobia. In response to countertransference feelings originating from the therapist's own internalized homophobia, some gay therapists may feel the urge to disagree with the patient's negative feelings about being gay. Similarly, because of a wish to comfort a patient in distress, the heterosexual therapist might wish to reassure him prematurely that it is all right to be gay. The most helpful response at this point is usually to acknowledge that the patient is experiencing difficulty in accepting himself because he feels people who matter to him do not seem to accept him, and that, as a result, he may not feel it is all right to be open about his identity. In this way, the therapist can help the patient to work through the internalized homophobia at his own pace. It may also be helpful for the therapist to acknowledge directly previous advances made by the patient in understanding and overcoming his internalized homophobia.

Special Considerations in Psychotherapy With Gay Men

As mentioned previously, most gay men who seek services from mental health professionals do so for the same reasons anyone might: to obtain help for the full range of mental disorders or for adjusting to interpersonal, work, or other social situations. Sexual orientation may be incidental in treatment with some of these men. However, for other gay men, the primary concern will relate to acknowledging, accepting, or adjusting to their sexual orientation.

The risk for antigay and heterosexist bias in psychotherapy with gay men is high. One study (Committee on Lesbian and Gay Concerns 1990) identified 25 different ways in which bias can affect psychotherapy in association with assessment, intervention, identity, intimate relationships, and therapist expertise and education. The therapist should be informed about the detrimental effects of inappropriate and negative assumptions made about patients based on their sexual orientation.

There are some special issues in psychotherapy with gay men about which the therapist should be aware. Hancock (1995) identified six treatment issues for gay men and lesbians: coming out, antigay and other prejudice, relationship issues, the concerns of gay and lesbian youth, gay and lesbian parenting, and family of origin concerns. Stein (1993) also described problems involving sexuality and sexual dysfunction, concerns related to race, age, and other forms of diversity, and special health issues, including HIV infection and AIDS and alcohol and substance abuse. Finally, Cohen and Stein (1986) identified several themes in psychotherapy with lesbians and gay men, including the following:

1. Identity for the gay man or lesbian involves a fundamental experience of difference from the mainstream heterosexual culture.
2. Coming out is a process that occurs over time in a nonlinear fashion.
3. Any individual who struggles to develop a healthy gay or lesbian identity will experience both positive and negative feelings as part of this process.
4. A patient's internalized homophobia has meaning in itself but also frequently is expressed in association with other conflicts concerning such issues as intimacy, dependency, and aggression.
5. The sexuality of gay men and lesbians may be a difficult area to explore for both patient and therapist.

Many of the special issues and considerations relevant to psychotherapy with gay men are discussed in a number of other chapters in this volume. In this section, the following topics are explored in greater detail: assessment of sexual orientation and internalized homophobia, understanding lifestyles, the impact of gender, and the influence of diversity.

■ Assessment of Sexual Orientation and Internalized Homophobia

Careful and complete assessment of sexual orientation is an essential first step in psychotherapy with gay men. While many clinicians continue to view sexual orientation as being essentially dichotomous, either homosexual or heterosexual, with a small number of individuals being bisexual, a number of scales and models have been developed that allow a more in-depth and complex assessment of the various dimensions of sexual orientation (Kinsey et al. 1948; Shively and De-Cecco 1977; Klein et al. 1985; Coleman 1987b). Components of sexual orientation described in these models include sexual attraction, sexual behavior, sexual fantasies, emotional preference, social preference, self-identification, and lifestyle; for many men, these components may be quite variable at different points in their lives. For example, some men who report strong homosexual desire and behavior may have previously been in heterosexual marriages and participated exclusively in heterosexual sexual relations. Other men may be involved in same-sex sexual relationships but do not identify themselves as being gay, do not participate in a gay lifestyle, and have social preferences for interactions with women or heterosexuals. It is important to understand where each man locates himself on these several dimensions of sexual orientation.

There may be a tendency on the part of the therapist to assume that discrepancies between the various components of sexual orientation invariably represent a lack of full achievement of a gay identity or perhaps a way station on the path to complete consistency on all of the dimensions. However, individual variation is much greater than this, and development does not always follow a linear path to some theoretically ideal end point. Factors such as level of characterological and object relations development, past experiences, and available personal, community, and social resources will significantly influence the progression of individual men along any developmental pathway. It is not the role of the therapist to judge a patient's progress in coming out or acquiring a gay identity or to have some expectation that the patient will achieve a certain lifestyle or type of relationship; rather, the therapist should help the patient to achieve those outcomes that are most satisfying and adaptive given his particular desires and resources.

Assessment of the form, extent, and direct influence of internalized homophobia is also important in working with gay men in psychotherapy. Although there are no existing scales of internalized homophobia that have been applied to psychotherapy, evidence for the effects of negative views of self resulting from the internalization of society's antihomosexual and heterosexist beliefs and attitudes may be pervasive. Direct devaluation of homosexuality and gay people, refusal to participate in gay community activities, limitation of academic and career achievements, lack of success in intimate same-gender relationships, and a variety of psychiatric symptoms such as anxiety, depression, and self-destructive acting-out behaviors may all directly result from internalized homophobia. Identification of the particular sources and expressions of internalized homophobia in each man is essential if these factors are to be understood and overcome through work in psychotherapy. The following case illustrates the importance of careful understanding of both the dimensions of sexual orientation and the expressions of internalized homophobia:

■ Case Example 2

Mr. B, a 40-year-old gay man, presented for psychotherapy with complaints of episodic depression, consisting of apathy, social withdrawal, feelings of hopelessness, and a sense of loss of meaning in his life, over the past 3 years. Further exploration of his concerns revealed the belief that his work as a successful small business owner was a sign of his lack of success because he saw his work as stereotypically "gay." Even though he enjoyed his work, he felt that it was not worthwhile. He reported that he began his work after failing out of college and at a time when he was just coming out as a gay man. In talking about these feelings, he came to understand that he had connected his lack of success in college and then beginning his own business with his homosexuality and the negative reactions he experienced after disclosing that he was gay.

Mr. B's depression had begun shortly after the death of his closest friend, a heterosexual woman, from cancer. He missed this friend a great deal and was still grieving for her, and had few other women friends. Discussion of the meaning of this woman in his life and the nature of his friendships with both women and men helped him to work through this significant loss and to understand his personal preference for a lifestyle that includes emotional attachments with both men and women.

This patient had viewed his work through a lens of internalized negative feelings about being gay that had resulted in part from negative reactions of others to his homosexuality. Awareness of these feelings came about as the result of a depressive episode that involved components of his sexual orientation other than sexual desire or behavior, specifically, his emotional and social interactions with women. Exploration of the meanings associated with this aspect of his sexual orientation helped him to explore and work through his reactions to the death of his woman friend. When he ended therapy, he had achieved renewed esteem in relation to his work, had returned to college, and had improved social interactions within his friendship network.

■ Understanding Lifestyles

Although lifestyle was identified above as a component of sexual orientation, it should also be recognized as a significant independent factor in work in psychotherapy with gay men. "The gay lifestyle" is some-times employed as a term that is synonymous with being gay or lesbian; however, this use is inappropriate because it implies that there is a single lifestyle, or way of living, associated with being gay or lesbian. Reference to "the gay lifestyle" is often connected with many stereo-types that reflect societal images of contemporary urban gay men, in-cluding such characteristics as high frequency of sexual relationships, use of drugs and alcohol, going to gay bars, dressing in certain styles of clothing, inability to be in relationships, and absence of interactions with women and children. In fact, however, gay men are involved in a wide range of types of lifestyles, and it is essential for the therapist to understand and respect the particular lifestyle of the individual man who is in therapy.

Making assumptions about sexual, relationship, social, or other life-style patterns based solely upon the existence in a man of sexual desire for or behavior with other men or upon declaration of a gay identity is never helpful. Thoughtful inquiry about the various aspects of lifestyle will convey an understanding and respect for the autonomy and indi-viduality of each patient. While knowledge of gay communities and their practices can help inform the therapist about the experiences of his or her gay patients, this knowledge should never be used as a substitute for exploration of the particular work, relationship, recreational, and other preferences and patterns that constitute the lifestyle of a given patient. Premature assumptions about how a patient lives his life based upon stereotypes of gay men and their lifestyles, even when these stereo-types may be positively valued, will dehumanize and objectify the pa-tient and may serve to further isolate and dissociate him from any interior experience of validation or specialness in relation to being gay.

◾ Impact of Gender

The most basic difference between homosexuality and heterosexuality is the gender of the person for whom one feels erotic attraction and desire. The fact that male homosexuality involves sexual and romantic relationships between two men, who share a similar gender socializa-tion, serves to shape much of the quality of the interactions between the two men as well as many of the reactions by others and by the society in general to these relationships. Masculine and feminine gender at-tributes are largely defined in opposition to each other in Western society, and gender socialization is different for boys and girls (Gilligan 1982), creating different relational characteristics for men and women. In general, men express higher degrees of autonomy, separateness, competition, aggression, and other attributes associated with being masculine. While individual men, including gay men, may not behave in a stereotypically masculine fashion, on the average, men will possess these traits more than women and, as a result, two men in a relationship with each other can be expected to display a more masculine style of relating than two women or a man and a woman in a relationship (Forstein 1986).

The extent of masculinity and rigidity of gender role experienced by a gay man can influence his capacity for intimacy and the degree of separation and individuation he is capable of experiencing in relation to another man. Flexibility in expression of gender role characteristics in both partners may provide the best basis for a successful intimate relationship between two men; but some men may attempt to mimic traditional heterosexual gender role differentiation, with one partner portraying more feminine and the other more masculine characteristics. The absence of visible role models of vital and successful gay male couples contributes to the difficulty men have in learning how to relate intimately with each other. Because male socialization in our society involves being taught that anxiety and stigma are associated with sexual and emotional attachments between men, gay men not only have to overcome masculine characteristics that work against intimacy in general but also have to surmount explicit prohibitions on such relationships with other men. Psychotherapy with gay male couples is discussed in more depth in Chapter 28 by Cabaj and Klinger; however, problems in forming and maintaining satisfying relationships due to gender socialization constitute a significant area of concern for individual gay men presenting for psychotherapy, and the dynamics underlying these concerns must be understood by the therapist.

Another gender-related issue for some gay men in psychotherapy is dealing with past or present experiences of gender nonconformity. Concerns may involve the traumatic consequences of stigma or violence directed against them as children or adolescents because of gender nonconforming behavior or current anxiety about being perceived as less masculine or as effeminate as a result of being identified as gay. These concerns may be particularly prominent in the early stages of coming out when disclosing sexual orientation to others and may reflect an aspect of internalized homophobia that devalues male homosexuality by associating it with the feminine and then projects this attribution onto others. Incidents of verbal or physical harassment that involve, for example, calling a gender nonconforming boy a sissy or a girl and a gay man a faggot serve to teach and reinforce these derogatory associations between male homosexuality and femininity and constitute acts of verbal abuse against both gay men and women. The therapist must display sensitivity and neutrality in working with the gay male patient who is uncovering past experiences of abuse related to his gender role characteristics or who is exploring current associations between his gender role and gay identity. The confounding of gender role and sexual orientation in many psychoanalytic discussions of homosexuality (Friedman 1986) has further contributed to the confusion of many therapists working with gay men on issues of gender. Therapists who were taught about homosexuality from such biased theoretical perspectives may themselves further strengthen the stigma of both gender role and sexual orientation experienced by their gay male patients. The following case provides an example of how gender role issues may present during psychotherapy with a gay man:

■ Case Example 3

Mr. C, a 50-year-old gay man, entered psychotherapy because of preoccupation with concerns about aging and sexual performance. During the course of treatment he recalled numerous painful incidents of being teased and ridiculed at school as a child. Following recall of these incidents, he reported to the therapist that when he came out as a gay man he had cross-dressed as a woman and had performed as a drag queen. He felt shame and embarrassment when he told the therapist about these events, but gentle exploration of this period of his life led to the realization that his performance—his pretending to be a woman—had helped him to master his fear that he actually was a woman because he was gay and had enabled him to assume a more adaptive and comfortable gender role presentation as an adult.

If the therapist had sided with the patient's negative view of his gender experimentation as a young adult, the reparative aspect of this behavior would have remained hidden and the stigmatized association between his gender role and his sexual orientation would have once again been reinforced. The therapist who works with gay men must be able to hold judgments about gender and sexuality in abeyance, support the patient while together they explore the complex mosaic of gender identity, gender role, and sexual orientation that makes up his sexuality, and be available to provide a new and affirming perspective on the patient's efforts to heal an often wounded sexual identity.

■ The Influence of Diversity

The gay community, like other groups that are stigmatized and discriminated against in American society, is often portrayed as homogeneous, as though all gay individuals are the same. In reality, of course, gay men are as diverse a group as any other collection of individuals. Certain characteristics, such as race, age, and class, serve to define major subgroups of gay men, who may differ from each other as much as they differ from other groups in society. In some instances, for example, for gay men of color, these characteristics serve as the basis for dual identities that may be difficult to integrate. These men often suffer further discrimination both as members of racial groups within the gay community and as gay men within their communities of color. The therapist must appreciate how interwoven the experience of sexual orientation is with these other important characteristics that conjointly influence sexuality and identity. Descriptions of selected types of racial and ethnic diversity among gay men and lesbians are explored further in Chapter 33 by Jones and Hill; Chapter 34 by Nakajima, Chan, and Lee; Chapter 35 by Gonzalez; and Chapter 36 by Tafoya.

The era he grew up in, his age when he came out as a gay man, and the length of time since he came out will significantly affect a gay man's experience of being gay. Comparing a 50-year-old man who grew up in the 1940s, 1950s, and 1960s and came out when he was 20 years old with a man who grew up at the same time but did not come out until he was 45 years old will often demonstrate a vast difference in perceptions of reactions by others to their homosexuality and of their gay identities. Similarly, comparing those 50-year-old men with a 20-year-old man who has just come out will illustrate additional wide gaps in experience related to their sexual orientation.

Two primary factors determine these discrepancies: the differing social climates in relation to homosexuality at the times the men grew up, came out, and lived as gay men, and the interaction between general developmental maturation and ages of coming out and acquiring a gay identity. Each decade since the 1940s has brought a very different set of responses to homosexuality in American society, and the social structures and culture associated with being gay have considerably altered during the same period of time. While extreme negative attitudes have persisted throughout this time, in general, the visibility of homosexuality and the possibilities for acknowledgment and acceptance as a gay man have increased considerably. Thus, negative societal attitudes about homosexuality and gay people continue to produce internalized homophobia in gay men, but the pervasive psychological destructiveness of these attitudes has undoubtedly diminished during the past 50 years. The therapist working with gay men must understand the specific effects of familial, interpersonal, and broader social reactions to an individual man's homosexuality in order to appreciate the impact of these reactions on his development.

With respect to the interaction of general developmental progression with coming out and acquiring a gay identity, the overlap or discordance between levels of identity formation and ego development and of coming out as a gay man will reciprocally influence each other, consistent with the biphasic development of gay men described by Malyon (1982b). Thus, for example, the gay man who acknowledges his homosexuality and comes out as a teenager will have a different set of developmental tasks concerning establishing intimacy as a young adult than the man who comes out at age 45 and had previously either avoided intimate relationships or had adapted by creating a heterosexual persona. While both men may be dealing with the early stages of acquiring a gay identity, they will have gone through very different life courses. The need to consider such age-specific developmental factors highlights the diverse set of issues that must be dealt with in psychotherapy with gay men.

Summary

Several aspects of psychotherapy with gay men have been described in this chapter, including the effects of childhood and adolescent development involving experiences of difference and stigma; the important role of acknowledgment and acceptance in therapy with these men; and a variety of special considerations in therapy with gay men. Although gay men generally present with the same problems as other patients, they often enter psychotherapy with particular treatment issues related to their sexual orientation. In this chapter, the need to understand how to assess the dimensions of sexual orientation and internalized homophobia, to appreciate the variety of lifestyles associated with being gay, to explore the impact of gender, and to investigate the role of other forms of diversity in gay men's lives is discussed. The therapist who works with gay men must be aware of all of these factors if he or she is to work respectfully and helpfully with these men.

References

Bell AP, Weinberg MS, Hammersmith FK: Sexual Preference: Its Development in Men and Women. Bloomington, IN, Indiana University Press, 1981

Bieber I, Dain HJ, Dince PR, et al: Homosexuality: A Psychoanalytic Study. New York, Basic Books, 1962

Cabaj RP: Homosexuality and Neurosis: Considerations for Psychotherapy. Edited by Ross MW. New York, Haworth, 1988, pp 13–23

Cohen CJ, Stein TS: Reconceptualizing individual psychotherapy with gay men and lesbians, in Contemporary Perspectives on Psychotherapy With Lesbians and Gay Men. Edited by Stein TS, Cohen CC. New York, Plenum, 1986, pp 27–54

Coleman E (ed): Psychotherapy With Homosexual Men and Women: Integrated Identity Approaches for Clinical Practice. New York, Haworth, 1987a

Coleman E: Assessment of sexual orientation. J Homosex 14:9–24, 1987b

Committee on Lesbian and Gay Concerns: Bias in Psychotherapy with Lesbians and Gay Men. Washington, DC, American Psychological Association, 1990

Cornett C (ed): Affirmative Dynamic Psychotherapy with Gay Men. Northvale, NJ, Jason Aronson, 1993

D'Augelli AR, Patterson CJ (eds): Lesbian, Gay, and Bisexual Identities Over the Lifespan. New York, Oxford University Press, 1995

de Monteflores C: Notes on the management of difference, in Contemporary Perspectives on Psychotherapy with Lesbians and Gay Men. Edited by Stein TS, Cohen CJ. New York, Plenum, 1986, pp 73–101

Forstein M: Psychodynamic psychotherapy with gay male couples, in Contemporary Perspectives on Psychotherapy with Gay Men and Lesbians. Edited by Stein TS, Cohen CJ. New York, Plenum, 1986, pp 103–137

Friedman RM: The psychoanalytic model of male homosexuality: a historical and theoretical critique. Psychoanal Rev 73:483–519, 1986

Gilligan C: In a Different Voice. Cambridge, MA, Harvard University Press, 1982

Gonsiorek JC (ed): Homosexuality and Psychotherapy: A Practitioner's Handbook of Affirmative Models. New York, Haworth, 1982

Hancock KA: Psychotherapy with lesbians and gay men, in Lesbian, Gay, and Bisexual Identities Over the Lifespan. Edited by D'Augelli AR, Patterson CJ. New York, Oxford University Press, 1995, pp 398–432

Herron WG, Kinter T, Sollinger I, et al: Psychoanalytic psychotherapy for homosexual clients: New concepts, in Affirmative Dynamic Psychotherapy With Gay Men. Edited by Cornett C. Northvale, NJ, Jason Aronson, 1993, pp 1–22

Hetrick ES, Martin AD: Developmental issues and their resolution for gay and lesbian adolescents. J Homosex 14:25–44, 1987

Hetrick ES, Stein TS (eds): Innovations in Psychotherapy With Homosexuals. Washington, DC, American Psychiatric Association, 1984

Isay RA: Being Homosexual: Gay Men and Their Development. New York, Farrar, Straus, Giroux, 1989

Kinsey AC, Pomeroy WB, Martin CE: Sexual Behavior in the Human Male. Philadelphia, PA, WB Saunders, 1948

Klein F, Sepekoff B, Wolf TJ: Sexual orientation: a multi-variable dynamic process. J Homosex 11:35–49, 1985

Malyon AK: Psychotherapeutic implications of internalized homophobia in gay men. J Homosex 7(2/3):59–70, 1982a

Malyon AK: Biphasic aspects of homosexual identity formation. Psychotherapy: Theory, Research and Practice 19:335–340, 1982b

Martin AD: Learning to hide: the socialization of the gay adolescent. Adolesc Psychiatry 10:52–65, 1982

Miller A: The Drama of the Gifted Child. New York, Basic Books, 1981

Miller A: For Your Own Good: Hidden Cruelty in Child-rearing and the Roots of Violence. New York, Farrar, Straus, Giroux, 1984

Ross M (ed): Psychopathology and Psychotherapy in Homosexuality. New York, Haworth, 1988

Shively MG, DeCecco JP: Components of sexual identity. J Homosex 3:41–48, 1977

Silverstein C (ed): Gays, Lesbians, and Their Therapists. New York, WW Norton, 1991

Stein TS: Overview of new developments in understanding homosexuality, in Review of Psychiatry, Vol 12. Edited by Oldham JM, Riba MB, Tasman A. Washington, DC, American Psychiatric Press, 1993, pp 9–40

Stein T, Cohen C (eds): Contemporary Perspectives on Psychotherapy with Lesbians and Gay Men. New York, Plenum, 1986

Troiden RR: Gay and Lesbian Identity. Dix Hills, NY, General Hall, 1988

25

Psychotherapy With Bisexual Individuals

David R. Matteson, Ph.D.

Most people think of sexual orientations as falling into two discrete categories: heterosexual and homosexual. Although perceiving from opposite perspectives, both heterosexual and gay and lesbian persons are likely to view these two orientations as "them" and "us." However, for self-affirming bisexual individuals, the division of human experience into these two categories makes no sense.

Like lesbians and gay men, bisexual persons belong to an invisible minority. But because of their heterosexual interests, they can more easily "pass," or maintain a "public identity" that is heterosexual. How-

Portions of this chapter are adapted from 1) Matteson DR: "The Heterosexually Married Gay and Lesbian Parent," in *Gay and Lesbian Parents*. Edited by Bozett FW. New York, Praeger, 1987b, pp. 138–161. Reprinted with permission of Greenwood Publishing Group, Inc., Westport, CT. Copyright 1987. 2) Matteson DR: "Counseling With Bisexuals." *Individual Psychology* 51(2):144–159, 1995. Reprinted by permission of Sage Publications, Inc.

ever, if they do so they will feel some incongruity. It is harder for them to affirm the gay or lesbian part of their experience if they keep it "in the closet." Thus the bisexual person's sexual identity and lifestyle are likely to be a bit more complex than those of the lesbian or gay man.

For purposes of this chapter, *bisexual* includes those who desire sexual relations with some persons of both genders, whether or not they have yet had sexual experience with both. (For a more complete definition and data regarding incidence, see Chapter 10 by Fox.) Persons with bisexual fantasies or experiences who seek counseling are likely to have either or both of two issues related to their bisexuality: identity issues, having to do with the struggle to identify themselves in relation to their sexual interests; and "systems" issues, having to do with how to "manage" a bisexual lifestyle. Identity and systems issues intertwine in the daily lives of most clients, but for conceptual clarity, it is helpful to treat them separately.[1]

"Coming Out" to Oneself: Therapeutic Issues

Anyone sexually attracted to persons of his or her own gender must struggle with societal taboos against homosexuality. In addition, many bisexual individuals find themselves at odds with the taboo against extramarital sex or multiple relationships. The pressure to conform to the heterosexual expectations of one's parents and peers leads many bisexual individuals into heterosexual commitments before they have explored their sexuality sufficiently to recognize and affirm the gay or lesbian component of their sexual orientation. The formation of a gay, lesbian, or bisexual identity is a difficult process because these are stigmatized identities and because models for these identities are usually not visible in the home, or even in the broader society.

Typically, it takes longer for bisexual individuals to identify themselves than for lesbians or gay men (Rust 1993a; Weinberg et al. 1994). The delayed coming out of bisexual individuals may be attributable to our society's dichotomous thinking about sexuality—the assumption

---

[1] Much of the material in this chapter has been previously published in Matteson 1987a, 1987b, and 1995. A longer version of this chapter (Matteson, in press) is being published in Firestein (in press).

that one is *either* gay *or* straight—and to the lack of social support for bisexual identity, as well as to the inherent complexity of this orientation (Matteson 1987a; Rust 1993a; Weinberg et al. 1994).

■ Lack of Social Confirmation for Bisexual Experience

Certainly the difficulty is aggravated by what sociologists call "marginality," the anomalous social position of individuals who are unable to find any clear group membership role because of straddling conventional social categories or boundaries (Paul 1988). Once a person has begun to explore homosexual experience, he or she will likely encounter some gay men and lesbians who believe that labeling oneself "bisexual" is a way of denying one's true identity as completely homosexual. Certainly bisexuality does serve as a temporary identity for some men (D. R. Matteson, unpublished observations, 1995) and women (Rust 1993b), but this is true for only a minority of bisexual individuals. Rust (1993b) has provided empirical documentation of lesbians' biphobia—their frequently negative or skeptical attitudes toward bisexual individuals. This author believes that biphobia is equally present in the gay male community. The personal struggles gay men and lesbians have undergone in shaping their own identities are often simplified by polarizing sexual orientation and defining themselves at the homosexual end of the polarity. For those who experienced attraction only toward persons of their own gender, this polarization fits their own experience. Therefore, it is hard for them to validate persons whose inner experience says, "I'm both!"

Because of this lack of social validation, often the most important intervention a counselor can make is simply to acknowledge that some people do feel attracted to persons of both genders. Persons who are just beginning to face their bisexuality often enter counseling because of their confusion. They may not need intensive counseling; they may only need confirmation that it is okay to accept the self that they are discovering. Permission-giving is often the first step in work with the bisexual client—and often it is the only "therapy" needed (J. Gochros 1989; Lourea 1985). H. L. Gochros (1978) quoted a client who said:

> I knew what I wanted, but was afraid to get what I wanted. What I got from you [the counselor] was the guts to do what I wanted to do. You got me thinking again about myself and my own needs. (p. 8)

■ Overcoming Homophobia and Biphobia

Part of becoming a healthy and congruent person is overcoming the judgments and evaluations of others that are not consistent with our own experience but nonetheless have been internalized. Positive models are very important for developing a positive lesbian, gay, or bisexual identity. Thus for clients in these invisible minorities who are comfortable doing so, it is advantageous to be seen by an openly gay, lesbian, or bisexual counselor (see Chapter 3 by Cabaj; Matteson, in press).

However, affirmation from a heterosexual counselor can also be a powerful facilitator of self-acceptance and can be supplemented by involvement in other gay-affirmative experiences described below, such as coming-out groups, in which the client can get to know persons who are comfortable with their minority sexual orientation (Lourea 1985; Paul 1988).

■ Affirming Exploration

It is important to respect each person's sexual orientation without judging it against either heterosexual or gay or lesbian standards. It is not uncommon to hear counselors, in talking about a client in the process of coming out or who is having difficulty coming out, sound as if they know what the right result should be. The therapeutic task is not to assign the person to a category, but to help the individual explore his or her own experiences and discover what scripts are externally imposed and need to be overcome. The development of sexual identity is not unlike the development of other aspects of one's identity, and reading a good review of identity research may be more useful for a therapist than following any particular theoretical model (Marcia et al. 1993). In modern Western society, where a highly individualized identity is important, exploration of alternatives—including experimenting with new life experiences—is crucial. The counselor can play an important role in giving permission for the client to explore, in assessing and reducing the risks involved and in working through fears and inhibitions that unrealistically restrain a client. As in any other therapeutic work, it is important to move at a pace consistent with the client's inner and outer supports.

When material arises that is new to the counselor, there is no harm in admitting areas of ignorance. When working with persons of minority groups, counselors need to be honest about their own lack of knowledge and to be open to new learning. There are a number of variables having a powerful influence on the type of lifestyle that fits a particular bisexual. Assessing these may be clarifying for both the client and the counselor, and may prevent either from drawing premature conclusions about the personal commitments the client can make. These include the following:

1. The role of fantasy in the individual's life: Can life decisions be sorted out by fantasy alone, or is real-life experience needed? Some clients become comfortable with a monosexual lifestyle once they have accepted and affirmed their bisexual fantasies.
2. The level of personal and social risk-taking the client can handle: One needs to differentiate psychological risks from physical dangers, such as the real risks of AIDS or the high incidence of gay-bashing, and from social consequences, such as being fired from a job. Is the client prepared to deal with the issues that may emerge with changes in his or her behavior or self-label (Nichols 1988)?
3. How much the client links, or distinguishes between, sex and intimacy: How open is the client to recreational sex? How open is he or she to intimacy with each gender? How important are each of these aspects of relationships to the client?
4. The importance of gender in choice of partners: Does the client feel a need for concurrent partners of both genders (at one extreme)? Or is gender simply not an important determinant of partner choice (at the other extreme)?
5. The level of the client's tolerance for ambiguity about self and for complexity in social relationships: Tolerance for ambiguity and complexity is necessary for successfully handling concurrent multiple relationships.

■ Grief

The coming-out process often involves dealing with grief, as the person recognizes that models and dreams that he or she has honored in the past will no longer work for him or her. The heterosexual model is so much a part of our cultural lore and our family upbringing that its loss must be acknowledged and grieved. Grief may become a counterpoint to the excitement of the new discovery of oneself.

■ Monogamy

Some bisexual individuals experience attraction as unrelated to gender—as a "continuum of sexual choices" (Shuster 1987, p. 62). For many of these, monogamy remains a comfortable option and sometimes an explicit value (Matteson 1987b, 1991). However, the majority of bisexual individuals, when they describe their ideal sexual relationships, desire more than one partner. Eighty percent of bisexual individuals say that the experience of sex is different with men than with women (Weinberg et al. 1994). Women often report desiring a partner of each gender because each fulfills different emotional needs (Blumstein and Schwartz 1977; Nichols 1988). Men who strongly desire concurrent male and female partners typically do so out of sexual needs. The salience of gender in sexual arousal may be connected with visual versus kinesthetic styles (Matteson 1987b). Persons who desire concurrent male and female partners rarely experience their bisexuality as a choice—it is not a question of desiring either male or female partners, but of longing for both. As a male research respondent put it, "It feels like I have two different kinds of horny" (Matteson 1987b, p. 140).

The desire for multiple partners is not easy to fulfill. Those who do have two ongoing relationships generally believe that the second relationship enhances their primary relationship and takes some of the pressure off the primary partner (Weinberg et al. 1994). Nevertheless, only one-third of bisexual individuals in the Weinberg et al. (1994) sample believed they had actually achieved that ideal at some point in their lives, and typically it lasted only 6 months or less. Several studies (Fox 1993; Rust 1992; D. R. Matteson, unpublished observations, 1995) have found that less than 20% of bisexual individuals were engaged in partnerships with both men and women at the time of the studies. Fox (1995) has suggested that bisexual individuals are constrained in their sexual behavior by the dynamics of their current relationships. Thus even those who desire concurrent relationships may live with only one ongoing relationship at a time in order to stabilize that relationship, limiting themselves to occasional uncommitted sexual relationships with persons of the other gender. Though many bisexual individuals do succeed in developing long-lasting relationships, on average their relationships seem less stable than those of homosexual or heterosexual individuals, at least in part because their partners are unable to handle their nonmonogamy (Weinberg et al. 1994).

▮ Sexual Orientation and Other Identities

Gender. Several important generalizations can be made about male and female differences in bisexual experience and development—even given the incredible range of differences within each gender and the fact that there is more overlap than difference between genders.

Perhaps because males in this culture receive more encouragement to explore sexually, men seem to act upon the homosexual component of their desires earlier, on average, than do women (Coleman 1981–1982). Further, usually men are first aware of their sexual attractions through fantasy, and they enter the homosexual or bisexual subcultures because of their sexual attractions. In contrast, women's first awareness of attraction to other women is usually prompted by a relationship (Coleman 1981–82; Dixon 1985; Weinberg et al. 1994). For many women, fantasies have not existed prior to a specific relationship and pleasurable behavior (Dixon 1985; Nichols 1988). Women often "fall in love with someone of an unexpected gender, and the power of that relationship pulls them to re-evaluate their identity" (Shuster 1987, p. 61). Even when sexual attraction to both genders is recognized, women's sexual identity may remain fluid, being defined in terms of particular relationships or social settings (Rust 1993a). Fluidity in sexual orientation or identity appears to be less common for men, who base their identity more on sexual desire.

Issues for those previously identified as gay or lesbian. The illusion that bisexuality is usually a "way station" to avoid facing one's homosexuality is so strong in gay culture that men who have acknowledged their gay identity are surprised when they meet a woman they find sexually exciting. Similarly, women who have been lesbian-identified may have great difficulty accepting that they may in fact be bisexual. This experience may throw their hard-sought identity into question. It is also painful for clients to realize that the gay or lesbian community, which had been so affirming during their exploration of same-sex attraction, fails to support them in this next step in their self-discovery (Silver 1992). Women whose commitment to the lesbian community had been partly based on feminist politics often experience a sense of having betrayed their community. In addition, the return to dating men often involves a profound culture shock, along with skepticism about finding a male partner who will support a genuinely equal relationship (Nichols 1988).

The earlier process of careful, step-by-step decisions about to whom to disclose their homosexuality is set in motion again as they consider sharing their bisexual experience with gay and lesbian friends. In larger cities where bisexual communities are emerging, at least some exploration of participation in that community might be encouraged, although there is no reason for the client to assume he or she must abandon participation in the lesbian and gay communities.

■ Finding Support Networks

Experiences in which one's differences do not require explanation or justification and are not a focus of attention—normalizing experiences—are important factors in the development of a positive self-image. It is important to help clients find their way to places where they can meet others with common interests as well as common sexual orientations. A huge range of interest groups, clubs, and social activities exists in larger cities; most large metropolitan areas have one or two groups specifically for bisexual individuals, often including a group for bisexual and gay men who are married. The easiest way to locate these groups is by calling the local gay and lesbian switchboard or hotline, which is usually listed in the phone directory under "gay." Safe settings in which clients can speak out confidently and naturally about their experiences help to identify internalized inhibitions and to distinguish them from realistic fears. This increases the chances that the lesbian, gay, or bisexual person will be able to speak out undefensively and with self-assurance in "heterosexual settings," breaking the conspiracy of silence and invisibility that is destructive to individual esteem and to the community as a whole (Martin 1993).

■ Coming Out to Others Outside the Gay, Lesbian, or Bisexual Community

Heterosexual therapists are often unaware of the damage done when bisexual individuals, gay men, or lesbians constantly hide their sexual identity. Most closeted gay men, lesbians, and bisexual individuals develop defenses allowing them to believe that being closeted is ego-syntonic, although in fact it consumes considerable emotional energy. The counselor can assist the client in planning the process of coming out in small steps taken at times when the client is feeling positive about himself or herself; for example, it is preferable to come out at work or school when one is feeling occupationally or academically secure (Gartrell 1984) and to choose the time one is ready to disclose to family or friends, rather than to do so reactively. Role-playing with the client can be helpful, both to plan how to come out to a particular person and to learn responses to handle intrusive questions when one is not yet ready to disclose. Because most bisexual individuals live much of their daily lives in the heterosexual world, it is also very freeing if they can come out to some of their closest heterosexual friends. Suggestions for assessing with whom to come out, and how, can be found elsewhere (Borhek 1983; Hamilton 1977; Muchmore and Hansen 1982).

Among bisexual men, one of the final residues of internalized homophobia is the fear of emotional intimacy with other men, which may continue long after fear of sexual intimacy has been overcome. Again, a peer support group, such as a men's consciousness-raising group, can be helpful in dealing with this concern.[2]

■ Summary of Skills Needed in Dealing With Identity Issues of Bisexual Clients

The therapist must be able to validate the client's experience of attraction to both genders; deal with grief that may emerge with the loss of one's former self-image and as a result of possible rejection by former friends and family; help the client find information on bisexuality that is not biphobic and develop support networks to overcome internalized biphobia; and recognize that there is no particular "outcome" in terms of a lesbian, gay, heterosexual, or bisexual identity that is appropriate. Nor is there a particular lifestyle (for example, staying married, living monogamously, divorcing, joining the lesbian or gay community) that is generally appropriate. The task is to create a lifestyle that fits the individual's unique needs and that seems authentic to his or her self-definition (Nichols 1988, pp. 240–242).

---

[2] NOMAS (The National Organization of Men Against Sexism) may be helpful. Their national office address is 2914 North Ridge East, #315, Ashtabula, OH, 44004.

Social Aspects of Bisexuality:
Issues in Counseling

▣ Systems Theory and Involvement of "Significant Others"

The therapeutic model presented here is one that confirms the naturalness of living out the sexual orientation that one discovers as one's own. A systems approach is particularly useful in working with clients who are still crippled by internalized homophobia, because it makes concrete the perspective that the problem did not originate from "inside" the client. Homophobia is a social disease, and the best cure is a social one (Matteson 1987b). In addition, just as parents of a gay, lesbian, or bisexual youth may best communicate their acceptance by actions such as encouraging their daughter or son to bring home her or his lover to meet them, one way the counselor may communicate acceptance of their clients' sexual orientation is by suggesting they invite their lover to some therapy sessions, when that is appropriate to the work being done. The counselor's unwillingness to involve the partner or partners as part of the assessment, or for a few sessions as part of the primary client's work, may communicate to clients that their present heterosexual or homosexual relationships are not valued by the counselor. A careful assessment needs to be made that considers the larger system (including all significant partners) before a commitment to individual work is made. Relationship issues (discussed in Matteson 1987b) should not simply be sidestepped, as often occurs with counselors unfamiliar with systemic work. If after assessment individual work becomes the primary contract, individual boundaries need to be respected, of course. With some clients, shifting back and forth between individual and couple formats can diffuse the work. But these considerations only accentuate the importance of a systemic assessment before individual work is decided upon as the treatment of choice.

The special issues of couples in which both partners are men or both partners are women are described in Chapter 19 by McWhirter and Mattison and Chapter 20 by Klinger. The focus here is on the issues that occur when a bisexual is a partner in a committed relationship that precedes his or her acknowledgment of bisexuality and on the issues that emerge when there are multiple partners.

Committed relationships. In the context of heterosexual marriage, the honest acknowledgment of the gay or lesbian component of a bisexual client's sexual orientation will usually lead to significant changes in the marriage; however, if the marriage has been one based on common values and genuine intimacy, it is possible that once the emotional reactions to the disclosure of one's bisexuality are dealt with, the couple can work out new contracts and agreements that will allow the relationship to continue (Latham and White 1978; Matteson 1985). Similar changes may occur with committed gay or lesbian couples when one partner realizes she or he is bisexual. H. L. Gochros (1978) described several stages in counseling with these "mixed orientation couples." Following the permission-giving stage and the ensuing exploration of options during the decision-making stage, the individual or couple typically move to the problems associated with settling into a new lifestyle.

The values—and risks—of triangulation in a lifestyle with dual or multiple relationships need to be understood for effective counseling. Scarf's (1987) writing, though not directed toward mixed-orientation marriages, is especially clarifying concerning both destructive and constructive triangles. The dual relationships of bisexual individuals may appear from outside as "the best of both worlds"; from inside, they are more likely to be a difficult balancing act. Typically, those who can maintain this lifestyle are those who enjoy complexity, have developed some particular skills at gauging tolerance levels of their partners, and find different aspects of their personalities fulfilled by their different partners. A common mistake bisexual individuals make in the period of exploration of multiple partners is to become so engrossed in the "balancing act" of meeting their heterosexual needs, their homosexual needs, and the needs of each of their partners, that they forget to spend time alone, to get "centered" in themselves. They run from end to end of the teeter-totter, when what they need is to focus on the center fulcrum.

In some instances a triadic relationship, an open arrangement in which three persons live together, can become mutually satisfying and stable. There is no empirical or theoretical reason to believe that dyadic relationships are more stable or healthy than triadic ones (Bowen 1978), although they certainly receive more social support and may be less complex.

With most committed couples, even when the communication skills of both partners are superior, a shift to an open relationship is possible only if clear agreements are made that the couple relationship is to remain primary (Weinberg et al. 1994). When one relationship becomes primary, the bisexual member tends to resign or adapt himself or herself to secondary relationships to satisfy the need or wish for a partner or partners of the other gender. (Some strategies for doing so are described in Matteson, in press.) Handling multiple relationships in the context of a heterosexual marriage, including when and how to bring in the third person in the triangle, is discussed in Matteson (1987a, 1987b).

The issue of balance is a central one in bisexual lifestyles that involve multiple partners, and needs acknowledgment (Green and Clunis 1989). Often what brings bisexual individuals to a counselor is that the balance has somehow destabilized, either intrapsychically—for example, as a result of a reduction in fear of being seen as lesbian or gay—or systemically—for example, because of the addition of a new partner. It is crucial to be alert to the therapist's effect on the balance, both in terms of which partners are seen and of the effect of therapy on the meaning of a particular relationship. For example, for some married bisexual individuals, the extramarital relationships have a mystique and excitement that are stabilizing factors for the marriage itself. Therapy may take some of the mystique out of the relationship, and thus unbalance the marriage. It is usually wise to work first with the couple in the primary relationship, seeing them together, and then to see each partner individually (and possibly with that partner's other partners) as they struggle to find a new balance for themselves as individuals and as a couple (Green and Clunis 1989).

A key issue in work with mixed-orientation marriages is the handling of jealousy on the part of monogamous partners. It is helpful to remember that jealousy is rooted in a sense of insecurity or fear of losing a relationship. The focus of counseling work concerning this issue, therefore, must be on the communication within the relationship in which one member feels jealous. To focus on the third person only repeats the pattern, rather than strengthening the threatened relationship. A constructive focus is on what the bisexual partner can do to clarify his or her commitment to the primary relationship.

Children.   The empirical literature makes it clear that children raised by gay or lesbian parents do not suffer personal deficits from this experience (Patterson 1992); it is reassuring for parents struggling with their own orientation to know this information. It is also clear that children find it easier to deal with their parent's sexual orientation if they learn of it prior to puberty, when their own sexuality matures and preoccupies them (Matteson 1987b; Patterson 1992). Unfortunately, when bisexuality has resulted in the dissolution of a heterosexual marriage, the bisexual parent may feel it necessary to delay disclosure to children until he or she is assured of protection of parental rights (Coleman 1989). The attitude of the court system in one's particular geographic area must be considered in this decision (Matteson 1987b; Martin 1993).

■ Summary of Skills Needed in Dealing With Systems Issues of Bisexual Clients

The therapist must be able to recognize the importance of relationship issues in the client's life; communicate acceptance of the client's choice of partners by including them in sessions when appropriate; explore with heterosexually married clients the option of staying in the marriage but reconstructing it to accommodate the new aspects of the bisexual client's identity; teach the client some of the strategies and skills needed to maintain multiple relationships; help the client with issues concerning balance and jealousy in multiple relationships; and assert the value of honest communication with children involved, as appropriate.

Counseling for Issues Not Related to Bisexuality

The most frequently stated criticism concerning professionals' work with bisexual individuals and their partners is that counselors are fixated on the uniqueness of the lifestyle and lose sight of other issues for which services may be sought. One woman, married to a bisexual man, described 3 months of counseling during which she was trying to resolve an issue with her daughter. After a resolution was achieved, the counselor expressed surprise at the mother's profound relief. The counselor had not believed that the husband-wife relationship could be stable and had assumed it was the underlying cause of the problem. Fortunately in this case, the counselor realized and admitted her own mistake.

Bisexual individuals may seek counseling for the same reasons that might prompt any other person to do so. These concerns can easily be overlooked by a counselor who is fixated on the bisexual issue. Assessment can be further compounded with clients who tend to use "bisexuality, or fear of being a 'latent homosexual', as a convenient scapegoat on which to hang all the things that go wrong in their lives" (Lourea 1985, p. 52), when in fact, personality or other problems exist that have no direct connection to the issue of bisexuality. There is no evidence of a higher frequency of personality problems or mental and social dysfunction among bisexual individuals (see Chapter 10 by Fox; Fox 1995), but such problems do occur and should not be overlooked.

Necessary Conditions for Conducting Ethical Therapy

Although many gay, lesbian, and bisexual counselors believe that the personal and political benefits of being "out of the closet" in our professional and other communities outweigh the risks, they also know that the risks are not simply phobic delusions; they are real. Although it may be appropriate to point out to the client the ways the closet is harmful, the decision as to when and where to risk disclosure belongs to the client and her or his intimates. It is especially important not to impose one's political views on the client.

Counselors may need to state their stance on some value issues about which they have strong feelings, alerting the client that objectivity may not be possible in those areas. Certainly if a counselor holds critical moral- or value-laden views regarding homosexuality, or homosexuality within a heterosexual marriage (Coleman 1989), it is appropriate to refer to a choice of other counselors and to clarify that the reason for the referral is due to the counselor's limits in working objectively with this situation. Because of the risk that clients will misinterpret a referral to mean they are being rejected or are "too sick to be helped," it is appropriate to own the problem with a statement such as, "There are counselors who are helpful with clients like you, but I am limited in this area and don't trust myself to work well with it."

"Duty to protect" laws in many states require counselors or therapists to protect others who are affected by the client's behavior. Legal and ethical issues are very unsettled when dealing with multiple relationships in this time of AIDS. Although in several states confidentiality is clearly limited when a specifically identified person is known to be in physical danger, it is not always clear how this limitation should be applied, as for example in the case in which the counselor knows that a client is engaging in unsafe sex and may potentially be exposing an unknowing spouse or partner to HIV. The issues and legal precedents are reviewed in Marks (1993).

■ Getting Accurate Information

It is important to know how to gather accurate information about the particular client. Many counselors inadvertently signal that information about heterosexual practices is of special importance to them. When asking about the client's history or his or her network of social support, the counselor should show interest in any person—female or male—for whom the client has had strong feelings. It is inappropriate to ask separate questions about heterosexual relationships, because such questions may be interpreted by gay, lesbian, or bisexual clients as manifesting a value judgment about the primacy of heterosexuality (Gartrell 1984). Questions regarding the etiology of same-sex feelings may imply that these feelings are pathological, suggesting that these feelings are a focus of concern in a way that heterosexual feelings are not. If exploration of sexual identity is an issue, the counselor should comment at some early point about cultural myths concerning homosexuality. Asking the client to describe his or her perceptions and fears about lesbians, gay, or bisexual persons is a good way to start identifying internalized homophobia and biphobia and gives an opportunity for the informed counselor to provide helpful, factual information (Gartrell 1984).

More complete information about bisexuality and bisexual lifestyles can be found in Chapter 10 by Fox and in Firestein (in press). However, direct personal experience with bisexual individuals is essential to overcome stereotypes. Attending workshops that permit some degree of personal interaction with leaders who identify as members of sexual minorities can be fruitful. Even better is to seek out members of different minority groups who one can get to know and respect as peers. Ideally, counseling students and therapists in training should first get to know members of a minority group as peers, allowing counselors a chance to learn about the special issues and perceptions of a minority, before accepting someone from that group as a client, with the complications of the "one up" position of the therapist inherent in clinical relationships. Someone who is in a mutual relationship as a peer is in a far better position to confront false assumptions and to help the counselor work through them. A grounding in cross-cultural psychology may help counselors to examine their cultural biases and avoid imposing them destructively on a client.

References

Blumstein PW, Schwartz P: Bisexuality: some social psychological issues. Journal of Social Issues 33:30–45, 1977

Borhek MV: Coming Out to Parents. New York, Pilgrim, 1983

Bowen M: Family Therapy in Clinical Practice. New York, Jason Aronson, 1978

Coleman E: Developmental stages in the coming out process. J Homosex 7:31–43, 1981–1982

Coleman E: The married lesbian. Marriage and Family Review 14: 119–135, 1989

Dixon JK: Sexuality and relationship changes in married females following the commencement of bisexual activity. J Homosex 11:115–133, 1985

Firestein B (ed): Bisexuality: The Psychology and Politics of an Invisible Minority. Newbury Park, CA, Sage (in press)

Fox RC: Coming out bisexual: identity, behavior and sexual orientation self-disclosure. Unpublished doctoral dissertation, California Institute of Integral Studies, San Francisco, CA, 1993

Fox RC: Bisexual identities, in Lesbian, Gay and Bisexual Identities Over the Lifespan. Edited by D'Augelli AR, Patterson CJ. New York, Oxford University Press, 1995, pp 48–86

Gartrell N: Issues in psychotherapy with lesbian women. Work in Progress #10. Wellesley, MA, Wellesley College, 1984

Gochros HL: Counseling gay husbands. Journal of Sex Education and Therapy 5:142–151, 1978

Gochros J: When Husbands Come Out of the Closet. New York, Haworth, 1989

Green GD, Clunis DM: Married lesbians. Women and Therapy (special issue: Lesbianism) 8:41–49, 1989

Hamilton W: Coming Out. New York, New American Library, 1977

Latham JD, White GD: Coping with homosexual expression within heterosexual marriages: five case studies. J Sex Marital Ther 4:198–212, 1978

Lourea DN: Psycho-social issues related to counseling bisexuals. J Homosex 11:51–63, 1985

Marcia JE, Waterman AS, Matteson DR, et al: Ego Identity: A Handbook for Psychosocial Research. New York, Springer-Verlag, 1993

Marks R (ed): Focus: A Guide to AIDS Research and Counseling. AIDS Health Project, University of California, San Francisco 8(April):5, 1993

Martin A: The Lesbian and Gay Parenting Handbook: Creating and Raising Our Families. New York, HarperCollins, 1993

Matteson DR: Bisexual men in marriages: is a positive homosexual identity and stable marriage possible? J Homosex 11:149–172, 1985

Matteson DR: Counseling bisexual men, in Handbook of Counseling and Psychotherapy With Men. Edited by Scher M, Stevens M, Good G, et al. Beverly Hills, CA, Sage, 1987a, pp 232–249

Matteson DR: The heterosexually married gay and lesbian parent, in Gay and Lesbian Parents. Edited by Bozett FW. New York, Praeger, 1987b, pp 138–161

Matteson DR: Bisexual lifestyles: what kind of "choice" is this? Invited presentation at annual conference of the American Association of Sex Educators, Counselors and Therapists, St. Louis, MO, May 1991

Matteson DR: Counseling with bisexuals. Individual Psychology 51(2):144–159, 1995

Matteson DR: Counseling and psychotherapy with bisexual and exploring clients, in Bisexuality: The Psychology and Politics of an Invisible Minority. Edited by Firestein B. Newbury Park, CA, Sage (in press)

Muchmore W, Hansen W: Coming Out Right. Boston, Alyson, 1982

Nichols M: Bisexuality in women: myths, realities, and implications for therapy. Women and Therapy 7:235–252, 1988

Patterson CJ: Children of lesbian and gay parents. Child Development 63:1025–1042, 1992

Paul JP: Counseling issues in working with a bisexual population, in The Sourcebook on Lesbian or Gay Health Care, 2nd Edition. Edited by Shernoff M, Scott WA. Washington, DC, National Lesbian and Gay Health Foundation, 1988, pp 142–150

Rust PC: The politics of sexual identity: sexual attraction and behavior among lesbian and bisexual women. Social Problems 39(4):366-386, 1992

Rust PC: "Coming out" in the age of social constructionism: sexual identity formation among lesbian and bisexual women. Gender and Society 7:50–77, 1993a

Rust PC: Neutralizing the political threat of the marginal woman: lesbians' beliefs about bisexual women. J Sex Res 30:214–228, 1993b

Scarf M: Intimate Partners: Patterns in Love and Marriage. New York, Ballantine Books, 1987

Shuster R: Sexuality as a continuum: the bisexual identity, in Lesbian Psychologies. Edited by Boston Lesbian Psychologies Collective. Urbana, IL, University of Illinois Press, 1987, pp 56–71

Silver N: Coming out as heterosexual, in Closer to Home: Bisexuality and Feminism. Edited by Weise ER. Seattle, WA, Seal Press, 1992, pp 35–46

Weinberg MS, Williams CJ, Pryor DW: Dual Attraction: Understanding Bisexuality. New York, Oxford University Press, 1994

26

Psychoanalytic Therapy With Gay Men

Developmental Considerations

Richard A. Isay, M.D.

H omosexual men have a predominant erotic attraction to others of the same sex. Their sexual fantasies are either entirely or almost entirely directed toward other men and have been so since childhood. Because homosexual behavior, like heterosexual behavior, may be inhibited, a man need not engage in sexual activity to be considered homosexual. Those who have homosexual contacts but, because of censorious social pressures, intrapsychic con-

---

This chapter is adapted from Isay RA: "Dynamic Psychotherapy With Gay Men: Developmental Considerations," in *American Psychiatric Press Review of Psychiatry*, Volume 12. Edited by Oldham JM, Riba MB, Tasman A. Washington, DC, American Psychiatric Press, 1993, pp. 85–100. Used with permission. Some portions are original to Isay RA: *Being Homosexual: Gay Men and Their Development.* New York, Farrar, Straus and Giroux, 1989.

451

flict, or both, are either unable to express or unable to accept that they are gay, are also homosexual. There are other men who may not even have conscious access to their homoerotic fantasies because they repress, suppress, or deny them. Their fantasies should become available to them during a properly conducted analysis or therapy, and the author also considers them to be homosexual.

What Is Homosexuality?

Investigations by psychologists over the years suggest that there is no greater psychopathology in gay men than in heterosexual individuals (Hooker 1957; Riess 1980). Psychoanalysis, in contrast to and despite such evidence, continues in general to remain committed to the conviction that homosexuality is always pathological. Homosexuality is seen ipso facto as a deviant form of sexuality because gay men do not reach the theoretical "normal" developmental end point of resolving the Oedipus complex by desiring someone like their mothers and identifying with their fathers.

Psychoanalysts have looked at the early childhood histories of gay men who have come to them as patients and isolated what seem to be environmental determinants of their desire for other men rather than for women as lovers. Some experts believe that the predilection for a same-sex love object is caused by a close-binding, hostile mother, who undermines her son's masculinity by blocking the development of his independence and thus interfering with the father-son relationship and inducing a fear of women. Others emphasize the role of an absent, weak, detached, or hostile father, who makes it impossible for the child to separate from his dominating mother.

Although these psychodynamic conceptions can be traced to Freud, he was in general much more open to the biological determinants of homosexuality than later psychoanalysts have been. He felt an obligation to stress environmental factors that psychoanalysts could investigate, because his major interest was in developing the clinical technique of psychoanalysis.

There is some suggestive evidence that there is a biological basis for homosexuality, as is generally assumed to be the case for heterosexuality. LeVay (1991) found a difference in nuclei in the anterior hypothalamus between heterosexual men and homosexual men who had died of AIDS. Although the study needs to be replicated with a diverse sample of healthy gay men, this finding does suggest a biological basis for male homosexuality.

Kallman (1952) found a concordance for homosexual behavior only slightly higher than normal in dizygotic twins, but 100% in monozygotic twins. Although this study has been criticized for its methodological flaws, another more recent study showed that the proportion of homosexual individuals was significantly greater in monozygotic twins than for either dizygotic twins or adoptive brothers (Bailey and Pillard 1991). Pillard and Weinrich (1986) demonstrated that gay men have significantly more homosexual or bisexual brothers (22%) than do heterosexual men (4%), and Hamer et al. (1993) discovered a gene marker linked to male homosexuality. These studies strongly suggest that homosexuality in men is both constitutional and heritable.

The author's own clinical observation of homosexual men over the past 20 years who have been in psychoanalysis or an analytically oriented therapy is that same-sex fantasies can be recovered from ages 3, 4, or 5 years, at about the same ages when heterosexual men recall opposite-sex fantasies (Isay 1986). These fantasies that are generally fixed and seem to start at such an early age also suggest a biological basis of male homosexuality.

From a clinical standpoint, it is helpful to view sexual orientation as biological. Because efforts to change homosexual behavior to heterosexual are injurious to the self-esteem of a gay man, and efforts to change core sexuality are futile, perceiving sexuality as constitutional permits therapists to understand and investigate the expression of a homosexual orientation with the same neutrality as they do heterosexuality.

The author's clinical work with gay men has brought him to the conviction that homosexuality is a nonpathological variant of human sexuality. The author has found no greater psychopathology in his gay patients than in his heterosexual patients. But unlike other psychoanalysts, the author works with gay men who are generally accepting of their sexuality.

The manner in which homosexuality, like heterosexuality, may be expressed is influenced by a variety of early experiences. For example, a boy who grows up with a dominant mother who uses him to fulfill ungratified needs of her own will have the same chance of becoming gay as he would if he were raised by a mother who ideally nurtures his growth and development. It is likely, however, that this child as an adult, whether gay or straight, will form intimate relations that are full of rage toward others, who in his mind threaten to engulf or bind him. Likewise, any child, heterosexual or homosexual, who has a distant, uninvolved, or unloving father will form relations with other men that are suffused with suspicion and rage. But a gay man whose father rejected him as a youngster may find that his erotic and intimate relations with other men are profoundly disturbed. He may be inhibited by a fear of rejection and by rage at the partner, who he believes will inevitably injure him emotionally.

Like all forms of love, homosexuality remains mysterious and eludes our total understanding. Like all forms of love, it is a longing for a lost attachment. That longing, for gay men, is usually for the father.

Childhood and Early Homosexual Identity

Most adult gay men will initially recall that their homoerotic attractions started somewhere between ages 8 and 13 or 14 years. Sometimes it is recalled as having "always been present." Gay men the author has seen in psychoanalysis or psychotherapy, although varying in their recollections of age at onset, report that starting from about ages 3, 4, or 5 years, they felt they were "different" from their peers. They saw themselves as being more sensitive than other boys; cried more easily; had their feelings hurt more readily; had more aesthetic interests; enjoyed nature, art, and music; and were drawn to other sensitive boys, girls, and adults. They reported that they felt like outsiders ever since those early childhood years.

Feelings of being different start at about the same time as same-sex erotic fantasies. As repression and denial begin to lift, adult homosexual men begin to recollect, like heterosexual men, that they had erotic fantasies from the very early age of 3 or 4 years. Most often the same-sex erotic fantasies centering on the father or the father surrogate initially make these children feel different from their peers. The child's perception of and response to these erotic feelings may account for such behavior as greater secretiveness than other boys, self-isolation, and excessive emotionality. Some gender-atypical traits may be caused by identification with the mother or a mother surrogate as a way of attracting the father's love and attention (Isay 1987). Other traits may be biological in origin (LeVay 1993).

Some of the behavior considered to be gender atypical for the 3-, 4-, or 5-year-old boy, such as his relative lack of aggressiveness, greater sensitivity, aesthetic sensibility, or compassion, may persist into adulthood. Other more overtly "feminine" behavior of some homosexual boys may disappear in adolescence and adulthood because of the pressure for peer socialization (Friedman 1988).

The following case illustrates how same-sex memories and fantasies from childhood are in the recesses of every patient's mind. They turn up eventually either as direct memories from childhood or as indirect memories that may be reconstructed from the transference or from current relationships.

> When the author first saw Mr. A in consultation, he was 32 years old and well muscled, but somewhat tight and rigid. He initially came to see the author because he felt lonely, anxious, and dissatisfied with his relationships with other men. He was moderately depressed and said he was distressed over the breakup a month before of a year-long love affair. He spoke easily of his homosexuality in the initial sessions, but although readily speaking of his attraction to other men, he also related how difficult it was to feel close to them.
>
> During the early hours of their work together, Mr. A spontaneously recollected that he had felt different from his peers during early childhood. He described this as "not liking to hit people or engage in rough stuff. I seemed more sensitive than other kids. I spent a lot of time playing the piano. I never liked being demanding." He did not enjoy participating in the activities and many of the games of his male peers, and he felt he was excluded because of this from some of their social activities.
>
> Mr. A's father was described as distant. Although his father always earned a good living, Mr. A looked on his father's work as demeaning. He accepted readily his mother's view that his father lacked ambition for not aspiring to managerial and executive positions, rather than the hands-on work that he always enjoyed. Mr. A's mother was clinically depressed during much of his childhood, but she was the dominant force in the family.
>
> Mr. A consistently treated the author with a striking indifference that suggested a need to deny that the author was of any importance to him. The author pointed out to him that he needed to keep the author and other men in his life emotionally distant, and over time he became more comfortable in expressing his warmth and curiosity. These changes in the relationship between Mr. A and the author helped him to become more open with others, and he soon met a new lover who was spontaneously and comfortably affectionate and tender.

It was during this period of generally increasing ease with his own affectionate and sexual feelings that Mr. A began to recall sexual fantasies that he had had when he was age 4 about muscular comic book heroes. As these sexual feelings became clearer, he became less preoccupied with feelings of having been different as a child. He had less need to protect himself from old erotic feelings that were now becoming increasingly acceptable.

He remembered that it was his father who would read him *Superman* and *Captain Marvel* comic books and that he felt warmth and pleasure while sitting on his father's lap. It became clear to both Mr. A and the author that Mr. A's sexual interest and excitement over muscular comic book heroes at age 4 were displaced and disguised expressions of his repressed sexual feelings toward his father. It appeared that there was a direct relationship between his becoming more aware of these erotic fantasies and feelings toward the father and his enhanced capacity for expressing warmth, tenderness, affection, and love toward other men as an adult.

One of the most interesting findings during the years of the author's work with many gay men has been the nature of this very early and powerful erotic attachment of males to their fathers. Many gay men report that their fathers were distant during their childhood and that they lacked any attachment to them. Reports vary from "My father was never around, he was too busy with his own job," to "I was victimized by my mother, who was always the boss in the family." Occasionally patients describe fathers who were present, but they portray them as having been uninvolved.

Gay men's memories of their fathers, like those heterosexual men have of their mothers, are often caused by the defensive distortion arising from the anxiety the adult feels about the early erotic attachment to the parent. Gay men distance themselves from their fathers in their memory to avoid recognition of this erotic attachment and of their sexual arousal in early childhood.

Mr. B started treatment with the author when he was age 24 because he was moderately depressed, a depression that stemmed in part from his loneliness. He had little conscious anxiety about his sexuality, feeling that he had "always been homosexual." He recognized that in early adolescence he had been attracted to certain teachers. His first sexual encounter was when he was about age 15. He had had a few short-term relations since that time, but those attachments never seemed to work out. If a man evoked his passion, he became disinterested in going out with him, feeling that there was something wrong or "lower class" about the sexual excitement.

At the beginning of treatment he recollected an incident that occurred when he was age 8 and was fondled by an older man. Initially he recalled this experience with great disgust, remorse, and anxiety, but during his third year of treatment he recollected that there had been some excitement during the encounter. A few weeks later, he began to recall the sexual arousal he had experienced when he first saw his father's penis. Thereafter Mr. B began to have more recollections of the fantasies he had had about his father when he was about age 3 or 4, and he gradually began to feel less inhibited and was more interested in having sexual contact with other men.

The sexual contact when he was age 8, frightening as it was, served as a screen for this early erotic interest in his father. As the repression and denial of his childhood recollections of erotic feelings gradually lessened, Mr. B's sexual fantasies became much more easily acknowledged. His sexual feelings in general became more readily and actively expressed.

Particular to the childhood of homosexual boys is that their fathers often become detached or hostile during their early years as a reaction to the child's homosexuality. The father usually perceives such a child as being "different" from other boys. This perception may lead to both the father's withdrawal and his favoring an older or younger male sibling who appears to be more sociable, more conventional, or more masculine. Some of the fathers of homosexual boys either consciously or unconsciously recognize that their sons have both a special need for closeness and an erotic attachment to them. These fathers usually withdraw because of anxiety occasioned by concerns about their own masculinity.

The withdrawal of the father is invariably experienced as a rejection and may be a cause of the poor self-esteem and the sense of inadequacy felt by some gay men. It is also an important reason why some gay men have difficulty forming loving and trusting adult relationships.

Mr. C was an articulate, intelligent, verbal, precocious child— marks of his difference in a family in which the parents were intelligent but uneducated. He also was "different" in many of the ways described earlier in this chapter. He thought that his first same-sex fantasies occurred "very early," but it was not clear how early.

Mr. C entered analysis in great conflict about his father, proclaiming his hatred for him. His life, he felt, had been scarred by his father's severe rejection. When Mr. C told his parents he was homosexual, his enraged father had proclaimed, "I always hated you." He was devastated at the thought that he could never win his father's love and attention.

During the course of analysis, it seemed clear that the father withdrew after a time of very early closeness. When a younger brother was born, the father shifted his interest from Mr. C to this new son. The way Mr. C now vented his hurt and anger was by subtly and at times not so subtly demeaning his father.

The father's rejection was extremely harmful to his son's sense of self-worth. It was largely responsible for the anxiety Mr. C felt whenever he met a man he liked. He anticipated that any relationship would wind up in disaster and rejection, like that with his father. This fear interfered with his capacity to form a close, loving, and responsive attachment to another man.

Although the author is emphasizing here the special importance of the relationship with the father, he does not minimize the importance of the primary attachment that any human being—heterosexual or homosexual, male or female—has with the early care-giving, nurturing mother. All relations, especially intimate ones, are profoundly influenced by the nature of this earliest relationship, most particularly by the sense of security and love, comfort, and caring, that affects self-esteem by conveying a sense of well-being to the child.

Those men who have a positive sense of themselves and their sexuality usually describe their mothers as having been "good enough." However, gay men may also be envious of and competitive with women, feelings that they are often not aware of and that originate in the rivalry with the mother for the father's attention. There is also often an underlying bond with women that is based on a mutual attraction to men as well as on other shared traits and interests.

Adolescence and Young Adulthood

Although every child enters adolescence with a burden of guilt from forbidden childhood erotic feelings and impulses, for the gay adolescent this developmental period may be particularly anguishing.

The consolidation and integration of sexual orientation, essential for a positive self-image, do not usually occur as early in homosexual adolescents as they do in heterosexual boys. Childhood paternal rejection, the internalization of society's prejudice, the wish to fulfill heterosexual cultural expectations, and the need for peer approval cause many homosexual adolescents to suppress or deny their sexuality with great vigor. Although many gay adolescents "know" from childhood that they are homosexual, the homosexual youth may develop many ways to deny and avoid this stigma.

Many gay adolescents, desiring to please their peers and fit in with their expectations, will attempt, despite recognition of their homosexual desire, to date girls and to have sex. These early forays into heterosexuality are usually without passion and are usually unsuccessful. Not having had the opportunity to experiment with his sexuality like the heterosexual adolescent, the homosexual youth may grow to feel that he will never be able to experience passion. During this period, when there are so many impediments to the integration of the sexual orientation because of peer pressure and societal bias, some gay youth may also begin to experiment furtively. Because sexual activity must be hidden and is usually outside of relationships, it is frequently found to be unloving and often ungratifying.

Casual sexual experiences outside of a relationship in adolescence make it difficult for many gay adults to reconcile their longings for affectionate relationships with the feeling that their sexuality is entirely an issue of lust. Sexual activities can grow ever more separated from warmth and affection as the young adult learns to believe that his sexuality is sick or bad.

The lack of positive role models for gay youth also may impede the gay adolescent's recognition of his sexuality. Those gay adults who are most easily recognized are usually those who are pointed out as being most effeminate and those portrayed by the media as being strange. Along with the lack of positive role models, such portrayals reinforce the gay youth's perception that he is immoral, sick, or weird. They add to the delays in recognition of sexual orientation and increase the likelihood that he will have a poor self-image and have difficulty in bringing loving, affectionate, and sexual feelings together into a relationship.

Effect of the AIDS Epidemic on Development

The AIDS epidemic has made it even more difficult for gay adolescents to consolidate and integrate their sexual orientation into a positive self-image. Some healthy young adults now perceive themselves as potential carriers of death, and others have become severely anxious about contracting the disease. The epidemic has caused some not to be able to express their sexuality and not to be able to perceive themselves as being gay because they feel that their sexuality is a mortal danger to themselves and others.

> The author first saw Mr. D early in 1984. He sought help because of severe inhibition in his sexual activity. Although attractive and intelligent, Mr. D believed that he was unattractive, especially his hips and buttocks. He would not remove his clothes in front of other men, and so he had no sexual contact during his first 2 years of college.
>
> When the author saw him for the first time at age 19, Mr. D readily acknowledged that he was gay. He had never had sex with a woman, and his sexual fantasies were almost exclusively homosexual. He was aroused by boys from his class, but he hated the idea of being attracted to anyone, finding it humiliating.
>
> As awareness about AIDS increased, Mr. D found reason to isolate himself further. The fear of contracting AIDS became a way of projecting his rage: He became convinced that someone was going to give him the disease. The author's efforts to help Mr. D understand that he was using the epidemic as a displacement of his own hostile impulses were largely futile. When the author pointed out to him that neither his current behavior nor his fantasies suggested that he was going to engage in unsafe sex, he became furious and accused the author of being unwilling to protect him from the illness, of exposing him to disease and death.

Most gay men, as their sexual desire becomes less repressed and less conflict-ridden, acquire greater responsiveness and more flexible homoerotic fantasies and behavior. When sexual behavior is inhibited, as it was in Mr. D, and the underlying causes of the inhibition are uncovered, there is then a freer expression of sexual feeling and behavior. Mr. D's anger at the author for supposedly encouraging him to engage in sexual behavior that might kill him gave the author an opportunity to help him understand something about the early roots of his sexual inhibition and rage. It also provided the author with the opportunity to acknowledge the real danger of AIDS and to educate him about safe sex.

This didactic attitude is not usual in a psychoanalyst or analytically oriented therapist. But the author does not wait for patients to tell him about having unsafe sex before he assumes an educational role—not when a fatal disease can be acquired through one such encounter. Helping patients first to clarify their conflicts and then suggesting caution may evoke further conflict about fantasies and desires. When this occurs, these conflicts must be further analyzed. But because of the grave risk, the author's intervention has generally been considered thoughtful and caring. If the risks were not so great, such efforts to educate might well be regarded by many patients as moralistic or controlling and would therefore likely be used in self-injurious ways during periods of negative transference.

"Coming Out"

As we have seen, the recognition and self-labeling of one's sexual orientation may be delayed in adolescence because of the poor self-image associated with paternal rejection, peer rejection, the internalization of social bias, and the lack of available, positive role models. Such self-recognition and then self-labeling as "gay" should begin in middle or late adolescence as part of the consolidation and integration of sexual orientation. Significant delays in this process beyond middle adolescence usually suggest self-esteem injury.

Coming out to other gay men usually follows self-labeling and self-recognition. Relationships with other gay men that are mutual and loving, both nonsexual and sexual, are essential to the healthy integration of a homosexual identity, helping to promote a positive self-image.

Coming out to gay men and being socially involved with them are necessary aspects of the integration of sexual orientation. They are ways of discovering those positive role models that are denied to gay youth in our society and of countering the social stigmatization and isolation that may occur during childhood and adolescence from early experiences with fathers and peers. However, the degree and nature of such socialization may be limited in our society by restrictive factors such as geography, vocation, and availability. A gay man in a rural area is obviously going to have much less opportunity for social contact with other gay men. Similarly, some gay men marry before they can identify themselves as being gay. If they do choose to preserve the relationship with a wife, they also may have less opportunity for continuing social relationships with gay men.

Psychotherapy With Gay Men

Gay men usually come to the therapist's office with the same problems as heterosexual patients do. They come with issues related to difficulties within relationships, problems in forming relationships, and problems related to work. In addition, many gay men seek assistance because of unconscious conflict about their sexual identity as a result of internalized homophobia. Therefore, it is essential that any therapist who works with gay men be knowledgeable about the kinds of developmental issues presented in this chapter. For no matter how determined a therapist may be to treat gay men in a nonjudgmental way, a belief that the only normal developmental pathway ends in taking the mother as a love object and identifying with the father will lead to interpretations and comments that convey bias and lack of understanding and will further undermine the self-esteem of the gay patient.

The author's perspective on the therapy of gay men is based on two convictions. First, gay men can live well-adjusted and productive lives with gratifying and stable same-sex relationships. This is an observation based on the author's clinical experience and on extensive personal observation. Nonetheless, although many experts believe this to be a self-evident proposition, most dynamically oriented therapists and psychoanalysts still contend that the same conflicts in the early lives of homosexual men that have caused their homosexuality have produced personality problems so severe that it is impossible for them to establish stable relationships and to live a reasonably happy life.

The author's second conviction is one established by clinical experience: The effort to change the sexual orientation of a gay man is harmful to him. Freud was not sanguine about the possibility of changing a homosexual to a heterosexual or about its usefulness. He stated, "In general, to undertake to convert a fully developed homosexual into a heterosexual does not offer much more prospect of success than the reverse, except that for good practical purposes the latter is never attempted" (Freud 1920/1955, p. 151).

The author's clinical follow-up of many gay men treated by other therapists has demonstrated that there may be severe emotional and social consequences in the attempt to change a man from homosexual to heterosexual. Although sexual behavior can be temporarily modified, by any variety of means, including transference compliance, the sexual orientation per se as determined by the persistence of same-sex fantasy life cannot be modified (Isay 1985), as illustrated in the following cases:

> When Mr. E consulted the author, he was 47 and the father of two adolescent girls. He had married in his late 20s, shortly after the completion of a 5-year analysis. Before the analysis he had had an active homosexual life, including a relationship with a young man whom he said was the only passion of his life. He had never enjoyed sex with women prior to his analysis and had *learned* [patient's emphasis] to enjoy sex with women during his analysis. Although sex with men was not specifically prohibited, the love affair was proscribed and sex with women was prescribed. There had been no homosexual sex since his marriage. He sought therapeutic assistance because of persistent depression, no zest for living, low self-esteem, apathy in his work, and no sexual relations since the birth of his last child. His masturbatory and other sexual fantasies were exclusively homosexual. He longed for the lost love of his youth.
>
> This man was a devoted father and husband. His wife knew nothing of his past homosexual life. He had no regrets over the change in his sexual behavior, except that he felt something was missing in his life—he called it a "passion." Mr. E was still homosexual: He had a conscious erotic preference for other men, still had an active homosexual fantasy life, and continued to long for the love of other men.
>
> Mr. E did not wish to resume analysis, but he did enter into analytically oriented therapy. He expressed a great deal of anger, which he had previously been unaware of, at his analyst for "manipulating" him. He grieved over having given up the passion that he spoke of so often. Over the course of 2 years of therapy, his life felt less burdensome as his depression decreased. He became more tolerant of his homosexual fantasies and impulses and was able to think of himself as homosexual. He never resumed sex with his wife, nor did he resume his homosexual life, because he felt it would disrupt his marriage.
>
> Mr. E always believed that his previous analysis had been successful. He had a wife and children from whom he gained enormous pleasure. He liked the conventionality, the relative lack of stress in his life, and his professional status. It became clear in our work, however, that the denial, repression, and unanalyzed acquiescence that had been necessary for him to achieve the renunciation of his homosexual behavior had affected his capacity to enjoy and achieve to the fullest extent possible, and that the failure to analyze these defenses and transference manifestations were in

part responsible for the depression that motivated his return for further treatment.

The next patient had had an analyst who, unlike the analyst of the previous patient, gave the appearance of being noncoercive, nonjudgmental, and not manipulative. Because the patient was not engaged in homosexual sex before or during his analysis, no apparent modifications in analytical technique or obvious violations of analytical neutrality were necessary to discourage such behavior. The observation afforded by the patient's subsequent long analysis suggested, however, that the analyst's social values had interfered with his patient's treatment. The author wants to illustrate with this case the ways in which the interpretation of homosexuality as a defense can convey the analyst's bias:

> Mr. F started his analysis when he was in his early 20s because of conflict about his homosexual fantasies and a lack of interest in girls. Homosexual masturbation fantasies and daydreams had persisted since before adolescence. When he entered analysis he had never engaged in homosexual activity, except for very occasional adolescent sexual play that was clinically insignificant. Throughout the analysis the analyst consistently interpreted the homosexual fantasies as a defense against assuming aggressive male roles, which included having heterosexual sex. The analyst's view implicitly and comfortingly conveyed to the patient that he was not really homosexual and that what appeared to him to be homosexuality and what he feared was homosexual could be analyzed and would disappear.
>
> Mr. F continued to have exclusively homosexual fantasies. Because of a powerful positive transference, however, he did engage in occasional sex with girls, although he was frequently impotent. Shortly after the termination of the analysis, he married. Sexual interest in his wife rapidly waned, and after several years of marriage, he began to have homosexual sex for the first time. When Mr. F came to the author in his late 30s, he was depressed, agitated, despairing, and confused. He was "wandering between two worlds" and wanted to find a way to bring them together.

The analyst's heterosexual bias was expressed largely and repeatedly in the interpretation of homosexual fantasy as a defense against fears of heterosexuality and of competition (i.e., as the unsuccessful resolution of oedipal stage conflict). When the author began to treat

Mr. F, it was clear that the patient had a need to feel enraged and to see his analyst as negligent and uncaring. Nevertheless, his perception of his former analyst's intolerance of homosexual behavior, which was expressed in the interpretation of Mr. F's homosexuality as a defense against heterosexuality, also seems to have been accurate. The analyst's inability to help the patient discover this aspect of his identity contributed to his later symptoms and to the painful social situation he found himself in at the beginning of his subsequent treatment.

In the preceding illustrations, each patient's transference wishes were unconsciously used by the analyst, because of the analyst's countertransference needs, to attempt to change the patient's sexual orientation. This, of course, made it impossible in these initial efforts for any of the patients to understand those essential conflicts that were expressed in the transference. For example, Mr. F had acquiesced to what he perceived as his analyst's wish for him to behave heterosexually out of an attempt to be the good sibling. His brother had been the actively rebellious one. Mr. F won his place by being acquiescent and agreeable. As a result of a longed-for love that he never received, Mr. F had not been rebellious as a child. His passivity and acquiescence expressed this deep longing for the love of both parents. Pleasing his analyst by attempting to be heterosexual, he could win a long-sought and always elusive love.

The exploitation of transference for hoped-for therapeutic gain is, of course, not new. Many of the gains of the brief analyses of the 1920s and the crisis-oriented and focal therapies today were and are in part based on such techniques. Those analysts who advocate, as mentioned earlier, the introduction of encouragement to overcome what they feel to be the homosexual's phobic avoidance of sex with women make conscious use of the transference for attempted therapeutic gain. The author's concern here, however, is with analysts' unconscious exploitation of transference wishes as an expression of their value system and countertransference, which add a measure of insidious conviction to the patient's long-standing belief in his being intolerable or evil.

Positive regard and affirmation must be provided by any therapists who work with gay men, just as they would provide such regard for a heterosexual who came seeking assistance. This regard and affirmation are necessary if there is to be an atmosphere in which the patient may safely project, witness, understand, and untangle the negative self-image he has acquired from childhood experiences and relationships, society's attitudes, and the lack of positive role models, as discussed previously. Therapists who cannot accept their patients as gay reinforce earlier images reflected in the patients' self-deprecatory, paranoid, masochistic, or sadistic attitudes that interfere with their capacity for more positive relationships and experiences.

> The author first saw Mr. G when he was a 19-year-old college junior. The author worked with him for 9 years, initially seeing him three times a week in psychoanalysis and then in twice-weekly analytical therapy. He had been in treatment with another analyst since his junior year in high school, but he had left him because he was feeling increasingly depressed and hopeless about ever being able to live a happy life. He "feared" that he was homosexual, because he felt "turned on" by other boys. His sexual fantasies, for as long as he could remember, had been almost exclusively about boys. He hated his homosexuality and wanted desperately to be heterosexual. He was distressed by the way he met other boys, which was in the restroom of his college library. He labeled himself alternately "a sissy," "sick," "sleazy," or "disgusting."
>
> In his first session he informed the author that he felt his mother would be devastated if she knew he was homosexual. He wanted to be straight for her, to live a conventional life, to give her the grandchildren that she so often said she wanted. It was she who also wanted him to go to a therapist at age 15, because of his lack of aggressiveness that made her believe he might be homosexual.
>
> Even though Mr. G felt little attraction to girls, he did occasionally date and attempt to have sex to please his peers and his mother. The sex was passionless and therefore not satisfying. In fact, it was a source of despair because it made him feel uncertain that he had the capacity to fall in love. Because he believed that his own needs and desires were unimportant to his parents, his attempts at heterosexual sex were also accompanied by a great deal of rage, which contributed to his distress.
>
> The author formed an early impression that Mr. G was homosexual because of his long-standing exclusively homoerotic fantasy life and his conscious desire for men. The author viewed his rejection of his homosexuality and his desire to be heterosexual as a symptom of his injured self-esteem.
>
> Whenever Mr. G had an anonymous sexual encounter in the restroom of his college library, he would spend hours admonishing himself for engaging in behavior that he believed despicable. At that time he could express his sexuality only in these encounters, which he felt were sleazy. The possibility of a romantic or lasting relationship was not something he thought possible at the beginning of analysis.

Anonymous or random sexual encounters are not necessarily a symptom of an inability to form intimate attachments in a gay man. Peer and parental pressure for heterosexual conformity and our society's unwillingness to permit gay youth to develop a system of courtship contribute to the need of some adolescents and adults to express their sexuality covertly. Restrooms and pornographic movie theaters or bookstores may also provide an opportunity to meet and talk with someone like themselves.

The author often inquired, therefore, about why Mr. G could not get more pleasure from these available, although limited, outlets for sexual contact. These questions implicitly acknowledged to him that the author affirmed his need to express his sexuality, an attitude that rapidly helped to improve his mood and sense of well-being. It was a first but important step in helping him to find more gratification in his sexual encounters, which led after about 2 years of analysis to his being able to acknowledge to himself that he was homosexual.

Just as the anxiety of a heterosexual man in his relations with women may evolve from repressed early erotic fantasies and desire for the mother, failures in intimacy of gay men such as Mr. G may be caused by the repression and denial of their early erotic attachment to the father. For some homosexual adolescents and adults, the recovery of these early erotic memories may lead to rapid resolution of inhibitions in sexual functioning or in difficulties with intimate relations. Mr. G's early childhood, however, made the recovery of these memories difficult. His mother had explicitly deprecated his father, making Mr. G's desire for closeness to him humiliating and his erotic feelings for him abhorrent. The withdrawal of both parents after a brother's birth and his father's favoring that sibling, who was 3 years younger, were added humiliations. For some time, therefore, Mr. G could remember his father only as a vague and unimportant person in his early life. Feelings and recollections emerged only after he could recall the pain, disappointment, and rejection he experienced from his father's withdrawal, as well as his intense rivalry with his brother. Then there was a gradual emergence of longing for the father and some vague recollection of early sexual feelings for him.

The importance of Mr. G's feelings for the author in the transference in helping him gain access to his early erotic feelings for his father cannot be overestimated. It was in the immediacy of his relationship with the author that he was able to reexperience his earliest fantasies toward his father, which had heretofore been repressed. Furthermore,

Mr. G gradually became more and more capable of experiencing warmth and affection both from the author and for the author. This contributed to making it possible for him to have both sexual and affectionate feelings for the men he was meeting.

Mr. G and the author terminated therapy after more than 9 years of working together. He was beginning a relationship with a man. Mr. G was very much in love, and this helped him further consolidate and integrate his sexuality into an increasingly firm and good sense of himself. Mr. G and the author both believed that he now knew himself well enough to work without the author on any difficulties that might arise.

An accepting attitude in which the therapist shows thoughtfulness, caring, and regard for patients is as essential in working with gay men as with heterosexual individuals. Although not underestimating the value of questioning, of uncovering, and of the usual interpretive work of any analytical or dynamically oriented therapy, the author would like to stress that an attitude of positive regard makes therapeutic work possible because it enables patients to express and analyze negative transference distortions from both the past and the present. It also has therapeutic value because it is through the interaction with the therapist that any patient should acquire a new, more positive, and more accepting self-image.

Summary

In this chapter, the author has suggested that it is not possible to change the sexual orientation of gay patients and that such efforts are not consonant with the growing empirical evidence that homosexuality in men is both constitutional and heritable. Explicit or implicit efforts to change homosexual behavior to heterosexual behavior usually have serious emotional and social consequences. Therapists can provide a neutral therapeutic experience only if they have knowledge of the particular developmental issues of gay patients and how these may differ from the experiences of their heterosexual patients. An effective dynamic therapy should help a gay man overcome those roadblocks that may have interfered with the development of healthy self-esteem and the capacity for sexual and emotional intimacy with other men.

References

Bailey JM, Pillard RC: A genetic study of male sexual orientation. Arch Gen Psychiatry 48:1089–1096, 1991

Freud S: The psychogenesis of a case of homosexuality in a woman (1920), in Standard Edition of the Complete Psychological Works of Sigmund Freud, Vol 18. Translated and edited by Strachey J. London, Hogarth Press, 1955, pp 145–172

Friedman RC: Male Homosexuality: A Contemporary Psychoanalytic Perspective. New Haven, CT, Yale University Press, 1988

Hamer DH, Hu S, et al: A linkage between DNA markers on the X chromosome and male sexual orientation. Science 261:321–327, 1993

Hooker E: The adjustment of the male overt homosexual. Journal of Projective Techniques 21:18–31, 1957

Isay RA: On the analytic therapy of homosexual men. Psychoanal Study Child 40:235–254, 1985

Isay RA: The development of sexual identity in homosexual men. Psychoanal Study Child 41:467–489, 1986

Isay RA: Fathers and their homosexually inclined sons in childhood. Psychoanal Study Child 42:275–294, 1987

Kallman F: A comparative twin study on the genetic aspects of male homosexuality. J Nerv Ment Dis 115:283, 1952

LeVay S: A difference in hypothalamic structure between heterosexual and homosexual men. Science 253:1034–1037, 1991

LeVay S: The Sexual Brain. Cambridge, MA, MIT Press, 1993, pp 97–103

Pillard R, Weinrich J: Evidence of familial nature of male homosexuality. Arch Gen Psychiatry 43:808–812, 1986

Riess B: Psychological tests in homosexuality, in Homosexual Behavior. Edited by Marmor J. New York, Basic Books, 1980, pp 296–311

27

The Negative Therapeutic Reaction and Self-Hatred in Gay and Lesbian Patients

Jennifer I. Downey, M.D.
Richard C. Friedman, M.D.

During the past 15 years, it has become progressively apparent that antihomosexual prejudice is a major factor leading to diverse pathological symptoms and syndromes in gay and lesbian patients. The most commonly used term for irrational antihomosexual attitudes at present is "homophobia." Coined in the early 1970s, the term has been criticized because most prejudice against gay and lesbian people does not seem to result from influences that usually lead to or are associated with phobias. Moreover, much prejudicial behavior results from social influences and not necessarily from unconscious irrational conflict, as suggested by the label "homophobia" (Herek 1991). So many patients, families of patients, and clinicians use the term "homophobia," however, that like the term "gay," it seems to have acquired its present meaning through common usage. The authors continue to use it in this chapter, although they acknowledge that the term usually does not refer to a phobia, as generally defined in psychiatric texts, and is not an all-inclusive label of antihomosexual attitudes.

Shortly after homosexuality as a diagnostic category was voted to be deleted from the DSM (American Psychiatric Association 1968) by the American Psychiatric Association in 1973, an important conceptual advance in clinical psychodynamic theory about homophobia was put forth by Malyon (1982). He pointed out that gay and lesbian patients are routinely raised in heterosexist, homophobic environments. He reasoned that because socialization of children depends on internalization of culturally sanctioned attitudes and values, the internalizations made by children who later become homosexual adults must be to a large extent antihomosexual. Malyon observed that negative internalizations in turn influence "identity formation, self-esteem, the elaboration of defenses, patterns of cognition, psychological integrity, and object relations. Homophobic incorporations also embellish superego functioning and in this way contribute to a propensity for guilt and intropunitiveness among homosexual males" (p. 60). Malyon concluded that biased socialization leads to "internalized homophobia."

The recognition that gay and lesbian patients tend to experience prejudicial judgments made about themselves as a result of childhood influences on their moral development suggested a therapeutic strategy. The psychoanalyst Franz Alexander (Alexander and French 1946) had earlier noted that patients with irrationally determined negative attitudes about themselves often responded positively to therapeutic experiences that corrected the cognitive distortions in an emotionally meaningful way. Malyon applied Alexander's model of the "corrective emotional experience" to the therapeutic situation of gay and lesbian patients. He reasoned that such individuals would benefit from therapeutic experiences that would "correct" the irrational ideas associated with guilt and shame about being homosexual. Until Malyon's contributions, most psychoanalytically informed clinical writings had hypothesized that the "etiology" of homosexual desires in gay and lesbian patients was pathological and that all other symptoms were of secondary significance. Malyon stressed the contrary formulation—that homosexual feelings in gay and lesbian patients are not pathological and that psychopathology in these patients results from the deleterious effects of biased socialization. He pointed out that internalized homophobia was not the only possible cause of psychopathology, however, because gay and lesbian patients are as likely to suffer from diverse psychopathological syndromes as are other patients. For example, the same etiological factors produce schizophrenia in gay men as in heterosexual men. On the other hand, although biased socialization does not cause schizophrenia, schizophrenic gay patients are affected by it, as are all gay patients.

The type of corrective emotional experience Malyon envisioned for gay and lesbian patients was one in which their gay identity was *affirmed,* not condemned. The therapeutic perspective embodying these ideas has come to be called "gay-affirmative" in the clinical literature. Gay-affirmative therapeutic strategies have since been of enormous use to countless therapists and patients (Corbett 1993).

As is true of all types and strategies of therapy, however, some patients seem unresponsive to gay-affirmative interventions. Although statistics regarding the proportion of such patients in groups of gay and lesbian patients have not been reported, the authors' clinical experience suggests that the phenomenon of failure to benefit from gay-affirmative treatment is reasonably common. The most important clinical subgroup, and the one the authors discuss here, consists of those who manifest variants of what Freud (1923/1978) termed the "negative therapeutic reaction."

As Freud acquired clinical experience with the novel treatment he called "psychoanalysis," he observed that some people seemed to actually get worse, not better, during the attempted therapy. In 1923 he wrote:

> There are certain people who behave in a quite peculiar fashion during the work of analysis. When one speaks hopefully to them or expresses satisfaction with the progress of the treatment, they show signs of discontent and their condition invariably becomes worse. One begins by regarding this as defiance and as an attempt to prove their superiority to the physician, but later one comes to take a deeper and juster view. One becomes convinced, not only that such people cannot endure any praise or appreciation but that they react inversely to the progress of the treatment. Every partial solution that ought to result, and in other people does result in an improvement or a temporary suspension of symptoms produces in them for the time being an exacerbation of their illness; they get worse during the treatment instead of getting better. They exhibit what is known as a "negative therapeutic reaction." (1923/1978, p. 49)

Freud observed that because the patient has profound guilt that is *unconscious,* he or she attributes the reasons for the symptomatic worsening to other factors:

> . . . as far as the patient is concerned this sense of guilt is dumb; it does not tell him he is guilty; he does not feel guilty, he feels ill. This sense of guilt expresses itself only as a resistance to recovery which it is extremely difficult to overcome. It is also particularly difficult to convince the patient that this motive lies behind his continuing to be ill. . . . (1923/1978, p. 50)

Later psychoanalytic clinicians, elaborating upon Freud's initial observations, described additional psychodynamic influences contributing to the negative therapeutic reaction, including the inability of the patient to accept the analyst as a good object and the role of envy in addition to guilt, particularly in patients with narcissistic personality disorders (Glick and Meyers 1988). In describing the negative therapeutic reaction, Freud (1916/1978) himself seems to have extended observations he had earlier made about a group of patients who were unable to tolerate success. Like the patients discussed earlier, those who develop the negative therapeutic reaction have difficulty allowing others to be helpful to them, and often undermine positive relationships.

Clinicians who have discussed the negative therapeutic reaction have tended to confine their observations to its manifestations during psychoanalysis. Psychoanalysis is only one of many forms of therapy, however, in which the negative therapeutic reaction occurs. Because the negative therapeutic reaction results from intense unconscious guilt, it is not restricted to any specific type of treatment.

Gay-Affirmative Psychotherapy: The Difference Between Supportive and Uncovering Approaches

The distinction between supportive and insight-oriented therapy is of fundamental clinical importance to contemporary psychoanalytically oriented psychotherapists. The authors' experience with patients in whom the negative therapeutic reaction has impeded treatment has been predominantly with those treated with supportive psychotherapy, rather than with insight therapy. The supportive therapist tends to confront actively the patient's distortions and to challenge them with reality testing. Psychoeducation is freely used, and coping with present problems is stressed. The therapy sessions are more structured than in insight-oriented therapy. Although associations may be explored, extended periods of free association are discouraged. Therapists often present themselves as real people, and might use themselves as role models. For example, a gay therapist might tell a patient struggling with conflict about "coming out," "I can understand your feelings well; they remind me of feelings I had before I came out." The patient's tendency to distort his or her perception of the therapist in keeping with the principle of transference is inhibited in supportive psychotherapy. The therapist's active efforts to assist the patient carry the message, in addition to the messages verbally expressed, that the therapist is different from the patient's family and therefore can be trusted.

Insight-oriented therapy is often called "uncovering" treatment because its goal is to make conscious conflicts that previously were warded off from awareness. The therapy sessions are much less structured and the patient is encouraged to associate freely and to say whatever comes to mind. Transference distortions are explored and interpreted. In contrast to supportive therapy, dream interpretation is carried out whenever possible.

A gay-affirmative stance may be present in both types of therapy. A gay-affirmative supportive therapist, however, would immediately and vigorously challenge his or her patient's negative beliefs about homosexuality. A homophobic gay patient's tendency to avoid sexual relationships might be labeled self-destructive. The positive aspects of coming out might be stressed, and the therapist might report numerous instances in which coming out and getting involved in sexual interactions led to enhanced self-regard.

On the other hand, an insight-oriented therapist who is gay-affirmative would explore the meaning of a homophobic gay patient's negative beliefs about homosexuality. Only after painstaking and detailed uncovering of the network of associations, fantasies, and memories triggered by the homosexual self-representation would the negative connotations attributed to being homosexual be interpreted. Some therapists use a mixture of supportive and insight-oriented techniques.

Difference Between Primary and Secondary Internalized Homophobia: Implications for Treatment

Descriptive psychiatrists in the 1970s (Woodruff et al. 1971) found it helpful to distinguish between primary and secondary psychiatric disorders, and this distinction may usefully be applied to internalized homophobia. The necessity for the distinction arose because of the frequent occurrence of several psychiatric disorders in the same individual. A disorder was considered primary if it became manifest earliest in development. Thus an adult patient with substance abuse, generalized anxiety, and depression would be considered to have primary depression if he or she manifested the onset of a depressive disorder first and developed substance abuse and anxiety later in development.

The authors believe that as a way of thinking about the motivations for self-destructive behavior in gay and lesbian patients, the primary and secondary distinctions have diagnostic and prognostic significance. As a general rule, patients with primary internalized homophobia seem to respond positively to supportive gay-affirmative psychotherapeutic interventions. These patients do not generally develop negative therapeutic reactions. Most patients with negative therapeutic reactions, in the authors' experience, seem to fall into the subgroup of those with secondary internalized homophobia. The authors discuss and elaborate upon this clinical point below.

At present antihomosexual bias is so pronounced in American society that it is safe to hypothesize that all children are exposed to its effects. These have been widely discussed and include a range of social responses from disapproval to violent attack of those believed to be homosexual. Both sexes begin to experience negative social input toward homosexual people well before adolescence. Among boys this input is likely to come from same-aged peers as well as from persons in the larger society (Friedman and Downey 1994). Girls tend to have more variable experience in this respect. The age range during which the earliest manifestations of sexual orientation reach awareness for many children overlaps with the age range during which the child is exposed to antihomosexual bias. Negative internalizations about one's homosexual orientation occur commonly for this reason, and many clinicians believe that they are ubiquitous, at least in the United States.

Given the intense, prolonged negative social input, it is understandable that many gay and lesbian individuals experience self-hate and engage in self-destructive behavior. Despite this situation and the fact that elevated rates of past depression and substance abuse in homosexual individuals have been reported, it is of interest that neither rates of current depression nor completed suicide have been demonstrated to be elevated among gay men and lesbians in the general population (Friedman and Downey 1994). Among gay and lesbian patients who consult psychotherapists, however, manifestations of internalized homophobia such as depression are very common.

No statistics are available concerning the prognosis of such patients. The authors' impression, however, is that when the internalized homophobia is primary and when major psychopathology is not present—that is, Axis I and II disorders as defined in the DSM-IV (American Psychiatric Association 1994) are not present—most patients respond favorably to supportive gay-affirmative psychotherapeutic interventions. Such patients do not report that the early phases of childhood (up to age 7 years) were characterized by parental abuse or neglect or by the type of psychic trauma that often leads to chronic severe psychopathology. In fact, during early childhood years, the caretakers of many children who later develop internalized homophobia seem to be nurturing and endow the child with a sense of positive self-regard. It is only later, when the child is exposed to extrafamilial influences, that self-hatred develops, usually as a result of defensive partial identification with aggressors.

Patients such as these with primary homophobia begin psychotherapy with the basic capacities to love and work preserved, although this might be difficult to ascertain initially. The favorable therapeutic outcome is associated with a sense of identity cohesion, increased pride in being gay or lesbian, and frequently, active involvement in the gay and lesbian subculture.

In contrast are a group of patients with a certain type of secondary homophobia. These are patients whose early childhood years were characterized by abuse, neglect, or severe psychic trauma. These patients experience self-hate long before they are exposed to negative social input about homosexuality. Harsh or neglectful early experiences with caregivers provide a template for later relationships during their lives. These patients often develop stereotyped repetitive intimate relationships in which they provoke abuse from others (Glick and Meyers 1988). This pattern is likely to be reenacted during psychotherapy.

Although these patients provoke hostile responses from others and also project their own angry feelings onto others, they have no awareness of doing so. In fact, they tend to see themselves as innocent victims involved with powerful, cruel external objects. They tend to be flooded by feelings of hostile depression and helplessness. The patients often believe that present suffering magically fends off threats of annihilation from dreaded unconscious objects incorporated during childhood.

Most patients with negative therapeutic reactions seem to come from this group. Because their manifestation may be homophobic symptoms, the underlying character pathology may not be immediately apparent. Patients with this type of secondary internalized homophobia are just as likely to attribute their psychic distress to self-hatred because of homosexual desires as are patients with primary internalized homophobia.

Recognizing Negative Therapeutic Reactions in Patients

The diagnosis of a negative therapeutic reaction is made when deterioration in the clinical condition of the patient immediately follows apparent solutions to life difficulties that emerge in the treatment situation or optimistic expressions by the therapist about the patient's progress. Although the reaction may occur in homosexual, bisexual, or heterosexual patients, the authors' focus in this chapter is on the first group. The pattern is repetitive. The worsening of the patient may be primarily expressed in the relationship with the therapist, in life outside the therapeutic relationship, or as is more usually the case, in both. Typically, the patient preserves an idealized image of the therapist, thereby conveying the message that the problem lies not in the therapist but in the patient. For instance, the patient may say, "You are so capable, warm, and understanding that I feel grateful to be involved with you. But there is something intrinsically defective about me." The therapist often finds the patient likable, even admirable, at the beginning of the relationship. The patient's humility (which hides an underlying tendency toward self-debasement) may be initially confused with true altruism. As the repetitive pattern of psychopathology unfolds, however, the therapist is likely to feel progressively more angry toward the patient. This hostile reaction may trigger feelings of guilt, particularly if the therapist does not realize that it is a response to the patient's controlling maneuvers.

Internalized Homophobia Resulting From Unresolved Childhood Traumatic Stress Reaction

■ Case Example 1

A gay man of 34 years had feelings of inferiority in dealing with older men in the workplace who were authority figures and whom he presumed to be heterosexual. When he felt that these men were evaluating his performance unfavorably, he experienced nausea and chest pain as well as disabling anxiety symptoms. Medical workup for the physical symptoms had been negative. Because the patient did not appear to have severe psychopathology, the therapist had used a supportive approach. He had emphasized that the patient's professional performance was superior and that the patient irrationally minimized this because he was gay. The therapist stressed that there was no need to think less of oneself for being gay and that there was actually no evidence that the men to whom the patient responded were in fact homophobic. The patient's response to this strategy was to become paralyzed by anxiety, and consultation was requested.

Review of the patient's history revealed that his father, who had been perfectionistic and hard-driving, had had a myocardial infarction when the patient was 8 years old. The father's career was cut short by his sudden illness, and although he survived, he became bitter that his ambitions had not been fulfilled. The patient had been present during his father's heart attack and had vivid memories of his father complaining of crushing chest pain and becoming diaphoretic and nauseated. Hovering for many hours at his father's bedside during the convalescence, he had experienced an intense sense of his father's loss of power and status as a result of the illness.

Later this patient's father remained hypercritical toward him—involved but unaffectionate—and the patient had conflicting feelings of anger at his father's controlling behavior and guilt to be angry with a man so debilitated. He also thought that his father might be more satisfied with him if he were more "macho"—better at sports and other interests such as military history enjoyed by the father. Years later, he decided that his father had really not loved him because he was homosexual.

Actually many of the patient's symptoms, including hypochondriacal worries about his heart and guilty ruminations that he did not deserve praise for performance successes, were not a result of internalized homophobia at all, but were rather due to a reaction to a traumatic event and its prolonged aftermath. The patient attributed the origins of his guilty conscience to being homosexual. The primary basis for his childhood guilt, however, was not the presence of early homosexual desire, but rather, angry feelings toward his father and the magical belief that he had caused his father's cardiac illness. These feelings and beliefs were disguised and condensed in the conscious perception of conflicted feelings about being gay.

Psychiatric Diagnosis of the Patient With Negative Therapeutic Reaction

The negative therapeutic reaction may occur in patients who have psychiatric disorders ranging over the entire spectrum. Its manifestations in a particular patient, therefore, depend on the symptoms of the basic disorders for which that patient seeks treatment. For example, the symptoms of a bipolar patient with an eating disorder and those of a somaticizing patient with hypochondriacal worries are quite different from each other. Nonetheless, the negative therapeutic reaction might worsen symptoms in both.

It is particularly important to recognize personality disorders when they are present in patients with negative therapeutic reactions. The symptoms of personality disorder may be subtle, and their worsening may easily be attributed to some other cause. For example, borderline patients who are involved in turbulent, painful intimate relationships may attribute the cause of their difficulties to traits of the partner. The tendency of such patients to deny and project their unconscious conflicts, coupled with their sense of urgency, may lend an air of plausibility to their complaints. It requires meticulous review of the therapeutic process to determine that the actual precipitant of symptomatic worsening is a negative therapeutic reaction and not at all a change in behavior of the partner.

Gender Differences in the Manifestations of the Negative Therapeutic Reaction

Because of gender differences based in biology as well as in rearing and in social circumstances, men and women with comparable levels of personality organization, and even similar psychiatric diagnoses and degrees of internalized homophobia, may present clinically in quite different ways. The most dramatic difference the authors have seen is the tendency of the female patient to respond to conflict and anxiety by seeking to fuse with the object, whereas the male patient is more likely to seek distance. The following cases illustrate this difference:

■ Case Example 2

> An emotionally needy woman with a borderline character organization and frequent bouts of depression had been talking with her female therapist about her yearning to find a partner with whom to share her life. Past relationships had ended with furious outbursts on the patient's part after provocations by her. The therapist noted that the patient had cut her hair in a comparable style to hers, had bought a similar necklace, and had taken to wearing similar clothing. At this point, the patient met a woman at a social event, had sex with her the same night, and arrived at her session 3 days later announcing that the two were in love and had decided to move to a distant city together. Careful history taking revealed that the patient actually knew very little about her new partner. Among the sparse information available, however, were the facts that the partner had difficulty holding a job, few vocational skills, a history of substance abuse and brief episodes of prostitution, and that she had moved frequently, never living in one place for more than a year. She presented herself to the patient as someone who had endured "hard times" and had put these behind her, but she presented no actual evidence that she had done so. The patient had already given her small sums of money and had tentatively agreed to provide more substantial financial support in the future. The patient herself, however, had limited economic means.

In this case the patient who yearned for closeness with her female therapist and was secretly angry and disappointed not to enjoy more intimacy with her, first created a physical resemblance, then sought out a surrogate female partner whose appropriateness as a match for her was questionable at best. This relationship was immediately formalized by the decision to share a residence and to sever connections with all persons currently in the patient's life, including the therapist. The therapist saw that the patient had enacted her self-destructive scenario (a replaying of early childhood events in which her mother rejected her for her more physically attractive sister) both in her outside life and in the transference, because her action was a parody of the search for intimacy she had been discussing with her therapist. The therapeutic relationship proved strong enough that the patient was able to remain in treatment and eventually to find a more appropriate life partner.

■ Case Example 3

A 35-year-old man with similar psychodynamics came for treatment of depression after his partner of 5 years died of a lingering illness. After he had established a relationship with his older male therapist, he began to have periods of severe anxiety during scheduled separations from him. He dealt with these episodes by cruising and engaging in sexual activity with partners he did not know and whom he never saw again. This was not a pattern of behavior he had ever engaged in before. The therapist was impressed with the self-destructive quality of this behavior, which developed in the context of a deepening tie between patient and therapist.

Whereas the female patient displaced a wish for intimacy with the therapist and translated it into action with an inappropriate partner, the man defended against such a wish by participating in repetitive, distant interactions with a variety of partners. These gender differences are quite typical.

Men and women are *equally* likely to engage in a variety of other defensive behaviors, however, while evincing a negative therapeutic reaction. Thus patients of both genders may devalue the object (either in the transference or outside the therapy), demonstrate explosive hostility, provoke the therapist's concern by making puzzling errors of judgment, forget appointments or even the past therapeutic work, and so forth.

Treatment

Sometimes the negative therapeutic reaction occurs in patients whose underlying Axis I and Axis II psychiatric disorders have not been adequately treated. When this is the case, the major psychiatric disturbances should be treated and the status of the negative therapeutic reaction subsequently reassessed.

Once the negative therapeutic reaction has been recognized as a clear pattern of behavior, the strategy of psychotherapy should be shifted from supportive to uncovering. If the therapist has been using both techniques, the balance should be shifted away from supportive. The therapist must be able to resist his or her impulses to reassure the patient, such as by enacting well-intentioned but misguided rescue maneuvers. Such interventions, for which the patient may express verbal appreciation, are likely only to make the situation worse. Rather, the therapist must explore with the patient the meaning of his or her behavior. Such exploration may be tedious and anxiety-provoking because the patient may simultaneously engage in dramatically self-destructive activities. If life and limb are immediately threatened, the security of the patient is more important than adhering to a strategy of exploratory psychotherapy. Absent such emergencies, the authors have found that carefully teasing out the multiple determinants of the patient's self-destructive and self-defeating behavior offers the best promise of true therapeutic improvement.

Relatively inexperienced gay or lesbian therapists who may only recently have worked through their own conflicts about their homosexuality may find it particularly difficult to withhold reassurance from patients whose apparent helplessness cries out for it. It may seem cold and counterintuitive to encourage exploration of motivation in the face of what appears to be intense anguish. Yet when the assessment of the patient has been accurately made, such an approach is not only warranted, but in the authors' view it is the only therapeutic strategy that offers the possibility of success. Maintenance of an attitude of hopefulness and a continuing desire to work with the patient while remaining tolerant of provocations and setbacks are perhaps the most important features of the therapeutic stance necessary to help these troubled people.

References

Alexander F, French T: Psychoanalytic Therapy. New York, Ronald, 1946

American Psychiatric Association: Diagnostic and Statistical Manual of Mental Disorders, 2nd Edition. Washington, DC, American Psychiatric Association, 1968

American Psychiatric Association: Diagnostic and Statistical Manual of Mental Disorders, 4th Edition. Washington, DC, American Psychiatric Association, 1994

Corbett C (ed): Affirmative Dynamic Psychotherapy With Gay Men. Northvale, NJ, Jason Aronson, 1993

Freud S: Some character types met with in psychoanalytic work (1916), in Standard Edition of the Complete Psychological Works of Sigmund Freud, Vol 14. Translated and edited by Strachey J. London, Hogarth Press, 1978, pp 309–333

Freud S: The ego and the id (1923), in Standard Edition of the Complete Psychological Works of Sigmund Freud, Vol 19. Translated and edited by Strachey J. London, Hogarth Press, 1978, pp 3–66

Friedman RC, Downey JI: Special article: homosexuality. N Engl J Med 331:923–930, 1994

Glick RA, Meyers DI (eds): Masochism: Current Psychoanalytic Perspectives. Hillsdale, NJ, Analytic Press, 1988

Herek G: Stigma, prejudice, and violence against lesbians and gay men, in Homosexuality: Research Implications for Public Policy. Edited by Gonsiorek JC, Weinrich JD. Newbury Park, CA, Sage, 1991, pp 60–80

Malyon AK: Psychotherapeutic implications of internalized homophobia in gay men. J Homosex 7:59–69, 1982

Woodruff RA, Guze SB, Clayton PJ: Unipolar and bipolar primary affective disorder. Br J Psychiatry 119:33–38, 1971

28

Psychotherapeutic Interventions With Lesbian and Gay Couples

Robert P. Cabaj, M.D.
Rochelle L. Klinger, M.D.

Research on lesbians and gay men has steadily increased since the early 1970s, when homosexuality was removed from the list of psychopathological disorders. Most of this research, however, has been about individual gay men and lesbians, rather than about couples. When researchers did ask questions about gay relationships, they often focused exclusively on sexual aspects and ignored issues of love and commitment (Saghir and Robins 1973; Weinberg and Williams 1975). The lack of recognition of gay male and lesbian couples can be traced in part to researchers' difficulties in finding, defining, and accepting healthy gay male and lesbian couples. Since the early 1980s, the professional literature on gay men and lesbians has steadily grown, with some of it concerning couples. However, much of this literature is based on the clinical experience of therapists, rather than on empirical study of gay male and lesbian couples (Berzon 1988; Decker 1984; Kaufman et al. 1984; Klinger and Cabaj 1993; Krestan and Bepko 1990; McCandlish 1982; Roth 1985; Slater and

Mencher 1991). Experience has shown that clinical samples are rarely representative of normative development. Therefore, the clinician should view much of the literature as a good starting point for clinical practice and future research but should expect changes as more empirical studies of gay male, lesbian, and bisexual relationships are completed.

The nature and characteristics of lesbian and gay relationships, including the numbers of gay men and lesbians in relationships and the demographics of such couples, are described in Chapter 20 by Klinger and Chapter 19 by McWhirter and Mattison. Gay men and lesbians form and maintain relationships for the same reasons as their heterosexual counterparts. Relationships satisfy universal human needs for love, companionship, growth, acceptance, and sexual expression. Kurdek (1992, 1995) has explored the satisfaction of gay men and lesbians in relationships, the longevity of relationships, and the motivations to stay together. Unlike heterosexual couples, however, gay male and lesbian couples usually lack external support for their relationships from such sources as the law, religion, and their families of origin. Gay men and lesbians also rarely get the chance to practice dating in adolescence as heterosexual individuals do; if they first "come out" later in life, they may experience the rapid ups and downs of falling in and out of love that usually occur in adolescence (Carl 1990).

It is important for the therapist not to impose his or her own ideas of what constitutes a relationship. Traditional marriage, based on ancient concepts of preserving property and bloodlines, involves a lifetime commitment to the same person. From this concept, assumptions are made that coupling is necessary for happiness or fulfillment and that long-term relationships are best (Carl 1990). This pattern is not necessarily true for all gay male or lesbian couples, or for all heterosexual couples for that matter. Many same-sex relationships closely resemble traditional heterosexual marriages—two people committed to each other and living together. However, many other configurations are seen in the gay and lesbian community, including couples committed to each other but not living together; individuals who see themselves as a couple, but who have more than one significant partner; or gay or lesbian relationships coexisting with heterosexual marriage. The pattern of commitment but separate living arrangements may be more common among gay male couples; in one study, more than half of gay men who stated they had a partner did not live with him (Jay and Young 1979). The best definition of a gay or lesbian relationship is made by the individuals who are involved in it.

Reasons for Seeking Therapy

Gay men and lesbians in relationships may seek therapy for reasons that are common to all couples or for reasons unique to people in same-sex relationships. Examples of universal reasons include communication difficulties, sexual problems, infidelity, excessive arguing, substance abuse, physical abuse, and help in staying together or separating. Even these familiar reasons, however, are influenced by the external and internal challenges faced by same-sex couples in a homophobic society. Some reasons to seek therapy specific to same-sex couples might be employment or other competition between the two individuals of the same gender; coming out as a gay or lesbian couple to family members or work colleagues; jealousy and envy regarding sexual experiences outside the relationship for couples that had agreed to have a sexually open relationship; and help in determining how to have a child in a same-sex relationship.

Specific psychological factors influence the presentation of gay men and lesbians in couples. Same-sex couples obviously consist of two women or two men, and the additive effects of female or male socialization produce unique issues in lesbian or gay male couples. For example, a growing body of literature has noted that women are generally socialized to be more relational than men (Chodorow 1978; Gilligan 1982; Miller 1976). Many therapists, combining this relational trait in women with their own clinical experience, believe lesbian couples have high levels of relatedness, which if excessive, may cause fusion or merger to be a common clinical presentation (Kaufman et al. 1984; Krestan and Bepko 1990; Roth 1985). Kurdek (1987), in studying nonclinical couples, however, did not find a higher level of relatedness or fusion among lesbian couples than among gay male couples. Parallel societal expectations for men emphasize independence and differentiation and may result in difficulties in forming intimate bonds and sharing in decision-making (see Chapter 24 by Stein and Cabaj).

Another factor unique to same-sex couples is the need for each individual to progress through the coming-out process and to confront his or her internalized homophobia. Difficulties in these areas for either or both partners can have profound effects on the functioning of the couple. Obviously, there is no parallel for heterosexual couples, who grow up in a world that supports their sexual orientation.

Several special therapeutic issues that affect gay men and lesbians individually and in couples deserve mention here. All the clinical issues are covered in greater detail in other chapters in this volume. The effect of HIV has been felt in some way by almost all gay men and lesbians. Many gay male couples have one or both partners with an HIV infection, and most gay male and lesbian couples know someone affected by HIV. It is therefore important to include inquiries about knowledge of HIV, safer sex practices, and serostatus in interviews with gay male and lesbian couples. Substance abuse and domestic violence are other common issues that prompt gay male and lesbian couples to seek therapy. In addition, therapists should be aware of the special issues facing bisexual men and women in relationships, and the particular concerns of gay men, lesbians, and bisexual individuals who are in relationships as adolescents, elders, or members of cultural or ethnic minority groups.

Evaluation and Assessment

■ Four Dimensions of Assessment

With the multiple factors described above to consider, an evaluation of a gay or lesbian couple can be a complex process. A thorough assessment is needed, however, to formulate the best treatment plan, if treatment is indeed recommended. To help simplify the process, the evaluation can be approached from a four-dimensional matrix that will clarify both societal and psychodynamic issues (Cabaj 1988). This assessment matrix is based on both the staging model for relationships, developed by McWhirter and Mattison (1984a), and the social exchange theory model, applied by Peplau (1991) to gay and lesbian couples.

First dimension—evaluation of the individuals.   The evaluator needs to determine the stage in the life cycle for each individual, on the basis of not just the age of the individual, but also on the level of life achievements and sense of comfort with self. In addition, cultural and ethnic factors will clearly have an influence; the evaluator needs to understand which factors are shared and which are different. Finally, the various personal psychological concerns for each individual need to be considered, including any psychiatric illnesses or personality styles that are notable. Great differences in ages, cultural or ethnic backgrounds, socioeconomic levels, occupational levels, and parental or marital status influence the internal dynamics, interactions, and life of the couple.

Second dimension—gay and lesbian development.   The evaluator also needs to determine the degree of coming out for each individual, the progress each individual has made in moving from self-awareness of being gay or lesbian to becoming comfortable with this awareness, and finally, to letting others know about it. The evaluation should also include an assessment of internalized homophobia, the level of personal comfort or discomfort each individual has with being gay or lesbian. Finally, the evaluator should know how "out" each partner is by ascertaining who knows about the individual's sexual orientation and in what context, and should also understand how out as a gay or lesbian couple the couple itself is.

Third dimension—staging the relationship.   As described in greater detail in Chapter 19 by McWhirter and Mattison, gay male couples can be viewed as progressing through a series of stages. Although discussed first for gay male couples (McWhirter and Mattison 1984a), the stages may also apply, with some alterations, to lesbian couples as well as to heterosexual and bisexual relationships (Cabaj 1988). Briefly, the stages can be summarized and characterized as the following:

Stage I: Blending, marked by merging, romantic love, equalization, and high sexual intensity and activity
Stage II: Nesting, marked by homemaking, compatibility, as well as ambivalence and decreased romantic love and sexual activity
Stage III: Maintaining, marked by reemergence of the individual, with risk-taking and increased conflicts but establishing traditions
Stage IV: Building, marked by collaborating, increasing productivity and independence but ability to count on partner
Stage V: Releasing, marked by trusting, merging of finances and possessions as well as taking the partner for granted
Stage VI: Renewing, marked by security, inward dwelling and remembering, and restoring the partnership

As described by McWhirter and Mattison (1984a), these stages and movement through them are quite fluid and somewhat tied to the longevity of the couple, but they are influenced as well by age, health factors, and social pressures. The individuals in a particular relationship will most probably move through the stages at different rates, leading to possible stage discrepancies. Thus the evaluator needs to assess what stage the couple is in and if the stage is appropriate for the time the couple has been together, and to note any differences between individuals in what stage of the relationship he or she seems to be.

Fourth dimension—external issues.   The evaluator should also consider external or additional influences and factors such as substance abuse, HIV-related issues, concerns about children, pressures from families of origin, married spouses, and financial problems.

◼ Assessment and Treatment Recommendations

Assessment of the couple and the individual partners through the use of these four dimensions will shape the treatment approach, treatment plan, and level of intensity of the intervention needed. Depending on the results of the evaluation, short- or long-term therapy, either supportive or insight-oriented, may be recommended (Forstein 1986); or a more limited intervention such as psychoeducational sessions may be all that is needed. It is not the therapist's role to determine whether a couple should remain together; therapy will not decide if two individuals should be coupled, but rather, it may help the couple to deal with some of the difficulties involved with intimacy, loving, and communication, allowing the individuals in the couple to decide whether they will remain together.

In beginning therapy or counseling, persons in all types of relationships usually need help with communication, and many may benefit from reading books that help them do some of the work on improving communication without the help of a therapist (Berzon 1988). Many couples report that they assume what the other person thinks or fears, and they may be afraid to ask or ascertain things directly. Often education about the stages couples go through or discussion about the compatibility of two people of the same gender with similar societal gender role expectations may provide sufficient treatment intervention (McWhirter and Mattison 1984b; Roth 1985), but the need for more intensive work to resolve conflicts around stage discrepancies or problems with merging of same-sex couples with similar gender role issues may require psychotherapy.

Because for most people the parental relationship serves as the primary and internalized model of how a couple functions, many gay men and lesbians find themselves in patterns similar to those in their families of origin, even when it was quite apparent to the individuals that those patterns were dysfunctional. It may be difficult for both the couple and the therapist to see these patterns, as it may seem counterintuitive to impose an opposite-sex model on a same-sex relationship (Cabaj 1988).

Diagnosis and Special Circumstances

The completed evaluation of the couple will help clarify the best treatment plan. There are some diagnostic concerns, however, that need to be considered before final treatment is planned and implemented.

▮ Concurrent Mental Illness

If the psychopathology of one of the individuals is severe enough, whether it be a DSM-IV Axis I or Axis II (American Psychiatric Association 1994) defined mental illness, that condition may require treatment first, before the relationship problems can be addressed. The same is true for active substance abuse by one or both partners. Because substance abuse seems to occur more frequently among gay men and lesbians than among their heterosexual counterparts (see Chapter 47 by Cabaj; Cabaj 1992), a same-sex couple is likely to present with substance abuse or a concern about the use of alcohol or other drugs. Psychotherapy without adjunct support through 12-step programs such as Alcoholics Anonymous, Al-Anon, or Narcotics Anonymous may increase the abuse and foster codependency and avoidance. Severe posttraumatic stress disorders or reactions to past sexual abuse of one partner may also need to be treated individually first in order to reduce symptoms and to allow the couple to undertake joint work.

▮ Domestic Violence

Domestic violence, defined as any pattern of behavior designed to coerce, dominate, isolate, or maintain control within a relationship, exists in some gay and lesbian relationships (see Chapter 48 by Klinger and

Stein). One survey of racially, ethnically, and geographically diverse women (Bradford and Ryan 1988) found that 22% of lesbians had been victims of domestic violence as adults, with half of these experiencing it at the hands of a lesbian partner. Among gay male couples, 15%–25% report domestic violence (Island and Letellier 1991). Abuse can take the form of physical violence, psychological harassment, sexual abuse and rape, destruction of property, and other forms of control, including economic and financial dependency on one partner. Couples treatment is generally not advisable when active battering is ongoing (Klinger 1991; Leeder 1988).

■ HIV Concerns

Individuals in relationships who are considering whether to take the HIV antibody test may present this issue during an evaluation of the couple. Partners need to decide whether one or both will be tested and, if both, whether they will be tested together. They will need to anticipate the impact on the relationship of learning that one or both are HIV-positive and to understand their motivations for being tested. This may occur at a time when men disclose sexual contacts outside the relationship, precipitating further problems in trust and communication. Newly formed couples may use taking the test as a type of bonding ceremony, or it may symbolize an expression of honesty and commitment in the relationship.

Discordant couples, in which one member is HIV-positive and one is negative, pose different challenges to the evaluator and therapist. The infected partner may constantly fear being left, or may be overly dependent or defensively counterdependent in relation to the uninfected partner. Conversely, the uninfected partner may be overly solicitous or may emotionally or physically abandon the infected person. Safer sex is crucial to discuss and negotiate with these couples.

■ Case Example 1

Mr. A and Mr. B met 6 months ago, started dating, and had a few very safe sex encounters (mutual masturbation). Both had tested HIV-negative over 1 year ago. They convinced each other of the need to be tested again, to allow more open and relaxed sexual interaction, and to herald the possible start of a committed relationship. The testing results, however, did not follow their expectations: Mr. A continued to test HIV-negative, but Mr. B now tested positive. The men sought psychiatric help as a couple to deal with this crisis. The evaluation helped them explore their fears, anger, and hurt, as well as their sense of betrayal, deception, and lack of trust. They decided, however, to remain together and to take care of each other, and they terminated therapy.

Acceleration or compression of the stages in gay male relationships can occur when HIV infection is present. This can sometimes be helpful in furthering intimacy, but at times it can also lead to missing essential stages or highlight dysfunction. For example, advancing infection in one or both partners can block the reemergence of the individual that occurs in the maintaining stage, or it can inhibit the independence associated with the building stage. The partners can then be drawn together prematurely, before they have established their individual identities. Psychotherapy may or may not be needed, depending on the nature of the HIV-related concerns presented by the couple. Referrals to support groups and caretaker support groups may be indicated in some instances (Walker 1991).

▪ Stage Discrepancies

The concept of stage development in relationships and the associated concept of stage discrepancy, which occurs when individuals in a relationship are at different stages, may also be useful for understanding the origins of conflicts (McWhirter and Mattison 1984b). Of particular importance are the transitions between stages, such as going from blending of the individuals in the early phase to the reemergence of the individuals in the later stages.

At the start of relationships, the early, intense feelings of love, romance, and intense sexual drive lead most individuals to blend or merge in some fashion. During this stage, the partners may seem ideal to each other, but as time goes by and as the intensity of the early love fades, the partners see each other more realistically. Individual needs and desires reemerge, along with differences and conflicts. These developments may be hard to understand, possibly being seen as signs of loss of love or of the end of the relationship. At this point, reasons for remaining together other than sex and passion become increasingly important; deeper love and building together are necessary if the relationship is to develop.

Individuals will progress through relationships at different rates. One partner may be ready to begin maintaining, that is, reemerging as an individual with his or her own personal needs, while the other partner may still be nesting or blending, feeling more merged or dependent. Each partner's level of maturity, stage in the life cycle, and ability to function as an independent individual influence these processes.

■ Case Example 2

Mr. C, a 38-year-old man, and Mr. D, a 27-year-old man, had been in a relationship for over 6 years. Mr. D decided to return to graduate school, and he began to notice a sense of strain and tension when he was with Mr. C. He felt that Mr. C lacked ambition and was possibly too dependent on him, as expressed by his wanting to know all about school and whether he was making new friends. They began to have fights, and sexual activity decreased from twice weekly to very infrequently. Mr. C asked for an evaluation as a couple because he was confused about why Mr. D suddenly seemed distant; he feared that the relationship had somehow ended without his awareness. The evaluation was brief, mainly clarifying the communication patterns and relationship expectations; the stage discrepancy model was described and was enthusiastically embraced by the couple. With this new understanding, the couple decided to try to work things out on their own.

■ Intimacy: Merger and Distance

Males in our society are taught, in general, to be independent and not to be very intimate. Two males, with culturally defined norms of "maleness," who are trying to deal with issues of power, control, intimacy, and boundaries within a relationship, may need help in trying to overcome these barriers. In contrast, lesbian partners may be pushed toward blending and merger, primarily as a result of opposite-gender socialization expectations. When partners give up their individuality, the ebb and flow of connection and separation present in true intimacy may become difficult or even impossible. Many gay male couples who have issues concerning how to remain close or how to increase compatibility after the nesting stage fades may need help with how to be intimate; in contrast, many lesbian couples who are unable to get beyond the blending or nesting stages may benefit from use of the specific technique of "distancing for intimacy" (Burch 1986, 1987; Kaufman et al. 1984) to help them achieve intimacy and independence while maintaining strong boundaries.

Treatment

Treatment of the lesbian or gay male couple begins after adequate assessment and diagnosis, as outlined above. On the basis of the clinician's assessment of the couple, traditional conjoint therapy with both members present may or may not be the best strategy. In some cases, individual, family, or group therapy may be more useful than couples treatment.

■ Individual Therapy

As noted above, individual treatment is indicated any time one person's psychopathology interferes with the couple's healthy functioning. Individual treatment or intervention is imperative under the following conditions: suicidal or homicidal ideation in either or both partners, the presence of domestic violence, and couples who have serious problems with merger. The following case illustrates the last situation:

■ Case Example 3

Ms. E and Ms. F have been in a committed relationship for 5 years. They are both attorneys at the same firm and work in close proximity. They had spent all their working and leisure time together. They presented for an evaluation as a couple after Ms. F became very attracted to a mutual friend, but she had not acted on the attraction. The couple described how they spent almost all their social and work-related time together, had not traveled independently since they met, and shared each other's clothes. Each partner tended to fill in answers for the other during the interview. Maladaptive merger was diagnosed and was explained to the couple, and individual therapy for each partner was recommended. At first they did not agree with the recommendation, wanting conjoint therapy instead, but eventually they agreed to try individual treatment. Over a 6-month period, slow but steady progress was made on each person's individuation, with subsequent improvement in the couple's functioning.

■ Couples Therapy

Before working with any couple, regardless of sexual orientation, the therapist needs to understand and be able to apply clinically theoretical models of family and systems therapy, including the approaches of Bowen (1978), Haley (1987), and Minuchin (1974). Systems theory views the couple as part of multiple interacting systems. Couples function most effectively in systems with clear hierarchies and boundaries. Often the couples therapist is called upon to reestablish boundaries and hierarchies between people in the system in order to enhance the couple's functioning (Minuchin 1974). The lack of societal recognition and legal supports for gay male and lesbian couples may make boundary issues particularly problematic for these couples. Failure of one or both partners to differentiate fully from their families of origin can also contribute to what Bowen called "triangulating" and to subsequent dysfunction in the couple (Bowen 1988). Case 3 provides an example of triangulating, in which Ms. F attempted to bring a third person into the couple.

Carl (1990) distinguished between symptom-oriented couples therapy, in which the couple presents with a symptom or problem such as HIV in one partner, and relationship-oriented therapy, which deals with interactional relationship issues in the couple. Most couples present with a symptom but may still benefit from relationship-focused couples therapy. Therapy may help the couple to stay together but may also help them to separate in an effective way with as few unresolved issues as possible. It is important for the therapist to remain neutral about the outcome to avoid being "triangulated" into the couple.

After assessing the couple's structure, outside influences, life cycle position, and family of origin issues, the therapist should intervene with the couple (Carl 1990). Interventions can include education, homework assignments, and practicing with new structures and strategies in the sessions. Case 4 is an example of interventions used with one gay male couple:

■ Case Example 4

Mr. G and Mr. H had been together for 12 years. They had begun living together when Mr. H was 18, after he had been forced to leave his parents' house after coming out to them. Mr. G was 15 years older than Mr. H. Until recently, Mr. G had supported Mr. H from his income as a regional sales manager, and Mr. H had worked only intermittently in jobs paying a minimum wage. However, 2 years before presentation, Mr. H had begun a career-oriented job and had been promoted rapidly. Mr. G initially presented individually with new-onset anxiety as Mr. H spent more and more time away from home on business. The therapist asked for Mr. H to accompany Mr. G on the next visit. In that meeting, it became clear that Mr. G was reacting adversely to the change in hierarchy and boundaries within the relationship, while Mr. H was thriving. This observation was presented to the couple. After some exploration, Mr. H felt strongly that he needed to leave the relationship to continue to grow on his own. The remaining therapy sessions focused on helping them to work through feelings and to end the relationship effectively.

■ Family Therapy

Family therapy with the couple and either families of origin, children, or both is indicated for some gay male or lesbian couples. Examples of situations in which family therapy may be prescribed include helping couples deal with blended family issues when children live with them; helping families of origin deal with their gay, lesbian, or HIV-infected offspring in same-sex relationships; and helping gay male or lesbian couples with children separate and negotiate visitation and custody in the absence of external support. Therapists need to be very aware of their own attitudes and countertransference in the clinically complex situation of family therapy with lesbians, bisexual individuals, and gay men.

■ Group Therapy

Group therapy is a powerful therapeutic tool that is often underutilized. Several types of groups may be indicated for gay male or lesbian couples. Support groups are often recommended for individuals and couples dealing with HIV. Also, when substance abuse is present, 12-step programs can be very helpful. Many metropolitan areas have gay 12-step programs, which are usually preferred by gay men and lesbians to general groups.

Many couples have multiple issues, such as a combination of internalized homophobia, substance abuse, and HIV issues. Therefore, an approach that involves a combination of treatment modalities is often used. For example, a combination of couples therapy, individual therapy for one or both partners, and 12-step treatment may be prescribed.

Outcome Studies and Future Research

As noted earlier, most of the literature on therapy with gay male or lesbian couples consists of reports from therapists' caseloads. Few of these couples are followed up after treatment to determine long-term outcome. At this point, no formal treatment outcome studies on psychotherapy with gay male or lesbian couples have been completed. This neglected area of study is probably a reflection of the low priority given to research about gay male and lesbian issues in couples therapy.

Empirical research is available on normal development of gay male and lesbian couples (Berger 1990; Kurdek and Schmitt 1986; Kurdek 1987, 1991; McWhirter and Mattison 1984a). Future empirical studies should focus on gay male and lesbian couples in treatment and the long-term outcome of couples therapy with them.

Conclusion

Although many gay and lesbian couples seek an openly gay or lesbian therapist, working with such a therapist provides no guarantee of success. The acceptance, openness, and nonjudgmental attitudes of the therapist—gay or straight—toward the gay male or lesbian couple, and not the sexual orientation of the therapist, are the most important factors determining successful psychotherapeutic work (Cabaj 1991). The clinician, of course, must have a basic knowledge of and experience with couples and family therapy and must have available the additional information and awareness the authors have described.

Gay men and lesbians have the same types and rates of emotional disturbances and mental illness as the general population, but the unique psychosocial stresses that gay men and lesbians experience may influence the presentation of their illnesses and symptoms, and they help shape the types of concerns that lead couples to seek help. The authors have described some of the unique issues for gay men and lesbians that will shape, and even challenge, work with gay and lesbian couples: two people of the same sex with same sex-role expectations; homophobia, both internal and external; and the developmental steps for gay and lesbian individuals and couples. Finally, the clinician needs to be aware of the influence that HIV infection and AIDS, substance abuse, family relationships, the presence of children, minority and cultural differences, and domestic and societal violence have on work with gay and lesbian couples.

References

American Psychiatric Association: Diagnostic and Statistical Manual of Mental Disorders, 4th Edition. Washington, DC, American Psychiatric Association, 1994

Berger RM: Men together: understanding the gay couple. J Homosex 91:31–49, 1990

Berzon B: Permanent Partners: Building Gay and Lesbian Relationships That Last. New York, EP Dutton, 1988

Bowen M: Family Therapy in Clinical Practice. New York, Aronson, 1988

Bradford J, Ryan C: The National Lesbian Health Care Survey. Washington, DC, National Lesbian and Gay Health Foundation, 1988

Burch B: Psychotherapy and the dynamics of merger in lesbian couples, in Contemporary Perspectives on Psychotherapy With Lesbians and Gay Men. Edited by Stein TS, Cohen CC. New York, Plenum, 1986, pp 57–72

Burch B: Barriers to intimacy: conflicts over power, dependency, and nurturing in lesbian relationships, in Lesbian Psychologies. Edited by the Boston Lesbian Psychologies Collective. Urbana, IL, University of Illinois Press, 1987, pp 126–141

Cabaj RP: Gay and lesbian couples: lessons on human intimacy. Psychiatric Annals 18(1):21–25, 1988

Cabaj RP: Overidentification with a patient, in Gays, Lesbians and Their Therapists: Studies in Psychotherapy. Edited by Silverstein C. New York, WW Norton, 1991, pp 31–39

Cabaj RP: Substance abuse among gays and lesbians, in Substance Abuse: A Comprehensive Textbook, 2nd Edition. Edited by Lowinson JH, Ruiz P, Millman RB. Baltimore, MD, Williams & Wilkins, 1992, pp 852–860

Carl D: Counseling Same-Sex Couples. New York, WW Norton, 1990

Chodorow N: The Reproduction of Mothering: Psychoanalysis and the Sociology of Gender. Berkeley, CA, University of California Press, 1978

Decker B: Counseling gay and lesbian couples. Journal of Social Work and Human Sexuality 2(2–3):39–52, 1984

Forstein M: Psychodynamic psychotherapy with gay male couples, in Contemporary Perspectives on Psychotherapy With Lesbians and Gay Men. Edited by Stein TS, Cohen CC. New York, Plenum, 1986, pp 103–137

Gilligan C: In a Different Voice. Cambridge, MA, Harvard University Press, 1982

Haley J: Problem-Solving Therapy, 2nd Edition. San Francisco, CA, Jossey-Bass, 1987

Island D, Letellier P: Men Who Beat the Men Who Love Them: Battered Gay Men and Domestic Violence. New York, Harrington Park Press, 1991

Jay K, Young A: The Gay Report. New York, Summit Books, 1979

Kaufman P, Harrison E, Hyde M: Distancing for intimacy in lesbian relationships. Am J Psychiatry 141:530–533, 1984

Klinger RL: Treatment of a lesbian batterer, in Gays, Lesbians, and Their Therapists: Studies in Psychotherapy. Edited by Silverstein C. New York, WW Norton, 1991, pp 126–142

Klinger RL, Cabaj RP: Characteristics of gay and lesbian relationships, in American Psychiatric Press Review of Psychiatry, Vol 12. Edited by Oldham JM, Riba MB, Tasman A. Washington, DC, American Psychiatric Press, 1993, pp 101–125

Krestan J, Bepko C: The problem of fusion in the lesbian relationship. Family Process 19:272–289, 1990

Kurdek LA: Sex roles, self schema and psychological adjustment in coupled homosexual and heterosexual men and women. Sex Roles 17:549–621, 1987

Kurdek LA: The dissolution of gay and lesbian couples. Journal of Social and Personal Relationships 8:265–278, 1991

Kurdek LA, Schmitt JP: Relationship quality of partners in heterosexual married, heterosexual cohabitating, and gay and lesbian relationships. Journal of Personality and Social Psychology 51:711–720, 1986

Kurdek LA: Relationship stability and relationship satisfaction in co-habitating gay and lesbian couple: a prospective longitudinal test of the contextual and interdependence models. Journal of Social and Personal Relationships 9:125–142, 1992

Kurdek LA: Lesbian and gay relationships, in Lesbian, Gay, and Bisexual Identities Over the Lifespan: Psychological Perspectives. Edited by D'Augelli AR, Patterson CJ. New York, Oxford University Press, 1995, pp 243–261

Leeder E: Enmeshed in pain: counseling lesbian battering couples. Women and Therapy 7(1):81–89, 1988

McCandlish BM: Therapeutic issues with lesbian couples, in A Guide to Psychotherapy With Gay and Lesbian Clients. Edited by Gonsiorek JC. New York, Harrington Press, 1982, pp 71–78

McWhirter DP, Mattison AM: The Male Couple: How Relationships Develop. Englewood Cliffs, NJ, Prentice-Hall, 1984a

McWhirter DP, Mattison AM: Psychotherapy for male couples: an application of the staging theory, in Innovations in Psychotherapy With Homosexuals. Edited by Hetrick ES, Stein TS. Washington, DC, American Psychiatric Press, 1984b, pp 115–131

Miller JB: Toward a New Psychology of Women. Boston, MA, Beacon, 1976

Minuchin S: Families and Family Therapy. Cambridge, MA, Harvard University Press, 1974

Peplau LA: Lesbian and gay relationships, in Homosexuality: Research Implications for Public Policy. Edited by Gonsiorek JC, Weinrich JD. Newbury Park, CA, Sage, 1991

Roth SA: Psychotherapy with lesbian couples: individual issues, female socialization, and the social context. Journal of Marital and Family Therapy 11:273–286, 1985

Saghir MT, Robins E: Male and Female Homosexuality: A Comprehensive Investigation. Baltimore, MD, Williams and Wilkins, 1973

Slater S, Mencher J: The lesbian family life cycle: a contextual approach. Am J Orthopsychiatry 61:372–383, 1991

Walker G: In the Midst of Winter: Systemic Therapy With Family, Couples and Individuals With AIDS Infection. New York, WW Norton, 1991

Weinberg MS, Williams CJ: Male Homosexuals: Their Problems and Adaptations. New York, Penguin, 1975

Lesbian, Gay, and Bisexual Families

Issues in Psychotherapy

Terry S. Stein, M.D.

Weinberg and Williams (1974) reported that during the 1960s, 71% of the gay men in their study were living with partners. Bell and Weinberg (1978) subsequently reported that in the 1970s, 82% of the lesbians they studied were living with another woman. In addition, estimates suggest that there are up to 3 million lesbian mothers (Pennington 1987) and more than 1 million gay fathers (Bozett 1987a) in the United States, who together have 6 million or more children (Bozett 1987a; Schulenburg 1985). Furthermore, like their heterosexual counterparts, all lesbians, bisexual individuals, and gay men have grown up in some type of family structure and continue to exist in networks of friendships and intimate relationships throughout their lives.

In her book *Families We Choose* (1991), Weston wrote that "claiming a lesbian or gay identity has been portrayed as a rejection of the 'family' and a departure from kinship" (p. 22). She described how this portrayal is undergirded by assumptions that lesbians and gay men do not have children or participate in long-term relationships and are invariably alienated from their biological families. The reduction of gay men and lesbians to only a sexual identity further serves to isolate them from social and intimate bonds. This line of reasoning has been used to create a political, legal, and moral opposition between homosexuality and the family. In spite of such negative and stereotypical portrayals, millions of lesbians, bisexual individuals, and gay men, in fact, live their lives as active participants in intimate relationships and family structures.

Lesbians, bisexual individuals, and gay men live and love within several types of family organizations in addition to couples, including divorced mothers and fathers, who may or may not have partners and may or may not be living with their children; single parents or same-gender couples who decide to have children; gay and lesbian children who are living with or relating to their parents; lesbian, bisexual, and gay individuals who are in heterosexual marriages or committed relationships and have children; extended biological families; and families of choice. In this volume the most basic type of gay and lesbian families, same-sex couples, are discussed in separate chapters (see Chapter 19 by McWhirter and Mattison and Chapter 28 by Cabaj and Klinger).

Problems and Stressors

A growing body of literature about the families of lesbians, bisexual individuals, and gay men (Barret and Robinson 1990; Bozett 1987b; Bozett and Sussman 1990; Slater and Mencher 1991; Patterson 1992) describes a consistent set of problems with which these families must contend. Although the research on the subject thus far has tended to focus on lesbian mothers and their children, similar problems arise for gay fathers and their children (Bozett 1987b). The concerns of gay and lesbian youth in their families have only recently begun to be identified (Boxer et al. 1991; Herdt 1989; Herdt and Boxer 1993); these concerns represent issues that are developmentally distinct from, but thematically parallel to, those presented by adult gay men and lesbians in their families.

Slater and Mencher (1991) discussed a series of recurrent stressors for the lesbian family, including challenges to their viability and lack of societal validation, persistent internalized homophobia, a need to negotiate private versus public identities, and a requirement for negotiation of roles. Each of these stressors acts on the lesbian family within a broader context of societal condemnation and oppression. Among lesbian couples, concerns about boundaries (Rohrbaugh 1992) and disclosure of sexual orientation (Levy 1992) are also widespread. In addition to the problems specifically associated with sexual orientation, these families must contend with the same issues confronting traditional families. For example, the effects of divorce by gay fathers or lesbian mothers who were previously in heterosexual marriages can be profound, and blended families present significant challenges to any family group, whether the parents are gay, bisexual, lesbian, or heterosexual.

The family therapy and family life-cycle literature has largely ignored the gay and lesbian family. Family theorists describe normative stages of development that are generally organized around having children and parenting, and family dynamics are assumed to exist within a larger society that validates, through laws, customs, and rituals, the inherent value and viability of the family and family relationships. In contrast, the societal context for the gay or lesbian family is one of condemnation and exclusion. DiLapi (1989) presented a "motherhood hierarchy" as a conceptual framework for understanding the stigmatization of lesbian mothers, who are at the bottom of the hierarchy; lesbians are viewed as inappropriate mothers because of the belief in an antilesbian mythology about characteristics attributed to lesbians that are inconsistent with motherhood. Thus gay and lesbian families must constantly interact with a larger society that either ignores or devalues them and frequently tries to destroy their connections by removing their children and controlling adult relationships.

■ Case Example 1

Ms. A, a lesbian mother who had custody of her children, was brought to court by her former husband because she had been living with her female partner for several years. Psychologists testified on behalf of the father that the children did not have any emotional problems and a psychiatrist brought in by Ms. A's lawyer as an expert witness testified that no evidence existed to suggest that the children would be harmed by living with their mother and her partner; in spite of these statements, the judge ruled that she would lose custody of her children if the partner continued to live in the home. After several unsuccessful appeals and actual removal of the children from the home, Ms. A and her partner were forced to buy a second home, in which the partner could reside, so that the children could continue to live with their mother.

Without visible role models and when confronted by a hostile society, many lesbian and gay families may turn inward and conceal their family relationships and individual identities from the outside world. The level of internalized homophobia on the part of lesbian, bisexual, and gay family members significantly influences the capacity for and nature of the response by a family to the stressors resulting from societal oppression. Having to interact with people at institutions such as schools and churches that require the presence of both parents of the same gender may arouse intense distress associated with fear of disclosure of sexual identity and of repercussions from outside the family. For many families, such concern may lead to a total denial to the external world of a gay or lesbian identity, and to dissonance between the public and private identities of the family.

One of the most challenging issues facing lesbian and gay families today is deciding whether or not to have children and, if children are desired, choosing how to have them. Options include adoption, becoming foster parents, artificial or arranged insemination, raising children from heterosexual marriages, and forming heterosexual relationships solely for the purpose of conceiving and raising children. The active construction of families by gay men and lesbians choosing to have children represents an assertive confrontation of their frequent disenfranchisement from families. Reflecting the importance of this increasingly prevalent phenomenon, April Martin has written a guidebook for these parents entitled *The Lesbian and Gay Parenting Handbook: Creating and Raising Our Families* (1993).

With respect to the children of lesbian and gay parents, Patterson (1992) concluded that no significant differences have been identified between the children of lesbian or gay parents and those of heterosexual parents in studies of characteristics related to sexual identity, personal development, and social relationships. Patterson acknowledged a number of methodological shortcomings in this body of research, which has thus far failed to examine the impact on child outcomes of process variables such as qualities of family interactions and relationships; however, she asserted that there is no evidence to conclude that children of gay or lesbian parents are in any way compromised in their development as a result of the sexual orientation of their parents. She called for the implementation of a new research agenda concerning lesbian mothers, gay fathers, and their children that poses questions related not to possible detrimental outcomes, but to potential desirable outcomes for the children in these families. The findings from the research on this topic clearly demand a reorientation of current public policy and legal practices, which frequently deny custody and parental rights to lesbian mothers and gay fathers.

Most gay men and lesbians recognize their homosexuality sometime during adolescence. Although homosexual behavior during adolescence does not invariably lead to adult identification as gay or lesbian (Remafedi et al. 1992), for teenagers who do adopt a lesbian, gay, or bisexual identity while still living with their parents, the ability to share their identity within the family of origin may have significant impact on self-esteem and development during young adulthood (Savin-Williams 1989). The reactions of the family following acknowledgment may help determine the expectations of these youth for consequences in the larger world of disclosure of their sexual orientation and may serve to shape their own views of their homosexuality.

■ Case Example 2

> A 16-year-old high school student informs his parents that he is gay. His parents are initially judgmental and rejecting of their son. He insists on seeing a gay-affirmative psychotherapist. Following several family sessions, the parents allow their son to enter individual therapy to increase his self-esteem and help him with longstanding symptoms of depression. Following individual therapy interspersed with periodic family sessions, the patient's signs of depressions are significantly improved, and his parents are more accepting of his homosexuality.

Regardless of the age of the child when the family learns that he or she is gay or lesbian, family members go through a process of adjustment to this information, which was labeled the "revelation crisis" by Strommen (1990). He described an initial reaction of many families to try to understand the gay or lesbian family member, which may unfortunately lead to endowing that individual "with an identity *constructed from the family's own stereotypes of homosexuality*" (p. 18). In addition, some families may negate the gay or lesbian child's previous role in the family and then experience "a sudden alienation from the homosexual member, a feeling that the homosexual member's previous identity is lost, and that the 'new' homosexual member is a stranger in their midst . . ." (p. 20).

Many parents, believing they have caused their child's homosexuality, experience guilt when learning about it; this guilt has been reinforced by mental health studies that erroneously blame parents and families for creating conditions that lead to homosexuality (see, for example, Bieber et al. 1962). Variables such as age, gender, geographic location, and type of religious affiliation may also affect the nature of family members' reactions to learning that someone in the family is lesbian or gay (Herek 1988). Long-term reactions tend to occur in stages that may lead to resolution and integration of the gay or lesbian family member into the family with a new identity (DeVine 1984).

Several resources are available to assist families who are struggling with these issues. Support groups such as Parents and Friends of Lesbians and Gays (PFLAG) may be helpful for some families. Publications that discuss the issues parents confront in learning to accept their lesbian and gay children may also be useful (Griffin et al. 1986; McDonald and Steinhorn 1993; Muller 1987; Fairchild and Hayward 1979). Finally, community agencies with programs designed for gay, lesbian, and bisexual youth, such as the Hetrick-Martin Institute in New York City and Horizons in Chicago, can serve as vital support groups for young people learning to manage their homosexuality within their families.

Clinical Implications

The recognition of lesbian, gay, and bisexual families and the greater variety of forms of these families create the need for two primary revisions in clinical practice. First, the theory and practice of family therapy needs to be expanded to encompass these nontraditional families, both by including them in existing conceptualizations of family dynamics and systems and by extending understanding and technique to respond to the special dynamics and concerns of these families. Second, the theory of development and behavior focused on the individual needs to be revised to incorporate the experiences of individuals in these nontraditional family forms. The assumption that all children grow up having two parents, one male and one female, who enact and model traditional gender roles, clearly needs to be abandoned and replaced by an appreciation for the variety of gender experiences people actually have while growing up in their families.

■ **Case Example 3**

> While in psychotherapy, Mr. B, a 50-year-old man, marries a woman 10 years younger who has three children, ages 10, 13, and 15. His own children from a previous marriage are older and married. Mr. B is concerned because of difficulties in relating to his stepchildren and reports that they have told him they do not need another father. Their father is gay and has been living with his gay partner since divorcing their mother several years ago. The children consider the gay stepfather to be their real stepfather and seem to resent the intrusion of an additional stepfather.

This case illustrates the type of problem related to homosexuality confronted by many families today, in which the reactions may not be directly antigay but involve complex issues related to the presence of gay or lesbian parents and children. A significant and specific need exists within psychotherapy to help families with lesbian and gay parents cope with stressors resulting from social opprobrium and to help them confront a homophobic society (Levy 1992); however, a broader mandate is to help foster in all family forms a greater capacity to deal with diversity and complexity that incorporates but is not limited to an appreciation of issues of concern to lesbian, gay, and bisexual family members. This appreciation must extend as well to the diverse attitudes and values concerning sexuality and homosexuality developed within the families of ethnic minorities (Morales 1990).

Now available in the literature are initial descriptions of a variety of approaches to dealing with gay and lesbian families within psychotherapy and family therapy (Baptiste 1987; Stein 1988; Ussher 1987; Weinstein 1992) and in special settings such as chemical dependency treatment programs (Shernoff and Finnegan 1991). The challenge for the future is to inform mental health professionals about these approaches and to ensure appropriate recognition and treatment of the unique set of dynamics and issues presented by these families.

References

Barret RL, Robinson BE: Gay Fathers. Lexington, MA, Lexington Books, 1990

Bell AP, Weinberg MS: Homosexualities: A Study of Diversity Among Men and Women. New York, Simon and Schuster, 1978

Bieber I, Dain HJ, Dince PR, et al: Homosexuality: A Psychoanalytic Study. New York, Basic Books, 1962

Boxer AM, Cook JA, Herdt G: Double jeopardy: identity transitions and parent-child relations among gay and lesbian youth, in Parent-Child Relations Throughout Life. Edited by Pillemer K, McCartney K. Hillsdale, NJ, Erlbaum, 1991, pp 59–92

Bozett F: Gay fathers, in Gay and Lesbian Parents. Edited by Bozett FW. New York, Praeger, 1987a, pp 3–22

Bozett FW (ed): Gay and Lesbian Parents. New York, Praeger, 1987b

Bozett FW, Sussman MB (eds): Homosexuality and Family Relations. New York, Harrington Park Press, 1990

DeVine JL: A systemic inspection of affectional preference orientation and the family of origin. Journal of Social Work and Human Sexuality 2:9–17, 1984

DiLapi EM: Lesbian mothers and the motherhood hierarchy. Journal of Homosexuality 18:101–121, 1989

Fairchild B, Hayward N: Now That You Know: What Every Parent Should Know About Homosexuality. New York, Harcourt Brace Jovanovich, 1979

Griffin CW, Wirth MJ, Wirth AG: Beyond Acceptance. Englewood Cliffs, NJ, Prentice Hall, 1986

Herdt G: Gay and Lesbian Youth. New York, Haworth, 1989

Herdt G, Boxer A: Children of Horizons: How Gay and Lesbian Teens Are Leading a New Way Out of the Closet. Boston, MA, Beacon Press, 1993

Herek GM: Heterosexuals' attitudes toward lesbians and gay men: correlates and gender differences. Journal of Sex Research 25:451–477, 1988

Levy EF: Strengthening the coping resources of lesbian families. Families in Society: The Journal of Contemporary Human Service, 73(1):23–31, 1992

Martin A: The Lesbian and Gay Parenting Handbook: Creating and Raising Our Families. New York, HarperCollins, 1993

McDonald HB, Steinhorn AI: Understanding Homosexuality. New York, Crossroad, 1993

Morales ES: Ethnic minority families and minority gays and lesbians, in Homosexuality and Family Relations. Edited by Bozett FW, Sussman MB. New York, Harrington Park Press, 1990, pp 217–239

Muller A: Parents Matter. Tallahassee, FL, Naiad Press, 1987

Patterson CJ: Children of lesbian and gay parents. Child Development 63:1025–1042, 1992

Pennington SB: Children of lesbian mothers, in Gay and Lesbian Parents. Edited by Bozett FW. New York, Praeger, 1987, pp 58–74

Remafedi G, Resnick M, Blum R, et al: Demography of sexual orientation in adolescents. Pediatrics 89:714–721, 1992

Rohrbaugh JB: Lesbian families: clinical issues and theoretical implications. Professional Psychology 23:467–473, 1992

Savin-Williams R: Coming out to parents and self-esteem among gay and lesbian youth. Journal of Homosexuality 18:1–35, 1989

Schulenburg J: Gay Parenting. New York, Doubleday, 1985

Slater S, Mencher J: The lesbian family life cycle: a contextual approach. American Journal of Orthopsychiatry 61:372–382, 1991

Strommen EF: Hidden branches and growing pains: homosexuality and the family tree, in Homosexuality and Family Relations. Edited by Bozett FW, Sussman MB. New York, Harrington Park Press, 1990, pp 9–34

Weinberg MS, Williams CS: Male Homosexuals: Their Problems and Adaptations. New York, Oxford University Press, 1974

Weston K: Families We Choose. New York, Columbia University Press, 1991

Sexual Orientation of the Therapist

Robert P. Cabaj, M.D.

The success of psychotherapy is influenced by many factors, including the training and experience of the therapist, the willingness or resistance of the patient to engage in the therapy, and the health and emotional state of both the patient and the therapist. The significance of an additional factor, the match of a patient with the therapist in terms of shared personal traits, continues to be debated, focused most often on gender, race, ethnic background, socioeconomic background, or educational level. Shared sexual orientation as a matching factor has received attention only in the last few years. The author explores this particular variable in this chapter and what possible influences it might have on therapy with gay men, lesbians, and bisexual individuals.

Psychotherapy Variables

In a review of whether, and how, psychotherapy creates change, a number of variables that may influence treatment have received attention (Carkhuff and Berenson 1967; Herron 1975; Oden 1974; Rogers 1957, 1962; Truax and Carkhuff 1967). Having established that some therapists are more effective than others, Carkhuff and Berenson (1967) listed the following characteristics of the therapist as having an influence on therapeutic effectiveness: empathic understanding, positive regard, genuineness, appropriate self-disclosure, spontaneity, confidence, intensity, openness, flexibility, and commitment. In addition, Guntrip (1969) clearly stated that the "patient and therapist need to be matched to secure the best results" (p. 328).

The variables of gender, race, and ethnicity have been well explored. In looking at the efficacy of treatment of African American patients, Jones (1978) concluded that African American patients preferred treatment by African American therapists, feeling better understood and accepted, and expressing a greater sense of rapport and willingness to open up in a session. In studying Latinos in psychotherapy, Roll et al. (1980) found that many situations and life adjustments were comfortable to the Latino patient but upsetting or confusing to the Anglo-American therapist. Psychoanalytic case studies have looked at the influence of gender in psychoanalysis (Chertoff 1989; Karme 1979). The literature on the cultural and societal expectations of gender roles has also examined the influences of gender on therapy (Chodorow 1978; Gilligan 1982; Mogul 1982).

Rochlin (1985) presented one of the first reviews of the influence of the sexual orientation of the therapist on therapeutic efficacy. Stein (1988) discussed several influences on psychotherapy for gay men and women, including the role of matching sexual orientations. Isay (1991) explored the impact of his more public openness about being a gay male psychoanalyst on his psychoanalytic therapy cases. Although formal research examining the effects of the variable of sexual orientation is not yet available, these articles, and the author's clinical experience, allow some speculations on the influence of the sexual orientation of the therapist on the psychotherapeutic process.

Self-Disclosure and Psychotherapy

The degree to which therapists intentionally reveal aspects of themselves depends partly on the psychotherapeutic technique used, the training background and model of psychological and psychodynamic understanding employed by the therapist, and the clinical setting. In traditional psychoanalytic psychotherapy, the therapist is often advised to be a "blank screen" and disclose little or no personal material to the patient. The purpose for such an approach is to let the unconscious material of the patient become accessible to the conscious ego without interference from the therapist. This model is adapted to other types of psychodynamic therapy, including supportive therapy, and allows the psychotherapeutic process to focus intensively on the issues and internal psychodynamics of the individual patient, with minimal outside influences. Whether such a blank-screen model is truly possible to follow is questionable; for example, photographs, degrees from schools and training institutes, skin color, gender, wearing a wedding ring, even a therapist's name, can reveal much about the therapist. A nonheterosexual therapist may not be able to preserve total anonymity regarding sexual orientation, depending on such factors as the characteristics of the local community—gay, lesbian, and bisexual people are often more visible to each other because they live in relatively small geographic and social circles—and the reputation of the therapist (Brown 1989; Gartrell 1992).

At the other end of the therapeutic spectrum are techniques and programs that promote the similarity of shared personal traits as the specific reason for certain patients to see particular therapists, for example, feminist programs devoted to treating only women, or Spanish-language clinics that focus on Latino and Latina patients. Similarly, a clinic or center dedicated to treating gay, lesbian, and bisexual patients often uses the fact that many of the therapists available are themselves gay, lesbian, or bisexual and, therefore, are presumed to be better able to treat gay, lesbian, and bisexual patients (see Chapter 42 by McDaniel, Cabaj, and Purcell).

The issues of self-disclosure for the therapist also occur in two other arenas that are of special interest to gay, lesbian, and bisexual patients. Substance abuse treatment programs often encourage disclosure of therapist characteristics because many of the therapists and counselors in such programs are themselves in recovery from substance abuse. Many such programs encourage self-disclosure on the part of the clinician, believing a therapist who shares patient characteristics can serve as a role model and inspiration for the patient; others promote keeping such information hidden or neutral to prevent setting up a model for the patient that could be a point of comparison or competition if sobriety is difficult to achieve. Gay-sensitive and gay-affirmative programs promote openness both about sexual orientation and about substance abuse as critical aspects of recovery from substance abuse in gay, lesbian, and bisexual patients (Cabaj 1992; see Chapter 47 by Cabaj).

Programs treating persons living with HIV infection or AIDS are often staffed by people who are themselves infected with HIV. Self-disclosure by staff in these settings can provide some patients with hope, but it can also confront patients with frustration and fear if the health status of infected staff members deteriorates (see Chapter 50 by McDaniel, Farber, and Summerville).

Being Open About Sexual Orientation in Psychotherapy

Two important questions for the therapist who works with gay men, lesbians, bisexual individuals, and transgendered persons are, Should the therapist self-disclose or be open about his or her sexual orientation? And would a patient be better treated by a gay, lesbian, bisexual, or transgendered therapist? Such openness may occur in several ways; for example, the therapist may frequent organizations, clubs, or businesses that cater to the gay community and thus be seen by patients; the therapist may be quite open about his or her sexual orientation with colleagues and be referred patients because of this sexual orientation; or the therapist may directly disclose his or her sexual orientation to a patient before beginning treatment or during a therapy session at an appropriate time.

Many gay, lesbian, and bisexual patients may wish to see a therapist who is also gay, lesbian, or bisexual. The patient may believe that he or she can avoid the overt effects of homophobia and more easily develop a sense of trust, safety, openness, and personal comfort with a gay, lesbian, and bisexual therapist. The patient may also believe that a gay therapist will share common experiences and know more about gay issues. Gay, lesbian, or bisexual therapists, in turn, may hold similar beliefs: that homophobia can be avoided, that a special rapport can be established quickly, and that a shared base of knowledge and experience exists when gay, lesbian, and bisexual patients and therapists work together.

Rochlin (1985) described how important knowledge about the "gay world" can be during therapy and suggested that gay consciousness-raising is an important aspect of doing therapy. He also describes the importance of openly gay, lesbian, and bisexual therapists serving as role models for people who do not have a visible place in our society.

■ **Case Example 1**

> Ms. A sought psychotherapy, and at the beginning of the first session, she demanded to know the sexual orientation of the therapist. She stated she was an open, self-accepting, and self-loving lesbian, who had experienced difficulties in obtaining psychotherapy in the past from therapists who were heterosexual or who refused to discuss their sexual orientation. The therapist did not initially answer the direct question, asking instead, what concerns the patient had about undertaking therapy if she did not know, or was not certain about, the sexual orientation of this particular therapist. Ms. A became angry, believing the therapist was playing a game. The therapist chose to be open about being a gay man, as he was well known in the gay community. The patient was visibly relieved, stated that she had in fact already learned that the therapist was gay, and felt self-revelation indicated gay affirmation, a lack of homophobia, and an acceptance of her being lesbian. The next several sessions focused on her immediate issues, but the theme of lack of acceptance and revelation of secrets returned when material was discussed that indicated a history of sexual abuse.

In general, conscious awareness of internalized homophobia and parallel heterosexism is an asset for the psychotherapist treating gay, lesbian, and bisexual patients (see Chapter 7 by Herek). Heterosexual therapists arguably cannot fully understand or personally experience internalized homophobia, although they may be able to recognize and confront heterosexism. The benefits of having direct knowledge about homosexuality and the issues that face gay people are obvious; such knowledge is not, of course, restricted to gay, lesbian, and bisexual therapists. Gay-sensitive therapy—treatment provided from a perspective that understands and accepts gay, lesbian, and bisexual concerns—and gay-affirmative therapy—treatment provided from the perspective that being gay, lesbian, or bisexual should be affirmed and that openness about sexual orientation should be encouraged—can be provided by heterosexual as well as gay, lesbian, or bisexual therapists.

Pitfalls are numerous facing a therapist who is open about his or her sexual orientation—from the perspective of the effect on the therapeutic process and not on the career or professional consequences for the therapist. The belief that the therapist and patient share values, experiences, and knowledge because they have the same sexual orientation may facilitate a false sense of trust and openness that is not derived from a shared therapeutic experience, which could be used in understanding transference and countertransference reactions. Many parts of the patient's life may in fact be avoided or not explored as a result of a conscious or unconscious collusion to sidestep painful material by assuming a mutual understanding of words or experiences. Because growing up gay, lesbian, or bisexual is a unique, personal experience, similar experiences on the part of the therapist and patient may lead to very different reactions. If these differences are ignored, important transferential and countertransferential feelings and reactions may not be expressed or explored—especially if they are negative—for fear of appearing homophobic or insensitive. Furthermore, if the patient believes the therapist, by being open about sexual orientation, is gay-affirmative, he or she may not feel comfortable in expressing doubts and fears about being gay, lesbian, or bisexual.

Keeping secrets or failing to explore certain material in therapy may lead to therapeutic impasses, with stalled or failed treatment, acting out (on the parts of both the patient and the therapist), and even eroticized transferences and countertransferences that may cross therapeutic boundaries and be acted upon (Brown 1989). In addition, a sense of competition can develop but not be expressed directly; for example, the patient may feel that he or she could never be as open, advanced, or successful a gay person as the therapist is perceived to be.

Openly gay therapists can function as important role models for younger people who are "coming out" (or for anyone who becomes aware of being gay, lesbian, or bisexual at any age), for persons who are in supportive therapy, and for those individuals who are participating in psychoeducational work. However, boundaries and roles in therapy can become confused when mentoring, friendship, or advisor roles are confounded. When the therapist and patient enter into friendship and their relationship becomes social and sexual, of course, the therapeutic relationship is destroyed (see Chapter 53 by Brown). Acting on sexual feelings or impulses between therapist and patient is always unethical.

■ Case Example 2

Mr. B sought therapy with concerns about coming out and accepting himself as a gay man. He was extraordinarily curious about the therapist, stating he had never met a gay professional and was very excited about meeting one. He explored his personal concerns, but

he kept repeating that he had not met anyone as special or as accomplished as the therapist and that he believed there were probably no such gay men available. He then demanded that the
therapist have sex with him because it would affirm that he was an
acceptable gay man and that he might somehow benefit from the
power that the therapist could pass along to him in the sexual encounter. The therapist made clear that therapy is a process that
uses words and not actions to explore feelings. The patient threatened that unless the therapist had sex right then and there, he
would leave therapy. The therapist again refused, in a firm but kind
way, and the patient stormed out of the room. He did not return
for subsequent treatment, but he did see the therapist in public
several months later. Although the therapist tried to walk away after a brief acknowledgment, the former patient insisted on speaking. He apologized about his behavior, saying he was too naive and
too overwhelmed by coming out at the time to try to find gay men
to meet on his own; once in therapy, he had come to believe that
by becoming lovers with the therapist, he could sidestep the
stresses involved in the coming-out process.

Internalized homophobia—the self-loathing or self-contempt a
gay, lesbian, or bisexual person absorbs from societal homophobia—is
a crucial variable in psychotherapy with gay men, lesbians, and bisexual
individuals. Just because therapists are open about their sexual orientation does not mean they have fully dealt with or confronted the internalized homophobia. A major part of psychotherapy for most gay,
lesbian, and bisexual patients is exploring, and trying to come to grips
with, the efforts of internalized homophobia. This author has observed
in his clinical practice of psychotherapy with gay clinicians that many
gay, lesbian, and bisexual therapists have not successfully completed
the task of dealing with the effects of their own internalized homophobia. In working with many gay therapists in supervision, this author
has seen the harm such unresolved internalized homophobia can have
on the therapeutic process, by slowing down the therapeutic pace, failing to acknowledge or reward progress, giving inappropriate advice on
the basis of their own experiences, intervening inappropriately in patients' lives, or projecting their own beliefs on patients concerning difficulties in forming relationships or being open about sexual
orientation with family, friends, or co-workers. The gay, lesbian, or bisexual therapist is at risk for overidentifying with patients of similar
sexual orientation (Cabaj 1991; see Chapter 53 by Brown). When thera-

pists cease to hear or see the patient as he or she really is, and project their own views and perceptions onto the patient, therapy becomes ineffective and potentially harmful to the patient.

Good supervision, a clear and strong knowledge base about gay, lesbian, and bisexual issues, respect for the challenging task of being a patient in psychotherapy, and if necessary, personal psychotherapy to deal with internalized homophobia are all safeguards against the potential problems discussed above. The openly gay therapist can have a special and beneficial impact on gay, lesbian, and bisexual patients who need understanding and acceptance for their sexual orientation, who are coming out, or who do not wish to have an unnecessary focus on sexual orientation interfere with other reasons for which they seek psychotherapy. In the best circumstances, the comfort and rapport that were described earlier in relation to ethnic minority patients working with therapists from the same ethnic minority group can result when patients and therapists who share a common sexual orientation work together.

Matching in Psychotherapy for Sexual Orientation

In the examination of the effects of the therapist and patient having the same or a different sexual orientation, several additional factors are worth discussing. First, heterosexual therapists can clearly work with gay men, lesbians, and bisexual individuals if they have the necessary knowledge and self-awareness (see Chapter 32 by Marmor). However, unexpected benefits and problems can also occur in such a combination. In seeking a gay-sensitive or gay-affirmative therapist, many patients may assume that the therapist to whom they were referred is also gay, lesbian, or bisexual, and many of the same problems described above resulting from assumptions by the patient about the therapist may occur, regardless of the actual sexual orientation of the therapist. The subject of the sexual orientation of the therapist may never come up in the therapy because of such assumptions, the difficulties in talking about anything sexual in our society, the belief that a patient should not ask too many questions of a therapist, or internalized homophobia and shame.

Some gay, lesbian, or bisexual patients may actually request a heterosexual therapist. Some such patients may believe they can avoid their erotic feelings with a heterosexual therapist, although others may be acting on internalized shame, guilt, and avoidance. In contrast, many gay people believe that no heterosexual person can ever truly accept and understand them, and thus they seek such acknowledgment and acceptance from a gay, lesbian, or bisexual therapist. Such a belief may be a reflection of the struggle the patients had with their parents, believing that the parents could never accept them as gay, lesbian, or bisexual. Conversely, since most parents are heterosexual, the acceptance and acknowledgment of a gay, lesbian, or bisexual patient expressed by a heterosexual therapist may be even more powerful and therapeutic in helping to correct the effects of the troubled parental interactions. Hoping that a therapist may somehow make up for the lack of heterosexual parental acceptance, some patients may not wish to know the sexual orientation of the therapist or may deny the obvious or easily learned sexual orientation of an openly gay, lesbian, or bisexual therapist.

Gay people, as well as heterosexual people, express homophobia and heterosexism. The request for a heterosexual therapist from a gay person may result from heterosexism, not only from internalized homophobia and self-doubt. Many gay men, lesbians, and bisexual individuals may believe that gay therapists are not as good as equally trained heterosexual therapists. Understanding the motivation for a particular referral or request for treatment can begin healing the damage caused by internalized homophobia and can be used as a step in recognizing and reducing its impact in interfering with the full functioning of the gay man, lesbian, or bisexual seeking treatment.

Conclusion

Questions about how open to be about sexual orientation in therapy and concerns about similarities and differences in patient and therapist sexual orientation raise complex issues; there are no clear guidelines or standards for resolution of these issues. Possible benefits of a therapist being open about his or her sexual orientation include a better rapport with the patient; a reduction in time spent in the therapy conveying basic information about being gay, lesbian, or bisexual; and a fostering of trust and safety in overcoming the harmful effects of internalized homophobia. The problems of openness about sexual orientation may involve overidentification of the therapist with the patient, unwarranted assumptions about sameness not based on presented material, a tendency to avoid internalized shame and other negative feelings, and the risk of blurring or even crossing the boundaries that are absolutely necessary for psychotherapy.

Because information about homosexuality and gay men, lesbians, and bisexual individuals is increasingly available, all therapists can learn about these issues even before seeing their first patients. Supervision is a vital and necessary part of all carefully and thoughtfully delivered psychotherapy, and it can be particularly important when there are concerns about boundaries in therapy. Homophobia and heterosexism are forces that both heterosexual therapists and gay, lesbian, and bisexual therapists can understand and address effectively. The acceptance and acknowledgment of a sexual orientation that is different from the majority and correction through psychotherapy of the negative effects of internalized homophobia require an open, sensitive, accepting, nonjudgmental, and nonpunitive therapist. Such a therapist can be heterosexual, gay, lesbian, or bisexual.

If a therapist recognizes that his or her internalized homophobia is interfering with the therapy or is manifesting itself in other aspects of the therapist's life, a consultation, supervision, or even a referral to another therapist is indicated (Cabaj 1988). The same interventions may be needed if the therapist is *too* accepting of the patient—that is, expressing an acceptance not based on actual material or knowledge about the patient—or is unwilling to explore the internalized homophobia of the patient. With appropriate precaution and awareness, effective and beneficial psychotherapy with gay, lesbian, and bisexual patients can be conducted by therapists of all sexual orientations.

References

Brown LS: Beyond thou shalt not: thinking about ethics in the lesbian therapy community. Women and Therapy 10:13–25, 1989

Cabaj RP: Homosexuality and neurosis: considerations for psychotherapy. J Homosex 15:13–23, 1988

Cabaj RP: Overidentification with a patient, in Gays, Lesbians and Their Therapists: Studies in Psychotherapy. Edited by Silverstein C. New York, WW Norton, 1991, pp 31–39

Cabaj RP: Substance abuse in the gay and lesbian community, in Substance Abuse: A Comprehensive Textbook, 2nd Edition. Edited by Lowenson JH, Ruiz P, Millman RB. Baltimore, MD, Williams & Wilkins, 1992, pp 852–860

Carkhuff RR, Berenson BG: Beyond Counseling and Therapy. New York, Rinehart and Winston, 1967

Chertoff M: Negative oedipal transference of a male patient to his female analyst during the termination phase. J Am Psychoanal Assoc 37:687–712, 1989

Chodorow N: The Reproduction of Mothering: Psychoanalysis and the Sociology of Gender. Berkeley, CA, University of California Press, 1978

Gartrell NK: Boundaries in lesbian therapy relationships. Women and Therapy 12(3):29–50, 1992

Gilligan C: In a Different Voice. Cambridge, MA, Harvard University Press, 1982

Guntrip H: Schizoid Phenomena, Object Relations and the Self. New York, International Universities Press, 1969

Herron WG: Further thoughts on psychotherapeutic deprofessionalization. Journal of Humanistic Psychology 15:65–73, 1975

Isay RA: The homosexual analyst: clinical considerations, in The Psychoanalytic Study of the Child, Vol 46. Edited by Solnit AJ, Neubauer PB, Abrams S, et al. New Haven, CT, Yale University Press, 1991, pp 199–216

Jones EE: Effects of race on psychotherapy process and outcome: an exploratory investigation. Psychotherapy: Theory, Research, and Practice 15:226–236, 1978

Karme L: The analysis of a male patient by a female analyst. Int J Psychoanal 60:253–261, 1979

Mogul KM: Overview: the sex of the therapist. J Psychiatry 139:1–11, 1982

Oden TC: A populist's view of psychotherapeutic deprofessionalization. Journal of Humanistic Psychology 14:3–18, 1974

Rochlin M: Sexual orientation of the therapist and therapeutic effectiveness with gay clients, in A Guide to Psychotherapy With Gay and Lesbian Clients. Edited by Gonsiorek JC. New York, Harrington Park Press, 1985, pp 21–29

Rogers CR: The necessary and sufficient conditions of therapeutic personality change. J Consult Psychol 21:95–103, 1957

Rogers CR: The interpersonal relationship: the core of guidance. Harvard Educational Review 32:416–429, 1962

Roll S, Millen L, Martinez R: Common errors in psychotherapy with Chicanos: extrapolations from research and clinical experience. Psychotherapy: Theory, Research, and Practice 17:158–168, 1980

Stein TS: Theoretical considerations in psychotherapy with gay men and lesbians, in Psychopathology and Psychotherapy in Homosexuality. Edited by Ross MW. New York, Haworth, 1988, pp 75–95

Truax CB, Carkhuff RR: Toward Effective Counseling and Psychotherapy: Training and Practice. Chicago, IL, Aldine, 1967

31

A Critique of Approaches to Changing Sexual Orientation

Terry S. Stein, M.D.

Approaches in psychotherapy to changing sexual orientation exclusively involve efforts to change homosexual and bisexual orientations to a heterosexual orientation (Nicolosi 1991) and largely deal with such changes in men, not in women (Adams and Sturgis 1977). Thus attempts to change sexual orientation parallel the focus of antihomosexual bias and heterosexism in American society: to stigmatize and ultimately to eliminate nonheterosexual forms of sexuality. The focus on change in men results not only from a greater emphasis on men in general in the psychological literature, but also from a stronger and frequently more virulent reaction to homosexuality in men than to homosexuality in women in our society. This differential reaction is due both to the greater rigidity of gender role requirements for men—and the resultant anxiety about gender variation in men—and to the devaluation of sexuality in women in general. As a result, psychological and moral techniques intended to alter sexual orientation, whether applied coercively or voluntarily, have been directed most consistently to men with homoerotic desire and behavior.

Several recent reviews of approaches to changing sexual orientation (Haldeman 1991, 1994; Murphy 1992a, 1992b; see Chapter 1 by Silverstein) comprehensively describe the types of conversion therapies, clarify the justifications for these therapeutic endeavors, and document the outcomes of such efforts. Murphy (1992b) described the following types of interventions to change sexual orientation: behavioral therapy, psychodynamic interventions, drug and hormone therapy, and surgery. In addition, Haldeman (1994) discussed a variety of religion-based conversion programs. All of these approaches assume that homosexuality is morally wrong, medically pathological, and socially undesirable and are based on the beliefs that erotic desire for someone of the same gender should be eliminated or redirected and that there are interventions that are effective in changing sexual orientation. Neither of these beliefs has been validated by empirical study.

Understanding Approaches to Changing Sexual Orientation

It is important to understand the conceptual and methodological approaches to sexual orientation conversion treatment. Many reports about these techniques have failed to describe certain important features of the interventions, including 1) why the attempt to change is undertaken, that is, the motivation on the part of both the therapist and the patient for attempting change (historically it has been assumed a priori in these approaches that a wish to change from homosexual to heterosexual is appropriate and desirable); 2) who seeks change, in terms of their preexisting sexual characteristics; and 3) what specific type of change these individuals are able to accomplish.

■ Why Change Is Attempted

The patient.　Gay, lesbian, or bisexual individuals may present to a therapist with discomfort about their homosexuality for a variety of reasons, including previous experience of antihomosexual bias; sexual inexperience or fear; trauma resulting from sexual abuse by a person of the same sex; or most commonly, a generalized, deeply held, internalized homophobia. In conversion therapies, all such individuals may be treated in the same manner and evaluated not in terms of the origins of the discomfort with their homoerotic wishes but solely through the lens of the assumed desirability of change. Before any type of treatment is offered to the person who wishes to change his or her sexual orientation, the motivation for change must be fully assessed.

The DSM-III-R (American Psychiatric Association 1987) states: "In the United States, almost all people who are homosexual first go through a phase in which their homosexuality is ego-dystonic" (p. 426). For most people who are disturbed about being homosexual—those for whom their homosexuality is ego-dystonic—the origin of their reaction lies in an internalization of negative societal views about homosexuality, or internalized homophobia. Internalized homophobia may express itself in young people through denial of being homosexual and identification with heterosexuality (Hetrick and Martin 1987), or through attempts to pass as heterosexual or to be assimilated into the predominant heterosexual culture (de Monteflores 1986). For some people, distress about being homosexual may be so strong that it leads to years of effort to eliminate entirely the homosexuality, the presumed source of the distress. Unsuccessful attempts to convert sexual orientation through psychotherapy are eloquently described in autobiographical reports by Howard Brown in *Familiar Faces, Hidden Lives* (1976), and by Martin Duberman in *Cures: A Gay Man's Odyssey* (1991).

In therapy with such individuals, therapists may ignore the actual origin of their distress, internalized homophobia in the form of conscious and unconscious agreement with society's derogation of one's sexuality when it is not heterosexuality, and this homophobia is often further strengthened during the course of such misdirected attempts to "treat" homosexuality (Martin 1984). The result may be analogous to the effects seen in the victims of cultural attitudes prescribing such practices as the binding of girls' feet in China: In an attempt to meet some societal ideal that is unnatural for a particular person, that individual's sexuality is suppressed and channeled until it is ultimately deformed.

Although all gay, lesbian, and bisexual persons experience negative feelings in relation to their sexual orientation as a result of living in a society that so profoundly denigrates variant sexualities, it is as difficult to imagine a persistent adaptive wish to alter one's sexual orientation as it is to conceive of a helpful desire to change one's height or eye color. Although such changes can be made under some circumstances and at great cost, they are usually cosmetic and reflect a desire to conform to some idealized standard of appearance, behavior, or beauty.

The therapist.   The motivation of the therapist who attempts to change a patient's sexual orientation is also important to understand, as it may influence the effect of such treatment on the patient. Often therapists argue that they are attempting to meet the stated needs and desires of the patient who is dissatisfied or unhappy with being gay, lesbian, or bisexual and is seeking a change in his or her sexual orientation. Although the conscious motivation of such therapists may be to help their patients, failure to assess the source of dissatisfaction and unhappiness and to explore the underlying internalized homophobia in such patients indicates several possible problems, including a lack of information about normative psychosocial development in gay, lesbian, and bisexual individuals, which involves regular and ongoing exposure to antihomosexual attitudes and behaviors leading to internalization of negative beliefs about the self (Malyon 1982); the presence of unconscious negative feelings about homosexuality; or simply a technical failure to complete an appropriate and thorough evaluation. Regardless of the source of a therapist's motivation to collude unreflectively with a patient's wish to change his or her homosexuality, the agreement by a therapist to undertake such an approach to treatment raises serious ethical concerns about the clinical functioning of the therapist (see Chapter 53 by Brown).

Arguments by therapists that the values and rights of persons who wish to modify their sexual orientation must be respected and responded to by offering them the opportunity to seek change through psychotherapy (Nicolosi 1991, 1993)—in the same manner that the plastic surgeon "corrects" the sagging skin of an aging person—fail to recognize the extent of the constriction of their freedom of choice experienced by individuals who have had a part of their identity so deeply stigmatized.

Other therapists who seek to change the sexual orientation of gay, lesbian, or bisexual patients are prompted to do so because of their beliefs that homosexuality is morally wrong or pathological (Nicolosi 1991, 1993; Socarides and Volkan 1991). Although such therapists also generally frame their approach to treatment in terms of the good of the patient, the fundamental reason for their effort lies in negative views about homosexuality. The therapist who holds such beliefs generally agrees with the patient who wishes to eliminate or redirect homosexual desire and behavior and offers him or her treatment with the hope of change. Interestingly, the views of these therapists do not always lead them to condemn gay and lesbian individuals who do not wish to change their sexual orientation or to argue against granting rights to these men and women (Kronemeyer 1980).

■ Who Seeks Change

The preexisting characteristics of individuals undergoing conversion therapy are rarely described in depth, and when such descriptions are offered, differences and difficulties within a sample may be ignored or condensed when outcomes are reported. One of the more egregious examples of such a presentation is a study of dissatisfied homosexual men reported by Masters and Johnson (1979). A large majority of the subjects in this study (45 of 54) initially ranged from 2 to 4 on the Kinsey scale (Kinsey et al. 1948) and thus were largely heterosexual or bisexual to begin with; any increases in heterosexual behavior as a response to treatment were clearly, for these men, no more than an augmentation of their already existing heterosexual capacity.

Determination of the preexisting and outcome sexual orientation characteristics of the person who seeks to change his or her sexual orientation requires careful evaluation of several behavioral, emotional, psychological, and social dimensions, all of which may vary considerably for some persons, without any external intervention such as psychotherapy, over the course of a lifetime (Klein et al. 1985). For example, an individual may alter the gender of his or her sexual partner without changing underlying desire, or a person may marry someone of the other sex but continue to have sexual interactions with persons of the same sex. The gender of persons with whom one interacts in social situations may have little or nothing to do with the gender of the person with whom one fantasizes about having sexual relationships. Full description of the preintervention and postintervention characteristics of these dimensions of sexual orientation is lacking in most reports of conversion treatments.

■ What Is Being Changed

With respect to the type of change that is sought, the therapist may respond by attempting to extinguish homosexual fantasies, feelings, or behavior, to replace homosexual with heterosexual practices or relationships, or to alter the fundamental sexual orientation of the patient. Although these are very different outcomes, they may, in the mind of the therapist and the patient alike, be viewed as similar or identical indications of change. In fact, however, for some persons change in sexual behavior or in the gender of one's primary partner may not indicate any change in underlying sexual desire at all.

In addition, studies of sexual orientation conversion report on different variables to indicate change, and they utilize a wide range of methods to assess change, including, for example, behavioral treatment techniques, self-report procedures, physiological indices, and techniques of self-monitoring and charting (Adams and Sturgis 1977). The lack of consistency in describing change makes comparisons of outcomes and determination of effectiveness extremely difficult. In their review of behavioral reorientation techniques used to modify homosexuality, Adams and Sturgis (1977) concluded,

> The results of these studies are difficult to analyze because the success criteria differed from study to study, authors frequently failed to specify the number or percentage of those achieving success, and there was rarely a breakdown of success according to the original subject characteristics or sexual patterns. (p. 1184)

Approaches to Changing Sexual Orientation

Efforts within the mental health field to change the sexual orientation of gay men during the past century can be described as behavioral, psychodynamic, religious, or biological. Specific techniques have included behavioral reinforcement and extinction, behavioral replacement through exercise and other types of "robust living" (Murphy 1992b, p. 502), psychotherapy, use of medications and hormones, surgery, education, hospitalization, and a variety of religious approaches. These techniques have been reviewed elsewhere (Haldeman 1991, 1994; Murphy 1992a, 1992b). Also for a description of contemporary religion-based approaches to changing sexual orientation see Chapter 52 by Haldeman.

Most of these approaches developed after the medicalization of homosexuality in the 19th century, when the word *homosexuality* itself was first used to describe same-sex attraction and when homosexual behavior began to be viewed as a sign of a medical disorder instead of as a failure of morality. During the following century, scientific views of homosexuality largely shifted, according to Bayer (1987), "from abomination to disease." Many religions continued to denounce homosexual behavior as a sin during this period (see Chapter 52 by Haldeman) and today are still associated with attempts to change homosexuality through moral condemnation and persuasion, for example, through the ex-gay movement (Pattison and Pattison 1980). Although there is no scientific validation of the effectiveness of religion-based conversion programs in changing sexual orientation, these programs do seem to encourage individuals to "become shamed, conflicted, and fearful about their homoerotic feelings" (Haldeman 1994, p. 225). However, even though attributions of immorality continued to be assigned to homosexuality during the period when it was considered a disease, significant attempts to study it scientifically were also undertaken (Kinsey et al. 1948; Hooker 1957).

Studies of homosexuality during the late 19th century were often focused on determining whether it was an acquired or an inborn trait, and by the mid-20th century, clinical reports began to concentrate on techniques for treating the "disease" of homosexuality. Although some researchers reported success with such techniques, particularly psychoanalytic (Bieber et al. 1962) and behavioral (Adams and Sturgis 1977) procedures, replication of results was rare, and identification of the "heterosexual bias" in the studies pointed out the underlying negative assumptions about homosexuality held by the researchers (Morin 1977).

The myriad attempts to change sexual orientation have produced little success. According to Haldeman (1994), "Evidence for the efficacy of sexual conversion programs is less than compelling. All research in this area has evolved from unproven hypothetical formulations about the pathological nature of homosexuality" (p. 223). Although the inaccuracies and false assumptions underlying the conceptualization of homosexuality as pathological have been carefully analyzed (Gonsiorek 1991), efforts to convert gay men and lesbians to heterosexual individuals persist nonetheless.

The most recent form of conversion therapy is designated "reparative therapy," described by the psychologist Joseph Nicolosi (1991) as a specific approach to individual and group therapy with the nongay homosexual man "who experiences a split between his value system and his sexual orientation" (p. 4). In the very titles of his two books, *Reparative Therapy of Male Homosexuality* (1991) and *Healing Homosexuality* (1993), Nicolosi has conveyed the view that homosexuality represents something that is broken or sick. In the introduction to his first book, Nicolosi (1991) straightforwardly reported his devaluation of homosexuality and of gay people in such statements as, "In reality, the homosexual condition is a developmental problem . . ." (p. xvi); "Taking a look at gay relationships, we see there are many inherent limitations in same-sex love" (p. xvii); and "it is legitimate to place higher worth on heterosexuality within the framework of one's value system" (p. xvii).

The essential elements of reparative therapy are a reinforcement of traditional gender roles and an encouragement of identification with a masculine figure, with the assumption that these conditions will lead to a change in self identification from homosexual to heterosexual. Nicolosi (1991) described his approach in the following manner:

> In relationship with a same-sex therapist, a client can find some of what he missed in the failed father-son bond. This is the way that a man absorbs the masculine—through answering the challenge of nonsexual male friendships characterized by mutuality, intimacy, affirmation, and fellowship. When he eroticizes a male relationship, a man is perpetually frustrated in absorbing the masculine. (p. 150)

So-called reparative therapy, like its predecessors, assumes that homosexuality is wrong, maladaptive, and pathological and perpetuates among both patients and the general public a pseudoscientific mythology of sexual orientation, prevalent in traditional psychoanalytic formulations of homosexuality (Friedman 1986), that confounds sexual orientation with gender identity and gender role, blames the victim for the effects of social opprobrium, and politicizes mental health by siding with the forces of social conformity. Seeming to respond directly to the provocative statement in the title of Gerald Davison's (1978) important article, "Not Can But Ought," which presented a proposal to terminate conversion therapy programs, Nicolosi and others who continue to try to change the sexual orientation of gay men ignore all contradictory findings about the efficacy and ethical soundness of their approaches. Davison (1978) stated,

> to urge that therapists desist from sex reorientation programs is not tantamount to exhorting them not to see homosexual individuals in therapy; indeed renouncing these widely used programs can help professionals focus on the problems homosexual individuals (and others) have, rather than on the so-called problem of homosexuality. (p. 170)

Now, almost 20 years later, the absence within sexual orientation conversion programs of a focus on problems that gay men, lesbians, and bisexual individuals have as a result of societal attitudes toward their homosexuality and the construction instead of homosexuality itself as the source of their problems remain one of the most potent techniques within contemporary American society for maintaining what Rich (1980) has called "compulsory heterosexuality." Ignoring scientific evidence contrary to their conclusions, denying reports that treatment for gay men, lesbians, and bisexual individuals that views homosexuality as pathological can produce harmful effects, and vociferously speaking out against gay-affirmative approaches to psychotherapy (Malyon 1982), the modern purveyors of conversion treatment create a significant risk for gay, lesbian, and bisexual mental health consumers.

Clinical Discussion

The negative impact on the patient of exposure to sexual orientation conversion therapy involves the exacerbation of the effects of existing internalized homophobia and further interruption of the development of an integrated gay, lesbian, or bisexual identity. For some patients, this can lead to a worsening of symptoms resulting from internalized homophobia and associated with increased self-hatred and self-destructive behavior, as well as to attempts to create unsuccessful and sometimes hostile heterosexual relationships. An example of the exacerbation of the effects of deeply held internalized homophobia is described in the following case example:

■ Case Example

Mr. A, a 45-year-old man, entered therapy because of signs of depression. He described a complicated psychiatric history with several previous episodes of depression beginning in adolescence, multiple medical problems, substance abuse, and efforts to deny his homosexuality since early adolescence. He reported that he had been arrested when in his mid-30s for having sex with another man in a public restroom. As a result of the publicity that followed from his arrest, he lost his job, and his wife of 12 years divorced him. Following these traumatic events, he became severely depressed and sought help from a psychiatrist, who told him that he was not homosexual because he had been married for so long and he was able to have sexual relations with a woman. The psychiatrist attempted to help the patient "convert" his lifelong homosexual desire and behavior—which had been kept secret from his wife until the time of the arrest—into a completely heterosexual adaptation.

Soon after beginning the reorientation treatment, the patient attempted suicide and was admitted to a psychiatric hospital. While hospitalized, he decided to terminate work with the psychiatrist, to enter Alcoholics Anonymous for his alcoholism, and to become actively involved in the local gay community. Following discharge, he was openly gay, remained largely asymptomatic, and continued to feel good over the next several years. At the time of reentering therapy for his current episode of depression, he was reluctant to see a therapist because he was afraid that he would again encounter someone who would try to change his sexual orientation. He deliberately sought out a gay-affirming psychotherapist who could respect the complex interactions between his recurrent episodes of depression, his sexual orientation, and the deeply held negative attitudes and affects resulting from his lifelong internalized homophobia.

Efforts to understand this patient can be approached from many perspectives and at different levels of psychological functioning, but this case is presented in order to illustrate the potential risk to some patients when their therapists incorrectly focus on homosexuality as the explanation for their problems, arbitrarily attempt to eliminate or redirect homosexuality to heterosexuality, and ignore a rigorous exploration of the sources and effects of internalized homophobia. This patient seriously attempted suicide, not following his arrest or his divorce, but after the intervention of a psychiatrist who reinforced the "homophobic incorporations . . . [that] contribute to a propensity for guilt and intropunitiveness" (Malyon 1982, p. 60) among gay men. Other, less vulnerable patients may simply remain in a self-destructive therapeutic relationship with a gay-negative therapist for years without any integration of their sexuality and capacity for intimacy. Still others may even be helped in circumscribed areas by a supportive and empathic therapist who views their homosexuality negatively, but the exploration of the patient's sexuality and other expressions of intimacy will be seriously truncated within such a negative therapeutic frame.

It is the responsibility of the mental health practitioner who interacts with a person in distress about his or her homosexual feelings, behavior, or identity to assess carefully and fully the origin and nature of this distress and to respond with a treatment approach that is respectful of the wishes of the patient, consistent with a knowledge of the complex developmental pathways for lesbians, gay men, bisexual individuals, and heterosexual individuals and the variety of possible outcomes of such development, and reflective of current psychiatric perspectives on homosexuality. The therapist must never impose his or her own values and choices on the patient. Furthermore, the therapist evaluating a person who is seeking to change his or her sexual orientation is ethically obligated to inform the patient both that homosexuality is not considered officially to be a mental disorder and that there is no valid evidence that change in sexual orientation is possible as a result of psychological intervention. Given these conditions, it is currently ethically indefensible for a therapist to agree to attempt to change the sexual orientation of a patient. Further research on this topic should shift from asking whether conversion treatments can be successful to determining scientifically the answer to the question, "What harm has been done in the name of sexual reorientation?" (Haldeman 1994, p. 225).

References

Adams HE, Sturgis ET: Status of behavioral reorientation techniques in the modification of homosexuality: a review. Psychol Bull 84:1171–1188, 1977

American Psychiatric Association: Diagnostic and Statistical Manual of Mental Disorders, 3rd Edition, Revised. Washington, DC, American Psychiatric Association, 1987

Bayer R: Homosexuality and American Psychiatry. Princeton, NJ, Princeton University Press, 1987

Bieber I, Dain HJ, Dince PR, et al: Homosexuality: A Psychoanalytic Study. New York, Basic Books, 1962

Brown H: Familiar Faces, Hidden Lives. New York, Harcourt Brace Jovanovich, 1976

Davison GC: Not can but ought: the treatment of homosexuality. J Consult Clin Psychol 46:170–172, 1978 de Monteflores C: Notes on the management of difference, in Contemporary Perspectives on Psychotherapy With Lesbians and Gay Men. Edited by Stein T, Cohen C. New York, Plenum, 1986

Duberman M: Cures: A Gay Man's Odyssey. New York, Dutton, 1991

Friedman RM: The psychoanalytic model of male homosexuality: a historical and theoretical critique. Psychoanal Rev 73:483–519, 1986

Gonsiorek JC: The empirical basis for the demise of the illness model of homosexuality, in Homosexuality: Research Implications for Public Policy. Edited by Gonsiorek JC, Weinrich JD. Newbury Park CA, Sage, 1991, pp 115–136

Haldeman DC: Sexual orientation conversion therapy: a scientific examination, in Homosexuality: Research Implications for Public Policy. Edited by Gonsiorek JC, Weinrich JD. Newbury Park, CA, Sage, 1991, pp 149–160

Haldeman DC: The practice and ethics of sexual orientation conversion therapy: J Consult Clin Psychol 62:221–227, 1994

Hetrick E, Martin D: Developmental issues and their resolution for gay and lesbian adolescents. J Homosex 14:25–43, 1987

Hooker E: The adjustment of the male overt homosexual. Journal of Projective Techniques 21:17–31, 1957

Kinsey AC, Pomeroy WB, Martin CE: Sexual Behavior in the Human Male. Philadelphia, PA, WB Saunders, 1948

Klein F, Sepekoff B, Wolf TJ: Sexual orientation: a multivariable dynamic process. J Homosex 11:35–49, 1985

Kronemeyer R: Overcoming Homosexuality. New York, Macmillan, 1980

Malyon AK: Psychotherapeutic implications of internalized homophobia in gay men. J Homosex 7(2–3):59–69, 1982

Martin D: The emperor's new clothes, in Innovations in Psychotherapy With Homosexuals. Edited by Hetrick E, Stein T. Washington, DC, American Psychiatric Press, 1984

Masters WH, Johnson VE: Homosexuality in Perspective. Boston, MA, Little, Brown, 1979

Morin S: Heterosexual bias in psychological research on lesbianism and male homosexuality. Am Psychol 32:629–636, 1977

Murphy TF: Freud and sexual reorientation therapy. J Homosex 23:21–38, 1992a

Murphy TF: Redirecting sexual orientation: techniques and justifications. J Sex Res 29:501–523, 1992b

Nicolosi J: Reparative Therapy of Male Homosexuality. Northvale, NJ, Jason Aronson, 1991

Nicolosi J: Healing Homosexuality. Northvale, NJ, Jason Aronson, 1993

Pattison E, Pattison M: "Ex-gays": religiously mediated change in homosexuals. Am J Psychiatry 137:1553–1562, 1980

Rich A: Compulsory heterosexuality and lesbian existence. Signs: Journal of Women in Culture and Society 5:631–660, 1980

Socarides CW, Volkan V (eds): The Homosexualities and the Therapeutic Process. Madison, CT, International Universities Press, 1991

32

Nongay Therapists Working With Gay Men and Lesbians

A Personal Reflection

Judd Marmor, M.D.

When the author began his psychoanalytic training in 1937, the prevailing view about homosexuality was that at the very least, it constituted a severe personality disorder, and at most, a dangerous perversion. In spite of Freud's unequivocal statement in his famous "Letter to an American Mother" (Freud 1951) that homosexuality "was nothing to be ashamed of, no vice, no degradation, (and) cannot be classified as an illness" (p. 736), his opinion that it represented a "certain arrest in sexual development" was seized upon by leaders and teachers of the psychoanalytic establishment as a justification for considering it a psychopathological condition that ought to be treated. In addition, there was a widespread tendency in the 1930s and 1940s for "experts" in the field, both at seminars and at scientific meetings, to describe their gay patients stereotypically in derogatory terms as possessing a wide variety of ego difficulties and sociopathological tendencies. Edmund Bergler (1956), who was widely regarded as a leading "homosexologist" in those years, described his homosexual patients as being "universally . . . masochistically provocative, injustice collectors, defensively malicious, flippant, rejecting of standards in nonsexual matters, and generally unreliable."

Nevertheless at the time, despite the fact that the author rejected the stereotyping and derogation, he was still influenced by the views of his psychoanalytic teachers, and he assumed that homosexuality did represent a developmental arrest as a result of early childhood relationships within the family and that it ought to be amenable to treatment. The gay men and lesbians who came to him for treatment in those years had feelings of unhappiness that they all attributed, largely or entirely, to their sexual orientation; and the author tried, in addition to exploring the presumptive early roots of their homosexuality, to encourage them to experiment with heterosexual relationships, on the assumption that if they could be enabled to overcome their "phobic feelings," they would ultimately be "cured." Most of those who tried did not succeed, and even those who were able to consummate heterosexual intercourse, uniformly reported that they did not obtain the same degree of satisfaction from them that they did from their same-sex relationships. A small minority of gay male patients who were bisexual to begin with and who were highly motivated to join the heterosexual mainstream were able, with treatment, to suppress their homosexual behavior and restrict themselves only to heterosexual relationships— even to get married and have children—but in every instance the author found that their sexual fantasy life continued to contain a strong homosexual orientation. In the case of lesbian patients, the situation was different in that those who were motivated to live a conventional heterosexual life were able to do so, inasmuch as their ability to participate in the sexual aspects of such relationships did not depend on their necessarily being aroused sexually (although some were, with the help of lesbian fantasies).

When, however, the "goal" of heterosexuality could not be reached with most of the author's gay male patients, he worked on helping them to accept themselves as they were, but always with the uneasy feeling that somehow or other he had failed them!

Over the years, as the author's experience and understanding broadened and as he followed the rapidly burgeoning research in the field, his conviction grew firmer that his psychoanalytic elders had been seriously mistaken. As the genetic and constitutional factors in homosexuality began to be clarified, the author no longer operated on the assumption that being gay or lesbian constituted a psychological fixation that was potentially reversible, and he began to take an increasingly active role, both in lectures and in writings (Marmor 1965, 1970, 1971, 1972a, 1972b, 1973, 1975, 1980), in the nascent movement to remove homosexuality per se from the category of mental illnesses in the influential *Diagnostic and Statistical Manual* of the American Psychiatric Association. This movement ultimately led to the historic 1973 decision of the American Psychiatric Association Board of Trustees to do so.

The author's activity also brought him into a highly rewarding association with Dr. Evelyn Hooker, whose important pioneering study of the psychological adjustment of male homosexual individuals (Hooker 1957) had deeply impressed him. Subsequently, the author had the privilege of working closely with her on the National Institute of Mental Health Task Force on Homosexuality and on the production of its ground-breaking report, which, though completed in 1969, was not published until 1972 (National Institute of Mental Health Task Force on Homosexuality 1972).

Another positive consequence of the author's taking a public stance on this issue was that a surprising number of his colleagues and social acquaintances began to identify themselves to him as being homosexual, and as a result, the author's understanding of the large group of closeted and nonpatient gays and lesbians—and of their essential psychological normalcy—broadened considerably. Thus the author's conviction of his new stance was powerfully reinforced.

Over those years there was also a gradual but notable change in the motivation that brought gays and lesbians into treatment with the author. The author no longer encountered the same degree of self-rejection among them that he had in the earlier years and their reasons for seeking assistance were no longer centered on achieving help toward a heterosexual adjustment. In most cases the reasons for their seeking help were not fundamentally different from those of the author's nongay patients—problems in their interpersonal relationships, difficulties in establishing long-term liaisons, career problems, and in more recent years, anxieties or consequences related to the AIDS epidemic. Problems of self-acceptance, however, still persisted, which is not surprising to the author in view of the fact that derogation and discrimination against gay men and lesbians continue to be prominent features of our society. The author's focus on the problem now, however, is on helping the patients to see that the core of the problem does not lie in their sexual orientation, but rather in the irrational homophobic prejudices of the social milieu in which they have developed. The fact that many gays and lesbians introject these prejudices is neither surprising nor unique. Similar self-rejecting introjections also exist among Jews, African Americans, and other minorities in our society. The need to eliminate such self-derogatory introjections among women has been a major focus of the feminist revolution also.

In view of the fact that many more gay and lesbian therapists are now "out of the closet," the question arises, in this contemporary context, of whether or not it is possible for nongay therapists to work as effectively with gay males and lesbians as gay therapists can. The author's conviction about this question is identical to that which he has always had about analogous issues as to whether male therapists can treat female patients as effectively as female therapists, or vice versa, or whether therapists of different ethnic, racial, or religious backgrounds from those of their patients can treat such patients as effectively as therapists with homologous backgrounds.

The author does not believe that a firm rule can or should be made with regard to this question. There can be no doubt, however, that for a nongay therapist to effectively treat gays or lesbians at this point in our history, he or she must be reasonably free of conscious or unconscious homophobic prejudice. (The question is open as to whether anyone, gay or nongay, who has grown up in a homophobic culture such as ours, can be *absolutely* free of residual traces of such prejudice.) The destructive consequences on gay and lesbian patients of the interactions with psychoanalysts and other therapists who were thus prejudiced have been repeatedly documented over the years. Anyone who has worked, as the author has, with gay patients who have been subjected to such therapies can vouch for the pain and suffering they have experienced, to say nothing of their enormous and fruitless expenditures of both time and money on efforts to change. Duberman (1991) has described such an experience in eloquent and moving terms in his book *Cures*.

Given an unprejudiced and accepting therapist, however, there is no inherent reason why he or she cannot adequately deal with the problems of gays and lesbians, just as empathic gay and lesbian therapists whom the author knows are able to work with nongay patients. The basic psychodynamic elements that make any psychotherapeutic interaction work are the trust and motivation of the patient and the integrity, warmth, knowledge, and genuineness of the therapist. This is not to deny that there are certain advantages in therapists sharing a common background with their patients, whether this be sexual orientation or racial, religious, or ethnic backgrounds. The patient's knowledge that such a common background exists often, but not necessarily, tends to foster a greater ability to trust and identify positively with the therapist. Indeed, such awareness often plays a part in the selection process that leads patients to seek out certain therapists in preference to others. At times, however, for various psychodynamic reasons, some patients may deliberately seek out therapists with different orientations or backgrounds from their own. This is apt to be particularly true in situations involving homosexual orientation in which patients have introjected antigay prejudices and are seeking for that reason to change their orientation. However, therapists who share these homophobic prejudices can only reinforce the patient's feelings of self-rejection with consequent antitherapeutic results.

Gay patients may also seek out nongay therapists for reasons pertaining to their idiosyncratic family dynamics. A nongay therapist can provide a corrective emotional experience as a warm and accepting father or mother surrogate for a patient whose parents were rejecting or lacking in understanding of them. By the same token, gay or lesbian therapists serve equally effectively as healing parent surrogates to nongay patients in need of similar corrective emotional experiences.

Nevertheless, for nongay therapists to work most effectively with gays and lesbians, it is helpful for them to make an effort to learn about, and understand more fully, the specific subcultural network systems— gay bars, social organizations, and so forth (Hooker 1965)—that may be available to their patients to facilitate their therapeutic progress and social interactions. Nongay therapists should also have a thorough understanding of gay and lesbian sexual practices and of techniques and methods of safer sex. The obverse of this may not necessarily be true for gay therapists treating nongay patients, inasmuch as heterosexual social networks are the ones in which most gays as well as nongays have grown up and have lived their daily lives. The subculture of gays and lesbians, however, is still a relatively segregated one and requires a special effort by nongay therapists to become knowledgeable about its many aspects.

In summary, it has been a source of deep satisfaction to me over the past five and a half decades to have witnessed the substantial advances in mental health understanding about gays and lesbians that have taken place and to have played some role in furthering that process. However, it would be an illusion to assume that the struggle is over. Unhappily in recent years, the AIDS epidemic has been interpreted by homophobic persons as a confirmation of their fears of homosexuality; various right-wing elements, having more or less lost the battle against abortion rights, now have cynically seized on the issue of trying to restrict the legitimate civil rights of homosexual individuals in order to further their political objectives. The role of a scientific approach in psychiatry and the other mental health disciplines in rebutting the outrageous and baseless attacks of these groups against gay men, lesbians, and bisexual individuals thus remains a vitally important and ongoing one.

References

Bergler E: Homosexuality: Disease or Way of Life? New York, Hill and Wang, 1956

Duberman M: Cures: A Gay Man's Odyssey. New York, Dutton, 1991

Freud S: Letter to an American mother. Am J Psychiatry 102:786, 1951

Hooker E: The adjustment of the male overt homosexual. Journal of Projective Techniques 21:18–31, 1957

Hooker E: Male homosexuals and their worlds, in Sexual Inversion: The Multiple Roots of Homosexuality. Edited by Marmor J. New York, Basic Books, 1965, pp 83–107

Marmor J (ed): Sexual Inversion: The Multiple Roots of Homosexuality. New York, Basic Books, 1965

Marmor J: Homosexuality and objectivity. Siecus Newsletter 6(2), 1970

Marmor J: Homosexuality in males. Psychiatric Annals 1(4):44–59, 1971

Marmor J: Notes on some psychodynamic aspects of homosexuality, 1969, in National Institute of Mental Health Task Force on Homosexuality: Final Report and Background Papers. Washington, DC, U.S. Government Printing Office, 1972a

Marmor J: Homosexuality: mental illness or moral dilemma? International Journal of Psychiatry 10:114–117, 1972b

Marmor J: Homosexuality and cultural value systems (abstract). Am J Psychiatry 130:1208–1209, 1973

Marmor J: Homosexuality and sexual orientation disturbances, in Comprehensive Textbook of Psychiatry, 2nd Edition. Edited by Saddock B, Kaplan H, Freedman A. Baltimore, MD, Williams & Wilkins, 1975, pp 1510–1520

Marmor J: Homosexual Behavior: A Modern Reappraisal. New York, Basic Books, 1980

National Institute of Mental Health Task Force on Homosexuality: Final Report and Background Papers. Washington, DC, U.S. Government Printing Office, 1972

SECTION VI

Differences and Diversity

Multicultural Identities and Communities

33

African American Lesbians, Gay Men, and Bisexuals

Billy E. Jones, M.D., M.S.
Marjorie J. Hill, Ph.D.

A frican American lesbians, gay men, and bisexual individuals stand painfully juxtaposed between the fear of cultural estrangement from the African American community and the fear of racial and ethnic alienation from the gay and lesbian community. They may be repeatedly placed in situations that call on them to choose between the two and declare their allegiance to one or the other. In essence, they must deal with the difficulties of living in a society that condemns homosexuality and condones racial prejudice. Far too little attention has been paid to the effects of dual discrimination.

In this chapter, the authors discuss the intrapsychic conflicts of African American lesbians, gay men, and bisexual individuals. They address what it is like to be a lesbian, gay man, or bisexual in the African American community, in white America, and in the gay, lesbian, and bisexual community. Finally, they explore the kinds of supports available to this minority within two minorities and the special issues affecting the treatment process.

Psychological Issues

■ Stereotypes

A unique set of stereotypes characterize America's view of African American lesbian and gay men. Lesbians are portrayed as man-hating, masculine butches preying on naive and unsuspecting heterosexual women. Gay men are seen as finger-snapping, wig-wearing, drag queens who work in beauty parlors. Although there undoubtedly are African American butch lesbians and effeminate gay men, these stereotypes are by no means typical.

Regrettably however, these stereotypical notions and the message they give have been accepted and internalized by far too many African American lesbians, gay men, and bisexual individuals. They create strong negative feelings about an individual's sexual identity and self-worth. Self-hatred can be a result of such internalized homophobia. To a certain extent, all gay men, lesbians, and bisexual individuals deal with internalized oppression, but it is particularly troubling for African Americans. It inhibits a person's ability to combat a frequently hostile, homophobic, and racist environment.

The result is that African American lesbian, gay, and bisexual people experience tremendous stress and anxiety. Many have serious concerns about both disclosure and living in an openly gay environment, their personal safety, success in relationships, and most recently, HIV. These stressors cause some African American lesbians, gay men, and bisexual individuals to keep their sexual identity hidden, but the failure to be open may come at a high intrapsychic price. "Closeted" African American homosexual individuals are viewed as socially immature, inept at relationships, and overly secretive and devious. Their suicide rate is significantly higher than that of their African American heterosexual counterparts (Bell and Weinberg 1978).

■ Identity Development

Identity development is a major task for all adolescents. Although there has been considerable research about the effect of race on identity formation in African Americans (Atkinson et al. 1979; Cross 1971; Parham and Helms 1981), and several models of sexual orientation identity formation (see Chapter 14 by Cass; Troiden 1993) have been described, little literature is available on gay and lesbian development among African Americans (Icard 1986; Loiacano 1993; Mays et al. 1986). However, a growing body of essays, poems, and novels addressing this topic clearly indicates that an African American identity significantly compounds the development of a positive, conflict-free lesbian or gay identity. This should not be misconstrued to mean that gay, lesbian, and bisexual African Americans have impaired identities, but rather that given the reality of racism and homophobia, positive identity development is a much more difficult task for these individuals.

Racism and Homophobia

Extensive literature has documented the effects of racism on African American people (Billingsly 1968; Boyd-Franklin 1989; Grier and Cobbs 1968; Guthrie 1976; Jones 1991; White 1991). Despite the universal consensus that African American gay men, lesbians, and bisexual individuals are subjected to racism, to date there has been little discussion as to how this may differ from the heterosexual's experience of racism. Moreover, sexual orientation, unlike variables such as skin color, gender, class, and educational levels, has only recently been considered as a variable in identity formation. The failure of researchers to pair sexual orientation with racial identity supports the myth that blackness and gayness are mutually exclusive. One consequence is that African American gay men, lesbians, and bisexual individuals seem to experience greater stress from racism because they are not supported by the African American community. In addition, African American lesbians, gay men, and bisexual individuals may experience an increased sensitivity to racial oppression.

The Impact of Sexism

A growing body of literature has assessed the impact of sexism on lesbians in general, and several authors (Loiacano 1993; Mays et al. 1986) have specifically addressed the impact of sexism on African American lesbians. These authors have indicated that these women occupy a minority status in both the lesbian and gay and the African American communities. However, it is interesting that in the Mays et al. (1986) study, African American lesbians reported more discrimination against them on the basis of race and gender than on sexual orientation. For these women, discrimination on the basis of being lesbian seemed to be strongly related to age, class, and gender role characteristics, with younger, lower class, and more masculine-looking women reporting greater discrimination.

Bisexuality

African American bisexual individuals clearly have some unique concerns. Largely as a result of the misperception that bisexual individuals are merely confused "fence sitters" who are unwilling to acknowledge their true gay or lesbian identity, bisexual individuals are often marginalized by people of all sexual orientations. Many African American bisexual individuals assume that they are more acceptable to other African Americans than are gay men and lesbians, and as a result they drive a wedge between themselves and this population. However, far too little is known about African American bisexual individuals, and more research is needed on both bisexuality among African Americans and on the impact of identifying oneself as openly bisexual to understand fully the experiences of these men and women.

The African American Community and Homosexuality

◼ Attitudes Toward Homosexuality

Like other ethnic groups, the African American community does not have a unified position on homosexuality; opinions range from acceptance to abhorrence. In addition, there is real doubt about the common assumption that African American people and their community are more homophobic than are other groups of people in this society (Hooks 1988). Nonetheless, several factors unique to the African American community do contribute to intolerant attitudes toward homosexuality, including religion, Eurocentric versus Afrocentric behaviors, and the existence of strong, predefined gender roles.

The Christian religion has historically been a strong spiritual, moral, political, and social force within the African American community, where it is commonly referred to as "the black church." In the main, the black church's position on homosexuality reflects the conservative religious belief that it is a sin, expressly forbidden in the Bible (Icard 1986; Peterson 1992). African American lesbians, gay men, and bisexual individuals must psychologically cope with the effects of this condemnation, which is a factor in explaining the feelings of diminished self-worth that exist among some African Americans lesbians, gay men, and bisexual individuals.

Myths and misconceptions in the African American community that homosexuality is purely a European phenomenon also contribute to this psychological problem of diminished self-worth. Afrocentric theorists contend that the historical roots of homosexuality emerged from Greco-Roman culture, arguing that the phenomenon did not exist in ancient African villages (Johnson 1981). However, even though there are only a few references to homosexuality in African villages in the past (Andreski 1970), the general lack of data or information about the subject should not be automatically equated with an absence of homosexual behavior historically. It may simply reflect nothing more than a lack of research on the topic of homosexuality in ancient cultures.

Another variation of homophobic theory among some Afrocentric theorists is the contention that white slave owners imposed homosexual practices on male slaves (Crouch 1979; Johnson 1981). This theory assumes that homosexuality is foreign to the African American experience and sends the message that African American gay men, bisexual individuals, and lesbians have identified with the white oppressor. Overt and covert racism in the homosexual community adds to the perception that homosexuality is a Eurocentric phenomenon and increases the special burdens placed on African American lesbians, gay men, and bisexual individuals.

Strongly defined gender roles within the African American community also present problems for African American lesbians, gay men, and bisexual individuals. Certain behaviors, mannerisms, and gestures are rigidly associated with a particular gender and, if exhibited by the other gender, are ridiculed. For example, African American males, particularly young males, are quick to label another male a "sissy" if he does not conform to expected gender manifestations.

Many of these gender stereotypes were first articulated by whites on the antebellum plantation, but they have endured and continue to be accepted in African American and white as well as gay and straight communities. Sexual images of African Americans have also been exaggerated to produce very stereotypical notions of sexuality (Weinberg and Williams 1988). The African American male is portrayed as extremely virile, with a large penis, and always ready for sexual intercourse. His feminine counterpart is a loose, highly fertile, Amazon-like woman with superior sexual abilities. These stereotypes damage all African Americans, but because these caricatures are premised on attraction to the opposite sex, they are particularly detrimental to lesbians, gay men, and bisexual individuals.

■ "Denial" of Homosexuality

Homosexuals and bisexual individuals are often rendered invisible by the larger African American community. Many African Americans find it inconceivable that these people even exist. However, the reality of the day-to-day experience of African Americans is different. Many interact with individual gay men and lesbians differently than with the African American lesbian and gay community as a whole. On a personal level, individuals are often related to in a warm, accepting manner as human beings, friends, or fellow church members. Even these relationships, however, are often premised on the unspoken supposition that the individual's sexual orientation should not be mentioned. Ironically, in almost all such cases the person's sexual orientation is known, but the straight individual will not speak about it, and the gay man or lesbian does not make his or her orientation explicit. Acceptance is permitted as long as the homosexuality is masked, rendering this essential aspect of identity invisible. The following case example illustrates this point:

■ Case Example 1

A 38-year-old African American lesbian who was in psychotherapy was invited to her partner's family home for Thanksgiving dinner, which on the surface appeared to be an act of affirmation and acceptance by the family of their 3-year relationship. However, during the session immediately following Thanksgiving, the client tearfully recounted how the day evolved: "Her parents, especially her mother, kept acting like we were barely casual friends. They kept dropping the names of old boyfriends and politely dismissing our relationship. What really made me angry was that my partner did not say or do anything." This woman's work over the next few weeks focused on ways of creating a safe haven when interacting within a hostile environment. She and her partner recognized that they had not discussed how to handle difficult circumstances within a family context. As a result, they decided to have their own Christmas Eve dinner and to drop in on the family only for dessert on Christmas Day.

■ Changing Attitudes

Attitudes about homosexuality in the African American community are changing, with greater ambivalence, tolerance, and acceptance. The African American media, which only a short time ago would not discuss homosexuality, now does so fairly and with little fanfare. Many African American political leaders have worked hard to include open lesbians and gay men in political coalitions. Most black civil rights organizations have gay antidiscrimination clauses in their bylaws and support gay rights issues. Openly gay groups now exist within the community and even within a few black churches.

The reasons for this attitudinal change come from within and outside the African American community. External reasons include changing attitudes in the larger society, the success of the gay rights movement, and new insights into the origins of homosexuality. Internally, the African American community has been deeply affected by AIDS, which has caused it to more often directly face the existence of homosexuality. In addition, African American lesbians, gay men, and bisexual individuals have become more vocal and have fought successfully for more acceptance. Finally, the existence of openly gay and lesbian African American role models has shattered myths and stereotypes about homosexual individuals. The following case example illustrates this issue:

■ Case Example 2

A 22-year-old African American lesbian recalled in a psychotherapy session how she "came out" to her favorite aunt. "I would go to Baltimore about every 2 months to visit my Aunt Pearl. On this particular occasion I invited my partner of 6 months to go with me. My mother thought it would be a problem to take a 'friend' and too upsetting for my uncle. I called my aunt, officially came out to her over the phone, and told her what my mother had said. My aunt assured me that both my partner and I were welcome to visit any time. My uncle was extremely gracious and supportive." In spite of their lack of experience with gay and lesbian culture, the patient's family was open and accepting.

The Homosexual Community and African Americans

■ A Minority Within a Minority

In spite of the perception of tolerance and diversity, racial discrimination is a pervasive problem among white gay men, lesbians, and bisexual individuals. Discrimination has been well documented in the literature (DeMarco 1983; Greene 1994; Icard 1986; Loiacano 1993; Pharr 1988). Lesbian and gay identified social groups, political organizations, and social services agencies often marginalize, or worse, hinder the full participation of African Americans.

Because white gay men, lesbians, and bisexual individuals are products of the larger society, it is easy to understand how racial discrimination became a part of their community. It is also easy to understand how discrimination against African American gay men, lesbians, and bisexual individuals would restrict the psychological benefits provided largely to whites by community participation. In fact, because of discriminatory practices, participation by African Americans in the gay and lesbian community may be anxiety-producing. This kind of stress may well be heightened because of alienation from the larger African American community. The resulting second-class, or perhaps third-class, citizenship is simply another contributor to low self-esteem and poor identity development.

Discrimination by the larger Anglo community can take a variety of forms. It is all too common for African Americans to be denied entry to a gay or lesbian club through a "carding process" (Peterson 1992). African Americans are simply asked to produce more pieces of identification than whites for entry. They may also be subject to biased service in a restaurant or bar frequented or owned by gay men or lesbians. Discriminatory practices based on race have also been identified in both employment and service in lesbian and gay agencies. Finally, a dearth of African Americans, as well as other people of color, lead major gay and lesbian organizations or serve on their boards of directors.

This overt and covert discrimination is damaging. It underscores and reinforces feelings of isolation and rejection and is particularly detrimental for young African American gay men, lesbians, and bisexual individuals. Although the trauma associated with coming out has been eased for white gay men and lesbians because of prominent role models in leadership positions, young African Americans have not benefited to the same degree. The problem is made more severe because those portrayed in gay-produced media are overwhelmingly white and male. African American gay men, lesbians, and bisexual individuals simply do not see themselves reflected in the larger gay community. The following cases illustrate this point:

■ Case Example 3

A 17-year-old African American gay youth complained bitterly in a lesbian and gay youth group that he was afraid of losing his identity as an African American. "My parents say this gay stuff is a white thing. All of my homeboys from the neighborhood are always putting down gay people. And when I come to programs for gay and lesbian youth, most of the adults are white. You white people are cool but I need to be with my own kind."

■ Case Example 4

A 32-year-old African American lesbian in treatment echoed these sentiments, "When I go to the Gay and Lesbian Center, I see primarily white gay men and lesbians. When I watch gay and lesbian programs on TV, I see almost exclusively white people. It really makes me feel invisible or worse; like accepting my sexual orientation is a betrayal of my race and heritage."

Therapy

■ Seeking Psychotherapy

A decision to seek psychotherapy is rarely a smooth or easy one, but it is particularly difficult for many African American lesbians, gay men, and bisexual individuals. Although there is a long-standing tradition in the African American community of seeking advice from others, it usually entails talking to a minister, relative, or friend. Until recently, those in the African American community have not sought assistance from a professional they do not know, and a variety of factors perpetuate this historical resistance to psychotherapy. First, psychotherapy is largely based on a Eurocentric (white), Freudian model. In addition, considerable stigma is attached in the African American community to both being a patient and not being able to cope with one's problems. When issues related to sexual orientation are added to these factors, the African American who could benefit from mental health services may experience overwhelming resistance.

Finding a suitable therapist is another problem for African American lesbians, gay men, and bisexual individuals. Questions about whether a therapist should be African American or white, gay or straight, male or female are all significant. As a rule, the authors believe that the most appropriate therapist is one who shares the patient's ethnicity, gender, and sexual orientation. Generally, there is a greater degree of interest, familiarity, and knowledge about the culture, gender, and sexual orientation issues held by therapists who share these same persuasions with the patient. There are, however, all too few African American therapists and far fewer African American therapists who are also gay, lesbian, or bisexual. It is quite possible that an African American gay male, lesbian, or bisexual seeking treatment will not be able to find the ideal therapist. The next best choice is generally a therapist who either shares the patient's ethnicity or sexual orientation or an individual with special training, knowledge, or sensitivity to the patient's cultural background and sexual orientation.

■ Psychotherapy Issues

In this chapter, the authors have focused on dual identity issues confronting African American lesbians, gay men, and bisexual individuals. They are the core issues that separate this population from the larger African American and gay and lesbian communities. Treatment must focus on issues resulting from the unique position of this minority within two minorities.

Therapists must be prepared to assist patients in uncovering and recognizing the inherent and particular conflicts involved in making primary and secondary identity choices. Patients also need help in understanding the justifiable anger produced by having to make such choices. Resolving the conflicts resulting from this choice is a key part of the therapeutic process. With therapy, a patient can decide whether he or she is more comfortable with a primary definition as African American or as lesbian, gay, or bisexual. The following case illustrates this conflict:

■ Case Example 5

A 40-year-old African American gay man was quite ambivalent regarding participation in the 1993 March on Washington, even though he had been politically active in the gay and lesbian community for several years. He could not decide if he should march with the Gay Men of African Descent or with ACT UP/NY. He thought it was important to be out, black, and proud; however, it was also important for him to show that not all AIDS activists are white. Although he went to the march, he ended up standing on the sidelines feeling guilty. He simply was unable to make a choice.

Therapists also need to work with patients on issues relating to diminished self-worth. The self-destructive behavior that being a member of two stigmatized communities can produce may lead to a variety of dysfunctional behaviors, such as an inability to start or maintain relationships, sexual dysfunction, compulsive sexual activity, or substance abuse. These problems for African American gay men, lesbians, and bisexual individuals may need to be addressed in therapy. Having helped to resolve these dilemmas, the therapist must assist the patient in integrating these adaptations into the personality and in reassessing self-worth.

References

Andreski I: Old Wives' Tales: Life-Stories From Ibibioland. New York, Schocken Books, 1970

Atkinson DR, Morton G, Sue DW: Counseling American Minorities. Dubuque, IA, William Brown, 1979

Bell AP, Weinberg MS: Homosexualities: A Study of Diversity Among Men and Women. New York, Simon and Schuster, 1978

Billingsly A: Black Families in White America. Englewood Cliffs, NJ, Prentice-Hall, 1968

Boyd-Franklin N: Black Families in Therapy: A Multisystems Approach. New York, Guilford, 1989

Cross WE: The Negro-to-black conversion experience: toward a psychology of black liberation. Black World 20:13–27, 1971

Crouch S: Clinches of degradation (review of Just Above My Head, by J Baldwin). Village Voice, October 29, 1979, pp 32–42

DeMarco J: Gay racism, in Black Men/White Men: A Gay Anthology. Edited by Smith MJ. San Francisco, CA, Gay Sunshine, 1983, pp 109–118

Grier WH, Cobbs PM: Black Rage. New York, Basic Books, 1968

Greene B: Lesbian and gay sexual orientation: implications for clinical training, practice and research, in Psychological Perspectives on Lesbian and Gay Issues, Vol 1. Lesbian and Gay Psychology: Theory, Research and Clinical Applications. Edited by Greene B, Herek GM. Thousand Oaks, CA, Sage, 1994

Guthrie R: Even the Rat Was White: A Historical View of Psychology. New York, Harper and Row, 1976

Hooks B: Talking Back. Boston, MA, South End Press, 1989

Icard L: Black gay men and conflicting social identities: sexual orientation versus racial identity. Journal of Social Work and Human Sexuality 4:83–93, 1986

Johnson JM: Influence of assimilation on the psychosocial adjustment of black homosexual men. Doctoral dissertation, California School of Professional Psychology at Berkeley, Ann Arbor, MI, University Microfilm International, 1981

Jones JM: The concept of race in social psychology: from color to culture, in Black Psychology. Edited by Jones R. New York, Harper & Row, 1991, pp 441–467

Loiacano DK: Gay identity issues among black Americans, in Psychological Perspectives on Lesbian and Gay Male Experiences. Edited by Garnets L, Kimmel D. New York, Columbia University Press, 1993, pp 364–375

Mays VM, Cochran SD, Peplau LA: The black lesbian relationship project: relationship experiences and the perception of discrimination. Paper presented at the 94th annual convention of the American Psychological Association, Washington, DC, August 1986

Parham TA, Helms JE: The influence of black students' racial identity attitudes on preferences for counselor's race. Journal of Counseling Psychology 28:250–257, 1981

Peterson JL: Black men and their same-sex desires and behaviors, in Gay Culture in America: Essays From the Field. Edited by Herdt G. Boston, MA, Beacon Press, 1992, pp 147–164

Pharr S: Homophobia: A Weapon of Sexism. Little Rock, AR, Chardon Press, 1988

Troiden RR: The formation of homosexual identities, in Psychological Perspectives on Lesbian and Gay Male Experiences. Edited by Garnett L, Kimmel D. New York, Columbia University Press, 1993, pp 191–217

Weinberg MS, Williams CJ: Black sexuality: a test of two theories. J Sex Res 20:197–217, 1988

White J: Toward a black psychology, in Black Psychology. Edited by Jones R. New York, Harper and Row, 1991, pp 5–13

34

Mental Health Issues for Gay and Lesbian Asian Americans

Gene A. Nakajima, M.D.
Yim H. Chan, M.D.
Kewchang Lee, M.D.

O nly in the last few years have Asians become visible as distinct groups in the lesbian and gay communities in North America, Australia, and western Europe. Many major cities such as New York, Sydney, and London currently have lesbian and gay organizations specifically composed of Asians. Coincident with the inception of such groups, several Asian American artists, writers, anthropologists, and other scholars have begun to write about the lesbian and gay Asian American experience. In the psychiatric and mental health fields, however, practically no literature concerning lesbian and gay Asian Americans has been published.

The authors thank Howard C. Rubin, M.D., Gust Yep, Ph.D., and Warren Ng, M.D., for their assistance.

Over the past decade, psychological and mental health differences between Asian Americans and people of other races have been described (Uba 1993). However, issues of sexuality, and in particular homosexuality, have generally not been explored, possibly as a result of the stigma attached to discussions of sex in most Asian American communities. In this chapter, the authors provide an overview of mental health issues facing lesbian and gay Asian Americans, from a lesbian- and gay-affirmative perspective.

There is great diversity in language, customs, immigration status, religion, acculturation to the majority culture, socioeconomic class, and lesbian, gay, and bisexual identification among Asian Americans. These differences affect their mental health treatment; accordingly, no generalizable treatment recommendations can be made, for example, both for a bisexual fourth-generation Japanese American woman and a recently emigrated gay man from Pakistan. In this chapter, the authors therefore provide therapists with a general knowledge base to enhance understanding and treatment of lesbian and gay Asian Americans.

The authors are East Asian American men who have a relatively high degree of U.S. assimilation and who have conducted therapy largely with Asian American gay men who are either of East Asian or Filipino origin; this chapter contains a bias toward those populations. Unfortunately, the authors are not familiar with any Asian American psychiatrists who have extensive experience treating lesbian or bisexual Asian American women. The authors also have not had any experience treating Pacific Islanders, and they are not discussed in this chapter. Because there is so little mental health research on the lesbian, gay, and bisexual Asian American populations, some of what follows is necessarily anecdotal and based on clinical experience. Future research and literature, it is hoped, will describe the experiences of treating a wider range of Asian American lesbians and gay men.

Homosexuality in Asia

Many of the attitudes concerning homosexuality among Asian Americans are derived from their countries of origin. There has been a long history of same-sex behavior documented in Asian countries. Many examples of same-sex male relationships are found in literature from preindustrial Japan, China, and India (Hinsch 1990; Lau and Ng 1989;

Saikaku 1687/1990; Schalow 1989). Most of the men in these writings are depicted as married to women but also have sex with men. The liaisons are usually with men from different social classes, age groups, or educational status. Saikaku (1687/1990), for example, in his *Nanshoku Okagami* (*The Great Mirror of Male Love*), depicted same-sex love relations between samurai men and boys and between merchant-class men and Kabuki actors. In 16th-century India, harems of young boys were kept by both Muslim and Hindu aristocrats (AIDS Bhedbav Virodhi Andolan 1993). There are fewer historical texts concerning lesbians in Asian countries. The depictions of lesbians are usually of women of the same class who assume stereotyped male and female gender roles (Lieh-Mak et al. 1983; Ruan and Bullough 1992). There are exceptions, though, such as the *Kama Sutra,* written by Vats Yama in the 4th to 5th century, which states that lesbian activity was observed in the Indian harems called "Anthaprera" (AIDS Bhedbav Virodhi Andolan 1993).

Coinciding with increasing contact with the West in the 19th century and increasing modernization, general suppression of sexuality, and in particular homosexuality, began in Asian countries. Two contributing factors were the importation of Christian moralistic attitudes toward, and psychiatric disease models of, homosexuality. Open expressions of homosexuality were therefore forced to go underground and became invisible to the public. This suppression of homosexuality remains particularly strong in eastern Asia and in the Communist-controlled parts of Asia. However, other Asian countries such as the Philippines and Thailand seem to be more open to homosexuality today (Whitman and Mathy 1986).

Currently, many Asians believe that homosexuality is much rarer in Asian than in Western countries. Despite a long history of homosexuality in Asian countries, a widespread belief persists that homosexual influences have recently been imported from the West. The current hostility toward homosexuality in many Asian countries has led some lesbian and gay Asian Americans to reject their origins. Others have attempted to reclaim their earlier homosexual traditions as a means of integrating their Asian American and gay identities.

In Asian countries the concept of same-sex love as a core identity, with a strict demarcation between homosexuality and heterosexuality, is much less prevalent than in the West. Asians who have sexual experiences with both genders may not identify as lesbian, gay, or bisexual, and many do not conceptualize themselves in terms of categories of sexual orientation. In many Asian countries, homosexuality, cross-dressing, and transsexuality are not strictly demarcated. Since a greater fluidity among sexual orientation, sexual behavior, and gender identity exists, it may be difficult for many people to distinguish homosexuality from cross-dressing. Cross-dressing is generally more widespread among gay men and lesbians in most Asian countries than in the West, and it has been institutionalized in traditional theater such as the Chinese Opera and the Japanese Kabuki for men and the Japanese Takarakuza theater for women (Robertson 1989). These Asian cultural traditions have been imported by immigrants to the West and may result in identity conflicts such as Manalansan (1996) described among gay Filipinos in the United States. In the Philippines, gay men who cross-dress, act effeminately, and emphasize passing as "real" women are called "Bakla." They generally perform the passive role in sex with a man who may not consider himself homosexual. Filipino gay men in the United States who are more assimilated and have adopted the mainstream gay white standards of masculinity may view effeminacy pejoratively and may distance themselves from what they consider to be Filipino, as opposed to U.S. gay culture. Manalansan (1996) also reported that the effeminate Bakla may reject assimilated gay Filipino American men because they are viewed as "mimicking white men and of having the illusion of being 'real' men" (p. 54).

Many other examples exist of cross-dressing and effeminacy in men in Asian countries, spanning what the West would consider transsexuality and homosexuality. The Hijras in India are a religious sect in which men surgically remove their penises and identify as women (Nanda 1984). In Indonesia, men who dress and act effeminately are called "Banci" (Williams 1990); in Thailand, "Katoey" (Puterbaugh 1990); and in Burma, "Acault" (Coleman et al. 1992). These Asian traditions of expressing homosexuality through effeminacy or cross-dressing may come into conflict with a current trend of gay male culture in North America, which prizes masculinity. This conflict may lead more assimilated gay Asian American men to reject their gay Asian traditions.

Although a more Western-influenced lesbian and gay culture is emerging in Asian countries, overt public expressions of homosexual love continue to be suppressed. Only in the last few years have lesbian and gay people in Asian countries organized civil rights organizations. The media have also demonstrated a greater willingness to depict homosexuality. For example, in 1993 two nominees for the Foreign Language Award of the Motion Picture Academy of Arts and Sciences went to a Chinese film (*Farewell My Concubine*) and a Taiwanese film (*A Wedding Banquet*), both of which portrayed homosexuality. In 1994 activists in Tokyo held the first lesbian and gay pride parade in an Asian country.

■ Philosophical and Religious Influences

There are many traditions and religions from Asian countries that affect Asian American lesbian and gay men, including Confucianism, Buddhism, Taoism, Hinduism, and Islam. In East Asia—predominantly China, Japan, and Korea—Confucianism influences many spheres of interpersonal conduct (Hong et al. 1993). Confucian cultures are patrilineal and emphasize ancestor worship and filial piety. Sons, particularly the first-born, are more important in Confucian cultures than daughters because they are responsible for continuing the family line. Therefore, homosexuality is viewed as a particular threat to the continuation of the family name. (Gay Asian American activists have recently made light of this tradition by selling T-shirts that state, "Queer 'N Asian, the Family Tree Stops Here.")

Traditionally, marriage has not been considered a romantic affair in most Asian countries and was often prearranged by family members. The role of marriage was to increase family kinship linkages and to fulfill expectations of continuing the family line. East Asian men are not expected to find romantic love in their marriages. Men, but not women, are theoretically free to find romantic interest with either men or women outside the marriage, as long as the appearance of having a heterosexual marriage and producing sons is maintained. In many Asian countries, gay men continue to have heterosexual marriages, but may have same-sex affairs on the side. In North America, arranged marriages among assimilated Asian Americans are not common; however, many gay people continue to accommodate their families by accepting a heterosexual marriage.

In Confucian-oriented cultures, emphasis is placed on scholarship, learning, and other nonphysical aspects of men. This emphasis comes in direct conflict with the value placed on the masculine appearance valued in mainstream American gay male cultures.

Confucian cultures generally place great importance on maintaining social harmony. Societal needs are elevated above individual needs. This emphasis creates pressure to conform to societal norms, and individual expression of sexuality is not tolerated. Lesbian and gay Asian

Americans must overcome the fear of breaking traditional societal boundaries that discourage "coming out." In accordance with the importance placed on social harmony, East Asian societies emphasize shame over guilt. As a result, not bringing disgrace to one's family, kinship, or company is vital to people from East Asian cultures. Because of the importance of "keeping face" or maintaining dignity, East Asian lesbians and gay men frequently feel compelled to maintain secrecy about aspects of their personal life of which society would disapprove. Pamela H. (1989) related, "Concern that family honor will be tarnished motivates many women to hide their lesbianism. This family shame factor reflects the tightness of many Asian American communities. . . . In fact the general Asian American community may be too close-knit for the closeted lesbian" (p. 287). However, there may be little guilt over sexual liaisons that no one, particularly one's family, discovers.

In many Asian countries such as Korea and Taiwan, Christianity has become widespread since World War II; many recent immigrants from those countries have converted to Christianity, and several have become fundamentalists who interpret the Bible literally and adopt the homophobic attitudes of many North American fundamentalists.

■ Psychiatric and Sexological Literature From Asia

Prior to Western influences at the end of the 19th century, homosexuality was not a topic of concern to physicians and scientists from Asian countries. However, European sexologists brought the scientific study of sexuality to Asian countries. Eventually, most Asian countries adopted a disease-oriented model of homosexuality.

Many Western travelers who went to Asian countries in the 19th century commented, usually disapprovingly, on widespread homosexual activity among Asians. European sexologists were intrigued by the seemingly more open atmosphere concerning homosexuality in Asian countries and started to write about it in the 19th and early 20th centuries. The first scientific journal devoted to homosexuality, the *Jahrbuch fuer sexuelle Zwischenstufen* ("Yearbook for Sexual Intermediaries"), which was published between 1899 and 1923 under the editorship of the first openly gay psychiatrist, Magnus Hirschfeld, contained several articles about homosexuality in Asian countries. These included an article by a Japanese professor at Berlin University about Saikaku

(Iwaya 1902) and an article about homosexuality in Japan. A 133-page monograph about homosexuality in East Asia appeared in 1906 called *"Das gleichgeschlectliche Leben der Ostasiaten: Chinesen Japaner Koreer"* ("The Same Sex Life of East Asians: Chinese Japanese Korean"), which was directly influenced by Hirschfeld's research on homosexuality as a "third sex" (Karsch-Haack 1906).

Despite the early 20th-century European sexological interest in Asian homosexuality, it has not been examined much in the Asian psychiatric literature. The existing literature has focused on psychoanalytic theories to explain the theoretically low incidence of homosexuality in Asian countries. Because traditional analysts thought male homosexuality was caused by an overly involved mother and a distant father, Western psychoanalysts might predict a greater amount of homosexuality in Asian cultures, where this pattern is quite common. In the Asian psychoanalytic literature, however, there are alternative and often contradictory ideas on the "etiology" of homosexuality. For example, Hsu and Tseng (1969) described how Chinese people resolve the oedipal complex:

> For boys there is less concern about developing signs of masculinity so that . . . a boy does not feel compelled to engage in sport. A girl does not have to be popular among boys to prove she is feminine. Chinese society distinguishes clearly the sexual role of man and woman. . . . The fact that family and society frown upon any person who does not dress properly according to his sex tends to eliminate bisexual tendencies, one of the factors which may favor the development of homosexuality. . . . Even though the mother-son relationship is very close, it is seldom sexualized so that it is not likely to develop into the 'double-bind' situation of maternal seductiveness along with maternal sexual restriction of the son, which is described as the usual prelude to the son's developing homosexual problems in Western culture. (p. 12)

Hahn (1970) noted that homosexuality was quite rare in Korea, with only eight gay and lesbian patients entering the Seoul National University Hospital between 1959 and 1969. He had an alternative explanation that the oedipal triangular relationship, and therefore, the negative oedipal complex does not occur in Korean families because the care of the child is primarily by the mother, and the male child does not have to compete with the father for his mother's attention. In a discussion of a case of a gay male Asian patient, psychoanalyst Doi had yet another explanation, postulating that a distant relationship with a mother was the partial cause of homosexuality (Jaschke and Doi 1989).

In 1993 the American Psychiatric Association Office of International Affairs polled psychiatric organizations from 125 countries about homosexuality; 34 countries responded (Hausman 1993). Those from China and India responded that most psychiatrists in their countries believe that homosexuality is a mental illness. Those from Korea, Taiwan, and Nepal responded that homosexuality is considered a curable sexual deviation but not a diagnosable mental illness. Because most psychiatrists in Asian countries continue to view homosexuality as a mental illness, family members of gay and lesbian Asian Americans may continue to encourage treatment to "cure" homosexuality. In 1994 OCCUR, a Japanese lesbian and gay civil rights organization, asked the Japanese Society of Neurology and Psychiatry to endorse officially the World Health Organization's position that homosexuality is not a mental illness. Only after a request by the medical director of the American Psychiatric Association did the Japanese Society respond that they had recently adopted ICD-10.

Gay- and lesbian-affirmative psychiatric treatment has only recently become available in Asian countries. As an example, at an international psychotherapy conference in Taipei in 1993, psychiatrists from the prestigious National Taiwan University gave a presentation on a coming-out group.

Lesbian and Gay Asian American Identity

As described by Cass (see Chapter 14 by Cass), lesbians and gay men go through stages when developing an integrated identity. Espin (1987), in her studies of Latina lesbians, noticed that ethnic minorities go through parallel stages in developing their lesbian or gay and their minority identity. Chan (1989), in an empirical study of Asian American lesbian and gay identity development, noted that lesbian and gay Asian Americans generally identify more strongly with their lesbian and gay identity than with their Asian American identity. Maria (1993) talked of her military experience as a young adult: "Those 3 years, the company of these women really helped me become more comfortable with myself . . . but throughout this time, my Indian self was basically dormant, trotted out when it suited me—usually when I figured that the exoticism of it would set me apart" (p. 205).

The process of embracing an Asian American identity may be particularly difficult for Asian Americans. Asian Americans often do not have much Asian American self-awareness and frequently go through a stage of believing that they are white—a phenomenon similar to internalized homophobia. For example, one participant in Hom's 1992 study of Asian lesbians (Hom 1992) stated, "If I ever saw Filipino dykes at the bar, I'd just shy away from them because I didn't want to be associated with them." Ahmed (1988) noted that every South Asian (people from the Indian subcontinent) "wants to be as white as possible or at least wants to be looked on as being fair . . . we are defining ourselves from a perspective as white people" (p. 5). Gay Asian American men may not interact among themselves because they view other Asian Americans as competition for the attention of potential sexual partners. Mangaong (1996) explained his experience of going to bars: "If there was another Asian in the bar, I tended to avoid him so as not to infringe on his cruising domain" (p. 108). Although the majority culture may expect Asian American gay men and lesbians to have common experiences and therefore to seek out the affiliation of other lesbian and gay Asian Americans actively, avoidance of other gay and lesbian Asian Americans is particularly common. It may be uncomfortable for an Asian American because such actions involve an acknowledgment, consciously or unconsciously, that he or she is an Asian American.

Frequently a crisis such as a severe breakup of a relationship or a severe illness brings forth issues related to personal identity, including culture and sexuality. Another subject in Hom's 1992 study (Hom 1992) stated, "At the age of 29, I checked into a treatment center; that's when I started sorting through what it meant to be a Filipina, being a lesbian, being a person of color" (p. 16). Gay Asian American men who become HIV infected may start seeking support of other Asian Americans for the first time, possibly because their peers may be understanding of particular family issues that arise in the context of death and dying.

■ Impact of Racism and Homophobia

Mainstream gay men and lesbians have generally ignored Asian American communities. Asian Americans rarely see themselves portrayed in the gay and lesbian media. Frequently Asian Americans are thought of as exotic, non-American, or foreign. Hom (1991) related her own experience:

> Once my Korean dyke friend and I were accosted by a white lesbian at . . . [a] lesbian bar. We are minding our own business, and . . . my vision is temporarily blocked by a woman with her hands in a prayer position, bowing and murmuring, "An-yo." We stared blankly at her and she asks if we understand Korean. . . . [I said,] "No, I've been colonized and led to believe that English is the only acceptable language. So much so that I cannot hold a decent conversation with my parents in Chinese." She went on to say that she had some Asian friends and that they were "just the cutest things; small and dainty like China Dolls." (p. 51)

Asian American men are often thought to be passive partners and sexually subservient. Fung (1991), in his examination of North American gay pornography, noted that the very few images of Asian Americans he found portrayed them as passive partners who only want to have sex with white men. Wat (1996) noted, "When a friend of mine finally convinced a drunken white man who had been forcing himself on him that he did not like playing the submissive role, the white man became disgusted and said, 'You have completely turned Americanized. Go back to Asia and learn to be Asian'" (p. 73).

Lesbian and gay Asian Americans tend to perceive the general Asian American community as homophobic. Chan (1989) found that lesbian and gay Asian Americans thought it was more difficult to "come out" to other Asian Americans and were more likely to participate in gay and lesbian groups than in Asian American groups. Lesbian and gay Asian Americans may also fear rejection from their families, which may be especially painful in light of the strong emphasis placed on the family in Confucian-oriented cultures. Asian American lesbians and gay men have difficulty forming an integrated identity because they may perceive rejection from both mainstream lesbians and gay men and the heterosexual Asian American community; at the same time they may avoid or be avoided by other Asian American lesbians and gay men. Ayyar (1993) stated, "The tug between the culture I share with my parents and the sexuality that is foreign to them has not abated within me. I feel loneliness and anger. . . . I feel angry at the Indian culture for not accepting who I am. I also feel angry at the West. . . . I feel that it has met my needs only sporadically" (p. 173). But recently, with the proliferation of lesbian and gay Asian American political and social organizations across the country, a more positive self-image and sense of awareness are emerging.

Relationship Issues

There appear to be few homoracial (same-race) relationships among Asian American gay men, and those that do occur are often among first-generation immigrants. Those in homoracial relationships are pejoratively called "sticky rice," a term referring to Asian Americans attracted to other Asian Americans. Asian Americans may have internalized the dominant culture's portrayal of Asian American men as unmasculine and undesirable. In the absence of visible, positive, gay Asian American role models, many may have allowed themselves to be defined and judged by criteria touted in the majority gay media. This dynamic may lead many Asian Americans to feel that their image of themselves and their sense of self-worth are dependent on the assimilation into and acceptance by the lesbian and gay majority communities.

Most gay Asian American men in relationships are probably involved with a partner of another race. Ideally, many Asian American men who are not interested in other Asian Americans would like to attract a partner who has had no prior interest in Asian Americans. However, a great number of Asian American gay men are involved with men who have exclusive interests in Asian Americans, have additional interests in other people of color, or are attracted to postpubescent adolescent boys ("ephebophilia"). Men with such interests are pejoratively called "rice queens." Stereotypically, a rice queen is an older non-Asian American man who may express his attraction to Asian Americans in terms of their youthful appearance, smooth skin, smaller body structure, passivity, and a perception of exoticness. These men frequently possess a sense of entitlement when interacting with Asian Americans, and they act in a manner that might be described as domineering, with a sense of privilege.

Asian Americans who are involved with the stereotypical rice queen may encounter disapproval from the Asian American gay community or from non-Asian American peers. The Asian American partner in an interracial couple may be perceived as a "banana" (yellow on the outside, white on the inside) and may be thought of as ashamed of his Asian heritage. There may be age, education, and income disparities between partners that are difficult to bridge. Such relationships, however, may reflect patterns in preindustrial Asian countries described above.

A common difficulty found in interracial relationships is stage discrepancies, in which one partner is at a different stage in the development of a relationship than the other. An Asian American in a relationship may also perceive that he has less power and feel that his partner could easily find someone else. The Asian American may desire a stronger commitment than his partner is comfortable with, which may lead to jealousy and frustration on the part of the Asian American partner.

Isay (1989) believes that interracial relationships may be stronger than homoracial relationships because there may be inherent differences between the two men that are likely to be complementary. McWhirter and Mattison (1984) also noted the positive aspects of having an age-discrepant relationship, such as a decreased need for direct competition.

Treatment Recommendations

Asian Americans are generally reluctant to seek mental health care, largely because of the stigma attached to mental health treatment. Asian Americans may have difficulty finding Asian American therapists, particularly when they must operate within the constraints of managed care; most Asian Americans who speak English have non-Asian therapists. Transference issues about race in therapy must be addressed by the therapist because the Asian American patient may be too uncomfortable to bring it up. Although most Asian Americans prefer Asian American therapists (Gim et al. 1991), many lesbian and gay Asian Americans refuse homoethnic therapists as a result of issues of confidentiality, internalized negative feelings about Asian Americans, or perceived homophobia in Asian American communities.

Therapists need to obtain an accurate history concerning Asian American identification, as well as a history of coming out. Particular focus may be placed on the question of whether the patient has any Asian American friends or avoids other lesbian and gay Asian Americans. Coming-out issues, particularly with regard to family members, are usually difficult for Asian Americans in light of the philosophical and religious influences described above. Because of cultural barriers, Asian Americans may seem to be coming out slowly, and great patience must be used in supporting and possibly directing an Asian American client through the various stages of lesbian and gay identification. Asian Americans frequently are pressured by their non-Asian American friends to come out to family members. It is particularly important to emphasize that it is not necessarily essential for the patients' development to come out to family members. Frequently language or other cultural barriers may make coming out to family members much more difficult for Asian Americans.

Asian Americans are frequently reluctant to enter therapy or support groups for fear of losing confidentiality. In addition, they may be reluctant to speak out or may feel like an outsider if they are the only Asian American in a group. In a mixed racial group, Asian American clients may feel competitive with the other Asian Americans. These issues must be addressed during the screening process before a referral is made for group therapy.

Family therapy may be underutilized in Asian American communities. It is essential to involve the family if possible in treatment, and the use of an interpreter is imperative if there are non-English-speaking persons in the family. Many therapists suggest that Asian Americans use Parents and Friends of Lesbians and Gays (PFLAG), but Asian American families are generally reluctant to attend such support groups. For example, in the Los Angeles chapter of PFLAG, only one Asian American family is involved (Hom 1996). This group made an unsuccessful attempt in 1993 to start a group for Asian American family members. However, a group solely for gay and lesbian Vietnamese and their families did form in Orange County, California (Carrier et al. 1992).

Making appropriate referrals to peer support groups or organizations may also be helpful for lesbian and gay Asian American clients. Many major cities have lesbian and gay Asian American organizations that can be divided into two types: Asian American-exclusive organizations and mixed racial organizations (Chua 1990).

Asian American-exclusive organizations generally have closed meetings, with only the social events open to non-Asian Americans. Most of these organizations address issues of racism and homophobia, and some have peer-led discussion groups or coming-out groups. Some organizations are for all members from the Asian diaspora, and others are ethnic-specific. South-Asians frequently form their own organizations because they feel that the general Asian American organizations ignore or are not aware of South-Asian issues. For example, in San Francisco, Trikone is a group for lesbian and gay South-Asians, and Shamakomi is a forum for South-Asian lesbians and bisexual women.

The ethnic-specific organizations may conduct their meetings in their ethnic language. Some clients may feel uncomfortable in all-Asian American settings and may not accept referrals to these organizations. Some of these organizations have the usually unfounded reputation of rejecting people in interracial relationships or recent immigrants.

There are social organizations for Asian American men with non-Asian American men, generally called "Asians and Friends." Many Asian Americans have complained that they are objectified at these meetings. These organizations may be problematic because some of them are dominated by stereotypical rice queens. These groups are useful for Asian Americans looking for non-Asian Americans who are interested in Asian Americans. They may be useful for people who need support for their interracial relationships.

Many therapists and lesbian and gay Asian Americans have little awareness of writings by lesbian and gay Asian Americans that may be useful for a better understanding of lesbian and gay Asian Americans. There are several anthologies that may be a resource for both therapist and patient (Chung et al. 1987; Leong 1994; Lim-Hing 1996; Ratti 1993; Witness Aloud 1993).

The authors end this chapter with a case that illustrates a few of the issues that have been outlined:

■ Case Example

Mr. A is a 27-year-old gay, Hong Kong-born, Chinese American man who was self-referred for individual psychotherapy after becoming increasingly depressed; the depression began shortly after he was passed over for a promotion as an accountant. Another stressor includes relationship problems stemming from difficulties expressing emotions and affection. He also fears that his parents will find out about his homosexuality.

Mr. A's sociocultural background instilled in him basic Confucian-based beliefs in the value of hard work, self-reliance, and frugality. His parents have always emphasized the importance of maintaining his role as reliable and dependable. The failure of a promotion at work has exposed his conflicts between his need to be perfect and in control and his self-image as weak, different, unassertive, and lonely.

Mr. A and his family immigrated from Hong Kong when he was 5 years old, and since then his parents have stressed the need to blend in with his environment and to become completely acculturated to mainstream American life. Mr. A has never felt comfortable with his Asian heritage. Although he has at times acknowledged his Asian background—during college he did some volunteer work in Chinatown—he feels more comfortable with mainstream white culture than with Asian American culture. He has no Asian friends, and the few friends he has are either heterosexual white colleagues from work or gay white friends of his partner. He admits being competitive with other gay Asians for white sexual partners and does not view other gay Asians as potential sources of support or friendship. Interestingly, when Mr. A sought therapy for his depression, he specifically requested an Asian therapist, perhaps because he wanted a therapist who would understand bicultural issues, particularly Asian family issues.

Mr. A believes that his parents consider homosexuality and the failure to marry and have children as shameful. He has never revealed his homosexuality to his parents and believes that he may cause his father's death by coming out to him because his father has a heart condition. His parents question the nature of Mr. A's relationship with his partner, but they have never communicated their suspicions directly. Mr. A keeps his Asian identity, which is closely tied to his family, completely separate from his gay identity. Although he has been out for over 5 years, he has few gay friends except those of his partner. His closest friends, his work colleagues, do not know of his homosexuality. His main contact with the gay world, besides his association with his partner, is through gay bathhouses and sex clubs.

Mr. A's partner is 13 years older than he and has a particular interest in Asian men. They have had a committed and open relationship for 2 years. His partner has expressed some interest in settling down and moving in together, but Mr. A does not feel ready for this more explicit commitment. The rejection of his promotion has exacerbated his feelings of inadequacy in relation to his partner, who is an established lawyer with a significantly larger income than his.

During the initial sessions, Mr. A appears to be ingratiating and superficially compliant. Later he engages in more competitive struggles and sees his therapist as uncaring and overbearing like his father. Sometimes Mr. A devalues the therapist's interpretations and suggestions. For example, when the therapist brings up the possibility of Mr. A contacting local gay Asian social groups, Mr. A feels that he was overcontrolling. In therapy Mr. A has had to confront his fear of intimacy with other Asian men and his need to be in a noncompetitive relationship with another Asian man. The therapist has used a cognitive approach, and the depressive symptoms have significantly lifted. Mr. A has also become more comfortable with his gay identity. He has considered telling his close friends at work about his homosexuality. In addition, he has become more in touch with his Asian identity. He has started to ask his father more about Hong Kong and has become more interested in the significance of holidays such as Chinese New Year. He has yet to explore in therapy his feelings about being a gay Asian and integrating his Asian background with his gay identity.

This clinical vignette highlights the cultural factors involved in psychotherapy with gay Asian Americans. Issues of extrapsychic and intrapsychic denial, bicultural identities, and Eastern religious and philosophical values all play an important role in the therapeutic process.

Conclusion

As health care reform continues, the need to focus resources on minority groups is receiving greater attention. Currently, little research is available on what mental health services or approaches are most useful for lesbian and gay Asian Americans. Most information, such as presented in this chapter, is anecdotal, and no research has been published that examines the impact of racism, sexism, and homophobia on mental health for lesbian and gay Asian Americans. Clearly, more research and studies are needed so that more information can be obtained about this understudied population.

References

Ahmed A, Islam S: Breaking the silence. Trikone, September 1988, p 5

AIDS Bhedbav Virodhi Andolan (ABVA): Homosexuality in India: culture and heritage, in A Lotus of Another Color. Edited by Ratti R. Boston, MA, Alyson Publications, 1993, pp 21–33

Ayyar, R: Yaari, in A Lotus of Another Color: An Unfolding of the South Asian Lesbian and Gay Experience. Edited by Ratti R. Boston, MA, Alyson Publications, 1993, pp 167–174

Carrier J, Nguyen B, Su S: Vietnamese American sexual behaviors and HIV infection. J Sex Res 29:547–560, 1992

Chan C: Issues of identity development among Asian-American lesbians and gay men. Journal of Counseling and Development 68:16–20, 1989

Chua S: Asian-Americans, gay and lesbian, in Encyclopedia of Homosexuality. Edited by Dynes WR, Johansson W, Percy WA. New York, Garland, 1990, pp 84–85

Chung C, Kim A, Lemesheusky F (eds): Between the Lines, An Anthology by Pacific/Asian Lesbians of Santa Cruz, California. Santa Cruz, CA, Dancing Bird Press, 1987

Coleman E, Cogan P, Gooren L: Male cross-gender behavior in Myanmar (Burma): a description of the Acault. Arch Sex Behav 21:313–321, 1992

Espin OM: Issues of identity in the psychology of Latina lesbians, in Lesbian Psychologies: Explorations and Challenges. Edited by Boston Lesbian Psychologies Collective. Urbana, IL, University of Illinois Press, 1987, pp 35–51

Fung R: Looking for my penis: the eroticized Asian in gay video porn, in How Do I Look? Edited by Bad Object-Choices. Seattle, WA, Bay Press, 1991, pp 145–168

Gim RH, Atkinson DR, Kim H: Asian-American acculturation, counselor ethnicity, cultural sensitivity, and rating of counselors. Journal of Counseling Psychology 38(1):57–62, 1991

H. P: Asian American lesbians: an emerging voice in Asian American community, in Making Waves. Edited by Asian Women United of California. Boston, MA, Beacon, 1989, pp 282–290

Hahn D: Sexual perversions in Korea. Journal of Korean Neuropsychiatry 9(1):25–34, 1970

Hausman KB: U.S. psychiatrists' views on homosexuality differ from colleagues' in other countries. Psychiatric Times, September 3, 1993, p 3

Hinsch B: Passions of the Cut Sleeve: A History of the Male Homosexual Tradition in China. Berkeley, CA, University of California Press, 1990

Hom AY: In the mind of an/other. Amerasia Journal 17:51–54, 1991

Hom AY: Family matters: a historical study of the Asian Pacific network. Unpublished master's thesis, University of California, Los Angeles, 1992

Hom AY: Stories from the homefront: perspectives of Asian American parents with lesbian daughters and gay sons, in Asian American Sexualities, Dimensions of the Gay and Lesbian Experience. Edited by Leong RC. New York, Routledge, 1996, pp 37–49

Hong W, Yamamoto J, Chang DS, et al: Sex in a Confucian society. J Am Acad Psychoanal 21:405–419, 1993

Hsu J, Tseng WS: Chinese culture, personality formation and mental illness. Int J Soc Psychiatry 16(1):5–14, 1969

Isay RA: Being Homosexual. New York, Farrar Straus and Giroux, 1989

Iwaya S: Nan sho k' (die Paederastie in Japan) [Pederasty in Japan]. Jahrbuch für sexuelle Zwischenstufen mit besonderere Berucksichtigung der Homosexualitaet 4:264–271, 1902

Jaschke V, Doi T: The role of culture and family in mental illness. Bull Menninger Clin 53(2):154–8, 1989

Karsch-Haack F: Das Gleichgeschlectliche Leben der Ostasiaten Chinesen Japaner Koreer (The Same Sex Life of East Asians, Chinese, Japanese, Koreans). Munich, Germany, Seitz and Schauer, 1906

Lau MP, Ng ML: Homosexuality in Chinese culture. Cult Med Psychiatry 13:465–488, 1989

Leong RC: Dimensions of desire–other Asian and Pacific American sexualities: gay, lesbian, and bisexual identities, and orientation, in Asian American Sexualities, Dimensions of the Gay and Lesbian Experience. Edited by Leong RC. New York, Routledge, 1996

Lieh-Mak F, O'Hoy KM, Luk SL: Lesbianism in the Chinese of Hong Kong. Arch Sex Behav 12:21–30, 1983

Lim-Hing S (ed): The Very Inside: An Anthology of Writing by Asian and Pacific Islander Lesbian and Bisexual Women. Toronto, Sister Vision Press, 1994

Mangaong G: From the 1970s to the 1990s: perspective of a gay Filipino American activist, in Asian American Sexualities, Dimensions of the Gay and Lesbian Experience. Edited by Leong RC. New York, Routledge, 1996

Manalansan M: Searching for community: Filipino gay men in New York City, in Asian American Sexualities, Dimensions of the Gay and Lesbian Experience. Edited by Leong RC. New York, Routledge, 1996

Maria: Coming home, in A Lotus of Another Color. Edited by Ratti R. Boston, MA, Alyson, 1993, pp 204–212

McWhirter DP, Mattison AM: The Male Couple: How Relationships Develop. Englewood Cliffs, NJ, Prentice-Hall, 1984

Nanda S: The Hijras of India. Med Law 3:59–75, 1984

Puterbaugh G: Thailand, in Encyclopedia of Homosexuality. Edited by Dynes WR, Johansson W, Percy WA. New York, Garland, 1990, pp 1288–1290

Ratti R (ed): A Lotus of Another Color. Boston, MA, Alyson, 1993

Robertson J: Gender-bending in paradise: doing "female" and "male" in Japan. Genders 5:50–69, 1989

Ruan FF, Bullough VL: Lesbianism in China. Arch Sex Behav 21:217–226, 1992

Saikaku I: The Great Mirror of Male Love (1687), translated by Schalow PG. Stanford, CA, Stanford University Press, 1990

Schalow PG: Male love in early modern Japan: a literary depiction of the "youth," in Hidden From History: Reclaiming the Gay and Lesbian Past. Edited by Duberman MB, Vicinus M, Chauncey G. New York, Meridian, 1989

Uba L: Asian American Personality Patterns, Identity, and Mental Health. New York, Guilford, 1993

Wat EC: Preserving the paradox: stories from a gay-loh, in Asian American Sexualities, Dimensions of the Gay and Lesbian Experience. Edited by Leong RC. New York, Routledge, 1996

Whitman FL, Mathy RM: Male Homosexuality in Four Societies. Westport, CT, Praeger, 1986

Williams WL: Indonesia, in Encyclopedia of Homosexuality. Edited by Dynes WR, Johansson W, Percy WA. New York, Garland, 1990, pp 597–599

Witness Aloud: Lesbian, gay, and bisexual Asian/Pacific American writings. Asian/Pacific America Journal 2(spring/summer), 1993

35

Latino Men, Latina Women, and Homosexuality

Francisco J. González, M.D.
Oliva M. Espín, Ph.D.

The term "Latino homosexuality" raises several important questions about what constitutes both Latino and homosexuality. In this chapter, the term "homosexual" is often used (rather than gay) because many Latinos in same-gender relationships do not self-identify as gay. "Latino" (rather than the federal government's category "Hispanic," referring to Spanish origins) is used to emphasize the broad racial and cultural background of this group (Alonso and Koreck 1993). Thus to write of Latino homosexuality is to invoke a fictional category that cannot possibly contain the diversity of motivations, behaviors, identities, and institutions that it purports to name.

The question of what we mean when we speak of "homosexuality"—whether acts, fantasies, affectional preferences, object choices, sexual aims, or identities—comes into sharp relief when we examine the cultural underpinnings of sexuality. A chapter on Latinos in a textbook of homosexuality places ethnic identification in the broader

583

matrix of sexual orientation. This conundrum of which comes first—orientation or ethnic identity—is critical for Latinos engaging in same-gender sex. The effect of culture on homosexuality is not simply embellishment and filigree; culture organizes and defines sexual orientation and sexuality in general (e.g., what is sexual and what is not), which in turn shapes specific possibilities for individual development (Herdt 1988, 1989).

Adding to the complexity of these theoretical concerns is the broad diversity of the Latino population in the United States. As defined by the U.S. Bureau of the Census, 22.42 million U.S. Hispanics encompass multiple races, most notably Native Americans, whites, blacks, and a substantial group of mixed racial heritage, including *mestizos* (Native American and white lineage) and *mulattos* (black and white lineage). Other national identifications are possible, each with its own complex history, politics, artistic traditions, and customs. Of Hispanics living in the United States, 64% are Mexican Americans, 14% are Central and South Americans, 11% are Puerto Ricans, and 5% are Cubans (National Commission on AIDS 1992). Hispanic individuals may speak English, Spanish, or Portuguese or indigenous languages or mixtures and variations of these, such as "Spanglish" on the East Coast of the United States or "Tex-Mex" in Texas (Anzaldúa 1990; Carballo-Diéguez 1989; Marín 1989). Latinos in the United States also comprise a wide socioeconomic spectrum, although most are poorer than average: 25% of Hispanic or Latino families live in poverty compared with 9.5% of non-Hispanic families (National Commission on AIDS 1992). In addition, the process of acculturation has a diversifying effect. Language, skin color, values and traditions, and the structure and role of the family all play critical functions in the degree of assimilation, separatism, or biculturalism compared with the dominant American culture. Latinos have dissimilar issues and concerns that are the result of their socioeconomic status and psychological identity. A recently immigrated, Spanish-speaking *mestizo* farm worker who occasionally has sex with other men but economically supports his wife and children still living in Nicaragua has different concerns from a third-generation, monolingual English-speaking, white, Mexican American lesbian activist, even though they are both Latino and homosexual.

This chapter is a place to start in working with and thinking about Latino men and women and their relationships to homosexuality. Rather than providing foreclosing answers, this chapter should allow the reader to pose salient questions. However, precisely because of the diversity of the Latino community, it is useful to identify certain key cultural institutions and values as points of reference. *La familia*, the Latino family, is the backdrop against which Latino homosexuality unfolds and the place to begin.

La Familia and Sexuality

The family plays a critical role in Latino culture, and "familism" stands as a core cultural value that transcends nation of origin and to some extent the effects of acculturation (Marín 1989). In contrast to white nuclear families, Latino families tend to be extended, with stronger ties to grandparents, aunts and uncles, and cousins (Marín and Marín 1991; Mindel 1980). Additionally, the strength of the Latino family has conferred a protective effect in the difficult process of acculturation and immigration. For less acculturated Latinos, familism is maintained by high levels of social support, a network of obligation, and a view of relatives as social referents for attitudes and behaviors. In more acculturated families, the perception of support remains the most salient characteristic, with obligations and referent functions diminishing (Sabogal et al. 1987). This view of the family as the primary social sphere has important implications for homosexual Latinos, as explained below.

The Catholic church, a significant influence on Latin culture, also can be seen as an adjunctive structure that supports traditional family dynamics and condemns homosexuality while promoting sexuality in the service of procreation (Tori 1989). Although folk religion often undercuts this Catholic hegemony and provides sanctuary and privilege for some homosexual practice (Bonilla and Porter 1990; Espín, in press; Fry 1986), for many homosexual Latinos the proscriptions of the church have been a source of anxiety and alienation (Carballo-Diéguez 1989; Cuadra 1991).

Finally, silence about sex and sexuality is another important dimension of the stereotypical Latino family (Díaz, in press). Relative rigidity of gender roles in which sexual positions are "prenegotiated" may contribute to this silence, as might the cultural script of *simpatía* in which frictionless, smooth social interactions are highly prized (Triandis et al. 1984). Whatever the underlying influences, Latinos appear to be quiet on sexual matters. Latinos, for example, report higher levels of sexual discomfort than non-Latino whites (Marín and Gómez 1994). Parents tend not to discuss sexual issues with their children, and partners with each other. According to the National Health Interview Survey (1990), of the Hispanic adults with children 10–17, only 57% (compared with 70% of whites) reported having talked to their children about HIV or AIDS (National Commission on AIDS 1992). Alonso and Koreck (1993) further argue that fear of stigma about homosexuality has contributed to the relative silence of the Latino community about AIDS.

Gender Roles: *Machismo* and *Marianismo*

Traditionally, sociologists have characterized the Latino family as rigidly patriarchal: machismo drives a dynamic of power in which the father is authoritarian, disloyal, and aggressive—the wife, demure and faithful. Recent reviews (Bonilla and Porter 1990; Staples and Mirandé 1980) have demonstrated a more egalitarian pattern of decision making and flexibility in the division of household tasks between husband and wife, but these reviews do not focus on sexuality or sexual roles where the concept of machismo remains central (Almaguer 1993; Díaz, in press; Marín and Gómez 1994).

We can say that machismo stands as a core organizer of Latino sexuality. *Machismo* refers to a code of virility and masculine conduct that prizes honor, respect, and dignity, as well as aggressiveness, invulnerability, and sexual prowess (Staples and Mirandé 1980). Carrier (1989a, 1989b) explains machismo as "a culturally defined hypermasculine ideal model of manliness" (p. 228) in which sexuality plays a major role. The stereotypical *machista* man views women as sexual conquests that validate his masculinity and continues to pursue sexual encounters even after marriage. Although these gender roles are softening, one recent telephone survey (Marín et al. 1993) of adults in three states found self-reports of extramarital relationships to be twice as high in Latino men as in non-Hispanic whites.

Women, correspondingly, are situated in a tense sexual dichotomy between whore and virgin/mother. Historical influences from the time of the Spanish conquest have emphasized the equation of women's virginity and family honor for Latina women (Espín 1984). Some authors use the term *"Marianismo,"* referring to the Virgin Mary, to describe a generalized attitude that promotes women's reticence on sexual matters as "purity" while typifying sexually open women as *putas* or whores (Espín 1987; Marín and Gómez 1994). *Marianismo* is the counterpart of *machismo*. The stereotypically good woman is expected to be the self-sacrificing mother who is ultimately subservient to men. These values of self-renunciation and sexual purity that conscribe traditional Latina femininity may foster negative attitudes about sexual behavior on the part of women, sometimes even within marriage (Espín 1984). Significantly, the classic *machismo/Marianismo* organization of gender operates not only between heterosexual partners but also informs how homoerotic desire plays out in Latino cultures.

Men, Gender Stereotypes, and Sexual Roles

For many Latino men, homosexuality is structured by sexual aim rather than sexual object choice and depends heavily on gender role (Almaguer 1993). In such a structure, sexual role takes precedence over sexual practice: being the penetrator is the defining act of masculinity, rather than having sex with a woman (Paz 1959). Conversely, passivity and being penetrated are associated with a feminine stance. Anal, penetrative sex is seen as a kind of displaced heterosexuality, in which the anus is equivalent to the vagina (Carrier 1985; Lancaster 1988). Desire might thus be conceived as heterosexual, even in same-gender interactions (as an interplay of the masculine and the feminine). In such a system, the passive role is most strongly denigrated by society, rather than the same-gender nature of the encounter. Stigma accrues not so much to a man being homosexual as to the man's being feminine (Almaguer 1993; Lancaster 1988).

■ *Activos* and *Pasivos*

Anthropologist Joseph Carrier, working in northwestern Mexico with *mestizo* men who engaged in homosexual behavior, postulated that sex role preference in these men remained relatively stable: "The sociocultural environment . . . gives rise to expectations that they should play either the insertee or the insertor sex role but not both, and that they should obtain ultimate sexual satisfaction with anal intercourse rather than fellatio" (Carrier 1977, p. 56). He concluded that active and passive sexual roles are distinct and consistent and that these roles correlate with identification as masculine or feminine. Additionally, he noted that effeminate men were socialized from early on (often after sexual encounters with older male relatives) to pursue the passive sex role with other men. More rarely some men engaged in both active and passive roles, earning the nickname *internacionales,* implying that such role fluidity was not indigenous practice. Even for these *internacionales,* Carrier postulated that sexual role is relatively fixed, decided by a mutual sizing-up of masculinity in the sexual encounter: the more masculine partner always playing the active, inserter role (Carrier 1977, 1985).

Other authors have described similar forms of "inverted" homosexuality, in which homosexual men are seen as having a woman within, among other Latino groups including Mexican, Brazilian, Nicaraguan, and Cuban men (Almaguer 1993; Alonso and Koreck 1993; Aráuz et al.; Arguelles and Rich 1989; Díaz, in press; Fry 1986; Lancaster 1988; Leiner 1994; Parker 1986; Taylor 1986). Although these descriptive studies have been extremely valuable, little quantitative data exist on sexual practice among Latino men who have sex with men. Data that do exist tend to be from research done in HIV prevention and cannot be seen as representative of this population as a whole. Nonetheless important features have emerged from these quantitative studies. Izazola-Licea et al. (1991), for example, investigated the relationship of sexual role (exclusively active, mixed behavior, or exclusively passive) and HIV risk behavior in their study of 660 gay and bisexual men in six Mexican cities. They found up to 32% of respondents reported exclusively active or passive role, with the majority practicing both roles. Homosexual men were more likely to be only passive than bisexual men, who tended to be more active.

■ Bisexuality

Carrier (1985) indicates that the major difference between bisexuality in the United States and Mexico is that "one drop of homosexuality" does not make a man totally homosexual, as long as the appropriate sex role is played. Studies from the HIV literature, in fact, show high rates of bisexual behavior. The Mexican Health Ministry found that frequency of bisexual practice in a cohort of 5,000 gay and bisexual men varied by community size: 67% of homosexually active men in small communities also reported having sex with women compared with 56% in metropolitan centers (García García 1991). The bisexual men tended to be less educated than the homosexual men, and the bisexual men in small towns were more likely than their urban counterparts to establish stable relationships with women and to have children. The story, however, may be different for more acculturated groups. In a United States survey of nongay or bisexual identified Mexican American and white undergraduates, Padilla and O'Grady (1987) found no significant difference between the two groups in same-sex contacts by frequency or number of partners.

Of critical importance here is the concept of identity. Although high rates of bisexual practice might exist, there is no indication that high numbers of Mexican men construct an identity around bisexuality. Many identify as heterosexual, in the masculine, penetrative role. Additionally, bisexuality may be a way of destigmatizing homosexual behavior. García García stated, "Bisexual activity among homosexual men is more frequent in groups where homosexuality per se is ostracized and where 'machismo' in its more flamboyant expression is looked upon as desirable" (p. 51).

Women, Acculturation, and Sexuality

Few studies exist in the research literature on HIV to document the sexual practice of Latino men, but the quantitative literature on women is practically nonexistent. However, a rich qualitative work exists that speaks to the subjective experience of Latina lesbians. Moraga (1983) and Anzaldúa (1987) described their struggles as both Chicanas and lesbians. In the social sciences, Amaro (1978) has spoken on the issue of "coming out" for Hispanic lesbians, and Espín (1987) and Escaserga et al. (1975) have studied other aspects of Latina lesbian lives such as identity development and attitudes toward psychotherapy. In general, however, the literature on Latina lesbians is scarce.

■ Invisibility of Lesbians

This scarcity may mirror the relative invisibility of lesbians in Latin culture, where only openly "butch" types are recognized as lesbian (Espín 1994). In a society where sexuality is often constituted in terms of the masculine, women who love women often remain unseen. This invisibility may protect some lesbians: because good Latina women are not supposed to be sexual, it may be more acceptable for lesbians to remain single and apparently asexual than it is for gay men to remain single. Families may justify an adult daughter not marrying because her job or educational level does not lend itself to marriage or may even encourage lesbian relationships as friendships that can support the *soltera* in her pitiful spinsterhood. Additionally *amistad intima,* or close friendship, that includes touching and constant companionship is more tolerated, even after marriage, between women than between men. Finally, because most Latina lesbians are single and self-supporting, their employment and educational level probably are higher than those of other Latinas, placing them in positions of leadership and advocacy in their communities (Espín 1984).

In a study conducted in the mid-1970s (Hidalgo and Hidalgo Christensen 1976–1977), about 50% of 61 Puerto Rican lesbians indicated their families suspected their orientation but treated them with "silent tolerance"; open acknowledgment of their lesbianism seldom occurred. This struggle against invisibility may explain why, in one qualitative study of 16 mostly immigrant and highly educated Cuban lesbians, Espín (1987) found that most of the women (11 of 16) would prefer to live among lesbians unfamiliar with Latino culture than to remain closeted among Latinos.

■ Immigration, Acculturation, and Gender Roles

Although not all Latinos are immigrants, many come from immigrant families. Immigration is a powerful process that influences the development of sexuality and sexual identity. Immigration and the subsequent acculturation process present different opportunities for women than for men (Espín 1994). Compared with most Latin American countries, the United States offers women greater freedom to explore gender roles and sexual behavior and presents new economic possibilities and challenges. Having left behind her formative psychocultural context, the immigrant woman must reorganize identity in a culture that presses with new societal expectations. Crossing the border may represent a metaphorical boundary crossing in personal development that allows homoerotic desires and identity issues to come to light (Espín 1994).

Although the need for such a reorganization of identity may be most striking in immigration, it is not limited to this process. Nonimmigrant Latina women also cross lines of demarcation imposed by class, generation, or sexism. Ethnicity and sexuality form an intricate braid, as Moraga (1983) makes clear:

■ **Case Example 1**

[For my mother], on a basic economic level, being Chicana meant being "less." It was through my mother's desire to protect her children from poverty and illiteracy that we became "anglocized"; the more effectively we could pass in the white world, the better guaranteed our future. . . . I took her life into my heart, but managed to keep a lid on it as long as I feigned being the happy, upwardly mobile heterosexual.

When I finally lifted the lid to my lesbianism, a profound connection with my mother reawakened in me. It wasn't until I acknowledged and confronted my own lesbianism in the flesh, that my heartfelt identification with and empathy for my mother's oppression—due to being poor, uneducated, and Chicana—was realized. My lesbianism is the avenue through which I have learned the most about silence and oppression. (pp. 28–29)

Homophobia

Strong familism, rigid sex roles, religiosity, and sexual silence may combine to strongly stigmatize homosexual behavior in Latino culture, because these factors tend to correlate with measures of homophobia (see Chapter 7 by Herek). Bonilla and Porter (1990) found Latinos to be less tolerant than non-Hispanic whites or blacks regarding approval of civil liberties for homosexuals (but not significantly different from whites) and more tolerant than blacks on moral disapproval of homosexuality. The small and presumably highly acculturated sample from this general social survey probably obscures more profoundly homophobic attitudes. Anecdotal homophobic sentiments are evident in Latino culture. Arguelles and Rich (1989) document homophobia in pre- and postrevolutionary Cuba, and Hidalgo and Hidalgo Christensen (1976–1977) in the Puerto Rican community. Tori (1989), reviewing 100 consecutive films in a Spanish-language movie house in Oakland,

California, found that the films sent a clear message to the audience that homosexuality is deviant, demeaning, and repugnant. Homophobia and gender role rigidity may have a mutually stabilizing effect on one another—in part by promoting the view of gay men as "women" or lesbians as "butch" (Ross 1983).

Identity Formation, Acculturation, and Difference

For Latinos sexual orientation and identity may be strongly correlated with gender identifications and sexual roles, but this does not fully explain homosexual identity in Latino communities. Latino homosexuality is changing. Under the influence of greater political organization, spurred in part by mobilization against HIV and the women's movement, homosexuality in Latin America may be shifting between gender-based identifications and more "gay" consonant forms that include switching sexual roles and greater political identification as homosexual (Alonso and Koreck 1993; Aráuz et al.; Carrier 1989a, 1989b).

■ *Locas, Mayates,* and *Bugarrones*

This shifting of identifications is nowhere more evident than in the spectrum of acculturation by Latino gay men in the United States. Using data from an unpublished study on AIDS prevention in the San Francisco Latino community, Almaguer (1993) and Díaz (in press) characterize these men along the lines of gay identification and level of acculturation.

Among the less acculturated, usually working class, Spanish-speaking men, two groups are evident. The first group is composed of men who have adopted an "effeminate gender persona" (Almaguer 1993), often drag queens, who take the *pasivo* role almost exclusively. They are sometimes referred to as *queenas* or *locas* (literally "crazy women") and tend to be attracted to men who identify as heterosexual. The second group of *mayates* or *bugarrones*—derogatory terms used in some of Latin America (Taylor 1986)—are heterosexually identified men who furtively have sex with other men. These men play the activo role and probably seek out encounters with other Latino men who follow the *activo* or *pasivo* script.

The more acculturated group is more likely to incorporate gay-structured homosexual identities and sexual practices, rather than the *activo-pasivo* system. This group includes largely assimilated men who identify with the dominant white gay community and retain only a marginal Latino identity as well as more biculturally identified men, who may structure their sexuality along gay lines but maintain contact with both the white gay and the emerging Latino gay subcultures.

These positions have not been similarly articulated for Latina women. However, a range of identifications is possible in which traditional Latin views of femininity and sexual roles intersect post-Stonewall lesbian conceptions of gender and sexuality.

■ Identity Formation and Difference

Cass and others have stressed the importance of recognizing sexual difference in the process of identity formation (see Chapter 14 by Cass). For Latino gays and lesbians (as for other ethnic minority groups), the difference from the majority culture is doubled because the individual is ethnic and homosexual. Developing a gay identity may come at the cost of losing cultural identity (Almaguer 1993). Especially for traditional Latinos, primary allegiance is often to the family. The focus of coming out may thus be on protecting the parents and extended family from pain and embarrassment, rather than on the anxiety and anger of being rejected (Díaz, in press). Homosexuality may become a token of the "acculturation wars" between the generations. Because the values of strong kinship ties, religion, and conformity to traditional gender roles may serve as a way of fending off assimilation, some parents may view "gayness" as a product of the erosion of traditional Old World values and a move toward the dominant culture (Tremble et al. 1989). Women may pay a higher price in this battle because women's gender roles (including sexuality and dress) are often rigidly controlled as a means of preserving cultural continuity amidst cultural dislocation (Espín 1994). Newman and Muzzonigro (1993), in a study on coming out in 27 minority youth (including 6 Hispanic youths), found that "high traditional" families were perceived to be more disapproving of the youth's gay identification than more acculturated families. So the process of developing a gay identity may involve temporarily (or permanently) setting aside identification as Latino to become homosexual or, conversely, deferring coming out.

■ The Latino Gay Community

Politically, the Latin American gay rights movement is young, dating only to the 1980s in most countries as a consolidated, organized front (Green and Asis 1993). Many Latino gay men and lesbians, struggling with repression and homophobia in their home countries, emigrate to the United States in search of greater personal freedom (Arguelles and Rich 1989; Espín 1994; Tori 1989). Once here, though, they often find economic hardship and racial discrimination.

The establishment of a powerful, organized gay community in the United States occurred in the 1970s through the mobilization of gay white men (Altman 1982); lesbians, even white lesbians, were often outsiders in this process. These men (usually economically independent) were able to establish separate gay ghettos in urban centers away from their families. For Latinos, however, the family has been a protective structure, a buffer against the socioeconomic and political pressure of immigration, acculturation, and racism. For more traditional Latinos, the family remains the primary referent system or social mirror. Thus identification with the gay community for Latino gay men and lesbians may be a costly move away from family and the underpinnings of economic, political, and cultural identity (Almaguer 1993; Espín 1984).

That Latinos do not support gay civil liberties also may help explain the difficulty the gay movement has had in getting established in Latino communities. Stronger ties to the family for cultural and economic reasons, silence in the family on sexual matters, and the negotiation of a double stigma of difference in identity development have all mitigated against the development of a consolidated Latino gay community. Nonetheless, most urban centers with a substantial Latino population have gay Latino subcultures, and in 1987 the National Latino/a Lesbian and Gay Organization (LLEGO) was formed.

Special Topics

■ HIV and Latino Homosexuality

In the United States, AIDS affects Latinos, especially Latino gay men, disproportionately to their representation in the population (Marín and Gómez 1994; National Commission on AIDS 1992). AIDS may be underreported among gay Latino men because many men who have sex with men do not identify as gay and because immigration status may affect the willingness to disclose sexual identity (Morales 1990; National Commission on AIDS 1992). Díaz (in press) has shown that even knowledgeable Latino gay men must surmount substantial psychocultural barriers to carry out safer sex intentions. Rotherham-Borus and Koopman (1991) have documented high-risk behavior in Hispanic and black gay and bisexual youth, despite accurate AIDS knowledge and positive beliefs about prevention. Latino HIV-positive men experience more stress with gay lifestyle issues than do non-Hispanic whites (Ceballos-Capitaine et al. 1990) and are less likely than whites to disclose their serostatus to relatives and lovers (Marks 1992). Difficulties with identification, a less powerful gay community, lower socioeconomic status, and acculturation issues may all conspire to complicate dealing with the epidemic.

■ Case Example 2

> Sr. B, a 28-year-old Guatemalan agrarian worker, immigrated to the United States with his wife and 2-year-old daughter seeking employment about 2 years before he was diagnosed HIV-positive in a community clinic where he sought help after developing wasting syndrome. He was unable to work, and his wife supported the family on a minimum wage salary. A demure, often reticent man, he waited months before revealing to his Spanish-speaking outreach worker that in addition to contact with a female prostitute in Guatemala, he had occasional homosexual contacts in the United States. He felt this was sinful, and he was reluctant to talk about it. "Gay positive" interventions were not useful, as Sr. B did not see himself as gay. General safe sex information and prevention strategies framed mainly for heterosexual sex were useful in allowing more dialogue about homosexual transmission modes.

Many authors have pointed to the need for culturally sensitive interventions for the prevention of HIV infection (Carballo-Diéguez 1989; Díaz, in press; Marín 1989; National Commission on AIDS 1992, 1993). These interventions must speak to the reality of Latino sexual practice and be sensitive to complex cultural issues, including the role of the family and preferred language.

▉ Substance Abuse

Rates of alcoholism and drug abuse tend to be high among gay men and lesbians (see Chapter 47 by Cabaj). Among Hispanics in the United States, degree of acculturation tends to correlate with higher frequency of alcohol consumption with more acculturation associated with more frequent drinking (Caetano 1987; Caetano and Medina Mora 1988). Latino gay and bisexual men may be at greater risk for drug and alcohol abuse given the multiple stressors reviewed in this chapter. For example, a study by Tori (1989) comparing homosexual Mexican American men residing illegally in the United States with control groups of heterosexual men living in the United States and homosexual men in Mexico showed that only homosexuality (not residency status) was associated with greater drug and alcohol use. Of note, homosexual men in the United States had high rates of inhalant use. Substance abuse has also been implicated as a risk factor for HIV in Latino gay men (Ramirez 1994). These data suggest the need for additional research in understanding the complex correlations between acculturation, sexual identity, and substance use.

Implications for Practice

Interventions with gay and bisexual Latino men and women can and should be formulated on multiple levels. In individual work with clients, practitioners should endeavor to educate themselves on the specific cultural and socioeconomic background of the individual because this background may strongly influence the issues and meanings of the work. Bilingual and bicultural practitioners are not immune from ignorance about other nationalities, cultural nuances, regionalisms, and slang (Carballo-Diéguez 1989). Within this informed context, non-Latino or nongay practitioners can often use their differences from the client to therapeutic advantage (de Monteflores 1986).

Acculturation issues will be a strong focus in negotiating the identity struggles of this group. Interventions should be appropriate to the degree of acculturation. A practitioner may want to encourage greater exploration of Latino identifications in a highly gay-acculturated client, for example, while providing a sense of security and positive mirroring for a Latino-identified client who is not out.

Family interventions also may have a role in mediating coming out or disclosing HIV status as perceived support from the family remains high even for highly acculturated Latinos. The practitioner (especially if Latino and an "insider") might facilitate the integration of difference between the gay client and the family by providing a culturally safe middle ground.

Some of the most significant interventions will need to occur at the community level in promoting education, furthering research initiatives, and establishing and maintaining centers that can offer culturally sensitive care and bilingual services (Ceballos-Capitaine 1990; Marín 1989; Morales 1990). A pressing need exists for more research about Latina lesbians to facilitate the development of culturally relevant programs and services. Finally, finding culturally syntonic ways to allow greater dialogue in the Latino community about homosexuality would greatly facilitate the difficult journey of self-discovery and affirmation for many Latino gay men and Latina lesbians.

References

Almaguer T: Chicano men: a cartography of homosexual identity and behavior, in The Lesbian and Gay Studies Reader. Edited by Abelove H, Barale MA, Halperin DM. New York, Routledge, 1993, pp 255–272

Alonso AM, Koreck MT: Silences: "Hispanics," AIDS, and sexual practices, in The Lesbian and Gay Studies Reader. Edited by Abelove H, Barale MA, Halperin DM. New York, Routledge, 1993, pp 110–126

Altman D: The Homosexualization of America, the Americanization of the Homosexual. New York, St. Martin's Press, 1982

Amaro H: Coming out: Hispanic lesbians, their families and communities. Paper presented at the National Coalition of Hispanic Mental Health and Human Services Organizations (COSSMHO), Austin, Texas, 1978

Anzaldúa G: How to tame a wild tongue, in Out There: Marginalization and Contemporary Cultures. Edited by Ferguson R, Gever M, Minh-ha TT, et al. Cambridge, MA, MIT Press and New Museum of Contemporary Art, 1990

Anzaldúa G: Boderlands/La Frontera: The New Mestiza. San Francisco, CA, Aunt Lute Books, 1987

Aráuz R, Sánchez AR, Sánchez AL, et al: Los homosexuales y la pre-
vención del SIDA en Nicaragua: ideas sobre la homosexualidad en
Nicaragua. Managua, Nicaragua, Fundación Nimehuatzin

Arguelles L, Rich BR: Homosexuality, homophobia, and revolution:
notes toward an understanding of the Cuban lesbian and gay experience, in Hidden From History: Reclaiming the Gay and Lesbian
Past. Edited by Duberman MB, Vivinus M, Chauncey G. New York,
New American Library, 1989, pp 441–455

Bonilla L, Porter J: A comparison of Latino, black, and non-Hispanic
white attitudes toward homosexuality. Hispanic J Behavioral Sciences 12:437–452, 1990

Caetano R: Acculturation, drinking and social settings among U.S.
Hispanics. Drug Alcohol Depend 19:215–226, 1987

Caetano R, Medina Mora ME: Acculturation and drinking among people of Mexican descent in Mexico and the United States. J Stud Alcohol 49:462–471, 1988

Carballo-Diéguez A: Hispanic culture, gay male culture, and AIDS:
counseling implications. J Counseling and Development 68:26–30,
1989

Carrier JM: "Sex-role preference" as an explanatory variable in gay
behavior. Arch Sex Behav 6:53–65, 1977

Carrier JM: Mexican male bisexuality. J Homosex 11:75–83, 1985

Carrier JM: Gay liberation and coming out in Mexico. J Homosex
17:225–252, 1989a

Carrier JM: Sexual behavior and spread of AIDS in Mexico. Med An-
thropol 10:129–142, 1989b

Ceballos-Capitaine A, Szapocznik J, Blaney NT, et al: Ethnicity, emotional distress, stress-related disruption, and coping among HIV seropositive gay males. Hispanic Journal of the Behavioral Sciences
12:135–152, 1990

Cuadra S: Lesbians and gays in Nicaragua: coming out of the closet.
Barricada Internacional August:32–33, 1991

de Monteflores C: Notes on the management of difference, in Contemporary Perspectives on Psychotherapy with Lesbians and Gay Men.
Edited by Stein TS, Cohen CJ. New York, Plenum Medical Press,
1986, pp 73–101

Díaz RM: Latino gay men and the psychocultural barriers to AIDS prevention, in A Plague of Our Own: The Impact of the AIDS Epidemic on the Gay and Lesbian Communities. Edited by Levin M, Gagnon J, Nardi P. Chicago, IL, University of Chicago Press (in press)

Escaserga YD, Mondaca EC, Torres VG: Attitudes of Chicana lesbians toward therapy. Master's thesis, Department of Social Work, University of Southern California, Los Angeles, CA, 1975

Espín OM: Cultural and historical influences on sexuality in Hispanic/Latin women: implications for psychotherapy, in Pleasure and Danger: Exploring Female Sexuality. Edited by Vance CS. Boston, MA, Routledge and Kegan Paul, 1984, pp 149–164

Espín OM: Issues of identity in the psychology of Latina lesbians, in Lesbian Psychologies: Explorations and Challenges. Edited by the Boston Lesbian Psychologies Collective. Chicago, IL, University of Illinois Press, 1987, pp 35–55

Espín OM: Crossing borders and boundaries: the life narratives of immigrant lesbians. Paper presented at the 102nd Annual Convention of the American Psychological Association, Los Angeles, CA, 1994

Espín OM: Latina Healers: Power, Culture and Tradition in U.S. Cities. Encino, CA, Floricanto Press (in press)

Fry P: Male homosexuality and spirit possession in Brazil, in The Many Faces of Homosexuality. Edited by Blackwood E. New York, Harrington Park Press, 1986, pp 137–153

García García MdL, Valdespino J, Izazola J, et al: Bisexuality in Mexico: current perspectives, in Bisexuality and HIV/AIDS: A Global Perspective. Edited by Tielman R, Carballo M, Hendricks A. Buffalo, NY, Prometheus Books, 1991, pp 41–58

Green J, Asis E: Gays and lesbians: the closet door swings open. Report on the Americas 26:4–7, 1993

Herdt G: Cross-cultural forms of homosexuality and the concept "gay." Psychiatric Annals 18:37–39, 1988

Herdt G: Gay and lesbian youth, emergent identities, and cultural scenes at home and abroad. J Homosex 17:1–42, 1989

Hidalgo HA, Hidalgo Christensen E: The Puerto Rican lesbian and the Puerto Rican community. Journal of Homosexuality 2:109–121, 1976–1977

Izazola-Licea JA, Valdespino-Gómez JL, Gortmaker SL, et al: HIV-1 seropositivity and behavioral and sociological risks among homosexual and bisexual men in six Mexican cities. Journal of Acquired Immune Deficiency Syndrome 4:614–622, 1991

Lancaster RN: Subject honor and object shame: the construction of male homosexuality and stigma in Nicaragua. Ethnology 27:111–125, 1988

Leiner M: Sexual politics in Cuba: machismo, homosexuality and AIDS. Boulder, Colorado, CO, Westview Press, 1994

Marín BV, Gómez CA: Latinos, HIV disease and culture: strategies for AIDS prevention, Chapter 10, in The AIDS Knowledge Base, 2nd Edition. Edited by Cohen PT, Sande MA, Volberding PA. Boston, MA, Little, Brown, 1994

Marín BV, Gómez CA, Hearst N: Multiple heterosexual partners and condom use among Hispanics and Non-Hispanic Whites. Fam Plann Perspect 25:170–74, 1993

Marín G, Marín BV: Research With Hispanic Populations, Applied Social Research Methods Series, Vol 23. Newbury Park, CA, Sage, 1991

Marín G: AIDS prevention among Hispanics: needs, behaviors, cultural values. Pub Health Rep 104:411–415, 1989

Marks G, Bundek NI, Richardson JL, et al: Self-disclosure of HIV infection: preliminary results from a sample of Hispanic men. Health Psychol 11:300–306, 1992

Mindel CH: Extended famialism among urban Mexican-Americans, Anglos and blacks. Hispanic Journal of the Behavioral Sciences 2:21–34, 1980

Moraga C: Loving in the War Years: Lo que Nunca Pasd por sus Labios. Boston, MA, South End Press, 1983

Morales ES: HIV infection and Hispanic gay and bisexual men. Hispanic Journal of the Behavioral Sciences 12:212–222, 1990

National Commission on AIDS: The Challenge of HIV in Communities of Color. Washington, DC, December 1992

National Commission on AIDS: Behavioral and Social Sciences and the HIV/AIDS Epidemic. Washington, DC, July 1993

Newman BS, Muzzonigro PG: Effects of traditional family values on coming out process of gay male adolescents. Adolescence 28:213–226, 1993

Padilla ER, O'Grady KE: Sexuality among Mexican Americans: a case of sexual stereotyping. J Pers Soc Psychol 52:5–10, 1987

Parker R: Masculinity, femininity, and homosexuality: on the anthropological interpretation of sexual meanings in Brazil, in The Many Faces of Homosexuality. Edited by Blackwood E. New York, Harrington Park Press, 1986, pp 155–163

Paz O: El Laberinto de la Soledad. Mexico, DF, Fondo de Cultura Económica, 1959

Ramirez J, Suarez E, de la Rosa G, et al: AIDS knowledge and sexual behavior among Mexican gay and bisexual men. AIDS Educ Prev 6:163–174, 1994

Ross MW: Femininity, masculinity, and sexual orientation: cross cultural comparisons. J Homosex 9: 27–36, Fall 1983

Rotherham-Borus MJ, Koopman C: Sexual risk behavior, AIDS knowledge, and beliefs about AIDS among predominantly minority gay and bisexual male adolescents. AIDS Educ Prev 3:305–312, 1991

Sabogal F, Marín G, Otero-Sabogal R, et al: Hispanic familism and acculturation: what changes and what doesn't? Hispanic Journal of the Behavioral Sciences 9:397–412, 1987

Staples R, Mirandé A: Race and cultural variations among American families: a decennial review of the literature on minority families. Journal of Marriage and the Family 42:887–903, 1980

Taylor CL: Mexican male homosexual interaction in public contexts, in The Many Faces of Homosexuality. Edited by Blackwood E. New York, Harrington Park Press, 1986, pp 117–136

Tori CD: Homosexuality and illegal residency status in relation to substance abuse and personality traits among Mexican nationals. J Clin Psychol 45:814–821, 1989

Tremble B, Schneider M, Appathurai C: Growing up gay or lesbian in a multicultural context. J Homosex 17:253–267, 1989

Triandis HC, Marín G, Lisansky J, et al: *Simpatía* as a cultural script of Hispanics. J Pers Soc Psychol 47:1363–1375, 1984

36

Native Two-Spirit People

Terry N. Tafoya, Ph.D.

Since 1987, there has been an annual gathering of Native lesbian, gay, bisexual, and transgendered individuals, who have alternated meeting in Canada and the United States. In these gatherings, there has been a deliberate effort to use the term "Native," rather than "Native American," because Native American excludes Canadian, Central, and South American Native people who have much in common. (Native American is used in this chapter when the specific research data are drawn from Native Americans, as opposed to Canadian Natives or other groups.) Although the term "indigenous people" is gaining in popularity, it is not frequently used within the Native American community as a point of self-reference. Through these gatherings, the term "two-spirit" has been sanctioned by those attending to describe themselves, going beyond "gay, lesbian, bisexual," or "transgendered." The latter terms are felt to be culturally biased in favor of non-Native concepts, which focus more on sexual orientation. Two-spirit is a term that can encompass alternative sexuality, alternative gender, and an integration of Native spirituality.

Two-spirit comes from the concept that one has both a male and a female spirit within. To be male means seeing through the eyes of a male. To be female means seeing through the eyes of a female, but to be two-spirit means seeing through both sets of eyes, and therefore being able to see further, or more holistically, than someone who is only male or female. This concept suggests why the two-spirit person is often associated with power and spirituality—having this "double vision" gave a greater potential for one to exist on a more integrated level. In general, everyone was regarded as having a male and female element within—in some tribes, this is why wearing the hair in two braids was common, to signify the balance one should seek between those inner principles. Two-spirit people were seen as naturally having that balance, as opposed to working to achieve it.

It is estimated that well over half of the surviving North American Native languages have terms for tribal members who were not considered completely male or female, but something else. Thus, the majority of Native communities had a concept of more than two genders (Roscoe 1987). For example, in describing Lakota formal categories of holy people, Powers (1986) includes

> the Winkte, variously translated as transvestite, hermaphrodite, homosexual, or more appropriately "would be woman." . . . Among the Lakota, Winktes . . . enjoyed a decided amount of prestige and high status. They were regarded as extremely sacred people who followed a particular lifestyle as a result of instructions received in visions. . . . (p. 188)

The Winktes are hardly unique among the various Native mythological and symbolic concepts of gender and its relationship to power and the "prestige and high status" accorded the position of the two-spirit. Although Walter Williams (1988) and other non-Native scholars have emphasized the sacredness and status of the two-spirit person in many Native nations, this conclusion may reflect agendas outside of the Native communities themselves. In reality, it may be far more likely that the two-spirit person was respected if he or she (English forces the use of inappropriate gender-based pronouns) was a good and valuable person, rather than because respect and honor were automatically accorded to someone with two-spirit status. An undesirable person was an undesirable person, and a valued person was a valued person, regardless of their sexual orientation or gender status. The advantage of the two-spirit person was the greater flexibility and the position of being a bridge between genders, sacred and secular, and Native and non-Native communities.

Unfortunately, because of the influence of over 500 years of European and European American oppression and repression, the stories of "those who are different"—the Winkte (Lakota), the Bote (Crow), the Kwid'o (Tewa), and other two-spirit people are often little known, even among many Native people themselves. In 1513, the Spanish "explorer" Balboa declared Native biological males who were "different" to be "sodomites," and let loose his dogs to have these "sodomites" ripped apart and killed (Goldberg 1992). "It should be remembered that this period was influenced by the Spanish Inquisition, where it was a norm to kill or maim an individual who held opinions different from the established European Orthodoxy" (Tafoya and Roeder 1996).

As a result of incidents like this, Native people learned very early not to discuss concepts of gender and sexuality because one could be killed for such discussion. A Native American woman from the Pacific Northwest talked about being reared by her grandmother, who was being interviewed by a linguist. The linguist gave her a small book of traditional legends from her community to distract her while he was interviewing her grandmother. To her surprise, her grandmother demanded the book back, telling her, "I don't want you reading that, because if I tell you these things in Indian, it's all right, but when you read it in English, it sounds dirty" (T. N. Tafoya, unpublished observations, 1994). This 1943 response is typical where many elders have maintained sexual references in their Native languages as a coping and survival skill, allowing the Native languages to cloak terms and concepts non-Native missionaries, teachers, and anthropologists might have found objectionable. Unfortunately, this has led in some cases to a Native internalization of the shame that non-Natives associate with sexuality, especially for those individuals who have lost their own language.

Historically, the most common term used to describe the two-spirit person was "Berdache." In a 1994 official statement to the American Anthropological Association, a group of Native and non-Native anthropologists and other scholars formally asked authors of introductory textbooks to update the terminology "Berdache" to "two-spirit" and to recommend that when the archaic term must be used for historical purposes, it should be written as "Berdache" [sic] (Jacobs et al., in press). This request is honored here. In other words "Berdache" has served as an overriding category that may well obscure significant and subtle categories within the hundreds of Native communities. For example, is "Lakota Berdache" (Winkte) precisely the same role as the "Crow Berdache" (Bote), or the "Tewa Berdache" (Kwid'o)?

In many ways "Berdache" is a misleading term. It is originally derived from a mid-Eastern term for "male sex slave," or catamite, a category brought back during the time of the Crusades by some Europeans (Angelino and Shedd 1955; Jacobs 1968). When French fur traders, missionaries, and explorers encountered Native people who were "different," they often used the word "Berdache" to refer to them. It has been suggested that in 19th-century French, "Berdache" had an implication of receptive anal intercourse (Williams 1988). This term is extremely limiting: it tends to exclude those individuals who were biologically female, rather than biologically male; it is of non-Native origin, and therefore often a word unrecognized by Native people themselves; it implies a specific behavior that is unsubstantiated in terms of what those who were, and are, "different" actually did, and do, sexually; finally, it confounds specific differences in sexual and gender-related activities and roles by subsuming them in an all-inclusive term.

Such attribution leads to a fundamental epistemological problem in cross-cultural issues of psychiatry—is depression exactly the same across cultures? Are there some psychiatric conditions that are unique to a specific culture (Becker and Kleinman 1991; Kleinman 1980, 1985; Manson et al. 1987)? Difference is not solely a function of place and ethnicity, but also a function of time. Just so, had this chapter been written before the 1970s, homosexuality itself would have been considered a psychiatric disorder, rather than a "normal sexual variation." The reality for researchers is that many historic documents consistently treated the "Berdache" as having a psychiatric disorder, reflecting the cultural bias of the non-Native writer, rather than the actual attitudes of the Native community itself (Devereux 1961).

Earlier synonyms for "Berdache" included hermaphrodite and transvestite, which reflect the perceptual limitations of the non-Native observer, rather than the perceptions of the Native communities. Interestingly enough, there is no evidence that "Berdaches" were actually hermaphrodites (a relatively rare physiological condition), based on physical examinations by non-Native physicians. The word transvestite, or cross-dresser, might also be inappropriate for individuals who dressed very specifically within their gender group, but were judged by non-Native observers who were unskilled in the nuance of a particular Native nation's fashion statement.

For example, "Finds Them and Kills Them," a famous Crow Bote, is shown in a historic photograph wearing clothing decorated with abalone disks sewn across the bodice. Women of the Crow and those of the surrounding cultural groups would wear clothing decorated with dentalium, cowry shells, elk teeth, or beadwork, but not abalone disks. "Finds Them and Kills Them" is, therefore, dressed as a Bote, not as a woman.

Cross-Cultural Issues of Sexuality

Because most Western thinkers are so automatically conditioned to conceptualize people as belonging to one of two genders, it may be difficult to perceive the true importance of culturally specific meaning related to classifications both of psychiatric concerns and of sexual orientation. Cross-cultural psychiatry often falls into a trap of simplistic reductionism—this equals that. For example, "Latisha" is the Sahaptin word generally equated to "depression," and "Bote" is the Crow word generally associated with "gay." Part of the basic training of a physician is awareness of differential diagnosis, where one sorts through a range of possibilities to find a specific diagnosis. If one is restricted by viewing binary concepts of gender as the only options, one may encounter serious limitations in understanding human sexuality from its broader human (versus European-American) perspectives. Imagine trying to understand all forms of affective disorders with only two categories.

Binary concepts of sexual orientation have caused tremendous confusion and frustration when attempting to place a patient into an available standard category where one "fits," much in the manner of Cinderella's step-sisters, who tried to shove their feet into a glass slipper that was not designed for them in the first place. One step-sister dealt with this by slicing off her toe, and the other by slicing off her heel. It could be suggested that a number of people who are "different" have attempted similar surgery on their sexual identity. If the only options are gay or straight, where does one place a biological male who desires being anally penetrated by a biological woman wearing a dildo?

As a further example, the Kinsey scale was designed for a survey focused exclusively on documenting specific sexual behaviors. Only much later were sexual fantasies investigated. When sexual fantasies are examined (Schwartz and Masters 1984), the results are fascinating. Among gay men, having sex with a woman is the third most common of the five most frequent sexual fantasies. For lesbian women, having sex with a man is also the third most common sexual fantasy. For heterosexual men, having sex with another man is the fourth most common sexual fantasy.

Thomas Szazz (1994) once suggested that, "In the animal kingdom, it's eat or be eaten—among humans, it's define or be defined." The common categories of gay or straight may be insufficient for understanding human sexual response. Freud (1910) himself wrote, "What is for practical reasons called homosexuality may arise from a whole variety of psychosexual inhibitory processes; the particular process we have singled out is perhaps only one among many, and is perhaps related to only one type of 'homosexuality'" (p. 101).

These ideas raise fascinating issues, because of the implication that the problems encountered are so culturally based within Western societies, generated by their epistemologies. As sexology critic Janice Irvine (1990) points out, the underlying recognition of only two sexual orientations, and the priority of heterosexuality, inform sexological practices in important ways:

> Categories of "natural" and deviant not only operate on the personal level to shape individual experience, but underpin the legal system as well. Whether a personal preference/orientation becomes a "sexual dysfunction," a "sexual deviancy," or a crime is a political decision often related to its status in the psychiatric community. (p. 104)

Weeks (1989) states that

> standard sexual classifications are not inborn, pre-given, or "natural" . . . these classifications are "striven for, contested, negotiated, and achieved often in the struggles of the subordinate to the dominate." (p. 207)

Research and Therapeutic Concerns

In sum, there may be great difficulties in discovering the most appropriate approaches to exploring non-European-based cultures, such as Native ones, because there may be fundamentally different ways of organizing and categorizing the world. The meaning of a particular behavior may be one thing in Western culture, and another in a non-Western society. For example, in general American culture, a firm handshake denotes strength and sincerity, and a non-firm handshake indicates a "cold fish" or a weak person. It has been suggested to businesswomen in America to use the more standard handshake, since historically, women were discouraged from displaying their own strength and confidence. For a number of traditional Natives, however, a strong handshake indicates that the person is attempting to dominate, rather than be reassuring, and is seen as threatening. Native handshakes tend to be very soft, with no firm grasping, and often are simply a touching of fingertips, with an upward lifting motion, rather than the pumping action of Westerners. Another perceived difference can be seen by the responses of a number of Native American cowboys when asked about their same-sex activities. They reported that they did not consider the sex they had with other men while "riding the range" (overnight herding of cattle) to actually be "sex," but rather a "sleeping aid" (T. N. Tafoya, unpublished observations, 1989).

The results of an Indian Health Service study of knowledge, attitudes, and behavior (KAB) associated with HIV/AIDS (administered to Native American cowboys and others at the 1989 National Indian Rodeo in Albuquerque, New Mexico) indicated that 22% of the Native American men surveyed had no sex partners, 8% had sex only with other men, 62% had sex only with women, and 3% had sex with both men and women (5% did not respond). Of the Native American women responding to the KAB study, 26% reported having no sexual partners, 65% had sex only with men, 4% had sex only with other women, and 1% had sex with both men and women (4% did not respond). Combining these figures, 11% of the Native American men describe having gay or bisexual behavior, and 5% of the Native American women describe having lesbian or bisexual behavior, well within the standard range reported in other ethnic groups.

In a study of interracial same-sex couples who had been together for at least 1 year, Native American partners reported a higher rate of heterosexual activity outside their primary relationships than any other ethnic groups (Tafoya and Rowell 1988). This finding is significant because of the stereotype that bisexual individuals are married men who have homosexual affairs outside their marriage. The results of this study suggest bisexual activity can work in both directions, as Native respondents in primary gay or lesbian relationships engaged in heterosexual activities.

Incidence of Sexual Abuse

In a three-state (Idaho, Oregon, and Washington) study of Native American adults (NW Portland IHS Portland Indian KAB Study,

unpublished study, 1989), 8% of the men and 9% of the women reportedly had their first sexual experience by the age of 10. On further
inquiry into their sexual experiences, a number of Native American
respondents asked the researcher if their "first sexual experience"
indicated their actual first experience or their first voluntary one.

The reason for this inquiry is that the extent of sexual abuse within
Native communities is a growing concern. Before the passage of legislation in the 1930s permitting Native American children to attend public schools, Native American students were required to attend federal
boarding schools, often being removed from their families of origin
and from their tribal communities by the age of 6. These boarding
schools had a devastating impact on Native American lives, deliberately
interfering with language, culture, spirituality, and sexuality. Required
attendance at boarding schools represented an attempt by the federal
government to "civilize the savages" by separating children from their
home environment. Although the majority of Native American students now attend public schools, as of 1994, fully 25% of these students
are still attending public boarding schools. Literally no community has
escaped the impact of these schools. Canadian Native people have had
similar experiences with boarding schools.

Traditional instruction regarding sexuality and gender concepts
was severely interrupted by attendance in these boarding schools, and
as a result, youth were not taught by their elders during the appropriate
developmental periods. Perhaps even more significant is the fact that
because the dormitory setting of boarding schools involved gender
separation, the first sexual experience for many young Native people
was with someone of the same gender. Additionally, missionaries, faculty, and school employees often sexually abused Native students, and
sometimes students dominated one another through sexual aggression.

Although no data documenting the full extent of sexual abuse, including intergenerational incestual abuse, are available, preliminary
research is very disturbing. For example, at a Native Wellness Conference in Canada, 340 out of 350 Native men attending reported being
sexually abused as youth (Tafoya 1994). In a workshop for sexually
abused men at a national conference dealing with Native Adult Children of Alcoholics in 1993, attendees reported variations of sexual
abuse—from boarding schools and churches, on reservations and in
urban settings, and perpetrated by older women and men, relatives,
older peers, and some individuals younger than themselves (T. N. Tafoya, unpublished observations, 1993). Anecdotal information from

Native chemical dependency counselors working in Native substance abuse treatment programs suggests a rate of sexual abuse ranging from 30% to 80% of both male and female clients.

For those Native individuals who identify as lesbian, gay, bisexual, or two-spirit, there are important clinical considerations indicating the need to question the impact of abuse on sexual orientation and answering the frequently asked question: if the abuse itself caused their same-sex orientation. Although the clinician must attend to the possibility of sexual abuse in lesbian, gay, and bisexual clients of all ethnicities, the high incidence of sexual abuse among many Native populations suggests it may be a more significant issue to explore in therapy with this population.

Ethnic Identity Versus Cultural Identity

It is estimated that before the passage of the Indian Child Welfare Act in the late 1970s, 25% of all Native American children were being reared in non-Native homes (Tafoya 1990). Thus, some of the Native patients treated by therapists may be ethnically Native, but may culturally more closely resemble their non-Native parents. Some Native patients may have as little exposure and experience with actual Native culture as most non-Natives psychiatrists. Some Native patients may resent a therapist focusing on his or her ethnic identity if the patient does not particularly claim the identity.

How one labels oneself is significant to the patient in terms of sexual identity, as well. Regardless of the terms a therapist may prefer, the most important issue is what the patient tends to call himself or herself. Some Native individuals may feel strongly that "two-spirit" is a term of empowerment, signifying a choice about how he or she wishes to be known. Other Native people may identify just as powerfully with being labeled lesbian, gay, bisexual, transsexual, transgendered, or queer, depending on their social-economic, regional, generational, or political attitudes. Some Native people reject the more standard classifications as being too culturally biased. Exploration in therapy of the meaning of a chosen term can be very productive.

In some Native communities, as in some Latino communities, one's sexual orientation is tied to behavior rather than to the gender of a partner. In other words, in some communities, a male will be considered heterosexual as long as he is engaged in an active, insertive "masculine" role. The gender of the partner is irrelevant for the "masculine" man, but a passive, receptive male partner would be labeled as homosexual. This labeling does not result from simple denial, because the entire community confirms the active partner as being heterosexual.

This alternative view of sexual orientation may pose a problem for lesbian or gay therapists who have invested a great deal of effort into the healthy and appropriate acceptance of their own sexual orientation and may automatically assume that non-European Americans should follow the same developmental process. Indeed many straight, lesbian, gay, and bisexual researchers and social scientists have established "homosexual development processes," with specific categories and stages (Diamond 1979; Miller 1986; Roof 1991; Troiden 1979; see Chapter 14 by Cass in this volume).

Although coming out is a key element of identity formation for many lesbian, gay, and bisexual non-Natives, a number of two-spirit Native people do not seem to have this type of experience, but report instead that their family "has just always known." Again, a Native patient statement that he or she has never had a formal coming out should not be viewed by the therapist as a denial of his or her sexual orientation, but should be seen within the context of cultural identity. For European-Americans, there is an emphasis on behavior determining identity, in contrast to the focus of many Native people on the core identity of a person. One engages in certain acts that confirm a European-American's membership in the newly acquired category; for many Native people, one is a member of a clan, an extended family, a tribe, or nation. What one does is irrelevant on certain levels, since that can always change. One's membership in the clan, family, tribe, or nation never changes, regardless of one's sexual behavior.

Clinical Considerations

In fundamental ways, Native patients need to be approached in the same manner one would approach any patient—with respect and with the attitude of a journey of co-discovery of how one's world view defines both problems and appropriate solutions. However, what is an acceptable and preferred solution for a non-Native person may not be an acceptable solution for a Native. For example, a Salish Native patient was involuntarily committed to a major Seattle hospital, following the death of her uncle. She had been committed because she had cut her hair, which was evaluated by a non-Native psychiatrist as symbolic self-mutilation with implication of suicidal ideation, and the psychiatrist had also classified her reports of knives around her door as hallucinations.

These findings were not signs of psychopathology, however. For many Native people, cutting one's hair at the death of a loved one is normative. In fact, there is peer pressure to do so as a public declaration of the grief process. As one's hair returns to its normal length in the months that follow, it is a concrete reminder of the healing process that is happening on a psychological and spiritual level. For many Native people living on reservations that have HUD housing, the quality of the construction is so poor that after a few years the locks stop working, and wedging butter knives around the door frame is common practice to "lock" the door at night. The Native patient was not hallucinating: there were knives around her door. The patient was certainly depressed. Her extended family had converted to fundamentalist Christianity and had rejected her attempts to honor her beloved uncle's wish to be buried with traditional Native ceremonies (T. N. Tafoya, unpublished observations, 1984).

Not all Native languages have the same terms that English provides to describe emotional states. Additionally, not all Native traditions emphasize insight as an important therapeutic factor and may focus instead on action-oriented interventions that match well with homework assignments in strategic styles of therapy.

In bilingual research, one can trace the influence of another language across three generations. Even if a patient can only speak English, if his or her parents or grandparents spoke a language other than English, this patient is not likely to process English in the manner of a native speaker of English. One of the most powerful cross-cultural signals indicating the first speaker is finished and another speaker can take a turn, is silence. In sociolinguistics, this is technically called "pause-time." For native English speakers, the average pause-time is approximately 1 second in duration. For other languages the pause-time may be considerably longer. For example, Athabaskan speakers from the largest Native language family in North America—including the Navajo and Apache of the American southwest, the Athabaskans of Alaska, and the Dine of Canada—have been documented as having a pause-time of approximately 1.5 seconds. This difference is long enough to interfere with conversations between English speakers and those with an Athabaskan influence, as they miscue one another.

In running support groups for Native and non-Native speakers, open discussion automatically allows those patients with the shortest pause-time to dominate conversation, leading to bias against those patients with the longest pause-times. Those with longer pause-time may be mistakenly viewed as passive-aggressive or withdrawn, when in reality, they never had an opportunity to say anything.

For a number of Native people, there may be a culturally sanctioned emphasis on nondirect forms of questioning and requesting. For example, a non-Native anthropologist (Farrer, unpublished observations, 1994) working with the Mescalero Apache people, found that if she asked directly where her collaborator was ("Where is Bernard?"), she got a different answer ("I don't know") than if she asked indirectly ("I wonder where Bernard might be?" . . . "I'm not certain, but if you show up at the trading post at two o'clock, you might find him there"). This style probably derives from the value in traditional cultures of saving face and protecting honor. To request something directly means one can be turned down directly. It is less risky to request something indirectly, because if one is turned down, then there is no honor lost, because one did not technically request it. In this way, a traditional culture may have many different ways of saying "no" without ever actually saying no. This communication style becomes a treatment issue when a therapist encourages patients to work with issues in a direct manner. This approach is not necessarily inappropriate, but the therapist may take for granted the ease of this particular style with a patient who has no real practical experience in its utilization.

Perhaps for many Native lesbian, gay, bisexual, transgendered, and two-spirit people, the sense of isolation from others who are also "different" can be just as powerful and painful an experience as it can be for non-Native people, especially if they are not sheltered and embraced by a family and community that has survived with many of its traditions of mutual tolerance and respect intact. For many Native people, the world is classified as "Native" or "non-Native." Much of the culture of the lesbian, gay, bisexual, and transgendered communities is based on non-Native values and principles, so Native people who are "different" may feel a strong sense of cognitive dissonance. For example, a person may ask, "Do I give up being a Native for being a lesbian?" For a number of European-American lesbians, gay men, and bisexual individuals, sexual orientation becomes the primary basis for identity. For the majority of Native people (and for other people of color), the primary basis for identity may remain the ethnicity.

Summary

It can be of great value to expose Native people to their own rich heritage of the two-spirit, with its connections to homosexuality, gender roles, and history. It should never be assumed that Native patients have had the opportunity to find out about their own traditions. Many Native communities communicate an expectation that one should look for role models of how one can act and think appropriately in contemporary settings. Some Native people are very conscious of how they can make sense of themselves in the context of their own people. In the words of Beth Brant (Personal Files 1993), a noted Mohawk lesbian writer,

> For what we do, we do for generations to come. We write not only for ourselves, but also for our communities, for our People, for the young ones who are looking for the gay and lesbian path, for our Elders who were shamed or mythologized, for all of life, including our relatives, who gave us our Indian blood and the belief system that courses through that blood.

Native concepts of gender and sexuality are in flux, as people begin for the first time in generations to decide for themselves how best to describe and define themselves. It remains to be seen whether the term "two-spirit" will end up as the label Native people continue to prefer. Richard LaFortune, a Yu'pik two-spirit, who was part of the working group addressing the American Anthropological Association, concluded that, "We are building a house in which we will not live" (Jacobs et al., in press).

Perhaps the most important gift Native people offer is an opportunity to go beyond Western binary consciousness that operates on the basis of opposition. The existence of two-spirit people speaks to the possibility that difference from the "norm" is not automatically pathological.

References

Angelino H, Shedd C: A note of Berdache. American Anthropologist 57:121–125, 1955

Becker K, Kleinman A (eds): Psychological Aspects of Depression. Hillsdale, NJ, Lawrence Erlbaum Associates, 1991

Devereux G: Mohawk Ethnopsychiatry and Suicide: The Psychiatric Knowledge and the Psychic Disturbances of an Indian Tribe. Washington, DC, Smithsonian Institution, Bureau of American Ethnography Bulletin, United States Government Printing Office, 1961

Diamond M: Sexual identity and sex roles, in The Frontiers of Sex Research. Edited by Bullough V. Buffalo, NY, Prometheus Books, 1979

Freud S: Leonardo da Vinci and a Memory of his Childhood (1910), in The Standard Edition of the Complete Works of Sigmund Freud, Vol 11. Translated and edited by Strachey J. London, Hogarth Press, 1974, pp 63–137

Goldberg J: Sodometries: Renaissance Texts Modern Sexualities. Stanford, CA, Stanford University Press, 1992

Irvine J: Disorders of Desire: Sex and Gender in Modern American Sexology. Philadelphia, PA, Temple University Press, 1990

Jacobs S: Berdache: a brief review of the literature. Colorado Anthropologist I:25–40, 1968

Jacobs S, Thomas W, Lang S: Two-Spirit People: Perspectives on Native American Gender and Sexuality. Urbana, IL, University of Illinois Press (in press)

Kleinman A: Patients and Healers in the Context of Culture: An Exploration of the Borderland Between Anthropology, Medicine, and Psychiatry. Berkeley, CA, University of California Press, 1980

Kleinman A, Good B (eds): Culture and Depression: Studies in the Anthropology and Cross Cultural Psychiatry of Affect and Disorder. Berkeley, CA, University of California Press, 1985

Manson S, Walker RD, Kirlahan DR: Psychiatric assessment and treatment of American Indians and Alaskan Natives. Hosp Community Psychiatry 38:165–173, 1987

Miller B: Identity conflict and resolution: a social psychological model of gay Familymen adaptations. Unpublished doctoral dissertation, Edmonton, University of Alberta, 1986

Powers WK: Sacred Language: The Nature of Supernatural Discourse in Lakota. Norman, OK, University of Oklahoma Press, 1986

Roof J: Polymorphous Diversity. Allure of Knowledge: Lesbian Sexuality and Theory. New York, Columbia University Press, 1991

Roscoe W: Bibliography of Berdache and alternate gender roles among North American Indians. J Homosex 14:3–4, 1987

Schwartz M, Masters W: The Masters and Johnson Treatment program for dissatisfied homosexual men. Am J Psychiatry 141:173–181, 1984

Szazz T: Bordercrossings: a conversation in cyberspace. Omni 16:2 1994

Tafoya T: Circles and cedar: Native Americans and family therapy, in Minorities and Family Therapy. Edited by Saba GW, Karrer BM, Hardy KV. New York, Haworth, 1990

Tafoya T, Wirth D: Native American Two-Spirit Men, in Men of Color: A Context of Service to Homosexually Active Men. Edited by Longres J. New York, Haworth, 1996

Tafoya T: The epistemology of Native healing and family psychology. The Family Psychologist 10:2, 1994

Tafoya T, Roeder K: Spiritual exiles in their own homeland: Native American gays and lesbians, in Addiction and Spirituality. Edited by Kus R. New York, Haworth, 1996

Tafoya T, Rowell A: Counseling gay and lesbian Native Americans, in The Sourcebook on Lesbian and Gay Health Care. Edited by Shernoff M, Scott WA. Washington, DC, National Lesbian and Gay Health Foundation, 1988

Troiden RR: Becoming homosexual: a model of gay identity acquisition. Psychiatry 42:362–373, 1979

Weeks J: Against nature, in Homosexuality, Which Homosexuality? Edited by van Kerkhof M. Amsterdam, Uiteverij An Dekker, 1989

Williams W: The Spirit and the Flesh: Sexual Diversity in American Indian Culture. Boston, MA, Beacon Press, 1988

SECTION VII

Learning New Paradigms

Training Mental Health Professionals

37

Teaching in Mental Health Training Programs About Homosexuality, Lesbians, Gay Men, and Bisexuals

Terry S. Stein, M.D.
Bonnie K. Burg, L.C.S.W., B.C.D.

I n 1973 the American Psychiatric Association removed homosexuality from its list of diagnoses of mental illness (Bayer 1987). However, clinical impressions of gay, lesbian, and bisexual patients often continue to reflect the biases of the past. The challenge of declassification is to move the perspective of homosexuality as pathology into the archives of psychiatric history and replace it with current understanding of homosexuality as a variation of normal development. Faculty in mental health training institutions hold the power to effect this change by their implicit and explicit choices about the content concerning homosexuality and lesbians, gay men, and bisexual individuals to be taught in courses, internships, and residencies (Humphreys 1983).

This chapter is based in part on Stein TS: "A Curriculum for Learning in Psychiatric Residencies About Homosexuality, Gay Men, and Lesbians." *Academic Psychiatry* 18:59–70, 1994. Used with permission.

The material taught in professional mental health training programs is easier to control than the surrounding attitudes and beliefs. Studies in the fields of psychology and social work show that bias against homosexuality as a normal variation is high among practicing and teaching professionals (Garnets et al. 1991; Humphreys 1983). Not surprisingly, research has demonstrated that the more homophobic the instructors, the less content on lesbian, gay, and bisexual issues is presented in their courses (Humphreys 1983). Training the trainers through seminars, in-service workshops, and curriculum development meetings is a prerequisite for inclusion of gay, lesbian, and bisexual course content (Newman 1989). Confronting institutional homophobia encourages normalization at all levels of the educational process.

Teaching about homosexuality and bisexuality in mental health training programs involves a unique set of issues related to the controversial and changing nature of our understanding about sexual orientation. Consequently, any proposal for teaching in this area must address such issues, including the influence on learning and clinical practice of negative attitudes about homosexuality and bisexuality and prejudice toward gay men, lesbians, and bisexual individuals; the difficulty in identifying faculty resources that results in part from prohibitions in many settings against faculty being openly gay, lesbian, or bisexual; problems related to potential discrimination against openly gay trainees and applicants; and persistence in some settings of theoretical positions that continue to equate homosexuality and bisexuality with psychopathology. Unaddressed, these factors may prohibit teaching about these important topics within many training programs, potentially producing an anti-intellectual learning environment as well as personally threatening situations for many gay, lesbian, and bisexual faculty and students. Such obstacles inimical to rigorous training and sound clinical practice must be confronted and surmounted if training is to be effective.

Rationale

Once homosexuality was redefined in 1973 as a variation in sexual orientation, the intellectual home for the concept significantly shifted to the social sciences, away from the mental health disciplines with their emphasis on mental illness and dysfunction. In the course of this fundamental paradigm shift, whole new topics integral to current concepts of homosexuality and bisexuality have emerged. The mental health disciplines must adopt the new perspective of normalcy and variation, and address and assimilate these new topics, which include the biological origins of sexual orientation (see Chapter 9 by Byne and Chapter 8 by Pillard); the normal development of homosexuality and bisexuality (Hetrick and Martin 1987); the emergence of contemporary gay, lesbian, and bisexual identities (Altman 1982); the cultural attributes of communities comprising gay men and lesbians (D'Emilio 1983); and the special mental health needs of gay men, lesbians, and bisexual individuals (Ross 1988).

On a national level, professional associations have mandated inclusion of gay and lesbian content into their respective training programs. Many recent publications in the fields of psychiatry, psychoanalysis, psychology, and social work, including the present volume, have reexamined homosexuality and bisexuality and begun addressing these topics (Coleman 1987a; Friedman 1988; Gonsiorek 1985; Isay 1989; Lewes 1988; Silverstein 1991; Stein and Cohen 1986).

Educational Objectives

The mental health disciplines represent a range of professional groups, including psychiatry, psychology, social work, counseling, and psychiatric nursing. While all of these professions uphold a similar code of ethics, there are certain distinctions among the disciplines that specify particular bodies of knowledge, skills, or emphasis in approach to patient populations. Psychiatry and psychiatric nursing share a foundation in medicine and pharmacology. Psychology has as its areas of specialization psychological testing and a broad spectrum of theory about human development and behavior. Social work has always seen part of its mission as serving the oppressed and minority populations with a goal of social change as an integral part of any intervention. Despite these differences, training in psychotherapy across all of the mental health professions derives fundamentally from a shared body of knowledge, skills, and attitudes applied by each profession in its particular theoretical context. Consequently, the authors can outline a comprehensive list of learning objectives regarding mental health knowledge, skills, and attitudes concerning homosexuality, lesbians, gay men, and bisexual individuals that can be applied differentially within the specific professions and training programs.

■ Knowledge

The student should be able to demonstrate an adequate understanding of the following:

◆ The definitions (DeCecco 1981), prevalence (see Chapter 4 by Michaels), and varieties (Bell and Weinberg 1978) of sexual orientation

◆ The history of homosexuality and bisexuality and their relationship to the mental health field (see Chapter 2 by Krajeski and Chapter 1 by Silverstein), including a critical exploration of the history of psychoanalytic ideas regarding homosexuality (see Chapter 11 by Drescher and Chapter 12 by Magee and Miller)

◆ The biological and genetic contributions to sexual orientation (see Chapter 9 by Byne and Chapter 8 by Pillard)

◆ Basic research findings about homosexuality and bisexuality (Gonsiorek and Weinrich 1991; McWhirter et al. 1990) and the types of bias in research in this field (Morin 1977)

◆ The effects of homophobia (Malyon 1985; Margolies et al. 1987), prejudice, and discrimination on gay men, lesbians, and bisexual individuals (see Chapter 7 by Herek), including the impact of antigay and antilesbian violence (see Chapter 48 by Klinger and Stein)

◆ The normal development (Bell et al. 1981) of gay men, lesbians, and bisexual individuals, including the impact of their sexuality on peer relations in childhood and adolescence; youth and adolescent development (see Chapter 16 by D'Augelli); "coming out" (see Chapter 14 by Cass); types of courting behavior (Remafedi 1987); and special issues in adult same-sex relationships (see Chapter 19 by McWhirter and Mattison and Chapter 20 by Klinger); and families (see Chapter 29 by Stein)

◆ The various lifestyles of gay men and lesbians (Herdt 1992) and the cultural characteristics of gay and lesbian communities (D'Emilio 1983)

◆ The clinical issues relevant to gay men, lesbians and bisexual individuals (see various chapters in this volume), including special approaches to assessment (Coleman 1987b; Klein et al. 1985), treatment, and disclosure of the therapist's sexual orientation (see Chapter 3 by Cabaj)

◆ The psychosocial origins and functions of homophobia when it occurs in patients, regardless of their sexual orientation (see Chapter 7 by Herek)

◆ The legal issues related to homosexuality and psychiatry (see Chapter 46 by Purcell and Hicks), including the role of the mental health professional in providing expert testimony in custody cases involving lesbian mothers and gay fathers

◆ The ethical issues relevant to homosexuality and the mental health field (see Chapter 53 by Brown)

◆ The concerns of gay and lesbian mental health professionals (see Chapter 3 by Cabaj)

▮ Skills

The student will demonstrate competence in the following areas:

◆ Working with gay, lesbian, and bisexual patients to do a comprehensive mental health assessment that leads to appropriate diagnosis, formulation, listing of problems, and design of treatment plans

◆ Relating history and clinical findings to the unique psychological and social issues confronting gay men, lesbians, and bisexual individuals

◆ Providing appropriate treatment for gay, lesbian, and bisexual patients, including psychotherapy informed by a value-free or neutral perspective on the development of sexual orientation (Mitchell 1978).

▮ Attitudes

Students should demonstrate in their behavior and demeanor that they are

◆ Aware of their own attitudes and values about homosexuality, bisexuality, gay men, lesbians, and bisexual individuals

◆ Able to be respectful and caring toward gay, lesbian, and bisexual patients and concerned about their special problems

◆ Committed to positive, ethical approaches to working with their gay, lesbian, and bisexual patients

Learning Experiences

■ Instruction

To achieve these educational objectives, it is recommended that mental health training programs attempt to infuse content about gay men, lesbians, and bisexual individuals into all relevant course work. Integration of this material throughout the course of instruction normalizes the life experiences of gay, lesbian, and bisexual persons and presents them in contexts where their sexual orientation is neither problematic nor the focus of clinical attention. Areas of special concern, such as the effects of prejudice, discrimination, and internalized homophobia, then become the necessary focus of clinical assessment and intervention.

Certain content on homosexuality and bisexuality can be effectively presented and discussed in a seminar format. The material presented in such a seminar should include

◆ Definitions and terminology related to sexual orientation, gay men, lesbians, and bisexual individuals
◆ The influence of negative attitudes in the form of homophobia, prejudice, discrimination, and stigmatization
◆ Research about homosexuality and bisexuality and problems in research resulting from bias
◆ The concerns of the gay mental health professional (coming out; role modeling)
◆ The development of homosexuality and bisexuality and gay, lesbian, and bisexual identities (growing up gay; gay, lesbian, and bisexual adolescents; family issues)
◆ Descriptions of lifestyles and relationships (same-sex relationships; alternative lifestyles; parenting and families; friends and support groups; subcultural issues)
◆ Concerns of gay men, lesbians, and bisexual individuals (fear of negative reactions by the mental health professional; effects of antigay and antilesbian violence; and common problems, such as alcoholism and other substance abuse, family and custody issues, sexual dysfunction, and AIDS/HIV infection)

◆ Special issues in psychotherapy with lesbians, gay men, and bisexual individuals (the gay adolescent; internalized homophobia; coming out; relationships; parenting; and transference and countertransference reactions)

◆ The advantages and disadvantages of various treatment settings, such as the use of gay and lesbian AA groups

Additional resources could include presentations by gay, lesbian, and bisexual individuals and by members of gay support groups and community organizations. Residents in urban settings also might visit gay community organizations.

■ Clinical Experiences

Ideally, mental health professionals should have the opportunity throughout their training to work with and follow lesbians, gay men, and bisexual individuals in a variety of clinical settings in which issues related to the patient's sexual orientation are not of primary concern. However, in part because disclosure of homosexuality and bisexuality in the health care setting is a sensitive issue, not all students will have this opportunity. At the very minimum, the authors recommend that all students have the opportunity to work directly in a clinical setting with at least one openly gay or bisexual male and one lesbian or bisexual female patient during their training program. This experience could include such activities as an assessment, formulation and identification of problems, and, when appropriate, development and implementation of a treatment plan.

In addition, students should have the opportunity to work with a gay, lesbian, or bisexual patient in psychotherapy over a period of time sufficient to identify the special issues for these persons and the potential problematic countertransference reactions for the student. While in general the problems of gay and lesbian individuals will not differ from those of heterosexual persons, it is important for the student to become familiar with the particular lifestyle and relationship concerns of gay men, lesbians, and bisexual individuals, and to understand how these concerns may influence the presentation of their problems. Whenever possible, additional elective time in clinical settings with larger numbers of gay, lesbian, and bisexual patients should be available for those students interested in working further with this population.

▓ Faculty Supervision

Students must receive supervision from qualified faculty who are knowledgeable and experienced in working with gay men, lesbians, and bisexual individuals and who represent positive attitudes and clinical approaches to these persons. The importance of visible, qualified, and respected openly gay, lesbian, and bisexual teachers and clinical supervisors cannot be emphasized enough. Similarly, gay, lesbian, and bisexual students should be able to discuss personal reactions resulting from their own sexual orientation without fear of wider disclosure or of supervisor disapproval. The sexual orientation of the supervisor for these students is not a major issue, as long as the supervisor's approach is sensitive and respectful. Residents' requests for openly gay, lesbian, or bisexual supervisors should be honored whenever possible.

Student and Program Evaluation

All students should be thoroughly evaluated to determine whether or not they have met the educational objectives related to learning about sexual orientation and gay men, lesbians, and bisexual individuals. Students should also have the opportunity to evaluate the effectiveness of their training about sexual orientation, gay men, lesbians, and bisexual individuals through written and verbal comments to the program training director, faculty supervisors, and seminar instructors. Overall program evaluation could also include measurement of gay, lesbian, and bisexual patients' satisfaction with student care, as well as other measures of quality of care delivered by students to this population, such as return rate and improvement.

Discussion

Reluctance to teach about homosexuality may necessitate curriculum evaluation to identify obstacles inherent in the present educational program. Some strategies are offered to assist in overcoming resistance to inclusion of material relevant to lesbians, gay men, and bisexual individuals:

◆ Faculty can obtain further information about what is currently being taught in other mental health training programs about sexual
orientation, gay men, lesbians, and bisexual individuals.

◆ Mental health training accreditation groups, by virtue of their
mandate, can facilitate introduction of this material by providing
up-to-date information for use in training programs, generating
new instructional materials about the subject, and inviting national gay and lesbian health and mental health organizations to
collaborate with training programs in educational efforts.

◆ Professional organizations can promote further education by
sponsoring educational workshops on sexual orientation, gay
men, lesbians, and bisexual individuals and by supporting political
activities aimed at stimulating concern for mental health issues
relevant to these individuals.

◆ Openly gay, lesbian, and bisexual professionals can support the
healthy aspects of being out by participating in their professional
organizations and serving as role models for students.

◆ Research about the negative effects of being closeted and of stigmatization can be undertaken to support greater visibility of lesbian, gay, and bisexual mental health professionals in the clinical
setting.

Such strategies will improve the likelihood that training will succeed, but cannot assure its success. Ultimately, the administration, faculty, and students in each mental health training program must be
willing to confront and surmount both their own internalized homophobia and the widespread contemporary American cultural prejudice
about homosexuality and bisexuality if the training goals are to be
achieved.

Conclusion

Implementing this training in mental health educational programs will
be neither a simple nor a straightforward undertaking. Homosexuality
and bisexuality are topics fraught with meaning for most individuals in
American society, for they touch upon deeply held religious, political,
moral, and personal beliefs. Thus, a list of educational objectives and
a description of courses and other learning experiences related to these

subjects, however carefully prepared and thoroughly presented, can serve only as a series of guideposts, which should in no way be confused with the journey itself. Training programs must nonetheless undertake this journey so that discussion of the full range of sexuality and sexual orientation can be reintroduced into mental health theory and practice to help practitioners more effectively care for gay men, lesbians, and bisexual individuals who seek treatment.

References

Altman D: The Homosexualization of America, the Americanization of the Homosexual. New York, St. Martin's Press, 1982

Bayer R: Homosexuality and American Psychiatry. New York, Basic Books, 1987

Bell AP, Weinberg MS: Homosexualities: A Study of Diversity Among Men and Women. New York, Simon and Schuster, 1978

Bell AP, Weinberg MS, Hammersmith SK: Sexual Preference: Its Development in Men and Women. Bloomington, IN, Indiana University Press, 1981

Coleman E (ed): Psychotherapy with Homosexual Men and Women: Integrated Identity Approaches for Clinical Practice. New York, Haworth, 1987a

Coleman E: Assessment of sexual orientation. J Homosex 14:9–24, 1987b

DeCecco JP: Definition and meaning of sexual orientation. J Homosex 6:51–69, 1981

D'Emilio J: Sexual Politics, Sexual Communities. Chicago, IL, University of Chicago Press, 1983

Friedman RC: Male Homosexuality. New Haven, CT, Yale University Press, 1988

Garnets L, Hancock KA, Cochran S, et al: Issues in psychotherapy with lesbians and gay men. American Psychologist 46:964–972, 1991

Gonsiorek JC (ed): A Guide to Psychotherapy with Gay and Lesbian Clients. New York, Harrington Park Press, 1985

Gonsiorek JC, Weinrich JD (eds): Homosexuality: Research Implications for Public Policy. Newbury Park, CA, Sage, 1991

Herdt G (ed): Gay Culture in America: Essays From the Field. Boston, MA, Beacon Press, 1992

Hetrick ES, Martin AD: Developmental issues and their resolution for gay and lesbian adolescents. J Homosex 14:25–44, 1987

Hildago H, Peterson T, Woodman JJ (eds): Lesbian and Gay Issues: A Resource Manual for Social Workers. Washington, DC, National Association of Social Workers, 1985

Humphreys GE: Inclusion of content on homosexuality in the social work curriculum. J Education for Social Work 19:55–60, 1983

Isay RA: Being Homosexual. New York, Farrar, Straus, Giroux, 1989

Klein TS, Sepekoff B, Wolf TJ: Sexual orientation: a multi-variable dynamic process. J Homosex 11:35–49, 1985

Lewes K: The Psychoanalytic Theory of Male Homosexuality. New York, Simon and Schuster, 1988

Malyon AK: Psychotherapeutic implications of internalized homophobia in gay men, in A Guide to Psychotherapy with Gay and Lesbian Clients. Edited by Gonsiorek JC. New York, Harrington Park Press, 1985

Margolies L, Becker M, Jackson-Brewer K: Internalized homophobia: identifying and treating the oppressor within, in Lesbian Psychologies. Edited by Boston Lesbian Psychologies Collective. Urbana, IL, University of Illinois Press, 1987

McWhirter DP, Sanders SA, Reinisch JM (eds): Homosexuality/Heterosexuality. The Kinsey Institute Series. New York, Oxford University Press, 1990

Mitchell SA: Psychodynamics: homosexuality and the question of pathology. Psychiatry 41:254–263, 1978

Morin SF: Heterosexual bias in psychological research on lesbianism and male homosexuality. American Psychologist 32:629–637, 1977

Newman BS: Including curriculum content on lesbian and gay issues. Journal of Social Work in Education 25:202–211, 1989

Remafedi G: Homosexual youth: a challenge to contemporary society. JAMA 258:222–225, 1987

Ross MW (ed): The Treatment of Homosexuals with Mental Health Disorders. New York, Harrington Park Press, 1988

Silverstein C (ed): Gays, Lesbians, and Their Therapists. New York, WW Norton, 1991

Stein T, Cohen C (eds): Contemporary Perspectives on Psychotherapy with Lesbians and Gay Men. New York, Plenum Publishing, 1986

38

Gay, Lesbian, and Bisexual Issues in Medical Schools

Implications for Training

Mark H. Townsend, M.D.
Mollie M. Wallick, Ph.D.

T he student bodies of U.S. medical schools, while not yet mirroring the country's population, have become increasingly diverse. In general, academic inquiry into the varied needs and views of this changed student population has lagged behind its emergence. Relatively few investigators have studied the impact of medical training on women and ethnic or racial minority students. By the same token, the effect these newcomers have had on medical schools has been understudied.

Similarly, little is known about the evolving relationship between lesbian, gay, and bisexual medical students and their training institutions. Although homosexual students were undoubtedly represented when medical student bodies consisted mainly of males of Northern European ancestry, the presence of openly gay and lesbian students is a more recent phenomenon. Even now, a key issue for these students is how "open" they can or should be.

The authors' knowledge about how current medical school curricula address both homosexuality and the care of gay patients is based in part on the reports of lesbian and gay students, because they are often willing observers and thoughtful critics. Medical schools have had to adapt to an unusual situation as homosexuality has evolved from a psychiatric diagnosis to an aspect of a patient's social history. It is not known whether the number of academic hours devoted to teaching about homosexuality has changed with its deletion from the *Diagnostic and Statistical Manual of Mental Disorders*. However, in the opinion of lesbian and gay students (Townsend et al. 1991), insufficient instructional time is allocated to the care of gay and lesbian patients.

In this chapter, the authors present information concerning both the expressed needs of lesbian, gay, and bisexual medical students and the services that medical schools direct toward them. In addition, the authors provide current perspectives on the academic treatment of homosexuality and the care of lesbian, gay, and bisexual patients.

The Medical School Milieu

Both female students and students from racial and ethnic minority groups often experience medical school differently than do students from populations not historically underrepresented. Lesbian, gay, and bisexual students differ from other underrepresented groups in that their presence is not immediately recognizable. These students, like lesbians and gay men everywhere, can choose to shield their sexual orientation from others to avoid social stigmatization and prejudice. The pressure to conceal this identity in medical school can be extreme and begins with the application process itself. Applicants are often unwilling to reveal their sexual orientation, fearing that their homosexuality may diminish their chance of acceptance. The effort to disguise one's sexual orientation can be dispiriting, because it involves omitting from view important relationships, activities, and accomplishments.

Once enrolled in medical school, lesbian, gay, and bisexual students find themselves in a milieu in which individual expression is discouraged. Medical student culture often dictates that students appear as similar as possible, at least superficially (Knight 1981). At the same time, competing demands from faculty, patients, family, and significant others may cause extreme stress (Dickstein et al. 1990; Vitaliano et al. 1988). Consequently, medical school can be a difficult place in which to embark on a journey of self-discovery such as the coming-out process (Martin 1991), because the student's solidifying identity as a lesbian or gay man can come into conflict with the professional socialization process emphasizing conformity. The result is that many gay, lesbian, and bisexual students do not come out and, instead, remain isolated and alone.

■ Support Services

In recent years, a growing number of support services have been directed toward lesbian, gay, and bisexual medical students (Tinmouth and Hamwi 1994). Townsend et al. (1991) reported that peer support groups—organized to provide social interaction, education, or both—are widespread and may take many forms. Groups may be student or university organized and may include students from one or several area schools. Some student groups are affiliated with chapters of national organizations, such as the American Medical Student Association (AMSA)—particularly AMSA's standing committee, Lesbian, Gay, and Bisexual People in Medicine—or the Gay and Lesbian Medical Association, the national, multispecialty organization for lesbian, gay, and bisexual physicians and their supporters.

All gay student groups, even local chapters of national organizations, are prone to wide swings in membership size as cohorts of medical students who may be quite "out" and known to one another graduate and move on. Students who follow either remain isolated or must begin the arduous process of forming a new network. Student isolation may be limited and the demise of support groups may be averted if faculty members refer gay students to one another or to gay faculty.

On the local level, one successful formula to ensure that students are aware of support services has been the appointment of an officially sponsored Student-Faculty Liaison for Gay and Lesbian Issues. Although such liaisons exist at only a handful of schools, they may be of great assistance to gay students by providing counseling and reassurance and by directing them both to peer and community support and to potential faculty mentors (Townsend et al. 1991). Although gay students appear to prefer that student-faculty liaisons themselves be gay, more important in their judgment is that the liaison be readily accessible and that students cannot be identified as gay merely because they are seen waiting outside the liaison's office.

In addition to providing peer support, lesbian and gay students are increasingly active in educating their heterosexual counterparts about homosexuality. A recent issue of "Pulse," the medical student section of the *Journal of the American Medical Association,* discussed issues related to gay and lesbian medical students and patients and included several articles written by lesbian and gay students (Crawford-Faucher and Lee 1994). At Temple University, members of Lesbian, Gay, and Bisexual People in Medicine, along with faculty and administrators, wrote, "A Community of Equals: A Resource Guide to the Gay and Lesbian Community," which is distributed to all students, residents, and faculty (Office of Student Affairs, Temple University School of Medicine, unpublished guidebook, 1992). The guidebook describes lesbian and gay services throughout the region and instructs students in how to provide more sensitive health care; it was subsequently adapted for use by several other medical schools. Lesbian, gay, and bisexual students may also be active in freshman orientation programs. At some schools gay students themselves participate in panel presentations in an attempt to increase awareness of gay issues.

▉ Barriers to Full Inclusion

The fact that lesbian and gay medical students are, in general, discouraged from revealing their sexual orientation imposes many barriers to their full inclusion in the medical school culture. One of the most potent barriers is that gay men, lesbians, and bisexual individuals are often presumed not to be present. This presumption can change only if gay students make themselves known—a daunting task, given that medical students often depend solely on their peers for companionship and support.

"Coming out" is made even more difficult by the circumscribed way lesbian and gay health care issues are treated in the medical school curriculum. Gay students receive little acknowledgment that their existence is important, much less that their concerns are relevant. Recently, one researcher (Tjia 1993) surveyed medical students at a national meeting and found that gay and lesbian students were more likely to have used mental health services and to have performed less well academically during the school year. Although perhaps not true of all gay and lesbian students, the results are nonetheless disturbing. A second researcher (Mosbacher 1993) found that being either closeted or openly gay while in medical school may exact an emotional price.

As has been mentioned, the role of sex, race, and ethnicity in medical training is an understudied area. Even less is known about the ways heterosexual and homosexual members of any given group compare regarding psychosocial adjustment, although the above-mentioned surveys (Mosbacher 1993; Tjia 1993) did indicate that heterosexuals appear to experience greater well-being in some ways. Women in medicine have, in general, reported less ability than men to form mentoring relationships (Abeshaus et al. 1993; Coombs and Hovanessian 1988), and it stands to reason that lesbian students may have even more difficulty finding lesbian physician role models. Again, the faculty should make certain that lesbian students have the opportunity to establish meaningful professional ties.

Regarding race and ethnicity, the fact that blacks, Native Americans, and Hispanics continue to be underrepresented in medical schools is frequently acknowledged (Petersdorf 1992; Watts and Lecca 1989). Members of these groups have also shown a higher rate of attrition than other medical students (Gupta 1991) and, along with women, appear to have more second thoughts about a medical career (Hadley et al. 1992). Gay minority students, whatever their ethnicity, are simultaneously members of another and often less evident group. Without accessible support, little is available to unite gay students from such diverse backgrounds, leaving them vulnerable to feelings of isolation. Furthermore, the existence of a gay support group alongside another organization that specifically serves minority students (e.g., the Student National Medical Association) may itself be conflictual: gay minority students may need to decide where to place their energy and, at times, their loyalties, because each group may have different aims.

Teaching About Homosexuality

A survey of gay and lesbian medical students regarding support services (Townsend et al. 1991) also explored the way in which the subject of homosexuality was addressed in the medical school curriculum. That inquiry was followed by a national survey of how faculty with responsibility for presenting information on homosexuality view the topic's academic treatment at their school (Wallick et al. 1992).

Although no significant differences were reported on the basis of class size or institutional affiliation, the mean number of curriculum hours allocated to the topic of homosexuality was significantly greater in the West than in other geographic regions. Table 38–1 summarizes the authors' overall findings, irrespective of region, regarding curriculum hours reported and instructional strategies most frequently used.

■ Panel Format, Exposure to Gays, and Small-Group Discussion

As indicated in Table 38–1, the most commonly reported instructional strategy was lecturing in human sexuality. The instructional methods tied for second place in order of usage were panel presentation and exposure to lesbians and gay men. The latter two approaches are combined at the authors' medical school (Louisiana State University School of Medicine—New Orleans) late in the fall semester of the freshman year. During the first 2 class hours, a panel of gay and lesbian physicians and a faculty member/parent of a lesbian share their life stories and are available to answer questions posed by students. The panelists present a view of lesbians and gays different from the stereotypic image often conjured up by many members of our society; they also serve as successful representatives of the medical profession and as attractive role models with whom to identify. Several researchers have found positive interaction with lesbians and gay men useful in reducing stereotypic attitudes (Bauman and Hale 1985; McGrory et al. 1990).

A highly interactive question-and-answer period is followed by a third hour of small-group discussion (eight or nine students with a department of psychiatry faculty member or resident as group leader) to deal further with the topic in "safer" surrounds and to allay any possible discomfort resulting from the earlier exposure. It has been demonstrated that, along with an educational component, focused group discussion is necessary to facilitate attitude change (Gallop et al. 1992). In addition to the strategies reported in Table 38–1, it is of interest that small-group discussion was another method frequently used.

To explore the possibility of group attitude change after the panel presentation and small-group discussion, the authors surveyed the

Table 38–1. Instructional strategies and curriculum hours devoted to teaching about homosexuality in 82 medical schools

Strategy in which homosexuality is addressed	Percentage and number of schools using strategy (N = 82)									
	In at least 1 year		In freshman year		In sophomore year		In junior year		In senior year	
	%	n	%	n	%	n	%	n	%	n
Lecture(s) on human sexuality	79.3	65	40.2	33	45.1	37	9.8	8	2.4	2
Meetings with gays and lesbians	40.2	33	19.5	16	20.7	17	2.4	2	0	0
Panel presentation on human sexuality	40.2	33	20.7	17	20.7	17	0	0	0	0
Case vignettes in psychiatry	31.7	26	3.7	3	9.8	8	20.7	17	4.9	4
Film	25.6	21	9.8	8	0	0	1.2	1	0	0
Lecture(s) on medical ethics	19.5	16	14.6	12	4.9	4	2.4	2	1.2	1
Case vignettes in physical diagnosis	19.5	16	2.4	2	13.4	11	3.7	3	1.2	1
Case vignettes in medicine	11	9	0	0	2.4	2	7.3	6	2.4	2
Panel presentation on medical ethics	9.8	8	6.1	5	3.7	3	0	0	0	0

Mean number of hours devoted (hours:minutes)

Total	Freshman year	Sophomore year	Junior year	Senior year
3:27	1:17	1:29	0:29	0:11

Note. In 1991, the authors surveyed appropriate faculty (mostly directors of medical student education in psychiatry) at all 126 U.S. medical schools to assess both the number of curriculum hours devoted to the topic of homosexuality and the instructional strategies employed in its academic treatment; faculty from 82 schools (65%) responded.

360 students in their school's 1991 and 1992 entering classes at the beginning, middle, and end of their freshman year, asking them to complete anonymously the Index of Attitudes toward Homosexuals (IAH) (Hudson and Ricketts 1980). As was reported for the authors' first cohort (Wallick et al. 1993), repeated administration of the IAH in both classes revealed a noteworthy reduction in group homophobic response, with the mean score of each class decreasing at midyear and continuing its downward movement at the end of the academic year. But in spite of the fact that 10% fewer students expressed a homophobic attitude at the end of the study, the group mean score on the IAH remained within the "low grade homophobic" range throughout each 8½-month period.

More striking was the apparent relationship between changes in the students' responses to individual items on the IAH and the content of the panel presentation. For example, the two items most closely paralleling the life situations of the panelists revealed the most immediate attitude change. In addition, five of the nine items with noteworthy changes over time involved learning that a family member, friend, or professional contact is gay. The authors concluded that students generalized the panel and small-group discussion to a variety of relationships, resulting in an overall diminution in group homophobic response. They are currently reevaluating their first cohort as the subjects begin their third-year psychiatry clerkship. With three-fourths of the class responding thus far, it appears that the group mean score on the IAH continues to be significantly lower than the prepresentation mean of the 1991 entering class.

In evaluating the authors' study of student attitudes toward homosexuality, they acknowledge that attitudinal change is multifactorial: it occurs throughout medical school, as a consequence of maturation, acculturation, and a multitude of environmental and educational influences other than exposure to a panel of gay and lesbian physicians followed by small-group discussion. A further limitation of the authors' attitudinal research is its lack of generalizability to other schools, especially those in other regions of the country. A reevaluation at Columbia University (McGrory et al. 1990) of an earlier study at the University of Mississippi (Kelly et al. 1987) of medical students' attitudes toward the acquired immunodeficiency syndrome and homosexual patients dramatically documented the impossibility of generalization: although the New York City researchers recognized potential differences in the students' demographic characteristics and in the extent of their interactions with gay men and lesbians as deterrents to direct comparison, the researchers' prediction of markedly contrasting attitudes at the two schools was proven accurate. In spite of the authors' inability to attribute causation and to generalize our findings, they are nonetheless pleased and encouraged by the lasting power of the earlier documented change.

▮ Other Instructional Approaches

In the authors' survey of medical schools (Wallick et al. 1992), only 1 of 82 respondents reported that gay and lesbian issues were "integral to most current teaching" (the expressed preference of the students in the authors' earlier survey [Townsend et al. 1991]). Eight faculty members indicated that the topic was totally absent from the curriculum, a finding both disturbing and identical in percentage to that reported by the students in the author's earlier survey. Twelve respondents reported the topic's treatment in association with HIV-related illness; in one case HIV was the only context in which homosexuality was addressed.

Regarding additional desirable ways in which the topic might be effectively presented, the faculty members' open-ended responses included "use of case material throughout the curriculum," "integration throughout the clinical years," and "inclusion in physical diagnosis and interviewing." One faculty member suggested the need for "an acceptable, less threatening way to teach [the topic]." The authors speculated that this apparent lack of comfort in discussing gay and lesbian issues might be due to a lingering association of homosexuality with deviance and psychopathology. Alternatively, the discomfort might be related to the frequent inclusion of homosexuality in instruction regarding HIV, thus linking homosexual identity—and not high-risk behavior irrespective of sexual orientation—with a frightening pandemic illness.

▮ Conclusions of Student and
Faculty Research

The major findings of the authors' study on medical school faculty opinion (Wallick et al. 1992) are remarkably consistent with those of their earlier research on student opinion (Townsend et al. 1991). It is likely that the marginalization in the curriculum reported in the two surveys trivializes the topic's importance in the minds of both faculty and students. Perhaps, in accordance with the students' recommendation (also made by three faculty members) that the topic be addressed across the entire spectrum of medical education, teaching about the care of homosexual patients should be wholly integrated throughout the curriculum—from the basic sciences through the full range of clinical experiences. Only in that way can faculty members' and students' sensitivity to and comfort with lesbian and gay issues be enhanced and stereotypic responses be countered.

■ Model Curriculum

Although courses on human sexuality at many schools include a brief homosexuality component, the only medical curriculum known to the authors that focuses exclusively on homosexuality is one proposed by the American Psychiatric Association Committee on Gay, Lesbian, and Bisexual Issues (Stein 1994). The curriculum includes objectives, suggested topics and content, instructional approaches, strategies to stimulate further teaching, and selected references.

Conclusion

Medical schools have only recently begun to identify and acknowledge key issues pertaining to homosexual and bisexual patients. At the same time, lesbian, gay, and bisexual students are becoming more visible within medical student bodies. These phenomena are not unrelated, because U.S. society itself is demonstrating an increasing awareness of homosexuality. The challenge for academic medicine is to be more sensitive than society as a whole to the needs of lesbian, gay, and bisexual providers, patients, and students.

References

Abeshaus DB, Epstein LC, Kane AB, et al: The status of women in medicine at the Brown University School of Medicine. R I Med 76:337–339, 1993

Bauman KA, Hale FA: Bringing the homosexual patient out: teaching the doctor's role. Med Educ 19:459–462, 1985

Coombs RH, Hovanessian HC: Stress in the role constellation of female resident physicians. J Am Med Wom Assoc 43:21–27, 1988

Crawford-Faucher AD, Lee FS (eds): Pulse (medical student section). JAMA 271:711–718, 1994

Dickstein LJ, Stephenson JJ, Hinz LD: Psychiatric impairment in medical students. Acad Med 65:588–593, 1990

Gallop RM, Taerk G, Lancee WJ, et al: A randomized trial of group interventions for hospital staff caring for persons with AIDS. AIDS Care 4:177–185, 1992

Gupta GC: Student attrition: a challenge for allied health education programs. JAMA 266:963–967, 1991

Hadley J, Cantor JC, Willke RJ, et al: Young physicians most and least likely to have second thoughts about a career in medicine. Acad Med 67:180–190, 1992

Hudson WW, Ricketts WA: A strategy for the measurement of homophobia. J Homosex 5:357–372, 1980

Kelly JA, St. Lawrence JS, Smith S Jr, et al: Medical students' attitudes toward AIDS and homosexual patients. J Med Educ 62:549–556, 1987

Knight JA: To wear the healer's mantle, in Doctor-to-Be: Coping with the Trials and Triumphs of Medical School. New York, Appleton-Century-Crofts, 1981, pp 39–56

Martin HP: The coming-out process for homosexuals. Hosp Community Psychiatry 42:158–162, 1991

McGrory BJ, McDowell DM, Muskin PR: Medical students' attitudes toward AIDS, homosexual, and intravenous drug-abusing patients: a re-evaluation in New York City. Psychosomatics 31:426–433, 1990

Mosbacher D: Alcohol and other drug use in female medical students: a comparison of lesbians and heterosexuals. Journal of Gay and Lesbian Psychotherapy 2:37–48, 1993

Petersdorf RG: Not a choice, an obligation. Acad Med 67:73–79, 1992

Stein TS: A curriculum for learning in psychiatric residencies about homosexuality, gay men, and lesbians. Academic Psychiatry 18:59–70, 1994

Tinmouth J, Hamwi G: The experience of gay and lesbian students in medical school. JAMA 271:714–715, 1994

Tjia J: Assessment of the effects of sexual identity confusion on academic performance. Paper presented at the annual meeting of the American Association of Physicians for Human Rights, Portland, OR, August 1993

Townsend MH, Wallick MM, Cambre KM: Support services for homosexual students at U.S. medical schools. Acad Med 66:361–363, 1991

Vitaliano P, Maiuro RD, Russo J, et al: A biopsychosocial model of medical school distress. J Behav Med 11:311–331, 1988

Wallick MM, Cambre KM, Townsend MH: How the topic of homosexuality is taught at U.S. medical schools. Acad Med 67:601–603, 1992

Wallick MM, Cambre KM, Townsend MH: Freshman students' attitudes toward homosexuality. Acad Med 68:357, 1993

Watts TC, Lecca PJ: Minorities in the health professions: a current perspective. J Natl Med Assoc 81:1225–1229, 1989

39

Issues for Gay Male, Lesbian, and Bisexual Mental Health Trainees

D. Lanette Atkins, M.D., D.V.M.
Mark H. Townsend, M.D.

L ittle has been written about the opinions and needs of lesbian, gay, and bisexual mental health trainees: psychiatry residents, psychology graduate students, and social work students. This chapter addresses the interpersonal and clinical issues that commonly affect gay and lesbian trainees. The authors discuss the events that typically accompany the transition into mental health training and, on its completion, into postgraduate training or the job market. The authors recently completed general psychiatric training (M.H.T.) and/or child and adolescent fellowship training (D.L.A.), and have long been members of the Association of Gay and Lesbian Psychiatrists; thus, this chapter includes many personal observations, as well as those of lesbian, gay, and bisexual colleagues.

Transition to Training

Even before beginning training, gay and lesbian trainees must face very difficult decisions that heterosexual trainees do not. One such decision is whether or not to be open about sexual orientation on the initial application to training programs. Often, applicants have been actively involved with gay and lesbian groups or projects before applying for graduate mental health training. The decision to list these on a curriculum vitae or application often creates much anxiety, because this information may result in some programs electing not to grant interviews to these applicants. On the other hand, omission of these activities often leaves out very important information concerning the applicant and may lead to the conclusion that the applicant is not well-rounded.

Applicants who choose to disguise their sexual orientation must again decide whether or not to discuss their sexuality during the interview process, as opportunities for self-disclosure often arise naturally. "Coming out" can benefit the applicant in a number of ways. The program's general stance on the pathology of homosexuality may be assessed, as well as the program's view of lesbian and gay trainees. Early self-disclosure also lessens the possibility that the students' or residents' sexuality will be discovered during training and somehow be used against them.

The number of psychiatric residents choosing to disclose their sexual orientation before accepting a position appears to be increasing. This decision may be influenced by the increased support and availability of others who have been in the same situation and by the fact that the number of available positions exceeds the number of applicants (Sledge et al. 1987), which may give applicants increased confidence that they will be accepted into a program in which they will feel comfortable. The presence of openly gay faculty and residents may also impact positively on one's decision to self-disclose.

Interpersonal Issues During Training

Graduate training is a stressful experience for all mental health trainees. The most significant issue of concern to psychiatric residents has been identified as limited time for social and recreational activities and for family and friends (Berg and Garrard 1980; Kirsling and Kochar 1989; Schwartz et al. 1987). Other stressors include lack of sleep, scarcity of study time, problems of self-confidence, and relationship disturbances. Higher stress was reported for those in the first year of psychiatric residency training, with depression being a common occurrence (Evans et al. 1986; Kirsling and Kochar 1989; Landau et al. 1986).

Yager (1974) reported that for psychiatry trainees a degree of personal and professional identity crisis is unavoidable, necessary, and indeed desirable in the process of professional identity formation. When trainees enter postgraduate training, the area of required competence is altered significantly. The new and unfamiliar tasks associated with beginning training raise questions of personal and professional efficacy. In addition to the stress associated with assuming responsibility for patient care, most trainees experience some loss of self-esteem and stature with acceptance of the student role (Kirsling and Kochar 1989; Scanlan 1972; Tischler 1972). Many trainees initiate a quest for external validation in response to these challenges. Gay and lesbian trainees may experience additional difficulties due to overt or covert bias against them by faculty. They may also avoid supportive interaction with faculty due to a fear of rejection. In addition, identity confusion may be complicated in some individuals by the stress of working through the process of accepting one's orientation.

Another significant stressor is that gay men and lesbians may feel that their personal relationships are not supported by their heterosexual colleagues. They may not feel comfortable including their significant others in activities intended to provide support and social interaction with others, and they may have little additional time for socializing. Gay and lesbian trainees may also be faced with the challenge of establishing a social support network in a setting where gay and lesbian communities are relatively invisible. Establishing such a network may be extremely difficult, especially in smaller towns.

Support systems need to be fostered during residency training (Landau et al. 1986). Social support of family and friends and time for relaxation have been well documented as affording some protection from stress and facilitating the ability to cope with crisis and adapt to change (Cobb 1976; Landau et al. 1986; Schwartz et al. 1987). Loss of friendships and support of close family members may significantly diminish the resident's ability to cope with stress when a geographic relocation has occurred (Kirsling and Kochar 1989).

A growing number of psychiatry training programs employ sensitivity or therapy groups for residents in which personal relationships may develop, enabling the formation of an important peer-support system (Berg and Garrard 1980; Russell et al. 1975). Through support groups, residents learn to deal with the stresses and conflicts of residency training, thereby enabling them to be more effective in both their professional and personal lives (Berg and Garrard 1980; Landau et al. 1986). Groups may be a positive experience in which members are able to share their personal lives and develop better understanding of each other so that they can provide more effective peer support. However, it will be difficult for some gay and lesbian trainees to receive the full benefits of such a group if they are unable to discuss their sexuality due to their own level of discomfort or fear of rejection by the group.

Administrators of training programs should take primary responsibility for developing support systems for trainees (Berg and Garrard 1980). When trainees are unhappy, faculty may be more likely to reach into the intrapsychic worlds of their protégés for explanations, rather than to blame external events, of which the faculty themselves are part (Yager 1974). The need for role models is great, and they should exist throughout training and perhaps well after training (Fleckles 1972; Kardener et al. 1970; Walfish et al. 1989). Faculty role models are important to the development of a resident's professional identity and can create an atmosphere in which one can learn to respect the diversity of colleagues (Yager 1974). Graduates have reported that the most important aspects of their residency training and professional development were their relationships with teachers and supervisory role models (Hales and Borus 1986). Access to gay and lesbian faculty may be limited, however, often due to the invisibility of these important role models.

Clinical Issues During Training

During their training, psychiatry residents, clinical psychology students, and graduate social work students are expected to become familiar with a number of therapeutic methods and to learn and apply a large and wide-ranging fund of knowledge. Mental health training is both time limited and structured, and little time is available to teach trainees to use their innate characteristics—sexual orientation, sex, race, and ethnicity—to therapeutic advantage. In fact, little is known about the complicated relationships between members of previously underrepresented groups and their training institutions.

Lesbian, gay, and bisexual trainees differ from members of other minority groups in that they can choose to shield their sexual orientation from faculty, peers, and mental health consumers. Gay residents and students must often take the initiative in making their issues known to supervisors and peers, because their colleagues may be unaware of their sexual orientation. They may be reluctant to speak up, in part, because of faculty who consider homosexuality an illness. In a recent survey of lesbian and gay psychiatry residents, more than one-fifth of respondents reported that their programs treated homosexuality as a disease (Townsend et al. 1993).

Mental health trainees have also reported that they consider instruction about care of lesbians, gay men, and bisexual individuals to be inadequate. One study of counseling psychology graduate students stated that most training programs provide little or no exposure to lesbian and gay patients or to their issues (Buhrke 1989). In a survey of clinical psychology Ph.D. and Psy.D. programs, both students and faculty reported that gay patients and their issues received a lower training emphasis than that accorded to other groups (O'Connor 1984). Almost one-third of the lesbian and gay psychiatry residents questioned in one study reported no exposure to formal instruction in homosexual patient care (Townsend et al. 1993). However, in a later survey of U.S. psychiatry residency training directors, almost all of them reported that some type of training in lesbian and gay issues occurred in their programs (Townsend et al. 1995). Although this discrepancy may be due to the different viewpoints of each group—for example, the training director may be more familiar than any one trainee with the entire curriculum—it appears that most mental health trainees receive insufficient instruction about the care of gay, lesbian, and bisexual patients.

Issues of self-disclosure are important for lesbian, gay, and bisexual trainees. Supervision to address the way a trainee's sexuality affects psychotherapy delivery is only possible if the trainee is forthcoming about his or her sexual orientation. It appears that the frequency with which trainees come out to colleagues is inversely proportional to status and seniority. For example, most lesbian and gay psychiatry residents in one study reported coming out to at least one other resident, but only half reported coming out to their training director, and just one-quarter reported coming out to their department chair (Townsend et al. 1993). Fewer still reported that they felt comfortable actually discussing lesbian and gay issues with their training director or chairperson. Sixty percent of this sample said they know of openly gay faculty; however, the researchers made no attempt to determine whether these faculty served as real mentors.

Coming out to faculty and peers is less controversial and encumbered by the ethical responsibility to maintain good therapeutic boundaries than is the decision to disclose one's sexual orientation to a mental health consumer. A gay resident or student who, for whatever reason, wishes to make certain his or her orientation is known must tell the patient directly. Approximately one-third of lesbian and gay psychiatry residents report this sort of disclosure, with a dramatic increase as training progresses (Townsend et al. 1993). Psychiatry residency training directors, on the other hand, tend to disapprove of this sort of disclosure, regardless of their program's reported stance on the pathology of homosexuality (Townsend et al. 1995). However, faculty may not know how frequently disclosure occurs and may be unaware of the presence of gay trainees. It is also likely that many gay psychiatry residents and psychology and social work students avoid discussing their sexuality with supervisors; these same gay trainees may also be unlikely to discuss aspects of their patients' homosexuality.

It is not solely the trainee's responsibility to initiate discussion on lesbian and gay issues. Given the high level of homophobia perceived by gay and lesbian trainees, faculty members must demonstrate a supportive and gay-affirming stance if they expect to provide thorough supervision. Otherwise, trainees may disguise the content of the therapy hour or seek forms of supervision outside of their programs. Many therapeutic issues relevant to homosexuality, which are important for the career development of both heterosexual and homosexual trainees and in the psychotherapy of lesbian and gay patients, are given inadequate attention in training.

Gender is an important factor in any discussion of lesbian, gay, and bisexual issues in mental health training, because gay men and lesbians can have very different experiences during training. Several studies demonstrated that women in medical training are, in general, subject to greater adversity than men: they are more likely to be harassed (Wolf et al. 1991), to have their commitment to medicine questioned (Marquart et al. 1990), to lack mentoring relationships (Abeshaus et al. 1993), and to have second thoughts about a medical career (Hadley et al. 1992). In the study of psychiatry residents by Townsend et al. (1993), gay men were more likely than lesbians to be aware of lesbian and gay faculty or to be affiliated with medical support groups. In addition, men reported a greater ability to discuss gay issues with their training directors and more frequently perceived that their programs considered homosexuality to be a normal condition. In light of these findings, training directors should place increased emphasis on working to integrate lesbians more fully into their programs and to facilitate satisfying mentoring relationships for these women.

Further Training

For gay, lesbian, and bisexual psychiatry residents and psychology and social work graduate students, the transition to postgraduate and fellowship training parallels earlier transitions in many ways. Decisions regarding disclosure of sexual orientation are once again in the forefront, especially if one is applying for a position working with children and adolescents or for further analytic training.

Significant homophobia can become evident when one is contemplating working with youth (Slater 1988). Many people continue to fear that homosexual adults may influence their children to become gay or lesbian (Mallon 1992). Others believe that homosexual individuals are likely to sexually assault children. These misconceptions may result in prejudice and discrimination against gay and lesbian trainees, which may cause them to continue to hide their sexual orientation (Mallon 1992). For these reasons, the decision to be open about one's sexual orientation may be difficult to make when entering child and adolescent training.

In contrast, if one feels comfortable with the decision to disclose his or her sexual orientation, being openly gay may provide many opportunities to serve as an essential role model for gay and lesbian youth and to assist colleagues in becoming familiar with their issues (Slater 1988). Due to the unique needs of gay and lesbian youth, it is important that informed professionals be in a position to address issues and advocate for these youth. It is also important to support inclusion of educational curricula that address the needs of lesbian and gay youth.

The decision to pursue psychoanalytic training also brings up issues related to self-disclosure. There has been long-standing conflict between the American psychoanalytic community and the gay community (Cornett and Hudson 1985). Only recently have analytic training programs begun to accept openly gay and lesbian applicants and to show concern over the public perception of psychoanalysts as homophobic and discriminatory (Roughton 1993). The belief that lesbians and gay men suffer from early and severe developmental defects that prevent them from being good analysts remains a stumbling block to psychoanalytic training in some institutes (Cunningham 1991; Flaks 1992). Once accepted, psychoanalytic candidates in institutes that emphasize the pathology of homosexuality may feel compelled to remain closeted, which may also negatively impact the candidate's own analysis.

Employment

The decision to conceal or reveal sexual orientation when seeking employment is as complicated as it is when applying for graduate school or residency. Again, this decision depends on both the individual's comfort with his or her own orientation and on the perceived institutional biases against disclosure. Once the gay therapist begins employment, however, self-disclosure issues do not lessen. By the same token, many lesbian and gay mental health workers, especially those involved in group practices, discover that it is they who must advocate on behalf of gay patients. Often, they must confront these challenges at a disadvantage if during training they did not acquire sufficient experience in openly and positively expressing their homosexuality.

Conclusion

Many of the concerns of gay, lesbian, and bisexual mental health trainees are similar to those of trainees in general. However, often these trainees feel the need to conceal their sexual identity and, as a result, are less able to advocate for their unique needs. Lesbian and gay faculty may also be closeted and, as such, unavailable for mentoring. In addition, gay, lesbian, and bisexual students and residents are often presumed not to be present by the heterosexual majority. Despite the risks of stigmatization and prejudice, the authors believe that trainees who arc open about their sexual orientation generally have a richer educational experience than those who remain closeted.

A number of interventions can be made to enhance the training experiences of gay, lesbian, and bisexual mental health trainees. Programs must take responsibility for initiating discussion on lesbian and gay issues. Curricula should include information on the unique issues of gay, lesbian, and bisexual people. Administrators of training programs need to take primary responsibility for developing support systems for trainees. Faculty members must demonstrate a supportive and gay-affirming stance if they expect to provide thorough supervision. Increased emphasis should be placed on working to integrate lesbians more fully into training programs and to facilitate satisfying mentoring relationships for women. Role models should exist throughout training as well as after training.

Administrators, faculty, and trainees must all work together to ensure that gay, lesbian, and bisexual trainees have the best possible experience during this time of professional development.

References

Abeshaus DB, Epstein LC, Kane AG, et al: The status of women in medicine at the Brown University School of Medicine. R I Med 76:337–339, 1993

Berg JK, Garrard J: Psychosocial support in residency training programs. Journal of Medical Education 55:851–857, 1980

Buhrke RA: Female student perspectives on training in lesbian and gay issues. The Counseling Psychologist 17:629–636, 1989

Cobb S: Social support as a moderator of life stress. Psychosom Med 38:300–314, 1976

Cornett CW, Hudson RA: Psychoanalytic theory and affirmation of the gay lifestyle: are they necessarily antithetical? J Homosex 12:97–108, 1985

Cunningham R: When is a pervert not a pervert? British Journal of Psychotherapy 8:48–70, 1991

Evans CL, Tamburrino MB, Franco KN, et al: Is internship really the worst? Journal of Psychiatric Education 10:113–119, 1986

Flaks DK: Homophobia and the psychologist's role in psychoanalytic training institutes. Psychoanalytic Psychology 9:543–549, 1992

Fleckles CS: The making of a psychiatrist: the resident's view of the process of his professional development. Am J Psychiatry 128:1111–1115, 1972

Hadley J, Cantor JC, Willke RJ, et al: Young physicians most and least likely to have second thoughts about a career in medicine. Acad Med 67:180–190, 1992

Hales RE, Borus JF: A reexamination of the psychiatric resident's experience in the general hospital. Gen Hosp Psychiatry 8:432–436, 1986

Kardener SH, Fuller M, Mensh IN, et al: The trainees' viewpoint of psychiatric residency. Am J Psychiatry 126:1132–1138, 1970

Kirsling RA, Kochar MS: Suicide and the stress of residency training: a case report and review of the literature. Psychol Rep 64:951–959, 1989

Landau C, Hall S, Wartman SA, et al: Stress in social and family relationships during the medical residency. Journal of Medical Education 61:654–660, 1986

Mallon G: Gay and no place to go: assessing the needs of gay and lesbian adolescents in out-of-home care settings. Child Welfare 71:547–556, 1992

Marquart JA, Franco KN, Carroll BT: The influence of applicants' gender on medical school interviews. Acad Med 65:410–411, 1990

O'Connor MF: Clinical psychology graduate training and the gay minority. Dissertation Abstracts International 45(9), 1984

Roughton R: New committee to address issues of homosexuality. American Psychoanalyst 27:14–15, 1993

Russell AT, Pasnau RO, Taintor ZC: Emotional problems of residents in psychiatry. Am J Psychiatry 132:263–267, 1975

Scanlan JM: Physician to student: the crisis of psychiatric residency training. Am J Psychiatry 128:1107–1111, 1972

Schwartz AJ, Black ER, Goldstein MG, et al: Levels and causes of stress among residents. Journal of Medical Education 62:744–753, 1987

Slater BR: Essential issues in working with lesbian and gay male youths. Professional Psychology: Research and Practice 19:226–235, 1988

Sledge WH, Leaf PJ, Sacks MH: Applicant's choice of a residency training program. Am J Psychiatry 144:501–503, 1987

Tischler GL: The transition into residency. Am J Psychiatry 128:1103–1107, 1972

Townsend MH, Wallick MM, Cambre KM: Gay and lesbian issues in residency training at U.S. psychiatry programs. Academic Psychiatry 17:67–72, 1993

Townsend MH, Wallick MM, Cambre KM: Gay and lesbian issues in U.S. psychiatric training as reported by residency training directors. Academic Psychiatry 19:213–218, 1995

Walfish S, Stenmark DE, Shealy JS, et al: Reasons why applicants select clinical psychology graduate programs. Professional Psychology: Research and Practice 20:350–354, 1989

Wolf TM, Randall HM, Von Almen TK, et al: Perceived mistreatment and attitude change by graduating medical students: a retrospective study. Med Educ 25:182–190, 1991

Yager J: A survival guide for psychiatric residents. Arch Gen Psychiatry 30:494–499, 1974

SECTION VIII

Working With Gay Men and Lesbians in Different Clinical Settings

Lesbians in the Medical Setting

Amy Banks, M.D.
Nanette K. Gartrell, M.D.

Despite evidence that lesbian behavior is common-place, social judgments and heterosexism remain embedded in the medical community. Although homosexuality was eliminated from the *Diagnostic and Statistical Manual of Mental Disorders* in 1973 (American Psychiatric Association 1980), efforts to educate health care providers about lesbian health concerns have been insufficient, and there has been relatively little research on lesbian health care. This combination of heterosexual bias and inadequate training in lesbian health issues has made it difficult for lesbians to find appropriate health care.

Several studies suggest that many lesbians avoid traditional Western health care. Glasock (1981, 1983) reported that 55% of the 27 lesbians interviewed in her study were hesitant to use the traditional health care system. Yearly physicals were obtained by only 46% of 117 lesbians studied by Kelly et al. (1987); 53% of the women reported seeing a health care provider only when a problem arose. Robertson (1992), in a small study of 10 lesbians, found that none received routine health care. A look at lesbians' experiences as health care consumers makes the paucity of help-seeking more understandable.

For many women the path into the health care system begins in a family planning clinic. These clinics often overtly exclude women who do not need birth control, effectively eliminating the clinic as an option for lesbians who are sexually active exclusively with women (Whyte et al. 1980). Few clinics cater exclusively to gay and lesbian clients, and those that do are primarily located in major cities, making them unavailable to many lesbians.

Fear of discrimination as a result of "coming out" is a major obstacle to seeking care. Homophobia is prevalent in health care systems. Bradford and Ryan (1988) in a national study of 1,925 lesbians found that distrust of health care providers and financial limitations were the most frequent reasons for not seeking treatment.

When lesbians do reveal their sexual orientation to health care providers, negative responses range from refusal to treat to inappropriate or even abusive treatment. In one study of lesbians who were pregnant, 10% had been refused obstetrical care because of their sexual orientation (Harvey et al. 1989). McGhee and Owen (1980), Dardrick and Grady (1980), Glasock (1981, 1983), Smith et al. (1985), and Stevens and Hall (1988, 1990) all reported significant and wide-ranging negative reactions (27%–72%) from providers toward lesbians who have come out. Smith et al. (1985) noted that disclosure may stimulate embarrassment, rejection, voyeurism, mental health referral, coolness, and breached confidence on the part of providers. Stevens and Hall (1988, 1990) reported reactions of ostracism, shock, pity, invasive questioning, fear, embarrassment, mistreatment of partners and friends, breached confidence, rough physical handling, derogatory comments, and pathological assumptions from health care providers.

Undoubtedly as a result of such experiences, fewer than 50% of lesbians seeking health care come out to providers (Cochran and Mays 1988; Dardrick and Grady 1980; Glasock 1981, 1983; Johnson et al. 1981; Reagan 1981; Smith et al. 1985; Zeidenstein 1990). Harvey et al. (1989) interviewed 35 lesbian mothers and found that 91% had come out to their obstetrical providers. Although 79% felt that their medical provider had been supportive, 50% felt that the providers were ill informed and uncomfortable about caring for lesbians. When lesbians do not disclose their sexual orientation, they experience invisibility, assumptions of heterosexuality, irrelevant health teaching, insensitive questioning, sexist remarks, and improper treatment and diagnosis (Stevens and Hall 1988, 1990).

Financial limitations are another reason that lesbians avoid routine health care. Although Bradford and Ryan's survey (1988) indicated higher education levels among lesbians than among heterosexual women, lesbians had lower salaries than expected based on education. Like other women, lesbians are disproportionately uninsured and hold jobs that are of lower status, with lower pay, and with fewer benefits (Stevens 1993). Although a few U.S. companies are beginning to recognize same-sex couples and provide spousal benefits for significant others, this practice is still an exception to the rule. With limited incomes and limited insurance benefits, most lesbians are not prepared to pay out of pocket for the current high-tech health care.

Support systems within the lesbian community are poorly understood by many health care providers. Contrary to the stereotype of lesbians as isolated and lonely women, most actually have a diverse and strong support system. Bradford and Ryan (1988) found most lesbians to have more than two people they could count on for basic needs. They found that 60% of lesbians, like 62% of heterosexual women, were involved in a primary relationship with a single partner. They also found a general trend away from religion of upbringing toward religious communities more sympathetic to gay men and lesbians.

Because at least 20% of lesbians are not out to their families (Bradford and Ryan 1988), biological family members may not be primary supports. Many lesbians have been disowned or abandoned by families because of their sexual orientation. Lesbians often choose to build alternate families through strong friendships and community. These families of choice need to be respected and valued in times of personal illness by all members of a health care team.

Not surprisingly, lesbians tend to be creative in their attempts to have health care needs met. Lesbians seek treatment where they will not be stereotyped, and if such facilities are not available, they may go without help in order to avoid discrimination. Despite documented underutilization by lesbians of community health centers, school counselors, and hospitals, many do select alternative health practices—including herbal treatments, meditation, and prayer (Bradford and Ryan 1988). Johnson et al. (1981) surveyed 117 lesbians to determine their health care utilization patterns; they found that 38% of lesbians in urban settings and 56% of lesbians over 30 years old see private physicians for care, whereas 35% use alternative clinics. Among pregnant lesbians there has been an increase in the use of midwifery, homeopathy, and chiropractic care (Kenney and Task 1992).

Multiple studies of lesbians provide salient documentation of their desire to be treated by women providers, preferably lesbian (Johnson et al. 1981; Lucas 1992; Robertson 1992). Given the current level of homophobia within traditional health care systems, the number of lesbians needing treatment far exceeds the number of openly lesbian health care providers.

Attitudes of Health Care Providers Toward Lesbians

Homophobic attitudes toward lesbians are ubiquitous throughout the health care system. For instance, half of 110 gynecologists in Dade City, Florida, were not aware of ever having treated a lesbian patient, and only 9 had ever asked a patient directly about sexual orientation. Alarmingly, one-quarter felt they could identify a lesbian patient by clinical observation (Good 1976). Douglas et al. (1985) found homophobia scores of 91 registered nurses and 37 physicians in New York to be similar to those of the general population. Women scored higher on the homophobia scales then did men. Chaimowitz (1991) reported significant homophobic attitudes in 36% of family practice residents, 33% of psychiatric residents, and 26% of psychiatric faculty at a Canadian medical school. In a study of 119 medical students (Kelly et al. 1987), homosexual patients with the AIDS or with other life-threatening diseases were considered more deserving of illness and more deserving to die than heterosexual patients with equivalent illnesses. Additionally, 80 California psychologists rated gay and lesbian clients as less healthy than heterosexual clients with identical histories (Garfinkle and Morin 1978).

Fourteen (64%) of 22 East Coast nurses (Young 1988) indicated that they experienced feelings of pity, disgust, repulsion, unease, embarrassment, fear, and sorrow toward gay men and lesbians. Of these, only seven desired a change in attitude. A significant number of nurse educators in a midwestern study (Randall 1989) believed lesbianism to be unnatural (52%), immoral (34%), and illegal (19%). These educators also believed that lesbians transmit AIDS (20%), that lesbianism is a disease (17%), and that lesbians molest children (17%). A similar study of nursing students from the Midwest (Eliason and Randall 1991) found that 50% of the sample felt that lesbianism was unacceptable, 28% believed lesbians spread AIDS, and 15% thought lesbianism to be illegal.

Gay men and lesbians are often not welcomed within the disciplines of nursing and medicine. In a survey of 1,100 physicians (Matthews et al. 1986), 30% felt that qualified medical students who were gay should not be admitted to medical school. Over half felt that homosexual persons should be ineligible to practice pediatrics, and more than 40% reported they would stop referrals to a pediatrician or psychiatrist if they discovered that person to be homosexual. Eight percent of nurses in Randall's study (1989) felt that lesbians were unfit to be nurses.

Despite this growing body of research that documents the existence of homophobia among health care providers, little effort has been made to educate future and practicing physicians about homosexuality as a normal variant of human sexuality. Of the 65% of 126 U.S. medical schools surveyed (Wallick et al. 1992), only 1 reported that gay and lesbian issues were integral to its curriculum. Eight had no teaching in gay and lesbian issues, and the majority marginalized the teaching to a small component of their human sexuality curriculum. On the average, 3 hours and 26 minutes in 4 years of curriculum are spent presenting gay and lesbian issues to U.S. medical students.

Unfortunately, students are not likely to supplement their lack of education with up-to-date resources. In Whately's review (1992) of 14 health texts and 16 human sexuality texts, she found gay and lesbian images to be ghettoized and isolated. There was also an overrepresentation of gay social activism and an underrepresentation of the diversity in race, age, and ability that exists in the gay community. Finally, there are few representations of gay men and lesbians with children, despite a lesbian baby boom in the past decade.

Special Issues in Lesbian Health Care

■ Medical Care

Appropriate health care, particularly obstetrical-gynecological care, necessitates knowledge about lifestyles and behavioral practices of lesbians that differ from those of heterosexual women. Providers need more specific information regarding sexual practices when treating lesbians. The false assumption that all lesbians have had sexual contact only with women can lead to inadequate screening or health maintenance. Such assumptions also reflect insufficient education about the fluidity of sexuality over a lifetime. An open dialogue about sexual practices is essential.

There are no gynecological diseases that are unique to lesbians or that occur more frequently in lesbians than in heterosexual women (White and Levinson 1993). Vaginitis (primarily candidiasis) is the most common gynecological problem in lesbians. Nonspecific vaginitis, cervicitis, and trichomonas infections can be seen in lesbians as well. Yeast infections are found more often in bisexual women than in lesbians, but they can be passed between two women (White and Levinson 1993). Johnson and Palermo (1984) found that 50% of 117 lesbians had a history of vaginal candidiasis, a rate similar to that for heterosexual women.

Trichomonas vaginitis can be found in women who are sexually active only with other women. It can also be found in celibate and bisexual women. Fomites may be transmitted from person to person on vectors such as damp towels or underwear or through hand-genital contact. It is important that partners of infected clients be treated as well (White and Levinson 1993).

Sexually transmitted diseases—gonorrhea, syphilis, genital herpes, and chlamydia—are extremely rare in lesbians who are sexually active with women only (Johnson et al. 1981; Robertson and Schacter 1981). Routine screening of lesbians for sexually transmitted diseases is not thought to be cost-effective (Robertson et al. 1981). Pelvic inflammatory disease and hepatitis B are rare, and although human papillomavirus can be transmitted from female to female, the rate is also extremely low (White and Levinson 1993).

There have been few documented cases of HIV infection in lesbians who are sexually active with women only. As of June 1991, the Centers for Disease Control and Prevention reported that only 164 women fit this criterion. One hundred and fifty-two of these women had a history of intravenous drug use and the other 12 had blood transfusions before 1985, when HIV screening of blood donations was initiated (Chu et al. 1992). Peterson et al. (1992) studied 960,000 women in 20 large U.S. cities. Of these, 144 were found to be HIV positive and 106 of these women were interviewed. None reported that they had only had sexual contact with women since 1978.

HIV has been cultured in cervical and vaginal secretions, as well as from cervical biopsies taken throughout the menstrual cycle. Physicians should encourage lesbians to be tested for the virus and to use barriers in sexual encounters if they or their partners have not been tested or are known to be HIV positive (White and Levinson 1993).

A lesbian infected with HIV faces difficulties similar to those of a heterosexual woman infected with HIV. Diagnosis, drug trials, and controlled studies in HIV-positive women have been scarce. Women with HIV infection seem to die sooner than men infected with the virus. This may be in part due to insufficient education of health care providers concerning symptoms of immunosuppression in women: severe, persistent vaginal candidiasis, pelvic inflammatory disease, human papillomavirus infection, genital herpes, cervical dysplasia, and molluscum (Stevens 1993). Most alarming is that of these conditions only invasive cervical cancer is included in the 1993 Centers for Disease Control and Prevention diagnostic criteria for AIDS (Isselbacher et al. 1994).

Cancer screening in lesbians should follow standard guidelines for women based on an accurate history of individual risk factors. All women with a history of early first coitus with men, a history of human papillomavirus, or a history of herpes II virus are at an increased risk for cervical cancer. If a lesbian does not have these risk factors and has had minimal sexual contact with men, screening with Pap smears may be done at 18- to 30-month intervals (White and Levinson 1993).

Breast cancer is found more often in nulliparous women, women who are older than age 30 at first birth, and women who have not breast-fed. Although many lesbians may fit this profile, a growing number of lesbians are having children through alternative insemination or sexual contact with a man. Similarly, ovarian cancer may be seen more often in women who have not used oral contraceptives or in women who have not had children. While these conditions apply to some lesbians, general stereotypical assumptions should not be made. A thorough, specific history must be obtained for all lesbians. Screening can then be done based on documented risk factors and following guidelines provided for women in general (White and Levinson 1993).

■ Mental Health

Though sexual orientation is rarely associated with psychiatric symptoms (Whyte and Calpaldini 1980), the stress of social isolation, discrimination, and homophobia have a dramatic effect on mental health. Half of the lesbians in Bradford and Ryan's study (1988) had been verbally attacked for being gay; another 13% had lost jobs; and 6% had been physically attacked. In one university report, lesbians were twice as likely as heterosexual women to be victims of a sexual assault (White and Levinson 1993). Presently, lesbians and gay men are the group most victimized by hate crimes in this country (White and Levinson 1993).

Additionally, both physical abuse and sexual abuse appear to be prevalent in the lesbian population. Thirty-seven percent of the subjects in Bradford and Ryan's study (1988) had been physically abused at least once, and 41% had been raped or sexually abused at some point in their lives.

In general, health providers should be aware of the unique psychosocial stressors that lesbians experience living in a heterosexist culture. They should be alert to symptoms of depression and anxiety as a manifestation of these stressors. Providers should appreciate the risk of alcohol abuse and suicidality in their lesbian clients. If psychiatric symptoms are discovered during a routine health screening, a referral should be made to a lesbian-sensitive mental health provider or agency.

Bradford and Ryan (1988) reported that 21% of their subjects had sometimes or often thought about suicide and that 18% had actually tried to kill themselves. This rate is comparable to that seen in other high-stress groups such as medical students and physicians. There is a growing concern that gay and lesbian teenagers represent a larger-than-expected number of completed teen suicides (Paroski 1987).

To date, there is no evidence that alcohol dependence is a derivative of homosexuality (Mosbacher 1988), although various degrees of alcohol use are reported in the lesbian population. Johnson and Palermo (1984) reported that 25%–35% of lesbians have alcohol problems, a rate five to seven times greater than estimates for heterosexual women. A more recent study by Bradford and Ryan (1988) found that 31% of lesbians drank alcohol more than once a week. In a smaller study, Buenting (1992) found no difference in alcohol consumption between lesbian and heterosexual women. Health care providers should avoid assuming a casual relationship between the two and should include a thorough history of substance use and abuse in any health evaluation.

■ Parenting

Buenting (1992) reported no difference between the percentage of heterosexual women and the percentage of lesbians planning to have children. Lesbians' methods of having children are both creative and variable. Some lesbians raise children conceived with prior or current male partners and some adopt children. Most lesbians in the current lesbian baby boom have chosen alternative insemination.

As in other areas of health care, pregnant lesbians or those who wish to become pregnant are more apt to seek out nontraditional providers. Harvey et al. (1989) reported that one-third of a sample of lesbians preferred midwives over traditional obstetrician-gynecologists.

Health care providers need to obtain a thorough psychosocial history. The history should include the lesbian's definition of family and supports. Questions should be asked in such a way that information can be gathered about the diversity and creativity that the lesbian patient brings to her family and community.

■ Aging

Older lesbians, having grown up before the gay liberation movement, often are deeply closeted and unlikely to come out to others, including health care providers. Bradford and Ryan (1988) found older lesbians in their sample to be less involved in lesbian activities. It seems likely that the degree of outness and extent of self-acceptance have an effect on health and aging processes in lesbians. Deevey (1990) showed a correlation between excellent health and positive attitudes about being a lesbian. Quam and Whitford (1992) observed that lesbians who were active in the gay community felt better about aging, whereas those not involved in the gay community felt that being a lesbian made the aging process more difficult.

Quam and Whitford (1992), in their study of gay men and lesbians over 50 years old, found loneliness, health issues, and financial problems to be the most frequent worries. These concerns are similar to those of the general population. In addition, they found added burdens of the aging gay and lesbian population to be rejection by their children, homophobia from physicians, and discrimination because of their sexual orientation. An effective health care provider should make a special effort to identify aging lesbians and to break their isolation by providing them with acceptance, support, and referrals to community activities.

Recommendations

As Alcalay (1983) has stated,

> Health is related to the number of people in a social network, the frequency and integrity of contact with other members and the presence of family and friends within the network. (p. 86)

This important connection between health and relationships may be particularly significant in the lesbian population. Many lesbians are not out to close friends and family and are thus forced to interact unauthentically in these important relationships. Understanding this vulnerability is an important place to start in improving the health care of lesbians. Bradford and Ryan (1988) reported that the majority of their subjects welcomed the opportunity to be open with their health care providers about their lives, on the condition that they would be safe doing so.

To bridge this gap, health care providers must begin by questioning and thoroughly evaluating their current beliefs about homosexuality; they must avoid the assumption of heterosexuality and realize that any woman who enters treatment could be a lesbian.

From the perspective that lesbians exist as normal, healthy variants of the human population, much needed research on lesbians and their health care should be conducted. Research must encompass the diversity within lesbian culture rather than focus on the white, middle-class, educated lesbian group that is most easily accessible.

Education regarding lesbian health issues should encompass a growing research base, and it should be integrated in all aspects of health training. Training programs and health care environments need to be supportive of lesbian providers and to encourage them to be openly gay. Lesbian providers, in turn, serve as role models and educators within the health care system for both heterosexual and homosexual colleagues.

When all aspects of medical education include more instruction on lesbian health care, providers will be able to identify and to reach out to lesbian clients more effectively. Providers will be able to evaluate a lesbian's needs and assess their own limitations in treating such patients. If providers are unable to meet the needs of lesbian patients, such patients should be to referred to others who could appropriately care for them.

The first step is for individual providers to embrace and celebrate diversity. Only then will providers move beyond heterosexual assumptions to openness—in their behavior and in their words—so that lesbians can be included in the changing health care system, which promises adequate health care for all.

References

Alcalay R: Health and social support networks: a case for improving communication. Social Networks 5:71–88, 1993

American Psychiatric Association: Diagnostic and Statistical Manual of Mental Disorders, 3rd Edition. Washington, DC, American Psychiatric Association, 1980

Bradford J, Ryan C: The National Lesbian Health Care Survey. Washington, DC, National Lesbian and Gay Health Foundation, 1988

Buenting J: Health lifestyles of lesbian and heterosexual women. Health Care for Women International 13:165–171, 1992

Chaimowitz G: Homophobia among psychiatric residents, family practice residents and psychiatric faculty. Can J Psychiatry 36:206–209, 1991

Chu S, Hammett TA, Buehler JW: Update: epidemiology of reported cases of AIDS in women who report sex only with other women, United States, 1980–1991. AIDS 6:518–519, 1992

Cochran S, Mays V: Disclosure of sexual preference to physicians by black lesbian and bisexual women. West J Med 149:616–619, 1988

Dardrick L, Grady KE: Openness between gay persons and health professionals. Ann Intern Med 93:115–119, 1980

Deevey S: Older lesbian women: an invisible minority. Journal of Gerontological Nursing 16(5):35–39, 1990

Douglas CJ, Kalman CM, Kalman TP: Homophobia among physicians and nurses: an empirical study. Hosp Community Psychiatry 36: 1309–1311, 1985

Eliason MJ, Randall CE: Lesbian phobia in nursing students. West J Nurs Res 13:363–374, 1991

Garfinkle EM, Morin SF: Psychologist's attitudes toward homosexual psychotherapy clients. Journal of Social Issues 34(3):101–112, 1978

Glasock EL: Access to the traditional health care system by nontraditional women: perceptions of a cultural interaction. Paper presented at the annual meeting of the American Public Health Association, Los Angeles, CA, November 1981

Glasock EL: Lesbians growing older: self-identification, coming out and health concerns. Paper presented at the annual meeting of the American Public Health Association. Dallas, TX, November 1983

Good RS: The gynecologist and the lesbian. Clin Obstet Gynecol 19:473–482, 1976

Harvey SM, Carr C, Bernheine S: Lesbian mothers: health care experiences. J Nurse Midwifery 34(3):115–119, 1989

Isselbacher K, Braunwald E, Wilson J, et al: Harrison's Principles of Internal Medicine, 13th Edition. New York, McGraw-Hill, 1994

Johnson S, Palermo J: Gynecological care for the lesbian. Clin Obstet Gynecol 27:724–731, 1984

Johnson S, Guenther S, Laube D, et al: Factors influencing lesbian gynecological care: a preliminary study. Am J Obstet Gynecol 2:20–28, 1981

Kelly J, Lawrence J, Smith J, et al: Medical students attitudes towards AIDS and homosexual patients. Journal of Medical Education 62:549–556, 1987

Kenney J, Task D: Lesbian childbearing: couple's dilemmas and decisions. Health Care for Women International 13:209–219, 1992

Lucas V: An investigation of the health care practices of the lesbian population. Health Care for Women International 13:221–228, 1992

Matthews W, Booth M, Turner J, et al: Physicians' attitudes toward homosexuality. Survey of a California county medical society. West J Med 144(11):106–110, 1986

McGhee RD, Owen WF: Medical aspects of homosexuality. New Engl J Med 303:50–51, 1980

Mosbacher D: Lesbian alcohol and substance abuse. Psychiatric Annals 18:1 1988

Paroski PA: Health care delivery and the concerns of gay and lesbian adolescents. Journal of Adolescent Health Care 8(2):188–192, 1987

Peterson L, Doll L, White C, et al: no evidence for female-to-female HIV transmission among 360,000 female blood donors. J Acquir Immune Defic Syndr 5:853–855, 1992

Quam J, Whitford G: Adaptation and age-related expectations of older gay and lesbian adults. Gerontologist 32:367–374, 1992

Randall CE: Lesbian phobia among BSN educators: a survey. J Nurs Educ 28:302–306, 1989

Reagan P: The interaction of health professionals and their lesbian clients. Patient Counseling and Health Education 3(1):21–25, 1981

Robertson M: Lesbians as an invisible minority in the health services arena. Health Care for Women International 13:155–163, 1992

Robertson P, Schacter J: Failure to identify venereal disease in a lesbian population. Sex Transm Dis, April-June 1981, pp 75–76

Smith EM, Johnson SR, Guenther SM: Health care attitudes and experiences during gynecological care among lesbians and bisexuals. Am J Public Health 75:1085–1087, 1985

Stevens P: Lesbians and HIV: clinical research and policy issues. Am J Orthopsychiatry 63:289–294, 1993

Stevens PE, Hall JM: Stigma, health beliefs and experiences with care in lesbian women. Image 20:69–73, 1988

Stevens PE, Hall JM: Abusive health care interactions experienced by lesbians: a case of institutional violence in the treatment of women. Response to the Victimization of Women and Children 13(3):23–27, 1990

Wallick M, Cambre K, Townsend M: How the topic of homosexuality is taught in U.S. medical schools. Acad Med 67:601–603, 1992

Whately M: Images of gays and lesbians in sexuality and health textbooks. J Homosex 197–211, 1992

White J, Levinson W: Primary care of lesbian patients. J Gen Intern Med 8:41–47, 1993

Whyte J, Calpaldini L: Treating the lesbian or gay patient. Del Med J 52:271–280, 1980

Young EW: Nurses' attitudes toward homosexuality: analysis of change in AIDS workshops. Journal of Continuing Education in Nursing 19(1):9–12, 1988

Zeidenstein L: Gynecological and childbearing needs of lesbians. J Nurse Midwifery 35(1):10–18, 1990

Gay and Bisexual Men and Medical Care

William F. Owen, Jr., M.D.

M ost health care providers treating adult and adolescent patients will interact with gay and bisexual patients as well as patients who engage episodically in same-sex activity. Providers are often unaware of these encounters because societal stereotypes of gay men, lesbians, and bisexual people only apply to a small minority of gay and bisexual patients (Krajeski 1980). Marriage is also a poor marker for heterosexuality. A study by the Kinsey Institute (Bell and Weinberg 1978) found that 20% of gay men and 35% of lesbians had been married at least once. Another study (Fay 1989) found that many men who had reported occasional sexual encounters with other men had been married at some point.

Providers should be aware of the sexual orientation of their patients, not only to assess whether their patients may be at risk for certain diseases associated with sexual transmission, but also because sexual identity is a fundamental part of the lives of our patients. Just as forgetting to obtain a family or marital history would produce an incomplete profile of any patient, so too would ignoring sexual orientation result in a distorted view of the lifestyle and social and psychological supports of the gay or bisexual patient.

In this chapter, the author discusses the technique of obtaining a medical and sexual history from the gay or bisexual male patient. Topics include inquiring about sexual orientation, past medical history, history of sexual partners and practices, other lifestyle factors, gay identity issues, social support and family systems, and confidentiality. The author also reviews research about attitudes of gay and bisexual patients toward health providers and attitudes of health providers toward gay and bisexual patients.

Obtaining a Medical and Sexual History

The provider should attempt to obtain information about sexual orientation and sexual practices at the initial examination and to update it when the patient appears with acute complaints that might be associated with sexual activity.

■ Inquiring About Sexual Orientation

The provider may ask directly, "Are you gay, bi, or straight?" rather than using the more formal term "homosexual," because gay and bisexual patients generally feel a lot more at ease with the words "gay" and "bi." If the clinician feels the need to explain why he or she is asking this question, it may be introduced with a statement like, "We know that certain medical conditions, such as AIDS, may be related, in part, to a person's sexual practices."

Alternatively, one may ask the patient, "Have you ever had sex with men, women, both or neither?" Sexual orientation may also be included as part of a personal lifestyle inventory (Owen 1980): "Is there anything about your lifestyle, such as recent travel, diet, drug use or sexual practices, that might assist me to diagnose your medical problem?"

If a patient has a condition like pharyngitis, one may inquire whether he wants a culture to be sent for gonorrhea as well as strep testing. The response to this question may then be used as a springboard to further discussion about sexual orientation and sexual practices.

Verbal and nonverbal communication can impede the relationship between provider and gay and bisexual patients. A judgmental attitude may be conveyed if questions are phrased in a negative way: "You don't have anal sex, do you?" Rejection may be implied by displaying certain types of body language, for example, raised eyebrows, crossed arms, or reaching for the exam room doorknob (Maurer 1975).

■ Past Medical History Including Sexually Transmitted Diseases

In working with gay and bisexual men, the provider should inquire about sexually transmitted diseases. Specific diseases in the inquiry should include gonorrhea, chlamydial infection, herpes simplex, and genital warts, along with the site of infection; syphilis with results of titers after treatment; hepatitis A, B, and C, results of most recent hepatitis B antigen and antibody tests, and whether hepatitis A and B vaccines have been administered; enteric diseases, including shigellosis, *Campylobacter* infections, amebiasis, and giardiasis; and human immunodeficiency virus (HIV)-related conditions, including history of CD4 (helper T) cell levels, antiretrovirals, and medications to prevent opportunistic infections.

■ History of Sexual Partners

It is helpful to determine whether the patient currently has one regular partner or lover and, if so, whether they are in a "closed" (monogamous) or "open" relationship. Has the partner been tested for HIV? In order to assess whether the patient's risk for sexually transmitted diseases has changed over time, the provider may also inquire about the number of regular and nonsteady sexual partners, both male and female, over the past 24 months.

■ History of Sexual Practices

Gay and bisexual men employ a variety of sexual techniques and practices and are not restricted to either "insertive" or "receptive" roles. A history of specific sexual practices can assist the clinician in determining risk factors for the presence of sexually transmitted diseases and traumatic complications. The colloquial terms for these practices may be employed, if the provider feels comfortable doing so (Ostrow and Obermaier 1983). As an example, one may ask, "Are you into fucking, getting fucked, sucking, getting sucked, rimming, or fisting?" If a patient has anal-genital or oral-genital contact, additional questions should be asked about condom use and about contact with seminal fluid (cum) or preejaculate (pre-cum). The question may also be phrased in a more formal style: "When having sex, does your partner's penis come in contact with your anus?" or "Does your mouth ever come in contact with your partner's anus?"

Gay and bisexual patients will perceive the provider who is willing to discuss sexual practices as a supportive caregiver. The provider should view a frank and open discussion of specific sexual practices as an opportunity to educate gay and bisexual men, in a nonjudgmental manner, about risk reduction.

■ Other Lifestyle Factors

Questions about the elements of the food pyramid, vitamins and other dietary supplements, dietary fiber, and cholesterol will help the clinician get a general picture of the patient's nutritional status. An inquiry about use of drugs and alcohol will assist the provider in determining whether the patient may be at risk for complications related to these substances. The provider should ascertain the specific drugs used, including marijuana, stimulants (speed), and inhaled nitrites (poppers), along with the frequency and quantity of such use, the route of administration (oral, transnasal, intravenous), and whether such substances are taken in relation to sexual intercourse.

The importance of a regular exercise program, including aerobic exercise, should be discussed. Job satisfaction and occupational risks should be noted. Leisure time activities and hobbies should be determined, along with any special hazards associated with these activities. The mood of the patient should be assessed, including any specific life stresses. Physical abuse is a topic frequently neglected by health providers, but it does occur in both heterosexual and gay relationships, and questions about abuse should be considered. The duration and quality of sleep should be determined, because these can provide important clues to the presence of a variety of physical and psychological conditions.

■ Gay Identity Issues

Gay and bisexual men may consult their health care providers during the process of acquiring awareness of sexual orientation ("coming out"). The provider can assist gay and bisexual patients during this process by reassuring the patient that being gay or bisexual is a normal variant rather than a medical illness, by providing the patient with appropriate reading materials (Clark 1987), and by referring the patient, where indicated, to supportive therapists, local service agencies, and gay community organizations.

■ Social Support and Family Systems

In traditional family structures, emotional guidance in times of crisis often comes from other family members. Gay and bisexual men may receive such assistance from similar sources, for example, parents, children, and former spouses. Support may also come, however, from lovers, former lovers, or friends; in the case of gay and bisexual men with AIDS, it may come from volunteer gay community organizations.

Providers should be aware of alternative family configurations that are formed by some gay and bisexual men. Some men are celibate, some live in long-standing monogamous relationships, others have an open relationship, and still others have a series of sexual encounters. Some men are coparenting with single women and with lesbian couples. Other male couples are adopting children.

Patients should be asked whether they would like significant other persons included when discussing new health concerns or when decisions need to be made about the course of treatment. Patients should be encouraged to execute a durable power of attorney for health care. The power-of-attorney designee should be prepared to make health care decisions when the patient is incapable of doing so.

■ Confidentiality

Health care professionals have a responsibility to guarantee that knowledge of the sexual orientation of their patients remains confidential. Same-sex intercourse is still illegal in many jurisdictions and is a cause for discharge from the U.S. military. Although some jurisdictions have decriminalized homosexual activity between consenting adults, cultural and religious stigmas are still attached to homosexuality and bisexuality by many segments of our society. Being openly or even presumptively gay or bisexual has resulted in exclusion from certain fields of employment, in actual loss of jobs and housing, and in forfeiture of the freedom to immigrate to some countries. Homophobia, the irrational fear and loathing of gay men, lesbians, and bisexual persons, has led to violent behavior directed against gay and bisexual men and women for no reason other than perceived sexual orientation.

Many gay and bisexual patients, particularly those who are seropositive for HIV but asymptomatic, are also concerned about inadvertent disclosure of their HIV serological status. In small solo practices, providers can often remember the sexual orientation and serological status of their patients, but in larger group practices and in clinics it is sometimes necessary to communicate this information from one provider to another. Some clinicians have found it useful to agree informally on a coding system for this purpose, rather than writing the sexual orientation or the HIV antibody status directly in the medical chart. The provider and the patient should discuss the specific approach to documenting or withholding information about sexual orientation and HIV serological status on the medical record.

Attitudes of Gay Patients and Health Providers

Gay and bisexual men may underutilize health care services because they perceive some health care providers to be homophobic. Understandably, gay and bisexual men may be reluctant to seek treatment in locales where same-sex intercourse is illegal. A number of studies over the past decade have explored both the attitudes of health care providers toward gay and bisexual patients and the opinions of gay men and lesbians about their contacts with the medical care system.

■ Provider Attitudes Toward Gay Patients

The attitude of individual providers toward homosexuality has been examined in at least eight surveys over the past two decades. A 1970 survey of over 900 physicians in Oregon (Pauly and Goldstein 1970) found that physicians acknowledge fewer negative attitudes toward gay male patients (with 5% "always" and 10% "often" having attitudes that adversely affect treatment) than they attribute to "most physicians" (who were perceived by the surveyed physicians to have negative attitudes toward gay men in 35% of the cases). Many physicians (48%) in the Oregon survey acknowledged some degree of discomfort, however, in treating the medical problems of a person who "appears" to be a gay man.

A 1978 survey completed for the American Medical Association (Golin 1978) investigated the attitudes of over 200 physicians toward treatment of gay men. Most of the respondents (61%) had no negative feelings, but a significant minority (35%) revealed that they sometimes or often felt uncomfortable treating gay patients. In a finding that was parallel to the Oregon poll, a large majority of physicians in the American Medical Association survey (84%) felt that gay men hesitate to seek medical care because of physician disapproval. Another finding of this survey with implications for medical education is that 84% of the physicians felt that their training in human sexuality was inadequate.

A 1984 survey of nearly 1,000 members of the San Diego Medical Society in California (Mathews et al. 1984) revealed similar findings, with 60% of the respondents reporting no negative feelings, but 40% indicating that they often or sometimes feel uncomfortable treating gay patients. This survey also measured attitudes of physicians toward gay physician colleagues. Most physicians (70%) felt that qualified gay applicants should be admitted to medical school, but 29% believed that gay men and lesbians should not be admitted. Over 45% thought that gay men and lesbians should be discouraged from entering pediatrics, and 40% felt that entry into psychiatry should be discouraged. More than 40% of all physicians surveyed would stop referral to pediatricians and psychiatrists if they learned that their physician colleagues were gay.

In a 1985 survey of 239 house staff physicians and nurses at Beth Israel Medical Center in New York City (Wallack 1989), almost half of the respondents were found to be angry at the gay community and blamed homosexual promiscuity for causing the AIDS epidemic, whereas 18% of the doctors and 33% of the nurses believed gay men afflicted with AIDS had only themselves to blame. In fact, 6% of the respondents agreed that patients who chose a gay lifestyle deserved to get AIDS.

A 1988 telephone survey of 473 primary care physicians in New York City (Gemson et al. 1991) revealed that, although 71% had cared for a patient with AIDS and 90% had ordered the HIV antibody test, only 30% said they always or usually ask about the number of sexual partners and only 28% counsel new patients about reducing the risk of contracting AIDS. In this sample, 39% said they always or usually ask male patients about sexual orientation, and 36% agreed with the statement that "homosexual behavior between two men is just plain wrong."

A 1989 survey of 1,745 primary care senior residents in 10 selected states (Hayward and Weissfeld 1993) revealed that 16% felt that homosexuality was a mental disorder and 19% were unsure whether it was. One in five reported feeling uncomfortable around someone who is gay, and homophobia was strongly associated with unwillingness to provide AIDS care.

A 1990 mail survey of 1,121 physicians across the United States (Gerbert et al. 1991) indicated that, although 75% had treated one or more patients with HIV infection, 35% of the sample agreed with the statements, "I would feel nervous among a group of homosexuals" and "Homosexuality is a threat to many of our basic social institutions." Among physicians who had treated more than 10 patients with HIV in their careers, only 26% and 27%, respectively, agreed with these statements.

A 1992 survey of 2,545 randomly selected primary care physicians nationwide (Loft et al. 1994) found that only 49% asked about sexually transmitted diseases, 27% about sexual orientation, and 22% about the number of sex partners. One-fourth of physicians surveyed thought that their patients would be offended by questions about their sexual behavior.

A 1994 survey of 711 members of the Gay and Lesbian Medical Association, formerly known as the American Association of Physicians for Human Rights (Schatz and O'Hanlan 1994), revealed a widespread and alarming degree of antigay discrimination in medicine. A majority (59%) of physicians and medical students surveyed indicated that they have suffered discrimination, harassment, or ostracism from within the medical profession because of their sexual orientation. A vast majority of respondents (91%) reported knowledge of antigay bias directed toward patients. There were also reports of substandard treatment of lesbian, gay, and bisexual patients. Sixty-seven percent of respondents knew of lesbian, gay, or bisexual patients who received substandard care or were denied care because of their sexual orientation; 52% had observed colleagues providing reduced care or denying care to patients because of their sexual orientation; and 88% had heard colleagues make disparaging remarks about lesbian, gay, and bisexual patients.

These data suggest that negative attitudes toward gay patients are widespread among physicians. Providers who harbor stereotypes about gay and bisexual patients are often the same health care professionals providing medical care to these patients. It is imperative for all health care agencies to fight discrimination against gay and bisexual patients and providers through employee education, patient outreach, and support of openly gay physicians. As managed care plans become an ever-increasing factor in our health care delivery system, it is essential for these plans to identify providers who are knowledgeable about gay, lesbian, and bisexual health issues and to allow gay and bisexual patients to select these providers.

■ Gay Patient Attitudes Toward Providers

It is important for providers not only to become familiar with the clinical aspects of the conditions that may affect gay men, but also to become comfortable in eliciting a complete sexual history from their patients. Emotional stresses arising from the traditional moral and social stigmas associated with homosexuality may lead gay patients to conceal their sexual orientation from their physicians (Dritz 1980).

In a survey of over 500 residents of San Francisco, 83% of whom were gay and 9% bisexual (McGhee and Owen 1980), 73% of the gay and bisexual respondents reported that they had disclosed their sexual orientation at some time to a physician. Of those who had disclosed their sexual orientation, 42% perceived that their physicians reacted positively to this revelation, and 20% perceived a negative reaction. Of the gay and bisexual respondents who had never disclosed their sexual orientation to a physician, 33% said that they feared disapproval, 47% thought that disclosure was not important, and 20% gave other reasons for withholding this information.

In another survey of over 600 men responding to a questionnaire in a gay community newspaper (Dardick and Grady 1980), only 49% indicated that they disclosed their sexual orientation to their primary health care provider. Those who did not reveal sexual orientation were less likely to have been checked for sexually transmitted diseases and were more likely to be dissatisfied with their health care.

Another study of 604 gay men attending public and private clinics for sexually transmitted diseases in Sweden, Finland, Ireland, and Australia (Ross 1985) indicated that individuals who were reluctant to disclose their sexual orientation in the clinic were also likely to conceal their orientation from most people, to expect the most negative reaction to their homosexuality, to believe in more conservative sex roles for men and women, to report themselves as more bisexual, and to have had no previous sexually transmitted diseases. This study also suggested that gay men who are reluctant to disclose their sexual orientation are most likely to be reassured by empathy, explicit discussion and expressed acceptance of homosexuality and bisexuality, reiteration of confidentiality, and avoidance of questions that assume the sex of the sex partner.

In a study of HIV-positive and HIV-negative gay and bisexual men participating in the Multicenter AIDS Cohort Study in Baltimore and Los Angeles and of gay and bisexual men with AIDS at Johns Hopkins Hospital (Kass et al. 1992), 18% of men with symptomatic HIV disease reported being refused treatment by a doctor or dentist on the basis of a known or suspected HIV-related condition, compared with 5% of seropositive but asymptomatic men and 1% of seronegative men. However, many participants volunteered that they had deliberately sought care from gay practitioners to avoid discrimination problems, which could have resulted in underreporting.

These data suggest that gay and bisexual patients require provider-patient relations that are marked by trust, acceptance, and understanding. Many gay and bisexual patients fear insufficient diagnosis and treatment, but paradoxically, some patients are reluctant to be the first to raise the topic of sexual orientation with their providers. This barrier may be overcome, in part, by educating both providers and gay and bisexual men about the medical aspects of homosexuality and bisexuality and about the importance of the sexual history as part of a complete diagnostic evaluation.

Conclusion

Because clinicians cannot determine readily which patients are gay or bisexual, it is important to ask about the sexual orientation of all patients. The process of inquiry itself may enhance the relationship with the gay or bisexual patient because it indicates to him that the provider is sensitive to, and nonjudgmentally concerned about, his health care needs.

A history of past sexual partners, specific sexual practices, and location of sexual contacts should be obtained because this may assist the clinician in determining risk for a variety of conditions associated with sexual activity. Other factors that may contribute to a healthy or unhealthy lifestyle should also be assessed, such as use of drugs and alcohol, diet and nutrition, exercise, and concerns about sexual identity and sexual dysfunction. Providers should become familiar with the sources of emotional support used by the gay or bisexual patient, whether traditional sources such as members of the patient's nuclear family or nontraditional sources such as lovers, close friends, or gay community organizations.

Homosexual activity is still illegal in some jurisdictions and is attached to cultural and religious stigmas even in areas where it has been legalized. Unauthorized disclosure of the HIV antibody status of patients has led to discrimination in employment, housing, and medical care. For these reasons, providers should be aware of the issue of confidentiality as it applies to documentation of sexual orientation and HIV antibody status in medical records.

Surveys of physicians indicate that a substantial minority feel uncomfortable among gay and bisexual men and that a majority of physicians do not ask their patients about sexual orientation. Perhaps sensing this discomfort, many gay and bisexual patients either do not disclose their sexual orientation to their physicians or else seek care with openly gay health care providers. Health care organizations, including managed care plans, should develop programs to combat discrimination against gay and bisexual patients and providers through education of employees and professional staff, as well as outreach to gay and bisexual patients.

Trust, acceptance, and understanding are the hallmarks of a positive provider-client relationship. If care cannot be provided to gay and bisexual patients for personal reasons, the health care professional should refer these patients to understanding, competent providers or to clinics that can provide comprehensive care.

References

Bell AP, Weinberg MS: Part IV: a concluding overview, in Homosexualities: A Study of Diversity Among Men and Women. New York, Simon and Schuster, 1978, pp 217–231

Clark D: The New Loving Someone Gay. Berkeley, CA, Celestial Arts, 1987

Dardick L, Grady K: Openness between gay persons and health professionals. Ann Intern Med 93:115–119, 1980

Dritz SK: Medical aspects of homosexuality. New Engl J Med 302:463–464, 1980

Fay RE: Prevalence and patterns of same gender sexual contact among men. Science 243:338–348, 1989

Gemson DH, Colombotos J, Elinson J, et al: Acquired immunodeficiency syndrome prevention: knowledge, attitudes and practices of primary care physicians. Arch Intern Med 151:1102–1108, 1991

Gerbert B, Maguire BT, Bleecker T, et al: Primary care physicians and AIDS: attitudinal and structural barriers to care. JAMA 266:2837–2842, 1991

Golin CB: Fever chart: MD's assess problems in treating gays (Impact section). American Medical News, October 27, 1978, p 2

Hayward RA, Weissfeld JL: Coming to terms with the era of AIDS: attitudes of physicians in U.S. residency programs. J Gen Intern Med 8:10–17, 1993

Kass NE, Faden RR, Fox R, et al: Homosexual and bisexual men's perceptions of discrimination in health services. Am J Public Health 82:1277–1279, 1992

Krajeski J: Identifying homosexuals by mannerisms. Medical Aspects of Human Sexuality 14(July):11, 1980

Loft J, Marder W, Bresolin L, et al: HIV prevention practices of primary care physicians—United States: 1992. MMWR 42:988–992, 1994

Mathews C, Kessler L, Booth MW, et al: Physician attitudes toward homosexuality. West J Med 140:290–291, 1984

Maurer TB: Health care and the gay community. Postgrad Med 58:127–130, 1975

McGhee RD, Owen WF Jr: Medical aspects of homosexuality. New Engl J Med 303:50–51, 1980

Ostrow DG, Obermaier A: Sexual practices history, in Sexually Transmitted Diseases in Homosexual Men: Diagnosis, Treatment, and Research. Edited by Ostrow DG, Sandholzer TA, Felman YM. New York, Plenum, 1983, pp 13–22

Owen WF Jr: The clinical approach to the homosexual patient. Ann Intern Med 93(part 1):90–92, 1980

Pauly IB, Goldstein SG. Physicians' attitudes in treating male homosexuals. Medical Aspects of Human Sexuality 4(December):27–45, 1970

Ross MW: Psychosocial factors in admitting to homosexuality in sexually transmitted disease clinics. Sex Transm Dis 12:83–87, 1985

Schatz B, O'Hanlan K: Anti-Gay Discrimination in Medicine: Results of a National Survey of Lesbian, Gay, and Bisexual Physicians. San Francisco, CA, American Association of Physicians for Human Rights, May 1994

Wallack JJ: AIDS anxiety among health care professionals. Hosp Community Psychiatry 40:507–510, 1989

42

Care Across the Spectrum of Mental Health Settings

Working With Gay, Lesbian, and Bisexual Patients in Consultation-Liaison Services, Inpatient Treatment Facilities, and Community Outpatient Mental Health Centers

J. Stephen McDaniel, M.D.
Robert P. Cabaj, M.D.
David W. Purcell, J.D., Ph.D.

Mental health clinicians have long acknowledged the importance of appreciating diverse cultural differences in patient populations. Understanding such differences (including sex, sexual orientation, ethnicity, age, and religion) is essential to offering appropriate mental health interventions and ensuring treatment compliance. The unique cultural aspects of the gay, lesbian, and bisexual communities must be sensitively and affirmatively addressed to deliver effective interventions in mental health settings. In this chapter, the authors highlight the treatment of gay, lesbian, and bisexual individuals in three different mental health settings: consultation-liaison (C-L) services, inpatient treatment facilities, and community outpatient mental health centers.

Consultation-Liaison Psychiatry

Worldwide, an increasing number of mental health care professionals are practicing on medical and surgical wards of hospitals to address the mental health needs of medically ill patients (Stotland and Garrick 1990). However, as these clinicians have discovered, this clinical setting requires approaches to diagnosis and treatment that differ from those used in many other clinical settings. In the general hospital, clinician and patient collaborate on a different basis than they do in the outpatient or inpatient psychiatric setting, two arenas where patients commonly initiate mental health treatment (Beebe and Rosenbaum 1975). For example, the C-L clinician generally has contact with the patient at the request of a nonpsychiatric physician; therefore, the patient does not usually directly choose to be diagnosed or treated by the C-L practitioner. Such conditions place the C-L clinician in a delicate situation requiring him or her to mediate between, and develop alliances with, the medical-surgical team, the hospital staff, the patient, and often the patient's family or friends. Developing and nurturing these alliances are crucial to deliver needed mental health care.

■ Consultation by Mental Health Professionals

Gay, lesbian, and bisexual patients, just like other patients, frequently require mental health consultation when hospitalized for medical-surgical reasons. Although the circumstances surrounding consultation for such patients may be no different than those for heterosexual patients, some consultations are directly linked to the medical provider's discomfort with nonheterosexual patients. This discomfort, which is a manifestation of homophobia, can sometimes be projected onto the patient and hospital staff. In the presence of a health care professional, many gay, lesbian, and bisexual patients may report feeling anxiety, shame, or guilt regarding their sexual orientation. Similarly, nursing staff may feel uncomfortable and nervous around gay, lesbian, and bisexual patients, particularly if treating physicians tend to openly disparage or judge negatively such patients based solely on their sexual orientation.

In these settings, C-L clinicians can be of immense value by validating the patient's feelings in an affirmative way, while also conducting a full evaluation for psychological morbidity. The positive connection established with an affirming mental health clinician, even for a brief medical hospitalization, can be a powerful experience and a potent means of relieving anxiety for many gay, lesbian, and bisexual patients. By offering to meet with the medical team and with the nursing staff involved in the patient's day-to-day care, the C-L practitioner can educate other providers about how to recognize and manage countertransference in the treatment of gay, lesbian, and bisexual patients. Moreover, the C-L clinician can play an important role in sensitizing medical staff to the negative impact of their homophobia.

The professional mediation the C-L clinician must practice in the hospital setting directly affects how he or she approaches patient care. For example, an important part of any consultation is the opportunity to meet with family and friends of the hospitalized patient. For many gay, lesbian, and bisexual persons, family does not necessarily mean biological family, but rather chosen or extended family composed of lovers, adopted children, and close friends. A clinician's ability to openly acknowledge this network not only strengthens therapeutic alliances by sending a clear message to medical providers and hospital staff that such relationships are indeed "family," but it also affords the C-L practitioner a rich source of collaborative psychosocial history. Family interventions are an essential treatment strategy in the C-L setting; therefore, recognizing nontraditional families is an absolute necessity. All too often, gay, lesbian, and bisexual patients are treated like single individuals with poor family ties, rather than coupled, socially integrated persons with well-developed social support systems.

▇ Liaison Activities by Mental Health Professionals

As the word "liaison" in consultation-liaison suggests, the C-L clinician does more than provide consultation. In addition, some clinicians work to become integral members of a medical or surgical team and to educate nonpsychiatrists about psychiatrically relevant aspects of patient care (Lipowski 1974). One liaison specific to the gay, lesbian, and bisexual community that has emerged over the past decade is the mental health team within settings treating patients with HIV disease. This type of liaison has important implications for gay, lesbian, and bisexual providers as well as for patients from these groups. Many academic, public, and private institutions across the country now have specialized mental health services for persons with HIV infection and AIDS. Many of the clinicians involved in these services are themselves openly gay, lesbian, or bisexual. In spite of many dire consequences, the HIV pandemic has provided a more open environment for gay men, lesbians, and bisexual persons to serve their communities professionally by taking the lead in mental health care delivery and research in this medical environment.

The effect of HIV and AIDS on C-L psychiatry has also involved the incorporation of specialized training regarding neuropsychiatric aspects of HIV infection. C-L clinicians have taken a leading role in both the recognition and management of neuropsychiatric sequelae of HIV infection. C-L clinicians are often the first to diagnose such conditions as HIV encephalopathy (AIDS dementia), organic mood syndromes, delirium, anxiety disorders, pain syndromes, and a host of other complications that may arise in HIV-seropositive individuals (see Chapter 51 by Ostrow). Similarly, HIV-seronegative gay, lesbian, and bisexual patients who present with comorbid psychiatric symptomatology attributed to a rational or irrational fear of HIV may be best managed by a C-L clinician skilled in understanding the profound effects HIV and AIDS have left on their communities.

The experience of C-L clinicians working with HIV and AIDS patients demonstrates how the expertise of these clinicians can be used for the education of other medical care providers. For example, many C-L clinicians have developed an appreciation for taking a thorough sexual history, a part of the medical evaluation that continues to be ignored, avoided, or minimized by many health care providers, possibly due to discomfort with the sensitive nature of the questioning. In a recent survey of physicians (primary care, surgery, and emergency medicine) in North Carolina (Weinberger et al. 1992), 40% reported not taking a sexual history and 34% reported not offering AIDS education to their new patients. Similarly, a 1981 study (Johnson et al. 1981) revealed that fewer than 1% of lesbians surveyed had been questioned by their doctors about sexual orientation, and a later study (Smith et al. 1985) found that 9.3% of lesbians had been asked.

Sexual history taking is an important teaching opportunity, particularly in academic settings where clinicians-in-training are part of the C-L team. In a recent survey of second-year preclinical medical students at one medical university in the Southeast, a majority reported feeling uncomfortable taking a sexual history from or working with nonheterosexual patients (McDaniel et al. 1995). Because such attitudes are likely to be found elsewhere in the country, addressing sexual history taking and integrating an appreciation of diverse communities should be key teaching objectives of C-L rotations.

■ Case Example

Mr. A, a 58-year-old male accountant, was hospitalized to evaluate persistent anemia and intermittent lower gastrointestinal bleeding. Within the course of his medical evaluation, he was found to have colon cancer and was scheduled for bowel resection and possible colostomy placement. Both his internist and surgeon became increasingly concerned about the patient's level of anxiety and ambivalence about treatment before surgery; therefore, the psychiatric C-L service was consulted.

A careful review of Mr. A's chart before his evaluation revealed little about his psychosocial history other than that he was single and a successful businessman. There was no mention of a sexual history or previous psychiatric history. His past medical history was significant for hypertension, which was well controlled on medication (β-blocker). There were numerous nursing notes expressing concern because Mr. A seemed "withdrawn" and apparently had no family visitors, only occasional "friends."

After the mental health provider explained the reason for a consultation, Mr. A openly acknowledged a growing anxiety about his situation. Although at first Mr. A's thought content centered on the implications of a diagnosis of colon cancer and his fears of surgery, he slowly became more comfortable relating the details of his life to an empathic listener. Full psychological evaluation revealed that Mr. A was a gay man whose lover of 18 years had died of AIDS 3 years earlier. Mr. A was HIV seronegative. He had begun a new romantic relationship 18 months earlier with a previous business colleague. He had been estranged from his family for many years because of their inability to accept his being gay. He had numerous gay friends who visited him frequently and provided him with "family support." Along with his fears of cancer and the accompanying memories of his spouse's death, he had anxiety related to the implications of having a colostomy and how such surgery might affect anal intercourse. He also volunteered that he had been impotent since starting antihypertensive medication several years earlier and would intentionally not take his medication if he anticipated sexual activity.

Diagnostically, Mr. A met criteria for an adjustment disorder with anxious mood and male erectile disorder. His anxiety symptoms responded to supportive psychotherapy pre- and postoperatively, which included education about his condition and upcoming surgery. Efforts were made to include his significant other in all treatment decisions, both with regard to his psychological treatment and his medical-surgical treatment. A brief inservice session was provided for the nursing staff about the unique challenges of working with gay, lesbian, and bisexual patients. As a result, his nurses made an effort to welcome his significant other and friends as part of his family. His surgery was uncomplicated with a good prognosis. A colostomy was not indicated. Postoperatively, his internist gladly changed his antihypertensive medications and his impotency resolved. Overall, his anxiety and fears dramatically responded to the therapeutic interventions, which had integrated his identity as a gay man with his role as a medical patient.

This case clearly shows the importance of affirmatively managing the care of gay, lesbian, and bisexual patients and how treatment may remain inadequate if such patients are not allowed to integrate their sexual orientation into their full identity. Mr. A's sexual orientation had not been addressed by his medical team before the psychiatric consultation. A thorough sexual history would have revealed not only that Mr. A was gay, but also that he was impotent and feared the sexual implications of a colostomy. Such history taking also would have revealed much about his psychosocial history, including the death of his spouse and his own fears of death from cancer. In a supportive medical setting, it is doubtful that Mr. A's anxiety would have escalated to the point of needing mental health intervention. This case exemplifies the multifaceted role of the gay-, lesbian-, and bisexual-sensitive C-L clinician.

Inpatient Psychiatric Treatment

The inpatient psychiatric unit is a setting that offers additional challenges to clinicians working with gay, lesbian, and bisexual patients. Historically, clinicians have generally ignored issues related to sexuality with inpatients. The following specific topics are addressed in this section: general issues regarding gay, lesbian, and bisexual patients in inpatient units; potential interventions to sensitize staff to the needs of gay, lesbian, and bisexual patients; special inpatient settings; and sexual orientation among severely and persistently mentally ill patients.

■ Gay, Lesbian, and Bisexual Patients on Inpatient Units: General Issues

Generally, it is safe to assume that the quality of gay-affirming mental health care a gay, lesbian, or bisexual patient receives in the inpatient setting is directly linked to the sensitivity of the staff to diverse sexual orientations. In spite of the American Psychiatric Association's 1973 decision to remove homosexuality from the list of mental illnesses (Bayer 1981), it is not uncommon to find mental health staff members who still believe that homosexuality is a form of psychopathology. In particular, this mistaken belief may surface in response to those patients who are hospitalized because of symptoms brought about by difficulties in coming out or who remain ambivalent about their sexual orientation. In such cases, conflict related to sexual orientation may be viewed as psychopathology, rather than as a symptom related to difficulties in achieving a normal developmental task for gay, lesbian, and bisexual persons. Some of the more common psychiatric presentations in patients experiencing conflict about their sexual orientation are anxiety disorders, mood disorders, substance use disorders, and adjustment disorders (Hanley-Hackenbruck 1988).

The way that hospital staff react to such patient scenarios may be powerfully corrective in the case of gay-affirming providers or very harmful in the case of providers who are negative or who have not analyzed their own feelings about differences in sexual orientation. Providers who lack sensitivity concerning gay, lesbian, and bisexual issues may be unable to address issues of sexuality or associated fears of HIV and AIDS.

Smith (1992) outlined important patient assessment and intervention strategies available to psychiatric nurses that may help gay, lesbian, and bisexual patients to more comfortably assimilate themselves into inpatient settings. An inpatient unit that affirmatively recognizes nontraditional families and manages sexual orientation issues effectively in the milieu, including during group psychotherapy and in other treatment modalities, will be able to provide appropriate treatment to gay men, lesbians, and bisexual persons. As is true for heterosexual patients, most psychiatric hospitalizations of gay men, lesbians, and bisexual persons have little to do with conflict over their sexual orientation. However, if inpatient facilities are unable to integrate gay, lesbian, and bisexual diversity into their treatment interventions, patients may become further burdened or inhibited by the need to constantly self-monitor their language and behavior and, as a result, limit treatment participation to avoid discussion about their sexual orientation.

■ Interventions to Sensitize Staff

Although there has been little systematic research on the effectiveness of various techniques for educating clinicians about gay, lesbian, and bisexual issues, a number of interventions exist to sensitize inpatient staff to the needs of gay, lesbian, and bisexual patients (Murphy 1992). Educational training, whether in the form of brief inservice sessions and case conferences or longer workshops and continuing education programs, may reduce homophobia among various health professionals. For example, formal HIV training workshops that have used pre- and postintervention evaluations have shown that education can reduce negative attitudes about persons with HIV, including negative attitudes about homosexuality (Goldman 1987; Johnson et al. 1990). Spencer and Hemmer (1993) outlined how mental health clinicians can decrease anxiety and increase comfort with gay, lesbian, and bisexual issues through self-exposure to gay, lesbian, and bisexual cultures and through active consultation about the clinical needs of such diverse communities.

As is the case with the general public, heterosexual health care providers may be more likely to hold positive attitudes toward gay, lesbian, and bisexual patients if they have had positive interpersonal experiences, such as knowing and working with openly gay, lesbian, and bisexual staff members or knowing such people in their private lives (Herek 1994). Similarly, the manner of handling clinical supervisions and approaching treatment plans for gay, lesbian, and bisexual patients may impact homophobic staff members in a positive way. In summary, a clear and consistent educational message that legitimizes gay, lesbian, and bisexual patients' sexual orientations should be given to the inpatient staff.

▇ Special Inpatient Settings

Inpatient settings that attend to the special needs of gay, lesbian, and bisexual patients are a fairly new entity in the mental health arena. The majority of these programs focus on the treatment of substance abuse, which for many gay, lesbian, and bisexual persons is closely coupled with homophobia and lack of self-acceptance. Increasingly, recovery programs are becoming sensitive to gay patients, that is, aware of, knowledgeable about, and accepting of gay people in a nonprejudicial fashion (Cabaj 1993). A few programs openly advertise themselves as gay affirming, actively promoting self-acceptance of a gay, lesbian, or bisexual identity as part of recovery. One such gay-affirming program, the Pride Institute in Eden Prairie, Minnesota, has reported significant increases in abstinence after addiction treatment compared with non-gay-affirming programs (E. F. Ratner et al., unpublished observations, April 1991). Growing professional awareness of the unique needs of gay, lesbian, and bisexual patients may encourage administrators in all inpatient settings to actively train their staff to become more gay sensitive and affirming.

▇ Sexuality and Severe and Persistent Mental Illness

A discussion of inpatient psychiatric settings is incomplete without addressing the population of persons with severe and persistent mental illness. Because of the nature of their illnesses, persons with severe mental illnesses occupy a majority of psychiatric beds. Such patients may be diagnosed with schizophrenia, schizoaffective disorder, bipolar disorder, chronic substance abuse disorders, organic mental disorders, severe personality disorders, or mental retardation. For many years the mental health field has treated these patients as though they were asexual, particularly those patients with psychoses. However, new research evaluating HIV risk behaviors in this population indicates that persons with severe mental illnesses are indeed sexual, and a significant number engage in homosexual sexual activity.

Several researchers (Cournos et al. 1991; Sacks et al. 1990) examined HIV infection rates of severely mentally ill men who reported having sex exclusively with men and found rates of 5%–25%. In a recent report Cournos and colleagues (1994) evaluated HIV risk behaviors in persons with schizophrenia and found lifetime rates of same-sex sexual activity to be 23% for men and 20% for women. Interestingly, all of these patients also reported past opposite-sex sexual activity. Another group of investigators (Susser et al. 1993) examined HIV infection rates in severely mentally ill men and found that 7% of study participants reported bisexual behaviors.

Thus, although such patients may not identify themselves as gay, lesbian, or bisexual, studies of sexual activity support the notion that a significant number of people with severe and persistent mental illness engage in same-sex sexual contact. Effectively working with such patients requires sensitive acknowledgment of their sexual activity and affirmation of their sexual behavior and orientations. If such patients do report being sexually active, it is important to probe their knowledge about safer sexual practices. A number of structured HIV-related sex education interventions have been described for this population (Cates and Graham 1993; Goisman et al. 1991; Meyer et al. 1992).

Outpatient Community Mental Health Centers

Like heterosexuals, gay men, lesbians, and bisexual persons are most likely to seek mental health care in private or public outpatient settings. The issues involved in psychotherapy with these men and women are covered in other chapters in this book (see especially Chapter 23 by Falco, Chapter 24 by Stein and Cabaj, and Chapter 25 by Matteson). The many factors involved in delivering comprehensive, sensitive, and unbiased care to this population in outpatient community mental health centers are the focus of this section.

The issues raised previously—comfort with taking a sexual history, understanding nontraditional family patterns, realizing how the presentation of some mental illnesses can be affected by coming out, educating staff about gay and lesbian concerns, and responding to the issues that gay, lesbian, and bisexual clinicians face in clinical settings— all apply to outpatient clinics. Some mental health centers open to the general population also openly provide treatment to gay men, lesbians, and bisexual patients. These centers must deal with a variety of additional concerns that may not face centers that are specifically dedicated to the care of gay men, lesbians, and bisexual persons.

Structure of Outpatient Care

All treatment settings see gay, lesbian, and bisexual patients, whether their sexual orientations are recognized or not. Consequently, all clinics need to be sensitive to how their staff welcome and greet clients, for example, by using intake forms that are neutral about marital status and sex of the partner or spouse. Clinics that offer special care for gay men, lesbians, and bisexual persons need to balance the comfort of such patients with the discomfort or awkwardness heterosexual clients may feel in sharing space.

Gay-, lesbian-, and bisexual-related items placed in waiting rooms, such as posters, reading material, and HIV and AIDS information, need to be carefully considered but clearly available. Dealing with the homophobia of some clients will require sensitivity on the part of staff and may involve a need for consultation on how best to respond; managing such situations can be a learning experience for both staff and clients. A gay and lesbian treatment center faces similar issues and must be careful to balance material relevant to the lesbian, gay, and bisexual patients with material focused on the families and friends of the patients.

Staffing patterns are important. Will staff be allowed to be open about their own sexual orientation? Will heterosexual staff feel comfortable working with clients who may assume they are also gay or lesbian? The role of the sexual orientation of the therapist is discussed in Chapter 3 by Cabaj. Both heterosexual and gay staff need periodic education about the concerns of gay, lesbian, bisexual, and transsexual persons; opportunities to discuss and process their own homophobia and heterosexism; support regarding limit setting, boundaries, ethical issues, and countertransference; and support groups to help prevent burnout, especially if there is an HIV and AIDS treatment program included (see Chapter 50 by McDaniel, Farber, and Summerville).

Local Politics and Community Issues

Financial issues, local politics, and the size of the gay and lesbian community in the area will influence both the structure of a clinic devoted to gay men, lesbians, and bisexuals and the delivery of care. Freestanding gay and lesbian clinics often must scramble for limited grants and foundation support to augment the revenues from direct patient care. Many of the activities provided, such as educational groups, support services, and case management, may not be covered by insurance. Many clients using these clinics have limited funds and insurance coverage. Some have been denied coverage as domestic partners of employed partners; others may have lost benefits and coverage after having been laid off or discriminated against because of HIV infection; and others may be unemployed or have limited employment as a result of internalized homophobia leading to limited career expectations and societal homophobia producing limited job opportunities (O'Hanlan et al., in press). Social services may be needed to help clients connect with governmental benefits or legal recourses. Therefore, other financial supports for these clinics are imperative.

The providers serving gay, lesbian, and bisexual patients at university medical centers, public health agencies, and larger private treatment centers need to compete with other programs and justify the need for care devoted to gay men, lesbians, and bisexual persons. Such providers may have to confront resistance from officials and administrators at these sites to care for this unique and different population; such resistance may result from disguised homophobia on the part of the administrators. Without strong advocates and supporters in administration and program planning who are themselves gay men, lesbians, and bisexual persons, in addition to heterosexuals (who may be seen as having no personal issue to promote), such clinics and programs may be very difficult to start and defend when budget cuts and program reductions are sought.

Federal Ryan White monies have been dedicated to paying for services for HIV-infected clients. Such money has allowed many gay and lesbian clinics to survive and expand services, even though it unfortunately continues to link gay and lesbian issues with AIDS-related concerns at a time when AIDS is clearly a much broader based concern. Additional Centers for Disease Control and Prevention monies have supported HIV prevention efforts, thus allowing some federally funded direct service for non-HIV-infected gay men, lesbians, and bisexual persons. Both sources of money, however, are limited and quite dependent on local and federal politics.

Local politics and local community issues affect the neighborhood or community acceptance of such treatment sites and possibly influence the availability of financial support from voluntary contributions. Development of treatment programs for gay men, lesbians, and bisexual persons may face opposition in communities that tolerate homophobia and have limited or no legal protections for gay men and lesbians. The local press may not carry advertisements for these services, and local politicians may not support funding efforts. Once such centers are established, clients may fear attending such an openly gay and lesbian program for fear of the reprisal from neighbors or employers.

An important justification for such programs and centers—especially in academic settings—is to train clinicians to be comfortable with and knowledgeable about gay, lesbian, and bisexual health care, as well as to encourage research on the treatment of gay men, lesbians, and bisexual persons. Such objectives can be embraced only by systems that are not mired in heterosexism or overt homophobia. If the care for gay men, lesbians, and bisexual persons can be seen as a humane, ethical, and mandated concern, not one that distracts from or denies care of others, most reasonable administrators, clinicians, and concerned private and governmental individuals will be supportive. In this book, Chapter 41 by Owen and Chapter 40 by Banks and Gartrell further support the need for such services.

To help clinics and treatment centers survive, expand, and create new services for underserved gay men, lesbians, and bisexual persons, a newly reorganized national gay health center group and gay and lesbian health foundation, the National Gay and Lesbian Health Alliance, was founded in 1994. Other national groups such as the Gay and Lesbian Medical Association and the Association of Gay and Lesbian Psychiatrists can serve as consultants and be helpful in such efforts. The Gay and Lesbian Medical Association supported the acceptance of a revised American Medical Association paper on gay and lesbian health care (American Medical Association 1994) and promotes the awareness of homophobia as a health hazard.

■ Specific Clinical Concerns

No one clinical service can serve all the needs of gay, lesbian, and bisexual patients. Certain specific clinical issues and concerns, however, are common in gay men, lesbians, and bisexual persons, and health care providers for these patients need to be aware of these concerns.

Confidentiality.   Providers must make confidentiality and security of records paramount concerns. The decision to be out about sexual orientation or about HIV status is a very personal choice, and what is recorded in a medical chart about these matters needs to be discussed with the client. Insurance companies, employers, and the government—if they have access to such information—may use such materials in ways that are not in the best interest of the gay, lesbian, or bisexual patient. Many clinics devise a code system or agree on abbreviations to convey information needed for clinical care (see Chapter 41 by Owen). All records must comply with state and federal requirements and legal rulings, of course, but extra sensitivity is required regarding the need for confidentiality about sexual orientation and HIV status.

Violence against gay men and lesbians.   With the increased awareness of violence directed at gay men and lesbians (see Chapter 48 by Klinger and Stein), many clinics now offer counseling for victims of such crimes. The Fenway Community Health Center in Boston, Massachusetts, has one such program, including case management and community outreach. The Fenway Community Health Center learned that cooperation with the police and with local politicians is absolutely necessary for continued clinical impact. A recovery program for victims should offer group support services in addition to individual counseling, because an attack may uncover memories and reactions to past attacks or abuse that require extra support. Clinics for gay men, lesbians, and bisexual individuals may become the targets for attacks by homophobic people; safe and secure access to the center or clinic is vital. Postings of advisories and warnings about dangerous areas near treatment sites will help.

Parenting issues.   There is increased awareness of lesbian and gay male couples who have children, as well as of single gay, lesbian, or bisexual people who either have children or take part in raising children. As a result, many clinics now offer support for clients who are or wish to become parents (see Chapter 21 by Kirkpatrick, Chapter 22 by Patterson and Chan, and Chapter 40 by Banks and Gartrell). Couples attempting to have children may need support for their efforts to get pregnant, support or education about alternative insemination options, advice about legal options, or support during the possible frustrations faced in adoption attempts. Centers should be encouraged to provide child care facilities or other options for parents. Families of origin of some gay men, lesbians, and bisexual individuals may seek help in their acceptance of the sexual orientation of their relative and can benefit from education, support, or therapy.

Substance abuse services.   Substance abuse has a major impact on gay men, lesbians, and bisexual individuals (see Chapter 47 by Cabaj). As a consequence of the destructive effects of substance use, many substance-abusing patients have limited resources or insurance and may seek help at publicly supported clinics or centers. Staff well trained in recognizing and treating substance abuse are crucial to any clinic that welcomes gay men, lesbians, and bisexual individuals. Some clinics have blended mental health and addiction treatment into one comprehensive program. Support and psychoeducational groups are also very helpful. Some centers can provide space for Alcoholics Anonymous, Narcotics Anonymous, or Al-Anon meetings, thus helping to build bridges with the community of men and women in recovery from substance abuse.

HIV education and prevention efforts.   Though HIV is not a gay illness, the largest group with HIV and AIDS in America is men who have sex with men. No gay, lesbian, or bisexual center should be without HIV- and AIDS-related programs that incorporate both prevention and treatment components. The many mental health issues faced by gay and bisexual men with HIV infection (see Chapter 51 by Ostrow) are often best addressed at a gay, lesbian, and bisexual mental health program.

Other special clinical concerns.   Some of the clinical issues that some gay men, lesbians, and bisexual persons face might be difficult to address at a traditional clinic, possibly out of fear of misunderstanding or bias. For example, some gay and bisexual men struggle with compulsive sexual behavior and might be embarrassed to admit to this concern; group therapy may be of some benefit for this problem. Lesbians or gay men who have strong sexual feelings for the opposite sex may feel embarrassed or too confused to be open about these feelings and may benefit from talking with others facing similar confusion. Bisexual men who have not disclosed their bisexual feelings or homosexual activities to their spouses may need help in talking about these issues or guidance in negotiating safer sex with their spouses.

Conclusion

Several examples of mental health care settings providing treatment to gay men, lesbians, and bisexual persons are discussed in this chapter. C-L clinicians play an important role in the delivery of mental health care to gay, lesbian, and bisexual patients. C-L practitioners have the opportunity to educate other health care providers, to mediate conflicts among medical staff, and to diagnose and treat mental health conditions within the challenges of a medical setting. Such opportunities allow C-L providers to become a part of and profoundly impact multidisciplinary teams providing health care to gay, lesbian, and bisexual patients.

The inpatient psychiatric unit is a setting where it is important to acknowledge the sexuality and the sexual orientation of patients. This is especially true for gay, lesbian, and bisexual patients, who may be struggling with self-acceptance of their sexuality in addition to contending with other psychological problems.

Some outpatient clinics have specific units or programs devoted to gay men, lesbians, and bisexual persons; most treatment sites provide services for this population and need to learn to be comfortable with these men and women. Setting up dedicated programs and delivering the best quality care to gay men, lesbians, and bisexual persons in any setting will inevitably raise the issues of homophobia and heterosexism, which in turn may deter gay men, lesbians, and bisexual persons from seeking help or limit the quality of care.

All health care settings must confront homophobia as a health hazard. Quality care depends on the education, sensitivity, and dedication of the staff in treating all patients. The creation of an atmosphere and attitude that allows gay men, lesbians, and bisexual persons to be open, self-accepting, and self-affirming is essential.

References

American Medical Association: Health care needs of gay men and lesbians in the U.S. Report of the Council on Scientific Affairs: 8-1-94, accepted in December 1994. Chicago, IL, American Medical Association, 1994

Bayer R: Homosexuality and American Psychiatry. New York, Basic Books, 1981

Beebe JE III, Rosenbaum CP: Outpatient therapy: an overview, in Psychiatric Treatment. Edited by Rosenbaum CP, Beebe JE III. New York, McGraw-Hill, 1975, pp 227–263

Cabaj RP: Substance abuse in the gay and lesbian community, in Substance Abuse: A Comprehensive Textbook, 2nd Edition. Edited by Lowinson JH, Ruiz P, Millman RB, et al. Baltimore, MD, Williams & Wilkins, 1993, pp 852–860

Cates JA, Graham LL: HIV and serious mental illness: reducing the risk. Community Ment Health J 29:35–47, 1993

Cournos F, Empfield M, Horwath E, et al: HIV seroprevalence among patients admitted to two psychiatric hospitals. Am J Psychiatry 148:1225–1230, 1991

Cournos F, Guido JR, Coomaraswamy S, et al: Sexual activity and risk of HIV infection among patients with schizophrenia. Am J Psychiatry 151:228–232, 1994

Goisman RM, Kent AB, Montgomery EC, et al: AIDS education for patients with chronic mental illness. Community Ment Health J 27:189–197, 1991

Goldman JD: An elective seminar to teach first-year students the social and medical aspects of AIDS. Journal of Medical Education 62:557–561, 1987

Hanley-Hackenbruck P: "Coming out" and psychotherapy. Psychiatric Annals 18:29–32, 1988

Herek GM: Assessing heterosexuals' attitudes toward lesbians and gay man: a review of empirical research with the ATLG scale, in Lesbian and Gay Psychology: Theory, Research, and Clinical Applications, Vol 1. Edited by Greene B, Herek GM. Thousand Oaks, CA, Sage Publications, 1994, pp 206–228

Johnson SR, Guenther SM, Laube DW: Factors influencing lesbian gynecologic care: a preliminary study. Am J Obstet Gynecol 140:20–28, 1981

Johnson JA, Campbell AE, Toewe CH, et al: Knowledge and attitudes about AIDS among first- and second-year medical students. AIDS Educ Prevent 2:48–57, 1990

Lipowski ZJ: Consultation-liaison psychiatry: an overview. Am J Psychiatry 131:623–630, 1974

McDaniel JS, Carlson LM, Thompson NJ, et al: Knowledge and attitudes about HIV and AIDS among medical students. J Am Coll Health 44:11–14, 1995

Meyer I, Cournos F, Empfield M, et al: HIV prevention among psychiatric inpatients: a pilot risk reduction study. Psychiatr Q 63:187–197, 1992

Murphy BC: Educating mental health professionals about gay and lesbian issues. J Homosex 22:229–246, 1992

O'Hanlan KA, Robertson P, Cabaj RP, et al: Homophobia as a health hazard. JAMA (in press)

Sacks MH, Perry S, Graver EH, et al: Self-reported HIV-related risk behaviors in acute psychiatric inpatients: a pilot study. Hosp Community Psychiatry 41:1253–1255, 1990

Smith EM, Johnson SR, Guenther SM: Health care attitudes and experiences during gynecologic care among lesbians and bisexual persons. Am J Public Health 75:1086–1087, 1985

Smith GB: Nursing care challenges: homosexual psychiatric patients. Journal of Psychosocial Nursing 30:15–21, 1992

Spencer SB, Hemmer RC: Therapeutic bias with gay and lesbian clients: a functional analysis. Behavioral Therapist 16(4):93–97, 1993

Stotland NL, Garrick TR: Introduction and overview of the historical basis of consultation-liaison psychiatry, in Manual of Psychiatric Consultation. Edited by Stotland NL, Garrick TR. Washington, DC, American Psychiatric Press, 1990, pp 1–22

Susser E, Valencia E, Conover S: Prevalence of HIV infection among psychiatric patients in a New York City men's shelter. Am J Public Health 83:568–570, 1993

Weinberger M, Conover CJ, Samsa GP, et al: Physicians' attitudes and practices regarding treatment of HIV-infected patients. South Med J 85:683–686, 1992

SECTION IX

Special Topics/Special Concerns

Clinical Implications of Sexuality and Sexual Orientation

Gay and Bisexual Male Sexuality

Eli Coleman, Ph.D.
B. R. Simon Rosser, Ph.D.

I n this chapter, the authors review the literature on the sexuality and sexual functioning of gay and bisexual men. It commences with a review of major studies of homosexual behavior, identifying common patterns of homosexual sexual behavior and sexual satisfaction. The latter section concentrates on sexual-functioning problems and disorders.

Homosexual Behavior

▪ Homosexual Behavior and Normative Sexual Functioning

The study of normative sexual functioning of gay and bisexual men is fraught with difficulties. On methodological grounds, obtaining a representative sample of gay and bisexual men is probably impossible, at least given current cultural and social circumstances and discrimination (Bell and Weinberg 1978). By necessity, our impressions of male homosexual behavior are formed indirectly from an amalgam of many studies with differing methodologies. Historically, defining homosexuality as pathological behavior led not only to issues of underreporting but also to biases in research into homosexual behavior as nonproblematic. As a consequence, sexual function and dysfunction in gay male couples, for example, have only recently been studied. Indeed, before the mid-1970s, the term "[latent] homosexual" appeared in the literature most commonly as an explanation for [hetero]sexual dysfunction, rather than as a description of the population under study.

In the last 50 years, the scientific study of male homosexual behavior has exploded. At least three major factors have influenced this development, each with its own line of inquiry. First, the importance given to social science in the 20th century led to the legitimization of sexological inquiry as a valid area of study and a redefinition of the boundaries of human sexual behavior (Kinsey et al. 1948). In the Kinsey tradition, a number of studies examined homosexual behavior within the wider context of human sexuality. Second, the birth of the modern gay liberation movement led to a number of studies investigating gay and bisexual men's lives and lifestyles, including sexual behavior (Jay and Young 1979; Klein 1993). Third, the HIV epidemic resulted in an unprecedented number of studies investigating male homosexual behavior from an epidemiological perspective, for example, the Multicenter AIDS Cohort Studies (Chmiel et al. 1987). Each of these lines of inquiry is built on a different philosophical basis, and they provide differing impressions of normative homosexual behavior.

■ Sexual Behavior of Gay- and Bisexual-Identified Men

Gay men, by definition, have acknowledged their gay identity and are in some stage of a coming-out process. It is inaccurate to presume that gay-identified men have engaged in exclusive homosexual behavior throughout their lifetime. Just as sex in a homosexual context appears relatively common in men identifying themselves as heterosexual, so some heterosexual history appears common in men identifying themselves as gay. Surveys in the 1970s and 1980s of gay men indicate that 10%–20% have been heterosexually married (Bell and Weinberg 1978; Ross 1983), and 43%–63% reported experiencing vaginal intercourse

(Rosser 1991). Bisexual men, by definition, acknowledge their bipotentiality of sexual arousal. This identity does not assume that they are engaging in equal quantities of same- and opposite-sex sexual activity. In one study of 53 bisexual-identified men, 22 (41.5%) reported no heterosexual sex in the previous 3 years (Rosser 1991).

Masters and Johnson (1979) studied the sexual patterns of heterosexual, gay male, and lesbian couples. They observed that the gay male and lesbian couples took more time for their lovemaking than the heterosexual couples and appeared to place less emphasis on rushing toward orgasm. Gay male couples were more likely to orchestrate their partner's orgasm, touching and caressing more parts of their body (including nipples, buttocks, and thighs), and teasing them to greater stimulation and intensity of orgasm. These researchers observed that gay and lesbian couples appear to have an advantage over heterosexual couples: partners in same-sex relationships appeared better able to intuit their partner's desires, were less focused on simultaneous orgasms, and were more engaged in mutuality ("my turn, your turn" type of sexual interactions).

As a result of the gay liberation movement, the greater visibility of gay- and bisexual-identified men has enabled a wide variety of homosexual behavior studies to be undertaken within the gay community. These range from sociocultural studies of bar and bathhouse culture in large American cities (Bell and Weinberg 1978; Levine 1979; Saghir and Robins 1973) to social and psychological studies of male couples (Blumstein and Schwartz 1983; Mattison and McWhirter 1984).

In the last 10 years, in almost every major city in the Western world, epidemiological studies of homosexual behavior have been conducted in the interest of better understanding the epidemiology of HIV (T. J. Coates et al., unpublished manuscript, 1988). In general, current incidences of sexual behaviors appear related to the risk of HIV transmission. Unprotected anal intercourse, the sexual behavior most likely to transmit HIV, has decreased within this population, at least outside of long-term relationships. Estimates of the degree to which protected anal intercourse occurs vary widely. Behaviors with low risk of HIV transmission are reported with high frequency, including deep kissing, mutual masturbation, and digitoproctic acts (Rosser 1991). Although transmission of HIV through unprotected oral intercourse (Rozenbaum et al. 1988) and transmission of hepatitis and other non-HIV sexually transmitted disease through oral-anal intercourse have been documented (Ross 1986), guidelines regarding the risk of these behaviors have varied widely across the United States and elsewhere. Thus, it is not surprising that studies of the prevalence of unprotected oral sex present widely varying estimates.

Brachioproctic acts (fisting), sadomasochistic sex (S and M), and urolagnia (water sports) have been widely discussed in terms of HIV risk reduction for homosexually active men. However, their low prevalence within most major studies of homosexual behavior suggests these behaviors are uncommon.

With the rise of HIV infection in the 1980s and 1990s, there has been an increased emphasis on sex within the context of a relationship. In contrast to the sexual revolution of the 1970s, coupling, monogamy, and celibacy for gay men have been promoted as healthy and have become more socially acceptable (Levine 1992). Ensuing debate has focused on how realistic such options are for gay men. Early studies of HIV identified U.S. urban gay men as having a high lifetime number of sexual partners (Chmiel et al. 1987; Melbye et al. 1984). McWhirter and Mattison's study of male couples (1984) and a comparative study of heterosexual, lesbian, and gay couples (Blumstein and Schwartz 1983) both identified a low prevalence of monogamy in male gay relationships.

Ross (1991) dismissed stereotypes of gay men as having thousands of partners as artifacts of atypical samples (for example, early AIDS cases). A more modest estimate of the median number of lifetime male partners for American gay men is fewer than 50 (Darrow et al. 1981), still higher than heterosexual and lesbian estimates. Some have attributed these findings to male biological and sex roles (McWhirter and Mattison 1984). However, others have pointed to social factors including political messages about recreational sex, embracing of erotic freedom, and social expectations of the sexual revolution (Levine 1979; developmental factors such as the coming-out process (Coleman 1981–1982); and the lack of institutional support for monogamy and the influence of marginalization, homophobia, and the illegitimacy attached to homosexual liaisons (Sinclair and Ross 1986).

Whatever the reasons for higher number of partners, one of the major shifts within gay culture has been the shift in social support away from polygamy toward monogamy. Behavior that in the 1970s was labeled liberating in the 1990s is associated with disease. Gay men's sexual attitudes appear diverse, from treating sexual behavior as recreational to reserving genital expression for a life-long partner (Rosser et al. 1994).

■ Sexual Behavior of Gay Male Couples

Some indices of sexual behavior show gay male couples to be more similar to heterosexual couples than to lesbian couples. In the first 2 years of a relationship, 67% of gay male couples, 61% of heterosexual couples, but only 33% of lesbian couples reported a high frequency of sexual activity, defined as three times or more a week (Blumstein and Schwartz 1983). Although the frequency of sexual activity declined for all types of couples during the 3rd to 10th years of a relationship, the number of gay male and heterosexual couples engaging in sexual activity three times or more a week was still higher than the number of lesbian couples (32%, 38%, and 7%, respectively).

Exclusivity of sexual contact.   Studies of gay male sexual behavior have consistently shown that the majority of gay couples have not been exclusively sexual within the relationship (Bell and Weinberg 1978; Blumstein and Schwartz 1983; McWhirter and Mattison 1984; Saghir and Robins 1973). In contrast to heterosexual couples and lesbian couples, gay male couples do not seem to place as great an emphasis on sexual exclusivity to define their love and commitment. Among gay men, emotional rather than sexual exclusivity appears to be the central tenet of relationship (Ross and Rosser 1988).

However, all these studies were conducted before or early in the HIV epidemic. During the period of fear and uncertainty about the avenues of HIV infection, many gay men and couples tended to be more exclusive in their relationships (Centers for Disease Control 1987). By the late 1980s, gay couples acknowledged that the AIDS crisis had had a significant impact on their decisions regarding sexual exclusivity (Berger 1990).

Relationships and safer sex behaviors.   Conflicting evidence exists regarding future trends in gay relationships. Although studies indicate 60%–80% of gay men do not engage in unprotected intercourse (Communication Technologies 1990; Rosser 1991), men in relationships appear less likely to use condoms (at least with their primary partners) than their single counterparts. Overall, safer sex practices among gay men may be declining, possibly due to boredom with safer sex practices and overexposure to messages regarding safer sex behavior (Centers for Disease Control 1992). However, the majority of committed gay couples continue to care for each other's health. At the same time, gay men are gaining confidence that sexual behavior within certain limits or parameters can be safe (in the sense of avoiding HIV infection or other sexually transmitted diseases). Thus, they are more comfortable with taking the risks of having sexual activity outside of their committed partnership.

Gay relationships appear further affected by sociopolitical factors, including movements to legally acknowledge partnerships and to grant them privileges equivalent to those afforded married heterosexual partnerships. In 1989, the Danish government legalized homosexual domestic partnerships. In 1994, Sweden followed suit. Other countries are considering such legislation. New Zealand, countries within the European Community, some Australian states, and some municipalities within the United States have enacted legislation recognizing gay partnerships to some degree. In addition, an increasing number of large corporations and institutions have adopted policies that provide similar benefits for same-sex couples and heterosexually married couples. This institutionalization of gay relationships is likely to lead to an increase in the number of gay men seeking committed relationships.

When these studies are viewed together, an overall impression of homosexual behavior emerges. It appears oversimplistic and inaccurate to dichotomize behavior into homosexual and heterosexual. Contrary to popular opinion, most male homosexual behavior occurs between heterosexually identified men (McConaghy 1993). Anal intercourse occurs in only about one-third of male homosexual encounters; fellatio and mutual masturbation are more common, even normative, for same-sex encounters (Rosser 1991). Most homosexually active men have engaged in vaginal intercourse, and most gay men have been in a committed same-sex relationship at some point in their lives. For many diverse reasons, recent years have seen a significant shift toward community support for gay relationships. As Ross (1991) notes,

> The central issue is to appreciate that homosexual individuals cover the same wide spectrum of humanity as heterosexual persons, and that the division of people into "heterosexual" and "homosexual" groups is arbitrary although less psychologically threatening. . . . The diversity of individuals who may be homosexual precludes generalization about them from the fact of their sexual orientation alone. (pp. 141–142)

Sexual Dysfunction and Disorders
Among Gay and Bisexual Men

In male homosexual behavior, the sexual dysfunctions include aversion to sex, hyposexual desire, difficulties getting or maintaining an erection, rapid ejaculation, inability to ejaculate, and pain during or aversion to anal intercourse. Sexual disorders include the paraphilias and gender identity disorders. Although the sexual dysfunctions and disorders listed in the *Diagnostic and Statistical Manual of Mental Disorders, 4th Edition* (American Psychiatric Association 1994) apply to gay men, there is a heterosexist bias in these definitions. For example, although terms such as "vaginismus" and "dyspareunia" have been coined to describe problems in peno-vaginal functioning, there are no equivalent terms that accurately differentiate problems in anal intercourse. Similarly, the only illustration of compulsive sexual behavior is a heterosexual man who has repeated sexual conquests and sees women as objects to be used.

Although few good studies of sexual dysfunction in gay men exist, sexual dysfunctions and disorders appear to be common concerns of gay and bisexual men and may be underreported. Indeed, in one study (Rosser 1994) of 200 gay men attending a sexual education seminar, 97.5% reported a sexual dysfunction over their lifetime and 52.3% reported current dysfunction concerns. This finding highlights the need for professionals to discuss sexual functioning with their gay and bisexual patients.

■ Organic Etiologies

Gay men are not immune to the effects of illness, psychological processes, medication (such as antihypertensives), or other disorders that interfere with natural sexual functioning. However, gay men with sexual dysfunctions are more likely than heterosexual men to adapt to the dysfunction or disorder through increased communication and flexibility, which are associated with gay male sexual interaction. Others may suffer quietly by avoiding sexual activity or relationships. These men seldom seek sex therapy to address their sexual dysfunction or disorder.

Although many sexual dysfunctions have been viewed historically as psychogenic in origin, organic causes have received increasing recognition. While it is difficult to separate physical and psychological causes of sexual dysfunction, it is important for the health practitioner not to overlook the possibility that these dysfunctions may have physical causes. Historically, homophobia in physicians led to inferior health care for gay men (Dardick and Grady 1980; Pauly and Goldstein 1970). Homophobic sentiments among physicians persist and may provide a further barrier to gay men seeking and receiving quality health assessment, care, and treatment.

The most obvious organic sources of sexual dysfunction are vascular and neurogenic conditions, diseases, and prescription drugs that interfere with normal physiological processes involved in sexual arousal and orgasm. Careful assessment is also needed to uncover problems involving alcohol or other drug abuse or dependency (Schaefer et al. 1988). In HIV-infected men, the immunocompromising effects of HIV or the opportunistic infections can lead to difficulties in sexual functioning. Healthy sexual functioning is rarely addressed in HIV-infected individuals, yet this is an important aspect of physical health and well-being. It is also important to recognize that a sexual dysfunction can be a first symptom of a more systemic disease process (for example, diabetes and cardiovascular illness). Although rare, a paraphilic condition could be indicative of some temporal lobe lesions or neuroendocrine disorder (Money 1986).

■ Intrapsychic Conflict

Developmental problems. Sexual dysfunctions and disorders can develop as a result of intrapsychic and interpersonal conflict (Kaplan 1974). Healthy psychosexual development appears to be a necessary ingredient for healthy adult sexual and intimate functioning (Erikson 1956). Disruption in this development through trauma in the family or through the cultural abuse that many gay men experience can lead to problems developing a positive and integrated sexual identity (Coleman 1981–1982). Paradoxically, the challenges posed by these problems may also lead some gay men to an increased awareness and appreciation of healthy sexuality.

Development of sexual identity and intimacy functioning depend on receiving love and nurturance during critical periods of childhood (Bowlby 1969). Individuals must possess a healthy and secure balance of separation and attachment. Gay and bisexual men whose identity and intimacy development have been compromised often have difficulty maintaining healthy sexual relationships because of separation and attachment anxiety and fears. These developmental problems can result in low self-esteem, shame, anxiety, depression, or difficulties in sexual or intimacy functioning.

Several models of identity development among gay men and lesbians have been postulated. Although identity development may be more diverse and idiosyncratic than suggested by the models, they are nonetheless empirically sound and clinically useful (Cass 1979; Coleman 1981–1982). Central to these models is the process of self-acceptance and "coming out." Coming out is not a singular event; it is a developmental process in which a number of developmental tasks are to be accomplished. Although fewer social barriers to sexual identity development exist today for gay and bisexual men and women, a gay, lesbian, or bisexual identity remains stigmatized. More and more, gay, lesbian, and bisexual individuals are able to achieve an integrated identity and, thus, are less likely to need psychological or psychiatric assistance with their identity development. As clinicians, the authors more often assist gay, lesbian, and bisexual individuals who, for whatever reason, are compromised in their mental health functioning. Resolution of their personality, psychological, or psychiatric disturbances allows these individuals to meet the challenges of the coming-out process.

Because society does not foster the sexual identity development of gay and bisexual men and women, difficulties in sexual and intimacy functioning can be symptomatic of the failure to develop a positive sexual identity (Coleman 1981–1982). Because difficulties in sexual functioning can be more easily avoided or minimized in nonintimate situations, such problems are more likely to be experienced in the context of intimate relationships and indeed may be characterized as an intimacy dysfunction (Coleman et al. 1992).

Other developmental issues, such as facing midlife and aging, affect gay men, bisexual men, and heterosexual men in similar ways. However, certain characteristics of gay culture and the effects of HIV may result in many gay men experiencing an accelerated emphasis on the aging process (Friend 1988). A frequent emphasis on youth and finding a new sexual partner has often put pressure on gay and bisexual men as they age. The deaths of so many young and middle-age gay friends from AIDS have put even more pressure on many gay men to deal with an accelerated aging process.

Fear of death and loss of loved ones are more salient issues at earlier ages to gay and bisexual men than to heterosexual men. Like soldiers in war and others experiencing multiple deaths, they may see themselves as "old at a time before one's chronological peers define themselves as old" (Friend 1988). However, there is also evidence to suggest that this accelerated aging process begins to pay off as many older gay men become more equipped to handle the developmental issues of aging (Friend 1988).

History of abuse and neglect.   Gay and bisexual men who were neglected or abused as children are more likely to have difficulty with the aforementioned developmental process (Coleman and Reece 1988). An integrated sexual identity may be more elusive as these individuals try to differentiate the consequences of their abuse from their sexual orientation. Sexual sequelae of abuse include sexual dysfunction in intimate relationships, hypoactive sexual desire, avoidance of sexual activity, unsafe sexual behavior, and compulsive sexual behavior. Emotional and physical abuse and neglect are almost universally found in gay and bisexual men suffering from a compulsive sexual behavior (Coleman 1991).

■ Interpersonal Conflict

Misunderstanding what is normal.   Gradual lessening of sexual interest is a natural consequence of both aging and being in a long-term relationship. As indicated previously, the "normal" frequency of sexual activity diminishes in long-term relationships. One cannot compare the excitement of a new relationship or a sexual adventure with the quality of a sexual relationship in the context of a long-term relationship. Each type of sexual encounter is a unique experience. Many problems of low sexual desire are due to unrealistic expectations, unfair comparisons, and desire discrepancies (Coleman and Reece 1988).

Sexual desire discrepancies.   Incompatibilities in sexual interest can be a problem in all types of relationships regardless of sex or sexual orientation. It is important for the clinician to differentiate normal desire discrepancies from discrepancies that stem from intrapsychic or intrapersonal conflict. Although the clinician should normalize these experiences as much as possible, they may indicate other problems that have not been addressed in one of the partners or in the relationship. The partner with high desire may have as much conflict as the partner with low desire.

Because many gay male couples are not sexually exclusive, issues of jealousy, possessiveness, competitiveness, and perceived or real health risks are more common among these couples. Couples may not have the communication skills to resolve these difficulties. In working with gay male couples, helping the couples communicate their feelings, desires, and values is an important vehicle for reaching resolution of these conflicts.

■ Case Example

Bill and Joe have been together for 15 years. Although they were monogamous in the first year of their relationship, they decided to allow extrarelational relationships under certain prescribed circumstances. As the HIV epidemic became a health threat, they decided to "close down" their extrarelational activities to protect their seronegative HIV status. They maintained a monogamous relationship for the next several years. Subsequently, Bill felt that he could have sexual encounters outside of the relationship as long as he practiced safer sex and did not tell Joe. Joe started to suspect Bill's extrarelational sexual activity and confronted him about this. Joe refused to have sex with Bill for fear that he might contract HIV or some other sexually transmitted disease. Distance grew between them, conflicts became more intense, and the couple were at the brink of ending their 15-year relationship before seeking therapy.

The therapist assisted the couple with talking through the issues in their relationship and helped them look at options for resolving their differences. The situation was resolved by the couple redefining their commitment to each other as allowing no outside unprotected oral or anal intercourse and improving communication so they could tell each other whenever sex took place and what types of sexual activity occurred. They also decided that they would always use condoms in their own sexual relationship during oral or anal sex.

■ Sociocultural Etiologies

Institutionalized homophobia and heterosexism as expressed through legal restrictions (or lack of legal protections), religious prohibitions (or lack of affirmation), and family or cultural intolerance (or lack of acceptance) of homosexuality may have direct influence on the development of a sexual dysfunction or disorder. Institutionalized homophobia and heterosexism, which exist in families, schools, health care, and other public arenas, have a negative impact on the self-esteem and sexual identity development of gay and bisexual men and women. The challenge of the coming-out process is to overcome the impact of these societal prohibitions and lack of affirmation. In treating sexual dysfunctions and disorders, the clinician usually has to address the developmental tasks of the coming-out process that may have only been partially resolved.

Conclusion

In this chapter, the authors have reviewed many aspects of gay and bisexual male sexuality. They hope that through dissemination of this knowledge the mental and sexual health of gay and bisexual men will be enhanced. By normalizing sexual experiences of gay and bisexual men, professionals have the opportunity to improve their patients' sexual health and decrease pathology. At the same time that we need to affirm the natural and normal differences of gay and bisexual men's sexuality, it is important not to ignore the common sexual dysfunctions or disorders experienced by these men. In the spirit of affirming the healthiness of gay and bisexual male sexuality, health care professionals may overlook the fact that some of these men experience sexual dysfunctions and disorders and that these need to be treated by the sensitive and experienced clinician.

References

American Psychiatric Association: Diagnostic and Statistical Manual of Mental Disorders, 4th Edition. Washington, DC, American Psychiatric Association, 1994

Bell A, Weinberg M: Homosexualities: A Study of Diversity Among Men and Women. New York, Simon and Schuster, 1978

Berger RM: Men together: understanding the gay couple. J Homosex 19:31–49, 1990

Blumstein P, Schwartz P: American Couples: Money, Work, Sex. New York, William Morrow, 1983

Bowlby J: Attachment and Loss, Vol 1. New York, Basic Books, 1969

Cass VC: Homosexual identity formation: a theoretical model. J Homosex 4:219–235, 1979

Centers for Disease Control: Self-reported changes in sexual behaviors among homosexual and bisexual men from the San Francisco City Clinic cohort. MMWR 36:187–189, 1987

Centers for Disease Control: Hepatitis A among homosexual men—United States, Canada, and Australia. MMWR 41:155–164, 1992

Chmiel JS, Detels R, Kaslow RA, et al: Factors associated with prevalent human immunodeficiency virus (HIV) infection in the Multicenter AIDS Cohort Study. Am J Epidemiol 126:568–577, 1987

Coleman E: Developmental stages of the coming out process. J Homosex 7:31–43, 1981–1982

Coleman E: Compulsive sexual behavior: new concepts and treatments. Journal of Psychology and Human Sexuality 4:37–52, 1991

Coleman E, Reece R: Treating low sexual desire among gay men, in Sexual Desire Disorders. Edited by Leiblum SR, Rosen RC. New York, Guilford, 1988

Coleman E, Rosser BRS, Strapko N: Sexual and intimacy dysfunction among homosexual men and women. Psychiatr Med 10:257–271, 1992

Communication Technologies: HIV-Related Knowledge, Attitudes and Behaviors Among Minneapolis/St. Paul Gay/Bisexual Men: Results from the First Population-Based Survey. San Francisco, CA, Communication Technologies, 1990

Dardick L, Grady D: Openness between gay persons and health professionals. Ann Intern Med 93:115–119, 1980

Darrow WW, Barrett D, Jay K, et al: The gay report on sexually transmitted diseases. Am J Public Health 71:1004–1011, 1981

Erikson E: The problem of ego identity. J Am Psychoanal Assoc 4:56–121, 1956

Friend R: The individual and social psychology of aging: clinical implications for lesbians and gay men, in Psychotherapy for Homosexual Men and Women: Integrated Identity Approaches. Edited by Coleman E. New York, Haworth, 1988, pp 299–323

Jay K, Young A (eds): The Gay Report: Lesbians and Gay Men Speak Out About Sexual Experiences and Lifestyles. New York, Simon and Schuster, 1979

Kaplan HS: The New Sex Therapy. New York, Brunner/Mazel, 1974

Kinsey AC, Pomeroy WB, Martin CE: Sexual Behavior in the Human Male. Philadelphia, PA, WB Saunders, 1948

Klein F: The Bisexual Option, 2nd Edition. New York, Harrington Park Press, 1993

Levine MP (ed): Gay Men: The Sociology of Male Homosexuality. New York, Harper and Row, 1979

Levine MP: The life and death of gay clones, in Gay Culture in America: Essays From the Field. Edited by Herdt G. Boston, MA, Beacon Press, 1992, pp 68–86

Masters WH, Johnson VE: Homosexuality in Perspective. Boston, MA, Little, Brown, 1979

McConaghy N: Sexual Behavior: Problems and Management. New York, Plenum, 1993

McWhirter DP, Mattison AM: The Male Couple. Englewood Cliffs, NJ, Prentice-Hall, 1984

Melbye M, Biggar RJ, Sarngadharan MG, et al: Sero-epidemiology of HTLV-III antibody in Danish homosexual men: prevalence, transmission and disease outcome. BMJ 289:573–575, 1984

Money J: Lovemaps: Clinical Concepts of Sexual/Erotic Health and Pathology, Paraphilia, and Gender Transposition in Childhood, Adolescence, and Maturity. New York, Irvington Publishers, 1986

Pauly IB, Goldstein S: Physician's attitudes in treating homosexuals. Medical Aspects of Human Sexuality 4:26–45, 1970

Ross MW: The Married Homosexual Man: A Psychological Study. London, Routledge and Kegan Paul, 1983

Ross MW: Psychovenereology: Personality and Lifestyle Factors in Sexually Transmitted Diseases in Homosexual Men (Sexual Medicine, Vol 3). New York, Praeger, 1986

Ross MW, Channon-Little LD: Discussing Sexuality: A Guide for Health Practitioners. Artarmon, Australia, MacLennan and Petty Ltd, 1991

Ross MW, Rosser BRS: Monogamy is. . . . Geni Med 64:65–66, 1988

Rosser BRS: Male Homosexual Behavior and the Effects of AIDS Education. New York, Praeger, 1991

Rosser BRS: Male homosexuality in Minnesota: a psychosexual study of safer sexual behavior, affect, and cognitions of Man-to-Man: Sexual Health Seminar participants. Report to the Minnesota Department of Health, 1994

Rozenbaum W, Gharakhanian S, Cardon B, et al: HIV transmission by oral sex. Lancet 1:1395, 1988

Saghir M, Robins E: Male and Female Homosexuality: A Comprehensive Investigation. Baltimore, MD, Williams and Wilkins, 1973

Schaefer S, Evans S, Coleman E: Sexual orientation concerns among chemically dependent individuals, in Chemical Dependency and Intimacy Dysfunction. Edited by Coleman E. New York, Haworth, 1987, pp 121196140

Sinclair KCP, Ross MW: Consequences of decriminalization of homosexuality: a study of two Australian states. J Homosex 12:112–119, 1986

Lesbian Sexuality

Sarah E. Herbert, M.D.

L esbian sexuality is a complex subject involving a knowledge of female sexuality as well as homosexuality. A description of lesbian sexuality is more difficult because there has been a general lack of attention to the subject of female sexuality, especially to the ways in which it may be qualitatively different from male sexuality. Furthermore, because lesbians are often an invisible minority, there is even less information available about them than about women in general. In this chapter, the available studies are reviewed for what they can tell us about normative aspects of lesbian sexual functioning. Consideration is given to qualitative aspects of sexuality as well as to the more typical quantitative aspects. Assessment and diagnosis of lesbian sexual dysfunction are also addressed. Suggestions for further research on this important subject are made.

Conceptualizing Lesbian Sexuality

Sexual behaviors, fantasies and arousal, emotional attachments, self-image, and self-definition of sexual orientation all need to be considered in addressing lesbian sexuality. Developmental aspects of sexuality, including how expressions of sexuality may change as the individual matures and evolves over a lifetime, are additional important variables. The degree of flexibility in sexual behaviors and choice of partner vary from individual to individual and may vary by sex.

Any discussion of lesbian sexuality must recognize that differences exist between men and women in psychosexual development. Lesbian psychosexual development must be viewed in the context of female psychosexual development, as well as in the context of homosexual identity development. The ways in which lesbians differ from heterosexual women, as well as how they differ from gay and heterosexual men, are considered in this chapter.

Studies on female sexuality show that in heterosexual relationships men and women differ widely in sexual characteristics (Hurlbert and Apt 1993). Women place more emphasis than men on the emotional characteristics of a sexual relationship; in particular, intimacy and closeness are highly valued by women (Hurlbert and Apt 1993; Nichols 1988). Therefore, sexual satisfaction in a woman appears to be less related to physical sexual variables and more to the quality of the relationship with her partner. In contrast, sexual intercourse and other aspects of physical sexuality are key aspects of male sexual satisfaction.

Unfortunately, much sex research and theory have focused on male sexuality as the norm, with an emphasis on investigation of objective sexual variables such as frequency of sexual activity, specific foreplay techniques, and orgasm (Ogden 1994). In this context, women may be viewed as functioning deficiently compared with men (Person 1980). More recently, there has been an interest in redefining female sexuality from the perspective of women's own experiences (Bernhard and Dan 1986). One way in which the perspective of women has been explored has been to look at sexuality in lesbian relationships. Lesbian sexual relationships may be viewed as reflecting essential characteristics of female sexuality, because they function without the confounding factor of male influence. In most heterosexual couples, male dominance persists and serves to confound information gathered about female sexuality from these relationships (Cass 1990; Hurlbert and Apt 1993; Kitzinger and Perkins 1993; Nichols 1987a, 1990). Therefore, studies of lesbian sexuality have given us important information, not only about lesbians' sexual experiences, but about the sexuality of women in general.

If lesbian sexuality reflects some essential traits of female sexuality, it is not clear whether these traits are determined by biological differences between the sexes or are the result of female socialization. Women masturbate and have sex less frequently than men, but these differences could be either the result of an inherently different desire for sex or the result of female socialization, which encourages women to deny or repress sexual feelings. Lesbian and heterosexual women grow up in the same culture, which in the United States has encouraged repression of sexual feelings and discouraged expression of genital sexuality in women. Thus, one might expect to see significant effects of female socialization in expressions of lesbian sexuality (Blumstein and Schwartz 1983). A high percentage of lesbian women in the couples' studies indicated that they would like to have sex more frequently. This suggests that the lower frequency of sexual interaction in lesbian couples does not reflect essential characteristics of female libido, but may have more to do with difficulties women have in recognizing and asserting their sexual needs.

An essential characteristic of female sexuality that becomes particularly noticeable in lesbian sexual relationships is the value put on nongenital physical contact. This contact is highly valued by most women, but for lesbian women it can be an end in itself. While heterosexual women value nongenital physical contact, they may report experiencing it less frequently because their male partners are likely to view it as a prelude to genital sexual activity. Sexual satisfaction in women has been found to be more related to emotional factors, particularly the quality of the relationship, than to physical sexual variables such as frequency of sexual interactions or orgasm (Hawton et al. 1994; Hurlbert et al. 1993; Leigh 1989; Schreurs 1993). This finding may help to explain why lesbians in relationships are as satisfied sexually as partners in gay male or heterosexual relationships, despite having a lower frequency of genital sexual activity.

Research Issues in Lesbian Sexuality

When research is done about a stigmatized group like lesbians, who are not readily visible, the difficulty of obtaining a representative sample is a major research problem. The largest samples of lesbian women in existing studies were recruited nonrandomly. Convenience samples from lesbian bars, women's bookstores, gay and lesbian community organizations, friendship networks, lectures about lesbian sexuality, and gay and lesbian publications have provided the majority of subjects. Despite the limitations, these existing studies have given us invaluable information about lesbian sexuality, and often they were completed at a time when lesbian subjects were even harder to identify due to greater societal stigmatization. Important aspects of lesbian sexuality that have not been well documented or studied include the sexuality of middle-aged, older, and minority lesbian women and the impact of the HIV on lesbian sexual practices. Future research on lesbian sexuality should sample a more diverse population of lesbian women of all ages, races, and social classes.

Another deficit in the current status of sex research is the way in which sexuality is conceptualized. Much sex research focuses on a model of sexuality that appears to be more geared toward men and emphasizes quantitative aspects of sexuality. Future research should use different paradigms to investigate the ways in which sexuality is experienced by women. Emphasis on qualitative aspects of satisfying sexual relationships among lesbians, as well as the previous quantitative work, would be one way to address this need.

What We Know About Lesbian Sexuality

Existing empirical studies of lesbian sexuality have investigated the following topics: the prevalence of same-sex experiences among women, age of awareness of same-sex attraction and arousal, heterosexual experience, types of sexual practices, satisfaction in sexual relationships, the extent of masturbation, and problems with sexual functioning.

■ Prevalence of Homosexuality and Bisexuality Among Women

Although many men and women have had some same-sex sexual experience, a smaller percentage live as gay or lesbian for a substantial period in their lives. The percentage of women who report some same-sex sexual experience varies considerably depending on the study (Janus and Janus 1993; Kinsey et al. 1953; Laumann et al. 1994). Kinsey et al. (1953) found that 17% of women had had some same-sex sexual experience, whereas only 4% of the women Laumann et al. (1994) surveyed reported same-sex experience since puberty. A much smaller percentage of women are estimated to be predominantly or exclusively homosexual or to self-identify as lesbian (Diamond 1993; Janus and Janus 1993; Kinsey et al. 1953; Laumann et al. 1994). In the Laumann et al. study (1994) only 1.4% of the women and 2.8% of the men actually were self-identified as homosexual or bisexual. The prevalence of homosexuality in women has been found to be about half that in men in most surveys (Diamond 1993; Kinsey et al. 1953; Laumann et al. 1994). Studies of 12- to 20-year-old adolescents identifying themselves as gay or lesbian show a much lower prevalence, but reflect similar sex differences, with boys endorsing a homosexual orientation twice as frequently as girls (Boxer et al. 1989; D'Augelli and Hershberger 1993; Remafedi et al. 1992).

The prevalence of bisexual behavior (2–5 rating on the Kinsey scale, where 0 = completely heterosexual and 7 = exclusively homosexual) was estimated by Kinsey et al. (1953) to be 4%–11% among women 20–35 years of age. More recent data indicate that the Kinsey estimates were probably too high, and the prevalence is likely 3% or less of women (Janus and Janus 1993; Laumann 1994). Determination of an individual's sexual orientation can be complex because an individual's self-identification may be at variance with his or her behavior (see Chapter 4 by Michaels). The inclusion of bisexuality in data on homosexuality makes the analysis of differences more difficult (Bressler and Lavendar 1986).

Kinsey et al. (1953) included a category for subjects who were not sexually aroused by individuals of either sex, which included up to 15% of the women studied. It is not clear whether the extent of the women subjects' lack of arousal reflected the repressive attitudes of society toward women's awareness of their sexual feelings at that time, or whether it was a persistent finding about a significant minority of women, because there is no recent research data on this subject (Diamond 1993).

■ Early Awareness of Sexual Orientation

Romantic emotional attachments, crushes, fantasies, dreams, daydreams, and sexual arousal are early psychological and sexual responses that may indicate to a girl or young woman her sexual orientation (Bell et al. 1981; D'Augelli and Hershberger 1993; Jay and

Young 1979; Saghir and Robins 1973). These responses are present in the history of most lesbian women, occurring initially in the preadolescent or early adolescent years. In contrast, a much smaller percentage of heterosexual women report these same-sex attachments and arousal (Bell et al. 1981; Laumann et al. 1994; Saghir and Robins 1973).

Homosexual arousal in lesbian women has been described as occurring initially in the context of a friendship or casual contact, not in association with a genital relationship as it has for many gay men (Saghir and Robins 1973). Homosexual arousal may occur by midadolescence for many lesbians, but a substantial number become aware of it later in adolescence or even during the adult years. This finding contrasts with the Kinsey et al. study (1953), which found that over a quarter of women had experienced homosexual arousal by age 30 years.

A demographic study of sexual orientation among adolescents (Remafedi et al. 1992) found that a very low percentage of subjects (2.6%) reported bisexual or homosexual fantasies. It was interesting to note that such fantasies were reported more frequently by girls than by boys (3.1% versus 2.2%). Adolescents with homosexual fantasies were considerably more likely to describe a homosexual orientation than adolescents with heterosexual or bisexual fantasies (Remafedi et al. 1992).

◼ Masturbation

Masturbation is often the earliest form of genital sexual activity in men and women. Kinsey and his colleagues (1953) found that only 62% of the women had masturbated at any time during their lives. Since the time of the Kinsey study, societal attitudes toward sexuality have become less repressive. In more recent studies, larger numbers of women in the general population have acknowledged that they masturbate (Hite 1976; Janus and Janus 1993; Laumann et al. 1994). However, there are still a significant number of women who do not currently masturbate or never have masturbated (Janus and Janus 1993; Laumann 1994). When men are compared with women, the percentage of men who have masturbated or currently masturbate is always higher (Janus and Janus 1993; Laumann et al. 1994; Saghir and Robins 1973).

Earlier studies indicated that a significantly greater proportion of lesbian women than heterosexual women reported self-masturbation (Kinsey et al. 1953; Saghir and Robins 1973). More recent studies have suggested that the differences between lesbian and heterosexual women do not appear to be as significant as they previously were. The differences still exist, however, with a higher percentage of lesbian women reporting masturbation compared with heterosexual women (Califia 1979; Hite 1976; Jay and Young 1977; Laumann et al. 1994; Loulan 1987). The Laumann et al. study (1994) found that 58% of women in the total population had not masturbated at all in the previous year. In contrast, the percentage of women with same-gender partners in the past 5 years who had not masturbated at all in the past year was about 30%, or about one-half that of women in general (Laumann et al. 1994).

Early Homosexual Experience

The earliest systematically collected data we have on same-sex sexual experience for women is that of Kinsey et al. (1953), which indicated that the number of women who reported sexual contacts with other females, whether or not they were erotically aroused, rose gradually from the ages of 10–30 years, then did not increase substantially. By age 40 years, 19% of Kinsey et al.'s female subjects had described such experiences. About one-half to two-thirds of the women who reported sexual contacts with other females had achieved orgasm. This meant that 4% of the women subjects had experienced orgasm in same-sex relations by age 20, 11% by age 35, and 13% by age 45 (Kinsey et al. 1953).

A recent study (Laumann et al. 1994) done with a sample randomly selected from the U.S. population suggested that a much lower percentage of the population has had sexual experiences with same-sex partners than previously thought based on Kinsey et al.'s pioneering studies (1948, 1953). In his review of studies done since those of Kinsey et al. (1948, 1953), including those from other countries, Diamond (1993) found that 2%–3% of the women studied had engaged in same-sex sexual activity since adolescence. Laumann et al. (1994) showed significant differences between men and women in the persistence of same-sex sexual activity from the teen years until the adult years. Very few women who reported sex with a same-sex partner between puberty and age 18 years did not also have sex with a woman after age 18. Almost half the men who had sex with another male before turning 18 did not continue to have sex with a same-sex partner after age 18 (Laumann et al. 1994).

Homosexual experience often begins later for lesbian women than it does for gay men. Only one-quarter of the lesbian women studied by Saghir and Robins (1973) had been sexually active before age 15 years. This finding was in distinct contrast to that for the gay men, three-quarters of whom had been sexually active before age 15 (Saghir and Robins 1973). Before age 20, about half of the lesbian women still were not sexually active with female partners. These sex differences in the age of onset of genital sexual activity between gay men and lesbians are similar to those for heterosexual men and women. A recent review reported that most American males have had intercourse by the age of 16–17 years and females by 17–18 years (Seidman and Rieder 1994). The age at which males and females become sexually active has been decreasing since the time of Kinsey et al.'s reports (1948, 1953); thus, there is likely to be a cohort effect on the ages of onset of sexual activity.

◼ Sexual Practices

A number of authors, beginning with Kinsey and his colleagues (1948, 1953), have attempted to define the nature of sexual relationships between same-sex partners (Bell and Weinberg 1978; Blumstein and Schwartz 1983; Califia 1979; Coleman et al. 1983; Hedblom 1973; Hogan et al. 1977; Hurlburt and Apt 1993; Jay and Young 1977; Loulan 1987; Rosenzweig and Lebow 1992; Saghir and Robins 1973; Schafer 1976, 1977). Sexual practices surveyed have included the following activities: kissing and petting, manual-genital contact, oral-genital sex, tribadism (or body contact), object-genital insertion, and others. The focus of much of this research has been on objective measures of genital sexual activity such as frequency of sex, frequency of use of different techniques in lovemaking, number of orgasms, and number of sexual partners.

In a large study of lesbian women selected from the convenience sample of women attending a sexuality lecture (Loulan 1987), the following sexual activities were reported by a majority of the subjects when they engaged in sex with a partner: hugging; snuggling; kissing all over body; touching, kissing, licking, and nursing on breasts; oral-genital sex; insertion of fingers or tongue in the vagina; and masturbation. Oral-genital sex was a component of the sexual relationship for about 70% of the lesbian women in this study (Loulan 1987). Cunnilingus has been reported to be a part of the sexual relationship for approximately the same percentages of lesbian and heterosexual couples; approximately three-quarters of both groups engaging in it sometimes, usually, or always when having sex (Blumstein and Schwartz 1983). The least frequent sexual activities (less than 10% of the time) reported by lesbian women were use of a dildo in the vagina, anal stimulation or penetration, spanking, bondage, group sex, and sex with men (Loulan 1987).

Sexual practices have not been looked at developmentally in many studies of heterosexual or homosexual individuals. In one very small study done over 20 years ago (Saghir and Robins 1973), manual-genital stimulation was the more frequent sexual practice in the adolescent years, and it increased in frequency until it was used by all the lesbian women studied by age 30 years. Oral-genital stimulation occurred less frequently in the adolescent years, but it increased in frequency throughout the young adult years so that it became as important as manual-genital stimulation for the lesbian women studied by age 30 years (Saghir and Robins 1973). There are almost no other data on developmental aspects of sexual relationships among lesbians.

The preferred method of achieving orgasm in partner-related sexual activities for lesbian women appears to be oral-genital sex or manual-genital stimulation (Califia 1979; Hurlbert and Apt 1993; Schreurs 1993). In a few older studies approximately one-third of lesbian women used tribadism, or body contact, as a means of achieving orgasm (Jay and Young 1977; Saghir and Robins 1973). A small study comparing lesbian and heterosexual women in couple relationships (Hurlbert and Apt 1993) found that self-stimulation was the preferred method for achieving orgasm for 56% of the lesbian women, compared with 24% of the heterosexual women. Surprisingly, in the same study (Hurlbert and Apt 1993), cunnilingus was identified as the preferred method of achieving orgasm for 41% of the heterosexual women, but for only 12% of the lesbian women. Coitus was the preferred means to achieve orgasm for only 21% of the heterosexual women (Hurlbert and Apt 1993). It is surprising that the preferred or most common means of achieving orgasm has not been investigated more frequently for lesbian women or for women in general.

■ Frequency of Sexual Activity and Orgasm

It has been suggested that lesbians always reach orgasm in their love-making (Sisley and Harris 1977), but this does not appear to be entirely true. However, only a very small percentage (2%–6%) of the lesbian women surveyed by a number of different investigators never achieved orgasm with lovemaking (Hogan et al. 1977; Jay and Young 1977; Loulan 1987). Infrequent orgasms resulted from lovemaking for another 13% in one study (Loulan 1987). More recent surveys of women, regardless of their sexual orientation, have shown that 12%–16% have orgasms infrequently or not at all during lovemaking (Hite 1976; Janus and Janus 1993). Thus, lesbians have a similar or possibly lower frequency of anorgasmia compared with heterosexual women (Schreurs 1993).

The one consistent finding in most studies of lesbian couples has been that they engage in sex less frequently than do heterosexual or gay male couples. This finding has been affectionately labeled "lesbian bed death" by women in the lesbian community. Blumstein and Schwartz (1983) reported a lower frequency of sexual relations at every stage and at every point in the lives of the lesbian couples compared with heterosexual and gay male couples.

Lesbian couples together 2 years or less reported a frequency of sexual relations closer to that of other couples. Seventy-six percent of lesbian couples together 2 years or less had sex once a week or more frequently. The comparable data were 83% for married heterosexual couples, 92% for cohabiting heterosexual couples, and 94% for gay male couples (Blumstein and Schwartz 1983). The frequency of sexual relations appeared to drop most precipitously after the first 2 years of a lesbian relationship compared with other couples. Only 37% of lesbian couples together 2–10 years were still having sex once a week or more, whereas about twice as many of the other types of couples continued to have sex that frequently (Blumstein and Schwartz 1983). A few studies of the frequency of sex without respect to partner status (Jay and Young 1977; Schafer 1977) suggest less discrepancy between lesbians and gay men. The most recent study (Laumann et al. 1994) did not find significant differences in the mean frequency of sex per month in the past year when women with same-gender partners were compared with all women subjects. These data were not grouped according to duration of the relationship, as they had been in the previous study of couples (Blumstein and Schwartz 1983).

The very limited data available on sexual relationships in older lesbian women (Kehoe 1988) suggest that the frequency of sexual activity diminishes with increasing age, as it does in heterosexual women (Hawton et al. 1994). In one study (Kehoe 1988) more than half of a sample of 100 lesbian women over age 60 said they had had no sexual experience with a woman in the past year. Sex, however, was considered an important part of a lesbian relationship after age 60 for almost three-quarters of this sample. Some, but not all, of the discrepancy between these findings may be due to a lack of opportunity for sexual interaction. Commitment and compatibility were considered more important than sex to most of the 43 women in the sample who were currently in a coupled relationship (Kehoe 1988). There was no attempt to provide a control group to see how heterosexual women of the same age compared with this sample of older lesbian women.

◼ Qualitative Aspects of Lesbian Sexual Relationships

Decreased frequency of sexual interaction does not appear to affect sexual satisfaction among lesbian couples. Most respondents in studies of lesbian sexuality (50%–84%) reported being completely or very satisfied with their sexual relationships (Coleman et al. 1983; Jay and Young 1977; Loulan 1987). When lesbians were dissatisfied with their current sex life, the reasons cited were relationship problems, orgasmic problems, partner incompatibility, and celibacy (Loulan 1987).

Significant differences have been found in the qualitative aspects of sexual relationships when women involved in same-sex relationships are compared with those in heterosexual relationships (Coleman et al. 1983; Hurlbert and Apt 1993). Lesbian women reported significantly higher degrees of interpersonal dependency, compatibility, and intimacy in their relationships compared with heterosexual women (Hurlbert and Apt 1993). The heterosexual women in this study reported significantly greater sexual desire and sexual assertiveness, more frequent sexual activity, and more positive feelings about sexual fantasy compared with lesbian women (Hurlbert and Apt 1993). It is interesting to note that both groups of women were equally satisfied with their relationships (Hurlbert and Apt 1993).

Initiation of sex is much more likely to be shared equally among same-sex partners, whether gay or lesbian. In contrast, it is much more likely to be the man who initiates sex if this role is not equally shared in the heterosexual couple (Blumstein and Schwarz 1983).

◼ Number of Partners

Studies reporting on number of sexual partners have shown that gay men have significantly more partners than lesbian women (Bell and Weinberg 1978; Schafer 1977). Over half of the lesbian women in two

different surveys reported 10 or fewer same-sex partners in their lifetime (Bell and Weinberg 1978; Coleman et al. 1983); the comparable
figure for gay men was only 3%–6% (Bell and Weinberg 1978). Monogamy was considered important by at least three-quarters of lesbian
women in most studies (Blumstein and Schwartz 1983; Peplau et al.
1982; Schreurs 1993). Heterosexual women and married men likewise
considered monogamy important, but only half as many gay men endorsed monogamy as important (Blumstein and Schwartz 1983).
Changes in attitudes and behavior have occurred among the gay male
and lesbian population in the past 20 years, and these data may not be
accurate today (Kurdek 1991).

■ Heterosexual Experiences

Many lesbian women have had substantial heterosexual arousal and experience. Heterosexual romantic attachments, fantasies, dreams, and
daydreams were experienced by one-third to one-half of lesbian women
in one small study (Saghir and Robins 1973). Over three-quarters of
lesbian women reported having had heterosexual intercourse at some
point in their lives, both before and after their first homosexual experience (Chapman and Brannock 1979; Jay and Young 1979; Saghir and
Robins 1973; Schafer 1976). Lesbian women have higher rates of heterosexual intercourse, previous marriage, and parenthood than do gay
men (Bell and Weinberg 1978; Saghir and Robins 1973). It has been
estimated that one-quarter to one-third of lesbian women have been
previously married, and approximately half of these women also have
had children (Bell and Weinberg 1978; Kirkpatrick 1994).

■ Summary

In summary, based on findings from existing studies, it is likely that
2%–4% of women have lived for a substantial period of their lives as
lesbians.The prevalence of homosexuality among women consistently
appears to be about half that among men. Women become sure of their
homosexual orientation at later ages than men and, much like their
heterosexual sisters, experience sexual relationships at a later age than
men. However, girls who are sexually active with same-sex partners
before age 18 years are much more likely to continue this activity than
boys who report same-sex partners before age 18.

Heterosexual women experience romantic attachments, arousal, or attraction to other women, but these experiences occur less frequently than they do for lesbian women. Masturbation occurs more frequently among lesbian women than heterosexual women, but the differences appear to have narrowed over the 40 years that these behaviors have been studied, paralleling societal changes in attitude toward masturbation. Compared with gay men, lesbian women have had more heterosexual arousal and experience, have been married more frequently, and are more likely to be parents.

Lesbians engage in a variety of sexual behaviors during lovemaking, but the preferred methods for achieving orgasm are manual-genital and oral-genital stimulation. Lesbians resemble heterosexual women in the subjective and objective aspects of their sexual relationships much more than they resemble heterosexual or gay men (Blumstein and Schwartz 1983). The major difference between lesbian couples and other couples is the lower frequency of sexual relations. The difference in frequency of sex does not appear to significantly affect sexual satisfaction among lesbians, with lesbians' sexual satisfaction being comparable to that of women in heterosexual couples.

Clinical Issues in Working With Lesbian Sexuality

■ Lesbian Sexual Dysfunction

Sexual dysfunction in lesbian couples has not been systematically investigated. However, judging from existing knowledge about lesbian sexuality, the ability to achieve orgasm and sexual satisfaction appears to be quite high among lesbians (Coleman et al. 1983; Hurlburt and Apt 1993; Loulan 1987; Masters and Johnson 1979; Nichols 1988; Schreurs 1993). Lack of intimacy and power imbalance in relationships have been postulated to contribute to sexual dysfunction in couples. These do not appear to be significant factors contributing to sexual dysfunction in lesbian relationships because intimacy and equality are very characteristic of lesbian relationships (Hurlbert and Apt 1993; Nichols 1988).

Sexual dysfunction can stem from a lack of knowledge about how the female body functions sexually, but this is less likely to occur in lesbian relationships because both partners are female. Primary anorgasmia is not a common problem among lesbians, but secondary forms, in which a woman might be orgasmic with self-stimulation but not with lovemaking with a partner, may occur more frequently (Masters and Johnson 1979; Nichols 1987a, 1987b, 1988). Situational anorgasmia affecting only one member of the lesbian couple was the sexual dysfunction treated most frequently by Masters and Johnson (1979). Desire problems, including decreased sexual desire, inhibited sexual desire, and desire discrepancy problems, are the most frequently cited reasons for lesbians seeking sex therapy according to sex therapists who work with them (Hall 1988; Nichols 1987a, 1987b, 1988).

Desire Disorders Among Lesbian Couples

Desire difficulties encountered by lesbian couples may be attributed in part to the nature of a relationship between two women. The terms "fusion" and "merger" have been used to describe the closeness, dependence, and togetherness seen in many lesbian couples. If genital sexuality represents a desire to "merge" temporarily, couples who are already merged or fused may not find such contact necessary (Nichols 1988). Such a couple might alternatively avoid sex as a way to achieve some psychological distance in their relationship (Nichols 1988).

Another explanation for the prevalence of desire disorders is that lesbian women may experience guilt about their sexual feelings, or they may repress their sexual desires. There may be more reason for lesbian women to experience guilt about their sexual feelings or to repress their sexual desire, given the general societal condemnation of homosexuality. Thus, internalized conflict about the acceptance of homosexual feelings may be the etiology of desire problems (Nichols 1988).

A third reason has been suggested to explain desire disorders among lesbian couples (Nichols 1988). Women frequently state that sexual desire is triggered by romantic stimuli. If these stimuli are the primary means of triggering sexual desire, a relationship between two women might have fewer ways over time to trigger desire, once the inevitably short-lived romantic phase has passed (Nichols 1988). Options for triggering sexual desire other than romance—such as physical attractiveness, a particular sexual technique, use of sex for recreation, or tension release—may be ignored or not recognized by lesbian couples (Nichols 1988). Thus, lesbian couples may become less sexual with time compared with heterosexual or gay male couples, or they may move on to another relationship where they can recreate the early romantic phase of intense desire (Nichols 1988).

■ Diagnosis and Management of Sexual Problems Among Lesbians

When a lesbian individual or couple presents with sexual problems, the clinician should complete an initial thorough assessment. Factors to consider in this assessment include interpersonal conflict in the couple, intrapsychic conflict in the individuals, physical illness, medications, psychiatric and substance abuse disorders, and the effects of societal rejection of homosexuality on the individual or couple.

The clinician may follow a traditional format for assessment of sexual dysfunction (Kaplan 1974; Masters and Johnson 1970), but must adapt these formats, which are based on a heterosexual paradigm, to include consideration of the specific concerns of lesbians (Hall 1988; Nichols 1988). Suggestions for adapting these formats have included a less authoritarian model, less attention to diagnosis of sexual problems involving vaginal penetration, and more concern about problems relevant to lesbian sexual experiences such as phobic avoidance of oral sex (Nichols 1988).

A model for assessment and treatment of sexual dysfunction in lesbians suggests that the following issues be addressed: 1) specific definition of the problem; 2) history of the problem for this couple; 3) history of the problem in other relationships for each partner; 4) each partner's assessment of the problem; 5) previous attempts to solve the problem; and 6) the reason for seeking help now (Nichols 1988). A detailed description of the last time the couple made love is crucial to this assessment, as it can give the therapist information about which techniques the couple uses, who takes the initiative, what each partner feels, and differences in perception of the same situation (Nichols 1988).

Differential diagnoses to consider once the assessment has been completed would be 1) a relationship problem manifesting itself as a sexual problem; 2) a desire discrepancy between the two partners; 3) avoidance of sex due to another sexual problem such as sexual aversion or phobias; 4) boredom and a need for sexual enhancement techniques; 5) a physical disorder or medication side effect; or 6) a psychiatric problem such as depression, posttraumatic stress disorder, or substance abuse (Nichols 1988).

Sexual expression may be inhibited in some lesbian couples as a result of the avoidance of behaviors regarded by the lesbian feminist community as reflective of stereotypic heterosexuality (Loulan 1987; Nichols 1987b, 1988). For example, a lesbian couple might avoid demands for more frequent sexual relations, vaginal penetration, use of a dildo, certain positions, pornography, or sadomasochistic activities because they are thought to reflect imitations of heterosexual behaviors or the degradation of women (Loulan 1987; Nichols 1987a, 1987b, 1988). A phobia about oral sex has been described as a common complaint in lesbians coming for sex therapy (Nichols 1988). Physical reasons for sexual dysfunction may include physical illness or side effects of medication. Recent research (Balon et al. 1993; Post 1994) suggests that 30%–40% of women report sexual side effects such as inhibited orgasm and decreased libido with the use of antidepressant medications.

Management of common sexual problems in lesbian couples may involve a number of different strategies. Sexual boredom can be overcome if couples can allow themselves to enjoy sex without having to be "politically correct" (Loulan 1987; Nichols 1987a, 1987b, 1988). This nonjudgmental focus can be positive when both members of the couple are willing to consider experimentation and when the greater breadth in lovemaking practices is not harmful to an individual or couple. Diagnosis and appropriate treatment of depressive disorders, phobias, or aversion may result in improved sexual interest and functioning. Some of the more classic systematic desensitization techniques may be used in treating aversion, phobias, and other anxiety problems interfering with sexual functioning. On the other hand, if the use of psychotropic medications is etiologically related to decreased libido or anorgasmia, a trial of a different type of medication or a lower dose might improve sexual functioning.

Couples' therapy is needed to address relationship problems that may be the basis for sexual dysfunction. Desire discrepancy problems can be normalized as something that may occur in couples of all sexual orientations. It is important for therapists working with lesbians to recognize that ongoing societal homophobia can have a significant negative impact on an individual woman's enjoyment of her sexuality and on the value a lesbian couple may put on their sexual relationship.

Conclusion

Lesbian sexuality has more in common with sexuality among heterosexual women than that among gay or heterosexual men. Intimacy, monogamy, and physical contact are similarly important for lesbians and heterosexual women. Lesbians report more frequent masturbation, less anorgasmia, and higher degrees of intimacy and compatibility in their sexual relationships than heterosexual women.

Lesbian sexual relationships can get into difficulty when there is rigid adherence to the belief that one partner should not dominate or be demanding, and neither partner is comfortable with taking the initiative sexually (Blumstein and Schwartz 1983; Nichols 1987a, 1987b, 1988, 1990). When the desire for sameness and compatibility limits the variety of sexual behaviors in which the couple can engage, the sexual relationship may suffer. Decreased frequency of sexual activity among lesbian couples does not appear to be a disadvantage because lesbian couples are as sexually satisfied as heterosexual and gay male couples (Hurlbert and Apt 1993).

References

Balon R, Yergani VK, Pohl R, et al: Sexual dysfunction during antidepressant treatment. J Clin Psychiatry 54:209–212, 1993

Bell A, Weinberg M: Homosexualities: A Study of Diversity Among Men and Women. New York, NY, Simon and Schuster, 1978

Bell AP, Weinberg MS, Hammersmith SK: Sexual preference: its development in men and women. Bloomington, IN, Indiana Univeristy Press, 1981

Bernhard LA, Dan AJ: Redefining sexuality from women's own experiences. Nurs Clin North Am 21:125–136, 1986

Blumstein P, Schwartz P: American Couples: Money, Work, Sex. New York, William Morrow, 1983

Boxer AM, Cook JA, Herdt G: First homosexual and heterosexual experiences reported by gay and lesbian youth in an urban community. Paper presented at the annual meeting of the American Sociological Association, San Francisco, CA, August 1989

Bressler LC, Lavendar AD: Sexual fulfillment of heterosexual, bisexual, and homosexual women. J Homosex 12:109–122, 1986

Califia P: Lesbian sexuality. J Homosex 4:255–266, 1979

Cass V: The implication of homosexual identity formation for the Kinsey model and scale of sexual preference, in Homosexuality/Heterosexuality: Concepts of Sexual Orientation. Edited by McWhirter D, Sanders S, Reinisch J. New York, Oxford University Press, 1990, pp 239–266

Chapman B, Brannock J: A proposed model of lesbian identity development: an empirical investigation. J Homosex 14:69–80, 1987

Coleman EM, Hoon PW, Hoon EF: Arousability and sexual satisfaction in lesbian and heterosexual women. J Sex Res 19:58–73, 1983

D'Augelli A, Hershberger SL: Lesbian, gay, and bisexual youth in community settings: personal challenges and mental health problems. Am J Community Psychol 21:421–448, 1993

Diamond M: Homosexuality and bisexuality in different populations. Arch Sex Behav 22:291–310, 1993

Hall M: Sex therapy with lesbian couples: a four stage approach, in Integrated Identity for Gay Men and Lesbians: Psychotherapeutic Approaches for Emotional Well-Being. Edited by Coleman E. New York, Harrington Park Press, 1988, pp 137–156

Hawton K, Gath D, Day A: Sexual function in a community sample of middle-aged women with partners: effects of age, marital, socioeconomic, psychiatric, gynecological, and menopausal factors. Arch Sex Behav 23:375–95, 1994

Hedblom J: Dimensions of lesbian sexual experience. Arch Sex Behav 4:329–341,1973

Hite S: The Hite Report. A Nationwide Study of Female Sexuality. New York, Dell, 1976

Hogan R, Fox A, Kirchner J: Attitudes, opinions, and sexual development of 205 homosexual women. J Homosex 3:123–136, 1977

Hurlburt D, Apt C: Female sexuality: a comparative study between women in homosexual and heterosexual relationships. J Sex Marital Ther 19:315–327, 1993

Hurlburt D, Apt C, Rabehl S: Key variables to understanding female sexual satisfaction: an examination of women in nondistressed marriages. J Sex Marital Ther 19:154–165,1993

Janus S, Janus C: The Janus Report on Sexual Behavior. New York, Wiley, 1993

Jay K, Young A: The Gay Report: Lesbians and Gay Men Speak Out About Sexual Experiences and Lifestyles, New York, Summit Books, 1979

Kaplan HS: The New Sex Therapy. New York, Brunner/Mazel, 1974

Kehoe M: Lesbians over 60 speak for themselves, chapter 4: lesbian relationships and homosexuality. J Homosex 16:43–52, 1988

Kinsey A, Pomeroy W, Martin C: Sexual Behavior in the Human Male. Philadelphia, PA, WB Saunders, 1948

Kinsey A, Pomeroy W, Martin C, et al: Sexual Behavior in the Human Female. Philadelphia, PA, WB Saunders, 1953

Kirkpatrick M: Middle age and the lesbian experience. Paper presented at the annual meeting of the American Society for Psychosomatic Obstetrics and Gynecology, San Diego, CA, February 1994

Kitzinger C, Perkins R: Changing Our Minds. Lesbian Feminism and Psychology. New York, New York University Press, 1993

Kurdek LA: Sexuality in homosexual and heterosexual couples, in Sexuality in Close Relationships. Edited by McKinney K, Sprecher S. Hillsdale, NJ, Lawrence Erlbaum, 1991, pp 177–191

Laumann EO, Gagnon JH, Michael RT, et al: The Social Organization of Sexuality: Sexual Practices in the United States. Chicago, IL, University of Chicago Press, 1994

Leigh BC: Reasons for having and avoiding sex: gender, sexual orientation, and relationship to sexual behavior. J Sex Res 26:199–209, 1989

Loulan J: Lesbian Passion. Minneapolis, MN, Spinsters Ink, 1987

Masters W, Johnson V: Human Sexual Inadequacy. Boston, MA, Little, Brown, 1970

Masters W, Johnson V: Homosexuality in Perspective. Boston, MA, Little, Brown, 1979

Nichols M: Lesbian sexuality: issues and developing theory, in Lesbian Psychologies. Edited by Boston Lesbian Psychologies Collective. Chicago, IL, University of Illinois Press, 1987a, pp 97–125

Nichols M: Doing sex therapy with lesbians: bending a heterosexual paradigm to fit a gay life-style, in Lesbian Psychologies. Edited by Boston Lesbian Psychologies Collective. Chicago, IL, University of Illinois Press, 1987b, pp 242–260

Nichols M: Low sexual desire in lesbian couples, in Sexual Desire Disorders. Edited by Leiblum S, Rosen RC. New York, Guilford, 1988, pp 387–412

Nichols M: Lesbian relationships: implications for the study of sexuality and gender, in Homosexuality/Heterosexuality: Concepts of Sexual Orientation. Edited by McWhirter D, Sanders S, Reinisch J. New York, Oxford University Press, 1990, pp 350–366

Ogden G: Women Who Love Sex. New York, Pocket Books, 1994

Peplau LA, Padesky C, Hamilton M: Satisfaction in lesbian relationships. J Homosex 8:23–35, 1982

Person E: Sexuality as the mainstay of identity: psychoanalytic perspectives, in Women: Sex and Sexuality. Edited by Stimpson C, Person E. Chicago, IL, University of Chicago Press, 1980, pp 36–61

Post L: Sexual side effects of psychiatric medications in women: a clinical review. Jefferson Journal of Psychiatry 12:75–81, 1994

Remafedi, G, Resnick M, Blum R, et al: Demography of sexual orientation in adolescents. Pediatrics 89:714–721, 1992

Rosenzweig J, Lebow W: Femme on the streets, butch in the sheets? Lesbian sex-roles, dyadic adjustment, and sexual satisfaction. J Homosex 23:1–20, 1992

Saghir M, Robins E: Male and Female Homosexuality. Baltimore, MD, Williams and Wilkins, 1973

Schafer S: Sexual and social problems of lesbians. J Sex Res 12:50–69, 1976

Schafer S: Sociosexual behavior in male and female homosexuals: a study in sex differences. Arch Sex Behav 6:355–364, 1977

Schreurs K: Sexuality in lesbian couples: the importance of gender. Annual Review of Sex Research 4:49–66, 1993

Seidman S, Rieder R: A review of sexual behavior in the United States. Am J Psychiatry 151:330–341, 1994

Sisley E, Harris B: The Joy of Lesbian Sex. New York, Simon and Schuster, 1977

Transsexuals

The Boundaries of Sexual Identity and Gender

David Seil, M.D.

Transsexualism, as defined in DSM-III-R, is "the persistent discomfort and sense of inappropriateness about one's assigned sex," and "persistent preoccupation for at least two years with getting rid of one's primary and secondary sex characteristics and acquiring the sex characteristics of the other sex" (American Psychiatric Association 1987, p. 76) in a person who has reached puberty. Gender identity disorder (GID), as defined in DSM-IV, is a broader designation inclusive of transsexualism, gender identity disorder of childhood, and gender identity disorder of adolescence or adulthood, non-transsexual type (American Psychiatric Association 1994). The term "transsexualism" is not used in DSM-IV, although it is still widely used in the scientific literature and common parlance. Gender dysphoria describes a subjective feeling of discomfort or distress about one's assigned anatomic gender and the appropriate gender role. Transsexualism is the extreme form of gender dysphoria, persistent in its presence and severely distressing. Patients who meet the criteria for transsexualism are those who hope for and request the relief of sexual reassignment surgery (SRS).

Historical Perspective

The occurrence of cross-dressing and cross-living throughout history is well documented (Garber 1992; Paglia 1991; Steiner 1981), as is the institutionalization of it in non-Western societies (Ackroyd 1979; Jani and Rosenberg 1990; Mihalik 1989). In spite of cultural evidence to the contrary, cross-dressing was generally considered a sign of homosexuality. The distinction between cross-dressing and homosexuality apparently was not clearly made in the scientific community until the work of Hirschfeld (1925). The term "transsexualism," which defined another group of patients, did not appear until 1949. However, after the well-publicized case of Christine Jorgensen in 1952 revealed that a surgical treatment for this condition existed, patients started to request SRS, and the interest and controversy about GID began.

By the mid-1960s, the study and surgical treatment of gender-related disorders was in full swing (Pauly and Edgerton 1986), and continued to be so for a decade and a half. Because SRS was relatively new, outcome studies did not appear until the late 1970s. The most influential of these concluded that "sex reassignment surgery confers no objective advantage in terms of social rehabilitation although it remains subjectively satisfying to those who have rigorously pursued a trial period and who have undergone it" (Meyer and Reter 1979). In spite of the confused message in this statement, this opinion matched the negative attitudes in the medical community toward SRS that had been reported in 1966 (Green et al. 1966). Medical centers that had been providing services that included surgeries stopped their programs. SRS in particular was targeted, and the emphasis returned to psychotherapy as the treatment of choice. As workers in the field put it, "We sense a growing fear of transsexualism" (Fleming et al. 1980).

This setback in the medical community did not deter the growth of an international gender community consisting of a variety of organizations, publications, and support groups for gender dysphoric people (Bolin 1988). In order to minimize the occurrence of unsatisfactory treatment results, the Harry Benjamin International Gender Dysphoria

Association (HBIGDA, P.O. Box 1718, Sonoma, California), formed to promote research and share information worldwide, developed standards of care (SOC) (Walker et al. 1990) to guide both patient and caregiver along the road of transition.

Although patients had been treated for almost two decades, no official diagnostic criteria for transsexualism appeared until the DSM-III (American Psychiatric Association 1980). Its inclusion under psychosexual disorders along with ego-dystonic homosexuality and the paraphilias reflected a lack of knowledge of the etiology of the disorder as well as its course and impact on society. DSM-III-R (American Psychiatric Association 1987) listed transsexualism under disorders arising in childhood, which was confusing because many patients do not come for treatment until they are adults. DSM-III-R attempted to contrast true transsexualism and gender identity disorder of adolescence and adulthood, non-transsexual type (GIDAANT). The progression of GIDAANT to transsexual GID was designated "rare," although transsexualism was listed as the "major complication" of GIDAANT (American Psychiatric Association 1987, pp. 74–78).

In DSM-III-R, patients were subtyped as being homosexual, heterosexual, and asexual, on the basis of the patients' genetic or anatomic gender. This strictly biological viewpoint is at odds with the patients' self-view, and was perhaps reflective of lack of knowledge regarding the origin and meaning of sexual object choice. It produced confusion in the therapist, and the patients found the labels offensive and at variance with their self-concepts (Bradley et al. 1991). This classification creates an interesting philological situation. As an example, two individuals with external female anatomy and living in the female gender role are sexually attracted to each other on the basis of female gender signals and become sexually active. One of them, however, is a postoperative genetic male. Under DSM-III-R classification, both are subtyped heterosexual, and this mating must be considered a variation of heterosexuality. Remarkably, no studies contrast the characteristics of the male partner of a genetic woman from those of the male partner of a postoperative male-to-female (MTF) (Steiner 1985). It is futile to label the former partner heterosexual and the latter homosexual. Clearly, humans are not erotically attracted to genetic structures. Instead, they form erotic attachments on the basis of visual and psychological cues. To attempt clarity around this issue, however, when necessary the author will refer to the genetic sex of the subject.

Diagnostic Criteria and Differential Diagnosis

The DSM-IV (American Psychiatric Association 1994) designates the following criteria for adult GID:

> A. A *strong and persistent* cross-gender identification. . . . In adolescents and adults, the disturbance is manifested by symptoms such as a stated desire to be the opposite sex, frequent passing as the opposite sex, desire to live as or be treated as the opposite sex, or the conviction that one has the typical feelings and reactions of the opposite sex.
>
> B. Persistent *discomfort* with his or her assigned sex or sense of inappropriateness in the gender role of that sex . . . . In adolescents and adults . . . manifested by symptoms such as preoccupation with getting rid of primary and secondary sex characteristics (e.g., request for hormones, surgery or other procedures to physically alter sexual characteristics to simulate the opposite sex) or belief that he or she was born into the wrong sex. (pp. 537–538, italics added)

DSM-IV specifies sexual attraction toward males, females, both, or neither, thus avoiding labels.

This broader, more inclusive diagnosis provides greater latitude for both the clinician and the researcher. Subjective reporting by the patient is necessary because no objective test exists, although the gender subscale on the Minnesota Multiphasic Personality Inventory (MMPI) has been used to study this population (Althof et al. 1983).

Two fairly distinct groups of patients with GID, primary transsexual individuals and secondary transsexual individuals, are described in the literature (Stoller 1968). The primary disorder develops directly from GID of childhood. An early age of onset (age 5 to 6), low sexual activity, lack of sexual arousal when cross-dressing, and generally a genetic same-sex orientation characterize the primary transsexual. Secondary transsexual individuals are older, may have had sexual relationships and marriages with members of the opposite biologic sex, and report at least a phase during which cross-dressing was sexually arousing. Sexual preference has more variability than in the primary group (Verschoor and Poortinga 1988). These are the two "common routes leading to gender identity disorder in adolescence or adulthood" (Bradley et al. 1991, p. 339).

Although distinctions between these two groups are consistently verifiable, they are not absolute. Most secondary transsexual individuals in a sample examined by this author (Seil, unpublished observations, February 1994) report being aware of the wish to be the other gender, and even feelings that they were the other gender, usually around age 5, the same age of onset as for primary transsexual individuals. They suppress the cross-gender feelings and wishes with a variety of defenses in order to adopt appropriate gender roles and may temporarily lose the earlier memories. Their experience of gender dysphoria is ego-dystonic, and this distinguishes them from the primary group.

Clinicians need to distinguish transsexualism from transvestic fetishism, in which a heterosexual male acts out sexual fantasies involving the wearing of female clothing, usually associated with masturbation (American Psychiatric Association 1994, pp. 530–531, 536). The diagnosis of transvestic fetishism includes a specifier "with gender dysphoria," although Stoller (1968, p. 188) felt that erotic arousal by cross-dressing clearly distinguished transvestic fetishism from transsexualism. Later studies designated cross-dressers who touched the penis during urination or masturbation or who obtained sexual gratification from the penis, regardless as to how such gratification was obtained, as not true transsexual individuals (Money and Lamacz 1984). Further conditions of gender conflict include gynemimesis, which describes a male who presents to society as a female, may take hormones, and may sexually prefer other males but does not seek SRS. The "she-male," by contrast, is a biologic male who maintains a hermaphroditic presentation for erotic purposes and may have received vaginoplasty without penectomy and/or orchiectomy (Blanchard 1993). Autogynephilia refers to men who are erotically aroused by the fantasy of having a female body or by obtaining female secondary sex characteristics. Whether these conditions are phases of gender transition or established erotic fixations is not known, because long-term case follow-ups are not reported.

Differentiating GID from the gender dysphoria that might occur in other conditions is essential for treatment planning. Patients with borderline personality disorder may have identity problems expressed as gender issues, but in transsexualism the identity disorder is consistent and unwavering over time. It does not only exist in fantasy and in fact must be a persistent preoccupation, as described. Some psychotic patients believe that they are of the opposite sex, and they deny awareness of their biologic sex, a detail that is never forgotten by the transsexual. Although high degrees of effeminacy in some homosexual men may or may not reflect GID, the desire to keep male genitalia is the distinguishing factor. The equivalent is true also for markedly masculine lesbian women. Transvestites may wish partial treatment for their secondary sex characteristics, but it should not be assumed that they are requesting SRS. Patients with obsessive-compulsive disorder may become obsessed with the idea that they are transsexual, but do not express unhappiness with their gender characteristics.

Prevalence

Transsexualism is a relatively rare disorder. In DSM-III-R, prevalence is reported as one per 30,000 for males and one per 100,000 for females (American Psychiatric Association 1987, p. 75). In the Netherlands in 1986, it was reported as one per 18,000 for males and one per 54,000 for females. (Many transsexual individuals are drawn to the Netherlands for treatment because care is covered by national health insurance [Eklund et al. 1988]).

Etiology

As the mechanism by which the subjective sense of gender develops is not clearly known, the etiology of gender dysphoria remains an open question. Research on gender focuses on prenatal hormonal or genetic influences or postnatal psychosocial conditions. Very few family and twin studies exist, perhaps reflecting the rarity of GID. Only 14 cases of familial occurrence are reported (Freund 1985, pp. 266–268; Hoenig 1985, p. 66). Researchers hoped to find a biological marker, but none has been found. A review of this issue is found in Hoenig (1985, pp. 46–61).

To study the development of gender dysphoria is to study the development of subjective and objective aspects of gender itself. Research focuses on the effects of prenatal hormones on the hypothalamic–pituitary areas, but the source and nature of these prenatal influences are an unsolved problem. Because a review of this work is beyond the scope of this chapter, the reader is directed to Money (1988, pp. 9–50) and Pillard and Weinrich (1987).

Later socialization affects the expression of gender even in laboratory animals who received hormones in utero (Money 1988, pp. 9–50; Pillard and Weinrich 1987). Using case study technique, psychoanalytic theorists have focused on the relationship with the mother, hypothesizing failure to separate from the mother as pivotal for male transsexualism, and a threatening symbiosis with the mother for the female transsexual (Horner 1992; Lothstein 1983, p. 247). Statistical studies report an absent, distant, or even rejecting father, as compared to heterosexual and homosexual controls, but not a pathologic relationship with the mother (Cohen-Kettinis and Arrindell 1990). Although transsexual and transvestite subjects report that the mother had hoped for a female child, which was not the case for the homosexual subjects, intrafamilial childhood environmental factors appear not to differ otherwise (Buhrich and McConaghy 1978). The relationship of childhood GID to later gender development is significant in that whereas most male children with GID later become homosexual, only a few male children with GID carry this disorder into adulthood (American Psychiatric Association 1994, p. 536; Green 1985; Zuger 1988). It would appear, then, that for most male children with GID, the disturbance is a phase of homosexual development, and for the rest, the onset of a lifelong condition. Psychosocial factors can influence gender expression, but not the internal experience of gender identity in the vast majority of cases. When etiology is unknown, psychogenic cause is often the default conclusion.

GID and the Gay-Identified or Gay-Sympathetic Therapist

As a group, transsexual individuals have a high incidence of psychiatric difficulties. Among those who have applied for services at gender identity clinics, a history of a suicide attempt was given by 19%–25% (Buhrich 1981; Dixen et al. 1984; Kuiper and Cohen-Kettinis 1988; Verschoor and Poortinga 1988). History of drug or alcohol abuse was obtained from 30% and of psychiatric hospitalization from 11%. Breast mutilation was attempted by 2.4% of the females, and genital mutilation by 9.4% of the males (Dixen et al. 1984). Additionally, in the author's sample of 121 cases (Seil, unpublished observations, February 1994), 48% have had multiple years of psychotherapy and 35% meet the criteria for psychiatric diagnoses other than GID and drug/alcohol abuse.

In general, patients with varying degrees of gender dysphoria believe that gay-identified or gay-sympathetic therapists have more empathy for their lifestyles, and if they are unable to find a therapist with expertise in gender dysphoria, they characteristically seek help from such therapists. The individual's self-designated sexual orientation may also strongly influence the choice of therapist. In one study, 33.2% of the males who seek transition to female, male-to-female (MTF), had already formed relationships with women and thus designated themselves as lesbian. In the female-to-male (FTM) population, 19.1% were in relationships with men, designating themselves as gay men (Dixen et al. 1984). In a review of the literature on this subject, 28%–56% of the preoperative males (MTFs) reported being sexually preferential to women, and 0%–13% of the preoperative women (FTMs) reported preference for men (Burns et al. 1990). In this author's sample noted above, 34% of the MTFs consider themselves lesbian or bisexual. The percentage of female-to-males (FTMs) who are attracted to males is considerably less, only 8%. All these patients are likely to be more comfortable with a gay-identified or gay-sympathetic therapist.

For those patients who have the goals of hormone and surgical treatments, the psychotherapist plays the pivotal role of diagnostician and evaluator ("the gatekeeper") who must give or withhold recommendations for these procedures.

The Course of Gender Identity Disorder

■ Primary or Ego-Syntonic Transsexualism

The course of primary transsexualism differs in important ways from that of secondary transsexualism. Primary transsexual individuals report continuous memories of declaring that they believed they were of the other gender or wished that they were from about the age of 5 or 6. The 5- to 6-year-old child may directly state the belief that he or she is of the opposite gender or express dismay about his or her anatomic gender. Probably because of negative responses to such statements, later expressions of gender dysphoria are more likely to be behavioral. Their play is more appropriate to the opposite gender, they cross-dress, and they choose opposite gender friends. Secretly praying for a gender change while they go to sleep is not uncommon. Cross-dressing begins and usually continues throughout childhood and adolescence in one form or another, perhaps secretly.

This cross-gendered behavior does not go unnoticed by parents and peers. Males in particular do not remember childhood as being pleasant. The presence of a gender conflicted male child causes great difficulty for parents who typically do not support this notion and try to make the child drop cross-gender expressions, even by using severe physical abuse. A few children may be taken to counselors, where the diagnosis of childhood GID will probably be made. Fewer females seem to have intrafamilial conflicts, and they may attain the niche of family tomboy, often to the delight of the father. The social pressures that are brought to bear on these children have little effect on ego-syntonic feelings, and childhood memories around the issue are readily available in both sexes.

As puberty begins, however, both sexes experience increased distress. Males view their developing genitals as not belonging to them or as disgusting. Automatic sexual responses that focus attention on the genitalia are extremely disturbing. Many report low or absent sexual drives. The obvious male characteristic of facial and body hair becomes another preoccupation. Females find their breast development disgusting and the menses a disturbing monthly reminder. Both sexes may attempt to resolve their gender confusion by adopting a homosexual orientation. Experimentation in this area can help clarify the gender issue, because although the great majority of transsexual individuals are sexually attracted to their own genetic sex, they also wish to be desired as, and thus validated as belonging to, a gender they do not externally possess. Because their homosexual partners view physical and psychological gender as one, transsexual individuals soon reach the conclusion that they are not homosexuals.

These adolescents do not develop defense mechanisms to suppress or help them cope with their gender dysphoria, and thus they experience distress in all areas of life. The adjustment of the female primary transsexual in adolescence appears better than that of the male primary transsexual. A masculine young woman can find an acceptable place in adolescent society, whereas the feminine male is more frequently ostracized, teased, and rejected both by peers and families.

Physical abuse is common, and isolation and avoidance of peer contact may be the only coping mechanism available. Without support in the home, these males tend to drop out of school and run away to the street where they are vulnerable to drugs, prostitution, and AIDS. They are virtually unemployable because of lack of education, skills, and appropriate appearance. They find themselves trapped in poverty and unable to obtain the treatment that would free them. Those fortunate enough to have the understanding and support of family may begin transitioning.

Transition into the opposite gender role seems easier for the primary transsexual than it is for the secondary transsexual in some ways. Socially, they have not built elaborate structures and networks based on their genetic gender which would have to be revised. Physically, incomplete masculinization in the males facilitates better results from hormone treatment. The female transsexual assimilates more readily than the male, because validating social responses will cue more from facial hair and deepened voice and less from physique. With few exceptions, both males and females are attracted to partners of their own genetic sex, and they readily form primary relationships. In the author's sample (Seil, unpublished observations, February 1994), 50% of both the primary MTFs and FTMs were in relationships at the time of evaluation for hormones. Usually the partner knows the situation of the transsexual, but sometimes partners do not know, even though the pair is cohabiting.

■ Case Example 1

A was an 18-year-old genetic male when she was referred for evaluation by her therapist at a local community mental health center. She was the only child of a single parent and was raised in a large extended family that was tolerant of her expressions of wanting to be female from about age 3. She liked to play with dolls, wore androgynous clothing and kept her hair long. In high school, she became a target for teasing and harassment by her peers, which led her to drop out of two different high schools during her senior year and to seek counseling. Upon psychiatric evaluation, A professed her feelings of being female. She thought her male genitals were "ugly" and that God had "given (her) the wrong body." She met the criteria for the diagnosis of transsexualism, and aside from situational anxiety there appeared to be no other mental disorder.

With the collaboration of her therapist, family, and school officials, the decision was made to begin A on female hormones and to re-enroll her as a female in a different high school to complete her senior year. When seen in psychiatric follow-up 1 year later, she was extremely happy. She had graduated with honors in school and had had male dates to two proms, neither date being aware of her genetic gender. In consultation with her therapist and family, her request for reassignment surgery was approved. When seen post-surgically, she had found employment as a female. Her integration into society had been completed successfully.

■ Secondary or Ego-Dystonic Transsexualism

Most secondary transsexual individuals report an awareness of gender dysphoria at about the same age, 5 or 6 years, but the wish to be the opposite gender is ego-dystonic. The defense mechanisms employed to lower distress about their gender issues, including denial, isolation, dissociation, and acting out, suppress the gender dysphoria and memories of it until puberty or later. Cross-dressing and cross-gender play, if these exist, become secret activities. A suppressed urge to cross-dress commonly reemerges at puberty as fetishistic transvestitism, but the abuse of substances to deaden undesirable gender wishes frequently begins then as a secondary line of defense. Men may enter a "hyper-masculine phase" (Brown 1988) and join the military, marry early and more than once, and choose masculine-identified occupations, such as truck driving, or adopt highly dangerous hobbies, such as car racing. The females may marry and bear children or try to compromise by becoming masculine lesbians. The secondary transsexual is so success-ful in developing the appropriate role that a later announcement of true gender identity often comes as a complete surprise to associates.

Under life stress, the defenses that have suppressed the gender issue may weaken, and the presence of GID can no longer be denied. Inevitably secondary transsexual individuals try to integrate the unwanted gender identity into their egos. Some patients begin to face it concurrently with becoming sober. Media presentations of transsexualism may tell them that what they feel has a name and that they are not the only ones. Patients discover that whatever cross-gender expression they can manage makes them feel less tense and happier. Cross-dressing loses its sexual excitement, and many commonly wear opposite sex undergarments. The men may surreptitiously remove body hair and begin female nail care. Men also may arrange weekends away or other alone times when they can fully cross-dress. Women bind their breasts as they begin to cross-dress.

As these patients clarify their internal state, they realize that they face painful choices. They can continue to experience the "persistent discomfort" of GID, or seek to relieve distress by beginning a transition. Whereas the primary transsexual may come to the office or clinic solely to obtain a recommendation for hormones or surgery, the secondary transsexual individuals seek ongoing treatment. They are aware that a gender change will cause many serious losses. Not many marriages survive the announcement that a spouse is transsexual. Partners feel betrayed and also fear that the transition of a parent may psychologically damage the children. The children themselves may reject the transsexual parent. The transsexual individuals in transition have no protection in the workplace, and many find themselves unemployed and unemployable because of the necessary interface with the public or because of discrimination. The secondary transsexuals must also deal with more confusion around their variable sexual orientations. The experimentation that could help clarify it is not feasible for many in early transition, and they typically avoid forming any intimate relationships.

Consequently, isolation, loneliness, and loss of family, job, and social support are not uncommon. Those who feel these losses would be too devastating seek help in living with the decision not to transition. Although secondary transsexual individuals may need to deal with serious losses and have more confusion regarding sexuality, they generally have more education and occupational experience, and thus are in a better economic position to subsist autonomously and even underwrite SRS.

■ Case Example 2

> B was a 44-year-old genetic male when she was referred for treatment from the psychiatric ward of a general hospital, where she had been treated following a suicide attempt. During a family meeting in the hospital, B revealed to her spouse that she had been secretly cross-dressing for many years in her workshop in the cellar, and that now she felt an urgent need to begin to transition to female. The spouse abruptly terminated the marriage and informed B that she would never see her only child, a 12-year-old son, again.
>
> B entered treatment for depression and began transition with

electrolysis and hormone therapy. After initial disbelief, her parents offered support, and she joined a gender support group. She prepared her managers at work and began living full-time as female. After the required year, she underwent reassignment surgery with satisfactory results. She then began to date males.

However, upon learning of the surgery, her former spouse increased financial demands in the form of damages. She was still not allowed to see her son. The initial tolerance at work appeared to wane, and she found herself passed over for promotion and assigned the least desirable duties. She again became suicidally depressed under these stresses and required multiple hospitalizations. Although now adjudicated permanently disabled secondary to depression, she has never expressed regret about her gender change.

Treatment

Currently, more than 19 gender identity clinics operate in the Western world to provide sound medical and psychiatric care. The Harry Benjamin International Gender Dysphoria Association developed guidelines for the caregiver and patient regarding the steps of transition in 1979. Most recently revised in 1990, these guidelines, called Standards of Care (SOC), are widely known by transsexual individuals and generally followed by workers in this field. The main points are as follows:

1. Hormonal sex reassignment should precede surgical reassignment, and requires a recommendation from a clinical behavioral scientist. The clinical behavioral scientist must ascertain that the patient meets the diagnostic criteria for a diagnosis of transsexualism as outlined in DSM-III-R (1987). The condition must have existed for at least 2 years, and that information is best obtained by professional contact with the patient for at least 3 months. The administration of hormones is considered diagnostic as well as therapeutic. If hormone therapy does not produce greater stability, the diagnosis is not transsexualism.
2. Surgical (genital or breast) reassignment will be preceded by a period of at least 12 months during which the patient lives full-time as a member of the opposite gender (called "the life test"). The recommendation for surgery must originate from the clinical be-

havioral scientist who has known the patient in a psychotherapeutic relationship for at least 6 months and must be supported by a second opinion of another clinical behavioral scientist who has personally examined the patient. At least one of the examiners must be of doctoral level.

The SOC also emphasizes ethical issues and recognizes that transsexual individuals may have financial and legal difficulties, and suffer "social, legal and financial discrimination not known, at present, to be prohibited by federal or state law" (p. 10). The SOC does not differentiate between primary and secondary transsexualism (Walker et al. 1990).

The major functions of the therapist and psychiatrist are three: selection of patients who are appropriate for transition to SRS, support of these patients through and following reassignment, and assistance to those patients with GID who are inappropriate for surgery, who continue to live in the initial gender role for whatever reason, or are unclear and hesitant about their gender identity (Pfafflin 1992, pp. 63–89; Lothstein 1983, p. 305). The therapist must not impose personal opinion about SRS. If a patient is seeking surgery, psychotherapy will not reverse GID (Stoller 1968, p. 249), and attempting to do so on the therapist's part would be contraindicated. On the other hand, the therapist must allow the patient to stop or turn back at any point, even if the therapist is convinced that SRS is the best treatment (Shore 1984). If the therapist cannot be objective, the patient must be referred elsewhere. Also, the therapist must be willing to work as a member of a medical team because other medical specialists are involved in reassignment (Asschemen et al. 1989; Money and Lamacz 1984).

The most difficult role of the psychotherapist is distinguishing between those patients for whom hormonal and surgical reassignment will produce increased stabilization and subjective relief and those for whom it will not (Pfafflin 1992, pp. 63–89). Criteria for appropriate candidates for reassignment include a high level of comfort of the long-term therapist in recommending reassignment, absence of concurrent major psychiatric illness, social and familial support, lack of ambivalence in the patient regarding reassignment, young age, and success at integrating as the new gender. Criteria for inappropriate candidates are the discomfort of the long-term therapist in making a recommendation, active major psychiatric illness, active drug or alcohol abuse, history of mutilation or multiple suicide attempts, ambivalence and confusion regarding subjective gender on the part of the patient, and

incomplete or unsuccessful legal and social integration as the new gender (Brown 1990). Because social and personal stability are factors in
producing a positive outcome of reassignment, psychotherapy
throughout transition can improve results (Lundstrom et al. 1984).

Those patients who continue to live in the original gender or cannot for various reasons begin or complete reassignment remain in ongoing distress, and psychotherapy can help them find compromises
and alternate routes of gender expression as well as strengthen defenses against gender dysphoria. Because GID intensifies for many patients when they face stressful situations, any increase in the individual's
capacity to master stress may lower gender dysphoria. Symptoms may
develop that require the administration of psychotropic medications.

Psychotherapy alone may have reversed GID in some reported
cases, but in those cases, the psychotherapy was intensive, placing it
beyond the reach of most patients (Lothstein 1983, p. 305). It is perhaps most effective in mild cases of gender dysphoria. Because GID
appears to be "immutable to the effects of psychotherapy" (Kuiper,
unpublished article, December 1993, p. 1), many patients view it sus-
piciously as the means by which the medical establishment tries to block
SRS. The younger transsexual individuals for whom transsexuality is
ego-syntonic may have resistance to accepting ongoing psychotherapy.
However, their vulnerability to the social difficulties of homelessness,
prostitution, drug and alcohol addiction, poverty, and AIDS puts them
greatly in need of psychosocial services. The therapist must also encourage them not to seek underground treatments.

Sexual reassignment treats GID only, and while most patients report satisfaction with the outcome, they have to cope with losses and
at times isolation (Kuiper and Cohen-Kettinis 1988). Postsurgical psychotherapy should be recommended for these individuals.

Because SRS has been a subject of medical controversy, evaluation
of its effectiveness as a treatment for GID is of great importance. Since
the 1960s, 70 follow-up studies have been published, and all but one
(Meyer and Reter 1979) conclude that SRS was a satisfactory treatment
for many patients. These studies approach outcome from four viewpoints: social functioning, psychological functioning, physical functioning, and personal satisfaction (Kuiper, unpublished article,
December 1993).

As early as 1981, Pauley concluded that "a positive response to sex
reassignment surgery is ten times more likely than an unsatisfactory
outcome" (1981). Personal satisfaction as measured by asking whether

or not the individual would do it again rates between 90% and 100% (Blanchard et al. 1985; Kuiper and Cohen-Kettinis 1988; Lundstrom et al. 1984). Studies that examine characteristics that may be predictive of the most postsurgical dissatisfaction list the following factors: alcoholism, drug addiction, heterosexual experience, married, older age, lack of family and social support, psychosocial instability, and, for males, attraction to females and a more masculine body appearance (Lundstrom et al. 1984; Pfafflin 1992).

Psychological functioning as measured on the MMPI has been shown to improve after surgery (Fleming et al. 1981; Mate-Kole et al. 1990). Those postsurgical patients for whom cross-dressing had retained a fetishistic component showed more disturbance on psychological testing than the others (Beatrice 1985).

The most direct indication that SRS is a successful treatment would be the absence of gender dysphoria after surgery, and that apparently is the usual outcome. In a review of the literature, Pfafflin (1992) found less than 1% of the postsurgical men and slightly more of the women exhibited gender dysphoria regarding their new gender orientation, as shown by behavior consistent with returning to the prior gender role. This persistence of gender dysphoria was related to poor surgical outcome, failure to complete the "life test" (living at least 1 year as the new gender presurgically), and poor differential diagnosis. MTFs attracted to males tend to have more positive outcomes than MTFs attracted to females (Blanchard et al. 1989). However, because the latter tend to be older, they are more successful occupationally after surgical reassignment (Johnson and Hunt 1990).

Conclusion

Gender identity disorder is a lifelong condition of unknown etiology with a predictable course. The population with this disorder, although small, may be encountered in the private office, the detoxification center, the prison, the emergency and medical wards, the courts, and the family service agencies. Although gender dysphoria may not be the presenting issue, recognizing its presence is basic to understanding the patient from the biopsychosocial point of view.

Sexual reassignment including hormone therapy and surgery has been shown to be an effective treatment for a large number of these patients who otherwise would exist in constant emotional distress and socioeconomic despair. For those patients for whom reassignment is not advisable or possible, psychiatric care can provide substantial relief.

Although gender identity disorder "causes clinically significant distress or impairment in social, occupational, or other important areas of functioning" (American Psychiatric Association 1994, p. 538), individuals with GID are specifically excluded from the Americans with Disabilities Act and thus do not receive its benefits or protection. Although a large body of evidence exists that treatments are available and successful in many cases, insurers, public and private, specifically exclude coverage for treatment on the grounds that the treatments are either cosmetic or experimental. The stigma and discrimination thus directed at individuals with gender identity disorder prevent relief for many of them and perpetuate their distress and impairment.

Gender identity disorder relates gender and sexual orientation in intriguing ways, and the study of this disorder may eventually bring light to the darkness surrounding the origins of gender expression and sexual orientation.

References

Ackroyd P: Dressing Up. London, Thames and Hudson, 1979

Althof SE, et al: An MMPI subscale (gd): to identify males with gender identity conflicts. J Pers Assess 47:42–47, 1983

American Psychiatric Association: Diagnostic and Statistical Manual of Mental Disorders, 3rd Edition. Washington, DC, American Psychiatric Association, 1980

American Psychiatric Association: Diagnostic and Statistical Manual of Mental Disorders, 3rd Edition, Revised. Washington, DC, American Psychiatric Association, 1987

American Psychiatric Association: Diagnostic and Statistical Manual of Mental Disorders, 4th Edition. Washington, DC, American Psychiatric Association, 1994

Asschemen H, Gooren LJG, Eklund PLE: Mortality and morbidity in transsexual patients with cross-gender hormone treatment. Metabolism 38:869–873, 1989

Beatrice J: A psychological comparison of heterosexuals, transvestites, preoperative transsexuals and postoperative transsexuals. J Nerv Ment Dis 173:358–365, 1985

Blanchard R, Steiner BW, Clemmensen LH, et al: Prediction of regrets in postoperative transsexuals. Can J Psychiatry 34:43–45, 1989

Blanchard R, Steiner BW, Clemmensen LH: Gender dysphoria, gender reorientation and the clinical management of transsexualism. J Consult Clin Psychol 53:295–304, 1985

Blanchard R: The she-male phenomenon and the concept of partial autogynephilia. J Sex Marital Ther 19:73, 1993

Bolin A: In Search of Eve. Boston, MA, Bergin and Garvey, 1988

Bradley SJ, Blanchard R, Coates S, Green R, Levine SB, Meyer-Bahlburg HFL, Pauly IB, Zucker KJ: Interim report of the DSM-IV subcommittee on gender identity disorders. Arch Sex Behav 20:333–343, 1991

Brown GR: Transsexuals in the military: flight into hypermasculinity. Arch Sex Behav 17:527–537, 1988

Brown G: A review of clinical approaches to gender dysphoria. J Clin Psychiatry 51:57–64, 1990

Buhrich N: Psychological adjustment in transvestitism and transsexualism. Journal of Sex Research and Therapy 19:407–411, 1981

Buhrich N, McConaghy N: Parental relationships during childhood in homosexuality, transvestitism and transsexuality. Aust N Z J Psychiatry 12:103–108, 1978

Burns A, Farrell M, Brown JC: Clinical features of patients attending a gender-identity clinic. Br J Psychiatry 157:265–268, 1990

Cohen-Kettinis PT, Arrindell WA: Perceived parental rearing style, parental divorce and transsexualism: a controlled study. Journal of Psychological Medicine 20:613–620, 1990

Dixen JM, Maddever H, Van Maasden J, et al: Psychosocial characteristics of applicants evaluated for surgical gender reassignment. Arch Sex Behav 13:269–277, 1984

Eklund PLE, Gooren LJG, Bezener PD: Prevalence of transsexualism in the Netherlands. Br J Psychiatry 152:638–640, 1988

Fleming M, et al: A study of pre- and postsurgical transsexuals: MMPI characteristics. Arch Sex Behav 10:161–170, 1981

Fleming M, Steinman C, Bocknek G: Methodological problems in assessing sex reassignment surgery: a reply to Meyer and Reter. Arch Sex Behav 9:451–456, 1980

Freund K: Cross gender identity in a broader context, in Gender Dysphoria: Development, Research, Management. Edited by Steiner BW. New York, Plenum, 1985, pp 259–324

Garber M: Vested Interests. New York, Routledge, Chapman and Hall, 1992

Green R: Gender identity in childhood and later sexual orientation: follow-up of 78 males. Am J Psychiatry 142:339–341, 1985

Green R, Stoller RJ, MacAndrew C: Attitudes towards sex transformation procedures. Arch Gen Psychiatry 13:178–182, 1966

Hirschfeld M: Die Transvestiten, 2nd Edition. Liepzig, Wahrheit, 1925

Hoenig J: Etiology of transsexualism, in Gender Dysphoria: Development, Research, Management. Edited by Steiner BW. New York, Plenum Press, 1985, pp 33–74

Horner AJ: In the affirmation of gender in male patients. J Am Acad Psychoanal 20:599–610, 1992

Jani S, Rosenberg L: Systematic evaluation of sexual functioning of eunuch-transvestites: a study of 12 cases. J Sex Marital Ther 16:103–110, 1990

Johnson SL, Hunt DD: The relationship of male transsexual typology to psychosocial adjustment. Arch Sex Behav 19:349–360, 1990

Kuiper B, Cohen-Kettins P: Sex reassignment surgery: a study of 141 Dutch transsexuals. Arch Sex Behav 17: 439–457, 1988

Lothstein LM: Female-to-Male Transsexualism: Historical, Clinical and Theoretical Issues. Boston, MA, Routledge and Kegan Paul, 1983

Lundstrom B, Pauly I, Walinder J: Outcome of sex reassignment surgery. Acta Psychiatr Scand 70: 289–294, 1984

Mate-Kole C, Freschi M, Robin A: A controlled study of psychological and social change after surgical gender reassignment in selected male transsexuals. Br J Psychiatry 157:261–264, 1990

Meyer J, Reter D: Sex reassignment. Arch Gen Psychiatry 36:1010–1015, 1979

Mihalik GJ: More than two: anthropological perspectives on gender. Journal of Gay and Lesbian Psychotherapy 1:105–118, 1989

Money J: Gay, Straight and In-Between. New York, Oxford Press, 1988, pp 9–50

Money J, Lamacz M: Gynemimesis and gynemimetophilia: individual and cross-cultural manifestations of a gender-coping strategy hitherto unnamed. Compr Psychiatry 25:392–403, 1984

Paglia C: Sexual Personae. New York, Vintage Books, 1991

Pauly IB, Edgerton MT: The gender identity movement: a growing surgical-psychiatric liaison. Arch Sex Behav 15: 315–329, 1986

Pauly IB: Outcome of sex reassignment surgery for transsexuals. Aust N Z J Psychiatry 15:45–51, 1981

Pfafflin F: Regrets after reassignment surgery, in Gender Dysphoria: Interdisciplinary Approaches in Clinical Management. Edited by Bockting WO, Coleman E. New York, Haworth, 1992, pp 65–89

Pillard RC, Weinrich JD: The periodic table model of the gender transpositions: Part I. A theory based on masculinization and defeminization of the brain. J Sex Res 23:425–454, 1987

Shore ER: The former transsexual: A case study. Arch Sex Behav 11: 377–385, 1984

Steiner BW: From Sappho to Sand: Historical perspective on cross-dressing and cross gender. Can J Psychiatry 36: 502–506, 1981

Steiner BW: Transsexuals, transvestites and their partners, in Gender Dysphoria: Development, Research, Management. Edited by Steiner BW, New York, Plenum, 1985, pp 351–364

Stoller RJ: Sex and Gender. New York, Science House, 1968

Verschoor AM, Poortinga J: Psychosocial differences between Dutch male and female transsexuals. Arch Sex Behav 17:173–178, 1988

Walker PA, Berger JC, Green R, et al: Standards of Care: The Hormonal and Surgical Sex Reassignment of Gender Dysphoric Persons. Palo Alto, CA, Harry Benjamin International Gender Dysphoria Association, 1990

Zuger B: Is early effeminate behavior in boys early homosexuality? Compr Psychiatry 29:509–519, 1988

Institutional Discrimination Against Lesbians, Gay Men, and Bisexuals

The Courts, Legislature, and the Military

David W. Purcell, J.D., Ph.D.
Daniel W. Hicks, M.D.

N umerous factors affect the mental health of lesbians, gay men, and bisexuals, including 1) internalized feelings about one's own sexuality; 2) reactions to the attitudes of friends, relatives, fellow employees, and other individuals; and 3) the impact of institutional attitudes manifested by the courts, legislatures, and the military, as well as political and religious organizations. Although historically the attitudes of both individuals and institutions toward lesbians, gay men, and bisexuals can be characterized as hostile and disapproving, some positive changes have occurred in the 25 years since Stonewall, the beginning of the movement for civil rights for lesbians, gay men, and bisexuals. Today, sharply conflicting views about sexual orientation share an uneasy existence in America (Editors-Harvard Law Review [HLR] 1989). The focus of this chapter is on the institutional attitudes in American society that may affect mental health, with principal consideration given to the courts, legislatures, and the military.

The manner in which lesbians, gay men, and bisexuals have been and continue to be treated by powerful societal institutions is not only the product of prejudice; the attitudes manifested by these institutions play a key role in perpetuating and giving rise to new prejudice by providing official sanction to individuals who hold hostile attitudes (Bersoff and Ogden 1991; Melton 1989). In essence, these institutional attitudes support the persistence of individual hatred, fear, and violence. Although many groups suffer from prejudice, lesbians, gay men, and bisexuals are unique because discrimination and intolerance toward them often are supported by religious, governmental, and social institutions (see Chapter 7 by Herek). Violence is a natural outgrowth of this pervasive institutional intolerance (see Chapter 48 by Klinger and Stein).

It is reasonable to assume that institutional ignorance and bigotry have a negative impact on the mental health of lesbians, gay men, and bisexuals, especially those most in need of social approval, such as adolescents or those first becoming aware of their sexual feelings, regardless of age. Potential role models for gay youth, such as school teachers, stay closeted because of fears about their jobs and safety. Because gay people are persecuted by the military and vilified by courts and legislatures, they have become severely stigmatized and viewed in terms of undesirable stereotypes (Melton 1989). This process reinforces both individual homophobia in all members of society and internalized homophobia in lesbians, gay men, and bisexuals.

It is important for mental health professionals to be aware that prejudice and discrimination against lesbians, gay men, and bisexuals still are rampant in many societal institutions and individuals. Creating a nonjudgmental, empathic environment and understanding some of the special mental health issues for these men and women are necessary skills discussed in other chapters. Therapists also can play a crucial role by educating their peers, colleagues, schools, and communities about human sexuality and by working toward removing discriminatory laws and regulations, as well as by helping to elect judges and legislators who are supportive. Finally, through both research and education, mental health professionals can help to rebut the myths upon which many policies and court decisions are based (Herek 1991).

Courts and Legislatures

Much of the material in this book is based on scientific findings; however, very different considerations prevail in the legal and political domains. Courts and legislatures are political bodies subject to the sentiments of the majority, which are seldom based upon scientific knowledge (Rivera 1991). Legislation enacted both locally and nationally often reflects half-truths, prejudice, and popular myths. Although generally these myths have been disproved by scientific evidence (Herek 1991; Patterson 1992), this evidence has failed to have much influence on public opinion, and hence on legislators. One role of the courts in reviewing legislation is to temper the severity of popular judgment by applying and construing the law reasonably. Unfortunately, judges often are as biased as legislators (Stoddard 1992).

▓ Sodomy Laws and the Criminalization of Homosexual Conduct

The hostility of the criminal justice system toward lesbians, gay men, and bisexuals is evident in the laws passed to prohibit same-sex contact. The history of the enforcement of sodomy statutes has been muddled by the fact that the term "sodomy" lacks either a fixed cultural or social meaning (Hunter 1992). Sodomy statutes originally were adopted from religious regulations that were meant to prevent all nonmarital and nonprocreative sex. Existing in every state until 1962, sodomy statutes were aimed almost exclusively at men (regardless of the gender of the sex partner), and nonprocreation was at the heart of the crime. Sodomy laws in some states still exhibit the original intent to prevent nonprocreative sex by prohibiting oral and anal sex, even between spouses. Although same-sex contact was not the primary target of original sodomy laws, and woman-to-woman contact was not even contemplated or regulated at that time (Hunter 1992), today sodomy statutes usually are thought of in conjunction with the prohibition of same-sex sexual contact.

In 1948, Kinsey and his colleagues noted that 95% of all American men were committing sexual acts that were considered criminal under various state "sodomy" statutes (Kinsey 1948). In 1962, Illinois was the first state to adopt the Model Penal Code (MPC), a document drafted by national legal scholars as a model for revising and standardizing state criminal codes. The MPC decriminalized private, adult, consensual sex regardless of the gender of the participants (Rivera 1991). Since 1962, over half of the states either have repealed their sodomy statutes as applied to same-sex contact and replaced them with the MPC or have overturned them through state court rulings. In 21 states, however, same-sex conduct is still a crime (Wolfson 1994), and in many cases a felony (DeAngelis 1992). Moreover, there continues to be resistance to removing criminal sanctions for same-sex conduct. For example, when Arkansas and Tennessee adopted the MPC, thereby repealing sodomy laws applying to homosexual and heterosexual conduct, both legislatures turned around and specifically recriminalized only same-sex contact (Rivera 1991). Today, 5 states criminalize homosexual sodomy only, whereas 16 states criminalize both heterosexual and homosexual sodomy (Wolfson 1994).

The state-by-state approach to repealing sodomy laws has led to piecemeal change. Many legal scholars, however, believe that nationwide invalidation of sodomy laws is possible because such laws violate the federal constitutional rights of lesbians, gay men, and bisexual individuals on two grounds: 1) private, adult, sexual conduct is protected by the "right of privacy," a constitutional doctrine that has been interpreted to allow individuals to define themselves and their intimate relationships without governmental interference; and 2) certain laws discriminate against lesbians, gay men, and bisexual individuals as a class in violation of equal protection principles (Bersoff and Ogden 1991). Right to privacy claims are based on the right to engage in certain *conduct*, sodomy for example, whereas equal protection claims are based on unequal treatment based on *status* or *class*, for example, the class of people interested in same-sex contact (Bersoff and Ogden 1991).

Right to privacy. The U.S. Supreme Court has identified two related interests that are protected by the right to privacy: first, citizens can avoid disclosing personal matters, which includes recognizing a privacy interest in the home, where the government usually may not intrude (Bersoff and Ogden 1991); and second, citizens can make certain intimate decisions related to marriage, procreation, contraception, family relationships, and child rearing without governmental intrusion (Editors-HLR 1989). Prior privacy case law led many legal scholars to believe that same-gender, private, consensual sexual conduct would be found to be protected when and if the Supreme Court ruled on the issue (Rivera 1991).

However, in 1986, the Supreme Court upheld, by a narrow 5 to 4 margin, the right of Georgia to enforce its sodomy laws to restrain homosexual conduct because of the "ancient roots" of such laws *(Bowers v. Hardwick 1986).* In the case, Michael Hardwick was arrested in his own bedroom in a private home having sexual relations with another adult male. The majority narrowly framed the issue, finding that there is no right to privacy to engage in homosexual sodomy, thereby ignoring the fact that Georgia's sodomy statute also applies to heterosexual individuals (Editors-HLR 1989). The decision stunned legal activists and scholars and led to almost universal criticism in major newspapers and legal journals (Rivera 1991). The four dissenting members of the Court vigorously argued that the majority was deviating from prior precedent by focusing on the act of sodomy rather than on the underlying right to freedom from governmental intrusion in one's own bedroom (Editors-HLR 1989). Since *Hardwick,* legal authorities agree with the dissenters that the case was decided wrongly because the Court ignored and misread precedent. This case shows that bias against lesbians, gay men, and bisexual individuals occurs even among the loftiest reaches of the legal system.

It appears that the court also misjudged public opinion. At the time of *Hardwick,* polls showed that most Americans believed a fundamental right of privacy should exist for adult, consensual sexual relations (Rivera 1991). Furthermore, Justice Powell, who voted with the majority, has stated since his retirement from the Court that his vote was a mistake (Bersoff and Ogden 1991). *Hardwick* may not stand the test of time, although reversal may not come soon. In the case of the African American struggle for civil rights, it took 58 years for the Supreme Court in *Brown v. Board of Education* (1954) to overrule its "separate but equal" doctrine from *Plessy v. Ferguson* (1896) (Bersoff and Ogden 1991).

Until it is narrowed or overruled, *Hardwick* will dominate the law on the governmental regulation of sexuality (Hunter 1992). Although sodomy statutes are seldom enforced, the fact that the Supreme Court found them to be constitutional often has been used since *Hardwick* to justify other forms of legislative or judicial discrimination (Editors-HLR 1989). In legal briefs in cases involving the civil rights of gay men and lesbians, the American Psychological Association has argued that sodomy laws harm public health and individual mental health because neither same-gender sexual orientation nor same-sex sexual contact is pathological (Bersoff and Ogden 1991). Thus, preventing the development of same-sex sexual orientation and deterring such sexual conduct are not proper mental health goals. Furthermore, the threat of criminal punishment for private sexual acts harms public health efforts to deter the spread of HIV (Bersoff and Ogden 1991).

Equal protection.   After it became clear that constitutional challenges to state sodomy laws were not receiving sympathetic treatment in the courts, a new round of litigation arose focusing on laws that discriminate against lesbians, gay men, and bisexual individuals as a class, regardless of their behavior (Editors-HLR 1989). "Equal protection" claims arise only when the alleged inequality is the result of governmental action that creates discriminatory classifications among a "suspect class" of people. The three criteria for suspect classification are: 1) a long history of persecution due to irrational stereotypes; 2) an inability to obtain relief from nonjudicial branches of government; and 3) immutability of the trait, which makes it impossible or highly unlikely for its members to escape the class (Rivera 1991). To date, only race, national ancestry, and alienage have been granted suspect class status, whereas gender and illegitimacy have been found to be quasi-suspect classifications (Bersoff and Ogden 1991). Lesbians, gay men, and bisexual individuals should be able to meet the three requirements for suspect classification, although the test of immutability is the most uncertain (Rivera 1991). Legal scholars, however, have suggested that sexual orientation does meet the immutability test (Green 1988), in part because recent evidence suggests that sexual orientation is highly resistant to change (Melton 1989) and is at least partially attributable to biological and genetic factors (Friedman and Downey 1993). In the future, equal protection claims are the most likely legal strategy for attacking institutionalized discrimination.

■ The Recognition of Same-Sex Intimate Relationships

Although the legal definition of family has been expanding, same-sex intimate relationships generally have not been included (Editors-HLR 1989). Historically, a prevailing assumption in society has been that same-sex relationships are not sustainable and that heterosexual relationships are superior unions (Herek 1991). Society continues to hold a heterosexist bias that values heterosexual unions and devalues all others (see Chapter 7 by Herek in this volume), even though the data show that same-sex and opposite-sex pairings are similarly diverse in both the forms they take and in level of psychological health (Peplau 1991; Blumstein and Schwartz 1983). In secular society, the state promotes and protects the institution of heterosexual marriage by outlining the benefits, rights, and responsibilities associated with it and generally undermines same-sex couples by not recognizing them as worthy of support or protection (Robson and Valentine 1990). Some churches perform the same role in the religious domain.

Because heterosexual marital units are used as the standard by which "family" is defined, lesbians, gay men, and bisexual individuals often find themselves severely disadvantaged by the legal system. For example, they usually cannot obtain health benefits for their partners, cannot take family leave or bereavement leave for a partner's illness or death, nor can they file a joint tax return, even if it would be beneficial (Rivera 1991). If a same-sex partner dies or is incapacitated by an accident, the other spouse has no inherent right to visit his or her partner in the hospital, to help in making life-changing decisions, or to collect workers' compensation benefits (Editors-HLR 1989). The potential result of these policies was seen in 1983 in Minnesota when the parents of a woman severely injured in a car accident refused to acknowledge her lesbian partner or to allow her any access to the injured woman, despite the fact that the two women had lived together for 7 years and had purchased a home together. Only after a 7-year court battle was the woman awarded guardianship over her injured partner (Lesbian made guardian 1991). In most cases, such problems can be avoided by formally executing a legal package of wills, medical powers of attorney, and housing agreements, but for those who do not have such foresight, the default in the legal system is to ignore the existence of same-sex relationships.

Increasingly, lesbians, gay men, and bisexual individuals have been seeking equal treatment of their relationships through legislation, including the right to marry. In the past 5 years, Sweden, Denmark, and Norway have expanded their definitions of marriage to include same-sex couples. Some municipalities, corporations, and universities now offer "domestic partners" benefits to same-sex couples. In most cases, these measures offer economic benefits to same-sex couples, but they do not erase most of the disadvantages inherent in the legal system. In Hawaii, the state supreme court recently held that the ban on same-sex marriages may violate the state's equal protection clause and sent the case back for trial. However, in response to the court's decision, Hawaii's legislators quickly passed legislation banning same-sex marriages (Gallagher 1994c; Henry 1994) and a few other state legislatures have followed suit. In New York, the highest court recently expanded the definition of "family" to include gay couples, when it held that the life partner of a man who died of AIDS was family, and thus he could not be evicted from the apartment that was in his deceased partner's name (*Braschi v. State Associates Co. 1989*). Thus, there appears to be increasing support for an expanded definition of "family" in some courts, but 64% of the American public still is against same-sex marriages (Henry 1994), a figure that likely affects legislators.

■ Family Law Regarding Custody and Visitation Rights

Lesbian, gay, and bisexual parents who seek custody or visitation rights in divorce proceedings often have their sexuality used against them. The standard used in most states to determine custody, "the best interests of the child," is ambiguous and highly subjective, thereby leaving judges with broad discretion to consider those facts they think are most pertinent (Falk 1989). Moreover, custody questions are matters of state law decided by judges, not juries, and these decisions are difficult to get reversed on appeal (Rivera 1991). Uninformed or homophobic judges can make a custody hearing very traumatic for a lesbian, gay, or bisexual parent. With visitation, there is a presumption that visits are in the best interest of the child and visits are denied only if they would harm the child. However, in some cases, courts have restricted visits with lesbian, gay, and bisexual parents to no overnight stays, not going to the home shared with a same-sex partner, and not being around the parent's friends. These limitations clearly diminish the visitation rights of parents living a long distance from their children and place a heavy burden on the parent-child relationship (Editors-HLR 1989).

The preliminary problem faced by many lesbian, gay, and bisexual parents in custody and visitation cases is that sexual orientation concerns tend to overshadow the other evidence that is usually relied upon in such cases (Falk 1989). Furthermore, often no attempt is made to link the parent's sexuality to the child's welfare. In such cases, courts talk generally about the "harm" of the environment without articulating with any specificity what the impact will be on the child (Falk 1980). Even when courts do try to establish a connection between a parent's sexual orientation and the child's best interests, they often rely on general myths about homosexuality and ignore expert testimony and research findings (Falk 1989).

A number of myths, disproved by social science research for the most part, are commonly evoked in child custody and visitation cases (Falk 1989; Rivera 1991). The myths concern a variety of topics including 1) the fitness of the parent (the belief that homosexuals are mentally ill and, thus, cannot be good parents or that lesbians are poor mothers because they are less maternal); 2) the nature of the parent-child relationship (the thought that children are likely to be molested by gay parents or friends or that gender role development will be impaired); 3) the possibility of social bias (the idea that these children will be teased and stigmatized because of the sexual orientation of their parent); and 4) the morality of the parent's lifestyle (the judgment that homosexuality is immoral so the parent is unfit to be a parent). If a judge subscribes to the "moral" view, the custody proceeding often becomes a trial of the parent's sexuality rather than an inquiry into the best interests of the child (Rivera 1991). For example, in an ongoing Virginia case, the trial judge awarded custody of a 2-year-old boy to his grandmother rather than to his biological mother, Sharon Bottoms, because she was living with her female partner, thus violating the state's sodomy law. The Virginia Court of Appeals overturned the lower court decision, but the Virginia Supreme Court reversed, awarding custody to the child's grandmother (Bull 1995a). In the process, the court overlooked the growing scientific evidence that reveals few differences between children raised by gay or lesbian parents as compared to heterosexual parents (Patterson 1992). Although the court found additional reasons other than sexual orientation to deny custody, it also made clear that being a gay or lesbian parent, by itself, was sufficient to deny custody because of the "social condemnation" attached to gay and lesbian relationships, which ultimately will harm the child (Bull 1995a).

Custody battles are inherently traumatic, but if the sexual orientation of one parent becomes an issue in the case, intrusive and upsetting cross-examination can be expected. Lesbian, gay, and bisexual parents are unlikely to be emotionally prepared for the ugliness of such a battle and the psychological scars can be long lasting, especially if the decision is adverse. Individuals who recently have come out or who lack a support system may be particularly at risk in such cases. Children also are likely to be victims in such custody battles because these cases tend to be highly charged and lengthy. In the meantime, the child and the parents are left in limbo as precious years pass. Familiarizing lesbian, gay, and bisexual parents with the myths that courts may rely upon can help them to be psychologically prepared to handle a custody fight.

■ Employment Rights

Whether sexual orientation will be considered during an employee's hiring, promotion, annual review, or severance is an issue with daily significance. Approximately 25% of lesbians and gay men report discrimination in employment (Editors-HLR 1989). Lesbian, gay, and bisexual employees worry about whether they should remain closeted to obtain and retain satisfactory employment (Rivera 1991), and many report going to elaborate lengths to hide their orientation at work. Negative mental health effects are likely when employees have to continually worry about discovery of their sexual orientation during the employment process. It also may lead individuals to scale back their employment expectations and to seek jobs only in fields thought to be more accepting.

Private employment. Most Americans are surprised to discover that, in many cases, employers can fire them for no reason (Editors-HLR 1989). However, this "employment-at-will" doctrine has been limited by three developments: 1) federal and state antidiscrimination laws, which limit the ability of employers to consider race, gender, age, national origin, and handicap; 2) collective bargaining agreements, which usually require "just cause" for discharge of union employees; and 3) express or implied contracts between the employee and employer, which may be found to limit the employer's discretion in firing an employee (Rivera 1991). Unfortunately, these developments have not limited an employer's ability to discriminate against lesbian, gay, and bisexual employees in the private sector (Editors-HLR 1989), although more recently labor unions on the national level have become more proactive in favor of these employees (Rivera 1991). Moreover, eight states have passed laws adding "sexual orientation" to the classes protected by at least some civil rights laws, although usually only public employment is protected. Public opinion polls show that a majority of Americans support equal job opportunities for lesbians, gay men, and bisexual individuals (62%), even if they disapprove of other civil rights for this group (Henry 1994). Congress currently is considering a bill that provides that employees cannot be fired based solely on their sexual orientation, but a recent conservative shift in Congress makes passage unlikely.

Public employment.   The three most relevant types of public (government) employment are the military (discussed separately below), the civil service, and jobs requiring security clearances. In civil service jobs, great progress has been made since the late 1960s, when employees first began challenging the government's right to fire them arbitrarily (Rivera 1991). In 1976, President Carter issued a new policy for federal employees stating that their private lives were not relevant to personnel decisions. At least nine state governors have issued executive orders and a number of cities and counties have passed laws banning discrimination against gay people in civil service jobs (Rivera 1991). In practice, however, court rulings indicate that federal employees still may be risking their jobs if they are not discreet about their sexual orientation (Editors-HLR 1989). Thus, even in this more friendly work setting, gay people continue to be burdened by having to monitor their behavior.

Lesbians, gay men, and bisexual individuals have had an especially hard time obtaining and retaining jobs that require a security clearance, as in the FBI or CIA, because of fear that the gay employee could be blackmailed about his or her sexuality. The assumptions behind this prohibition have been challenged, usually unsuccessfully, due to the great deference given by the courts to security concerns by quasi-military agencies like the FBI and CIA (Rivera 1991). However, in 1994, after a protracted lawsuit by a gay male FBI agent who was fired after many years of excellent service, the FBI agreed to stop discriminating on the basis of sexual orientation in hiring and firing (FBI pledges gay equality 1994). Similarly, just a week earlier, Attorney General Janet Reno announced a policy barring all Justice Department agencies from discriminating on the basis of sexual orientation.

The regulation of public school students and teachers.   In school settings, lesbian, gay, and bisexual students and teachers have different concerns and are affected by different legal doctrines, although both groups are faced with questions about their right to raise the topic of sexual orientation in public schools. The legal regulations imposed on students and teachers are important because many people first recognize same-sex feelings in high school and college. Moreover, the restriction on the free exchange of information about sexuality in school settings leaves many teenagers and young adults with no role models or sources of information, thus increasing their risk for poor mental health outcomes.

Public schools are a forum where two competing values collide: school as a forum for free speech versus school as a tool to instill society's mores and values (Editors-HLR 1989). Under "free speech" and "free association" principles of the U.S. Constitution, both state and federal courts have held that lesbian, gay, and bisexual college students, and to a lesser extent high school students, do have the right to meet, form formal groups, advocate, and socialize together (Rivera 1991). Lesbian, gay, and bisexual high school teachers have not fared nearly as well as students regarding their ability to discuss or to reveal their sexual orientation in school. Generally, courts have allowed teachers very little discretion to be open (Editors-HLR 1989). Courts balance the teacher's right to free speech versus the school's right to maintain an efficient workplace. Cases, which usually arise when a teacher challenges his or her firing, have tended to allow disclosure, speech, and participation in activities outside of school but have not allowed discussion or disclosure of sexual orientation in the classroom (Editors-HLR 1989).

■ Recent Trends in Judicial and Legislative Protections

Despite the overall hostility of the judiciary and legislatures, lesbians, gay men, and bisexual individuals have achieved some measure of civil rights and protections through federal and state hate crimes laws as well as state and city civil rights laws.

Hate crimes protections.   Lesbians, gay men, and bisexual individuals are a principal target of hate crimes, including verbal and physical assaults leading even to murder (see Chapter 48 by Klinger and Stein). In 1990, the federal Hate Crimes Statistics Act was passed, requiring law enforcement agencies nationwide to collect statistics on hate crimes against a number of groups, including crimes based on "sexual orientation." In addition, almost 40 states and the District of Columbia now have hate crimes laws, which elevate penalties for crimes committed because a person belongs to a certain class. Unfortunately, only 22 states and the District of Columbia include protection for sexual orientation in their hate crimes law (Boulard 1994).

Civil rights legislation.   To date, eight states—California, Connecticut, Hawaii, Massachusetts, Minnesota, New Jersey, Vermont, and Wisconsin—and numerous urban areas protect gay men and lesbians (and in some cases bisexual individuals and/or transgendered people) against some form of discrimination, usually in housing, employment, and education (Henry 1994). Although many lesbians, gay men, and bisexual individuals remain unprotected or only partially protected, these moderate advances have alarmed Christian right-wing groups, leading to backlash (Henry 1994).

Numerous right-wing groups have organized in a concerted effort to take the decision-making authority concerning civil rights based on sexual orientation away from the courts and to give that power back to the voters. These organizations have been trying to accomplish this through statewide ballot initiatives or repeal of local legislation. For example, in 1992, the citizens of Colorado passed Amendment 2, which amended the state's constitution to repeal civil rights protections based on sexual orientation in four Colorado cities and prohibited any other city from passing such civil rights protections. Although the district court judge found Amendment 2 unconstitutional and the Colorado Supreme Court agreed (Gallagher 1994b), the decision was appealed and the case will be heard by the U.S. Supreme Court in late 1995 (Morales 1995). Even if the Supreme Court finds that antigay initiatives are unconstitutional, conservative organizations already are pursuing other ways to deny equal rights to lesbians, gay men, and bisexual individuals in the areas of adoptions, foster parenting, and marriage (Bull 1995b).

The Military

The military is the largest secular institution in the United States with a clearly articulated policy of exclusion of gays and lesbians (Rivera 1991). Prior to World War I, there were no official policies concerning homosexuals in uniform, but persons engaging in homosexual acts were punished and discharged (Berube 1990). Nonetheless, anecdotal and historical evidence confirms that thousands of gay people have served honorably in the military throughout the history of the United States (Shilts 1993).

■ History of the Military Policy on Homosexuality

After World War I, psychiatrists were asked to devise interviews to screen recruits who may have mental illness, in response to the tremendous number of psychiatric casualties that had occurred. The interviews included diagnostic criteria for homosexuality, considered a mental illness at the time. Persons with "degenerative physiques" (feminine body types), "perverts," and "psychopaths" were excluded. These were the first written standards regulating the "condition" of homosexuality rather than homosexual conduct, although they were not routinely enforced (Berube 1990).

When the United States began preparations for World War II, homosexuality still was viewed as an illness. However, certain psychiatrists thought that homosexual applicants should be referred for compassionate treatment, not subjected to criminal prosecution. Although a few applicants were deferred from service due to confessed or alleged homosexuality, most homosexuals were not detected and went on to serve their country (Rivera 1991; Shilts 1993). Women also were extensively recruited for the first time during World War II, but screening for lesbians was rarely enforced due to the acute need for personnel (Berube 1990).

After World War II, the demand for troops decreased dramatically. Under the influence of the conservative McCarthy era, the policy that had been initiated to "protect" homosexuals was used to eliminate them from the military. Persons known or suspected to be homosexual were interrogated until they confessed; then they were asked to implicate others in exchange for lesser punishment. This led to massive "witch hunts" that ruined careers and resulted in dishonorable discharges (Shilts 1993). This method was used to keep the "homosexual problem" under control until the birth of the gay liberation movement.

After the 1969 Stonewall riots and the gay rights movement, lesbians and gay men in the military began challenging their superiors, refusing to accept their discharges, and going to court to protect their reputations and careers. In 1976, Leonard Matlovich, a decorated Vietnam veteran, openly declared himself to be gay, and he was immediately dishonorably discharged (Rivera 1991); he took the case to court and eventually won a cash settlement. However, in the majority of court cases brought by discharged personnel in the 1970s, judges generally deferred to the military policy based on national security concerns (Cooper 1993).

In the face of increasing court challenges and inconsistent application of the exclusionary policy among military branches, conservative Reagan administration officials drafted new regulations that explicitly declared that "homosexuality is incompatible with military service" (Department of Defense Directive 1981). These regulations gave more authority for discharge based on gay or lesbian "status," not just conduct. From 1980 to 1990, 16,919 service members were discharged for homosexuality, at a cost of $500 million for retraining and replacement, not including the costs of investigations or trials (United States General Accounting Office Report [USGAO] 1992).

President Clinton was elected in 1992 with the promise that he would lift the military ban against lesbians, gay men, and bisexual individuals. Clinton announced a plan to write an executive order removing the ban, but political reaction from the well-organized conservative right led him to investigate the issue further. Defense Secretary Les Aspin commissioned a special RAND National Defense Research Institute report which found that 1) public opinion was more against racial integration in the 1940s (61% against) than against homosexual integration today (21% against); 2) unit task cohesion would not be harmed by integration, even if social cohesion failed to develop between gay people and heterosexual individuals; and 3) all service personnel should adhere to equally high standards of conduct, regardless of sexual identity (DeAngelis 1993). However, Senator Sam Nunn, chair of the Armed Services Committee, who was opposed to removing the ban, structured the hearings so that it appeared that allowing homosexuals into the military would be a threat to national security. Ultimately, Nunn's committee recommended the "Don't Ask, Don't Tell" proposal, a compromise that President Clinton was willing to accept (DOD Memorandum 1993).

Under this policy, applicants to the military will no longer be asked questions about their sexual orientation; if gay men and lesbians do not mention their orientation, they will be allowed to serve in the military. Once admitted to the military, if gay men and lesbians mention their sexual orientation or behavior at work, this could be grounds for separation. Theoretically, witch hunts are less likely to occur because commanders must have credible evidence, not just suspicion or rumor, to begin an investigation about alleged homosexuality. However, what constitutes homosexual conduct is not well defined in the regulation; it may include nonsexual physical contact between two persons of the same sex or private conversation that may be overheard. Recent reports regarding enforcement of the new policy indicate that harassment of gay and lesbian personnel continues and that individuals have been discharged even when carefully following the new policy (Gallagher 1994a).

■ Challenges to the Military Policy

The same arguments that were used in an attempt to prevent integration by race and sex have been used to prevent lesbians, gay men, and bisexual individuals from serving in the military, including perceived threats to national security, unit morale, and unit cohesion. However, a number of reports over the years have shown convincingly that discrimination against lesbians, gay men, and bisexual individuals in the military has no rational basis. The Crittenden report, commissioned in 1957 but suppressed for several years, found that gays and lesbians do not pose an increased security risk (USGAO Report 1992). Recent reports from top military leaders lend support to the fact that gay troops perform well and are not security risks (USGAO Report 1992). In 1988, the military commissioned a report by the Defense Personnel Security Research and Education Center (PERSEREC), which was suppressed until congressional pressure led to its release. The PERSEREC Report revealed that gay men and lesbians were rated in their job performance as equal to or better than their heterosexual peers (Dyer 1990). One of the authors (D. W. Hicks, unpublished observations, 1994) reports that many lesbians, gay men, and bisexual individuals are fairly open about their sexual orientation in their units and serve with no problems or disruptions. Moreover, in other countries, where sexual orientation is not reason for exclusion from the military, there have been no major problems in military functioning (USGAO Report 1992). Furthermore, paramilitary organizations such as police and fire departments also have effectively integrated openly gay persons without major difficulties, with training and desensitization (Herek 1993).

Increasingly, the courts are being used to challenge the exclusionary policy and the underlying assumptions on which it is based (USGAO Report 1992; Stoddard 1992). Although each case is decided on its individual merits, the predominant message from the courts in their rulings has been that, due to the unique nature of the military, the armed forces should be allowed to have their own special requirements and restrictions, which could include the exclusion of gay men and lesbians. Recently, however, judges have challenged the rationale for the exclusion and have asked for more definitive evidence to support its continuation. For example, the cases of sailor Keith Meinhold, Annapolis cadet Joseph Steffan, and Colonel Margarethe Cammermeyer—all of whom openly declared their homosexuality—are significant because all were ordered back to duty or awarded commissions on court orders (Caplan 1994). Some of these cases are currently in appeal, but the current trend is for some courts to view the discharge of highly trained, competent troops, based solely on their sexual orientation, to be legally suspect. In the short term, the positive publicity about these cases may be more important than whether the suit actually is won, but in the long term, for the policy to end, Congress must believe that it no longer serves a valid purpose or that public opinion no longer supports it (Stoddard 1992).

■ The Role of Mental Health Professionals

The military policy on homosexuality does not foster a healthy environment of openness, honesty, and self-esteem for lesbians, gay men, and bisexual individuals. It is important for care providers to recognize that most active duty clients will not feel comfortable discussing sexual orientation issues because of fears of discharge if the information is not protected (Caplan 1994). Many people join the military in their late teens, before they are fully aware of their sexual identity. Moreover, the military environment is not conducive to an open exploration of sexuality; thus many such persons have never recognized or acknowledged their same-sex feelings. Mental health providers must be aware of these special circumstances in order to build trust, and they must work to establish strict confidentiality in order to create an atmosphere that allows safe exploration of sexual issues and the amelioration of the effects of internalized homophobia.

References

Bersoff DN, Ogden DW: APA amicus curiae briefs: furthering lesbian and gay male civil rights. Am Psychol 46:950–956, 1991

Berube A: Coming Out Under Fire: The History of Gay Men and Women in World War Two. New York, Free Press, 1990

Blumstein P, Schwartz P: American Couples: Money, Work and Sex. New York, William Morrows, 1983

Boulard G: The anti-twinkie defense. The Advocate, June 14, 1994, pp 33–38

Bowers v Hardwick, 478 US 186 (1986)

Braschi v State Associates Co., 544 NYS 2d 784 (Ct. App. 1989)

Brown v Board of Education, 347 US 483 (1954)

Bull C: Losing the war. The Advocate, pp 33–35, May 30, 1995a

Bull C: See you in court. The Advocate, p 18, April 4, 1995b

Caplan L: Don't ask, don't tell, marine style. Newsweek, p 28, June 13, 1994

Cooper MS: Equal protection and sexual orientation in military and security contexts: an analysis of recent federal decisions. Law and Sexuality: A Review of Lesbian and Gay Legal Issues 3:201–243, 1993

DeAngelis T: Kentucky high court repeals sodomy law. American Psychological Association Monitor, December 30, 1992, p 1

DeAngelis T: Report could help challenge DoD policy. American Psychological Association Monitor, December, 1993, p 28

Department of Defense (DOD) Directive Number 1332.14, sec. h.1, Enlisted Administrative Separations, 1981, revised 1982

Dyer K (ed): Gays in Uniform: The Pentagon's Secret Report. Boston, MA, Alyson Publications, 1990

Editors-Harvard Law Review: Developments in the law: sexual orientation and the law. Harv Law Rev 102:1508–1671, 1989

Falk PJ: Lesbian mothers: psychosocial assumptions in family law. Am Psychol 44:941–947, 1989

FBI pledges gay equality in settlement of lawsuit. The Atlanta Constitution, March 23, 1994, p A6, column 1

Friedman RC, Downey J: Neurobiology and sexual orientation: current relationships. J Neuropsychiatry Clin Neurosci 5:131–153, 1993

Gallagher J: Some things never change. The Advocate, pp 46–47, May 17, 1994a

Gallagher J: A victory in the courts. The Advocate, pp 41, February 8, 1994b

Gallagher J: The wedding is off. The Advocate, pp 24–27, May 17, 1994c

Green R: The immutability of (homo)sexual orientation: behavioral science implications for a constitutional (legal) analysis. Journal of Psychiatry and Law 16:537–575, 1988

Henry WA: Pride and prejudice. Time, June 27, 1994, pp 54–59

Herek GM: Myths about sexual orientation: a lawyer's guide to social science research. Law and Sexuality: A Review of Lesbian and Gay Legal Issues 1:133–172, 1991

Herek GM: Policy implications of lifting the ban on homosexuals in the military: testimony before the U.S. House Armed Services Committee, by the American Psychological Association, Washington, DC, May 5, 1993

Hunter ND: Life after Hardwick. Harvard Civil Rights-Civil Liberties Law Review 27:531–554, 1992

Kinsey AC, Pomeroy WB, Martin CE: Sexual Behavior in the Human Male. Philadelphia, PA, WB Saunders, 1948

Lesbian made guardian of her quadriplegic lover. The Atlanta Constitution, December 18, 1991, p A6

Melton GB: Public policy and private prejudice: psychology and law on gay rights. Am Psychol 44:933–940, 1989

Morales J: Cases closing. The Advocate, May 30, 1995, p 26

Patterson CJ: Children of lesbian and gay parents. Child Dev 63:1025–1042, 1992

Peplau LA: Lesbian and gay relationships, in Homosexuality: Research Implications for Public Policy. Edited by Gonsiorek JC, Weinrich JD. Newbury Park, CA, Sage Publications, 1991, pp 177–196

Plessy v Ferguson, 163 US 537 (1896)

Rivera RR: Sexual orientation and the law, in Homosexuality: Research Implications for Public Policy. Edited by Gonsiorek JC, Weinrich JD. Newbury Park, CA, Sage Publications, 1991, pp 81–100

Robson R, Valentine SE: Lov(h)ers: lesbians as intimate partners and lesbian legal theory. Temple Law Review 63:511–541, 1990

Shilts R: Conduct Unbecoming: Gays and Lesbians in the U.S. Military. New York, St. Martin's Press, 1993

Stoddard TB: Lesbian and gay rights litigation before a hostile federal judiciary: extracting benefit from peril. Harvard Civil Rights-Civil Liberties Law Review 27:555–573, 1992

U.S. General Accounting Office Report to Congressional Requesters: Defense force management: DOD's policy on homosexuality. GAO/NSIAD-92-98, P.O. Box 6015, Gaithersburg, MD, 20877, June 1992

Wolfson E: Fighting sodomy laws. The Lambda Update, LLDEF, 666 Broadway, Suite 1200, New York, NY 10012, Summer 1994

47

Substance Abuse in Gay Men, Lesbians, and Bisexuals

Robert P. Cabaj, M.D.

A lcohol and other drugs have a major impact on the lives of gay men, lesbians, and bisexual individuals. There is no solid agreement about the amount of alcohol and other substances used or the incidence of substance abuse in the gay, lesbian, and bisexual population. Most studies (Beatty 1983; Diamond and Wilsnack 1978; Lewis et al. 1982; Lohrenz et al. 1978; McKirman and Peterson 1989a; Mosbacher 1988; Pillard 1988; Saghir and Robbins 1973), reports (L. Fifield et al., unpublished observations, 1975; Lesbian and Gay Substance Abuse Planning Group, unpublished observations, August 1991), or reviews of surveys (E. S. Morales et al., unpublished observations, 1983; Weinberg and Williams 1974) and the experiences of most clinicians working with gay men and lesbians (Cabaj 1992; Finnegan and McNally 1987) estimate an incidence of substance abuse of all types at approximately 30%—with ranges of 28%–35%; this estimate contrasts with an incidence of 10%–12% for the general population.

A careful review of each report, however, demonstrates significant and persistent methodological problems, ranging from poor or absent control groups, to unrepresentative population samples (some studies gathered subjects only from gay and lesbian bars), to a failure to use uniform definitions of substance abuse or of homosexuality itself. Nonetheless, no matter where the sample was taken—urban or rural, various socioeconomic settings, in the United States or other countries—the rates are strikingly uniform, although there are some variations in use reported. For example, Stall and Wiley (1988) note greater substance use but no greater alcohol use in gay men compared with heterosexual men in San Francisco, whereas McKirman and Peterson (1989a) report that heavy alcohol use was not greater for gay men and lesbians compared with heterosexual persons sampled but did note that there were fewer gay and lesbian alcohol abstainers and a greater number of gay and lesbian moderate alcohol users.

A few surveys have focused on lesbian substance abuse, including one in the general population (J. Bradford et al., unpublished observations, 1987) and one in lesbian medical students (Mosbacher 1993). Both reports continue to indicate a high use of alcohol and other drugs in lesbians and a higher concern over a problem with alcohol and drug use than in similar heterosexual populations. Currently, no study specifically focuses on the drug or alcohol use of bisexual men or women, although many such people are included in some of the studies described above. Most of the ideas in this chapter can apply to bisexual individuals, because the focus is on the effects of external and internalized homophobia.

Alcohol abuse has been the primary focus of most studies. No specific studies of injecting drug use (IDU) and the gay population are currently available. The Center for Disease Control's (1994) quarterly reports on AIDS and HIV infections clearly indicate a subgroup of IDU gay and bisexual men, and one of the routes of HIV infection for lesbians is via injecting drug use.

Substance Abuse and Gay Identity Formation

Many factors contribute to the prominent role of substance use and abuse in gay men, lesbians, and bisexual individuals. At one point, American psychoanalytic psychiatry, for years focused on the etiology of male homosexuality, even postulated that homosexuality was a cause of alcoholism (Israelstam and Lambert 1983). Because homosexuality, repressed or not, does not cause alcoholism (Israelstam and Lambert

1986)—indeed, alcoholism and substance abuse are not "caused" by any psychodynamic or personality factor alone—other factors must be examined, the two most important being genetic and biological contributions and the psychological effects of homophobia, both external and internal.

New research continues to support, in great part, genetic, biological, and biochemical origins for the diseases of alcoholism and substance abuse. Similarly, there is continuing and growing evidence that homosexual orientation may have—at least in part—genetic, biological, and biochemical components (Pillard 1988; Pillard and Weinrich 1986; Pillard et al. 1982; see Chapter 9 by Byne and Chapter 8 by Pillard). Such parallel contributions to both sexual orientation and substance abuse have led to some speculation of a possible chromosomal link between the genetic contributions to substance abuse and sexual orientation. Such a direct genetic link between sexual orientation and the propensity to substance abuse, however, is unlikely. The studies just cited indicate that male homosexuality and female homosexuality may be different phenomena, with differing familial patterns; substance abuse appears to have equal incidence among gay men and lesbians.

Societal, cultural, and environmental factors, however, may lead to a greater expression of any genetic predisposition. By analogy, there has been an increase in the incidence of alcoholism in women since the beginning of the 20th century (Vaillant 1983). Although partially explained by better data collection, and awareness of the hidden homebound female alcoholic, the increase can also be explained by social factors. In the early 1900s, women were prohibited by societal pressures from drinking in public; as the social acceptability of drinking increased, more women drank, thus increasing the likelihood of exposure to alcohol, which is needed to trigger the genetic expression of alcoholism.

Gay men, lesbians, and bisexual individuals have faced great societal prohibitions, not only on the expression of their sexual feelings and behavior, but on their very existence. Societal homophobia could well have a parallel effect, leading to the higher degree of expressivity of the genetic potentials for substance abuse in gay men, lesbians, and bisexual individuals. Also, societies or cultures in turmoil or undergoing social change have higher rates of alcoholism (Cassel 1976; Vaillant 1983).

For most of the 20th century, societal pressures forced most gay people to remain "in the closet," hiding their sexual orientation or not acting on their feelings. Responding to societal expectations rather than personal desire, some gay, lesbian, and bisexual people may marry someone of the opposite sex and raise a family, creating a potentially stressful situation. Legal prohibitions on homosexual behavior, overt discrimination, and the failure of society to accept or even acknowledge gay people have limited the types of social outlets available to gay men and lesbians to bars, private homes, or clubs where alcohol and other drugs often played a prominent role. The role models for many young gay men and lesbians just "coming out" may be gay people using alcohol and other drugs, who are met at bars or parties. Continuing societal homophobia, as well as the impact of HIV on gay men, lesbians, and bisexual individuals, further add to the stress (Israelstam and Lambert 1989; McKirman and Peterson 1989b).

Some gay and bisexual men and women cannot imagine socializing without alcohol or other mood-altering substance. Gay men, lesbians, and bisexual individuals are brought up in a society that says they should not exist and certainly should not act on their feelings. Such homophobia is internalized. Many men and women have had their first homosexual sexual experiences while drinking or being drunk to overcome their internal fear, denial, anxiety, or even revulsion about gay sex. For many men and women, this linking of substance use and sexual expression persists and may become part of the coming-out and social and personal identity developmental processes. Many gay people continue to feel self-hatred; the use of mood-altering substances temporarily relieves but then reinforces this self-loathing in the drug withdrawal period. Alcohol and many other drugs can cause depression, leading to a worsening of self-esteem.

In addition, the stages of developing a gay, lesbian, or bisexual identity may be intimately involved with substance abuse. Although some substance abusers appear to have a genetic predisposition to substance abuse—supporting an illness model with psychosocial manifestations—not all people with such a genetic predisposition develop alcoholism or substance abuse in their lifetimes. Intrapsychic, psychological, and psychodynamic factors, influenced by psychosocial and parental upbringing, may lead certain people to turn to substance use and, therefore, potentiate a genetic predisposition for substance abuse.

The link between the psychodynamic forces in developing a gay, lesbian, or bisexual identity and the use or abuse of substances becomes clear in examining the early development and progression through the life cycle for a gay person from the perspective of the work of Swiss psychoanalyst Alice Miller (1981). As noted in Chapter 24 by Stein and

Cabaj, her description of how parents influence the emotional lives of their "talented" or different children has strong parallels with the development of a gay, lesbian, or bisexual identity. Parental reactions shape and validate expressions of children's needs and longings; parents reward what is familiar and acceptable to them and discourage or deemphasize behavior or needs they do not value or understand. Harm, of course, occurs when a parent is too depressed, preoccupied, or narcissistic to respond to the *actual* child and the *actual* needs and wants of the child. Children eventually learn to behave the way parents expect to get rewards and to hide or deny the longings or needs that are not rewarded.

Like Miller's examples, many gay and bisexual men and women are aware of being different early in life because they have affectional and sexual needs and longings that are different from others around them (see Chapter 15 by Hanson and Hartmann). Some male children who will grow up to be gay may desire a closer, more intimate relationship with father; this desire is not encouraged or even understood in our society (Isay 1989). The prehomosexual child learns to hide such needs and longings, creating a false self. Real needs are often suppressed or repressed and rejected as wrong, bad, or sinful. Dissociation and denial, therefore, become major defenses to cope with internal feelings. In addition, the studies of familial patterns (Pillard 1988; Pillard et al. 1982) indicate that gay men have a greater than usual chance of having an alcoholic father and, as adult children of alcoholics, may be even more skilled in denial.

■ Case Example 1

After sustaining a job loss that seemed to result from his employer discovering he was gay, Mr. A sought help in maintaining sobriety. He was able to use both individual psychotherapy and a support group to stay sober but revealed a deep depression that required medication. In discussing his life, he recalled knowing he was different and was clearly aware of attraction to men by age 5. However, he only fully came out to himself and others as a gay man at age 38, after years of social isolation. He remembered being a very active, friendly young child, in awe of his father's male friends; however, he never felt that he received attention or direct support from his father. He noticed how his father played with and interacted with his older brother, who played sports and talked about the girls in his class. Interpreting the lack of attention to himself—and the focus of father's attention and affection on the brother— as a prohibition against following his natural feelings and desires, he then withdrew and, as he developed, avoided all sexual activity in adolescence and early adulthood. He began to drink heavily in high school.

This case explores the psychology of being different and learning to live in a society that does not accept difference readily and how such an adjustment to being different shapes the sexual identity development as the child emerges from childhood and the latency period (de Monteflores 1986; see Chapter 24 by Stein and Cabaj). When he is rewarded for presenting a false self and ignored for presenting his true needs and feelings, the child may suppress his more natural feelings. In latency, many children who will become gay or bisexual—especially boys who are effeminate, fear other children, or feel very different— become more isolated. In adolescence, conformity is certainly encouraged, further supporting denial, suppression of gay feelings, dissociation, and splitting off of associated affect and behavior.

Because of the childhood experience of not being acknowledged or accepted for who they are, many gay men, lesbians, and bisexual individuals are especially sensitive to rejection and may expect it or even seek it out unconsciously; substance use helps many such people brace themselves for rejection by others and may make "living in the closet," with its built-in need for denial and dissociation, easier or at least possible. Substance use serves as an easy relief from negative feelings, can provide a degree of social acceptance, and, more importantly, reinforces what has come to be a comforting dissociation developed in childhood. Alcohol and other drugs can cause dissociation of feelings, anxiety, and behavior, thereby mimicking the emotional state many homosexual people had to develop in childhood to survive. The symptom-relieving aspects of substance use can serve to disinhibit what are experienced as forbidden behaviors, foster social comfort in bars, and, most importantly, provide comfort through the familiar experiences of numbing, dissociation, and isolation of feelings. The following case describes a woman with strong internalized homophobia and her attempts to overcome its repressive effects:

■ Case Example 2

Ms. B was raised in the southern part of the United States and was told that gay men and lesbians were evil disciples of the Devil and should be objects of ridicule and violent attacks. She became aware of her lesbian feelings in early high school but attempted to deny them to herself. She prayed to be allowed to be straight and even considered joining a church-sponsored program to change sexual orientation. She did begin to have sex with other women in college, but only when intoxicated. She would go through a period of disgust and self-punishment after every contact and increased her drinking to "help blot out the shame." She would then have another lesbian sexual experience after drinking enough alcohol. The cycle continued until she was referred to treatment by her employer, who was concerned about possible drinking on the job.

Special Treatment Concerns for Gay and Bisexual People

Treatment of gay men, lesbians, and bisexual individuals who abuse substances must focus on recovery both from substance abuse and from the consequences of homophobia. The emotional and psychological symptoms and reactive signs seen in people with internalized homophobia and those seen in substance abusers are very similar and can cause personal limitations—the so called "dual oppression" of homophobia and abuse (Finnegan and McNally 1987). These reactions include denial; fear, anxiety, and paranoia; anger and rage; guilt; self-pity; depression, with helplessness, hopelessness, and powerlessness; self-deception and development of a false self; passivity and feeling victimized; inferiority and low self-esteem; self-loathing; isolation, alienation, and feeling alone, misunderstood, or unique; fragmentation; and confusion. These close similarities make it difficult for gay men or lesbians who cannot accept their sexual orientation to recognize or successfully treat their substance abuse. Self-acceptance of one's sexual orientation thus appears to be crucial to recovery from substance abuse.

In the assessment of a gay man, lesbian, or bisexual person presenting for mental health services, clinicians need to be aware of the higher incidence of substance abuse in this population and, accordingly, routinely screen for symptoms of alcoholism or other substance abuse. In formulating a treatment plan for gay men, lesbians, or bisexual individuals determined to have a substance abuse problem, the personalized treatment plan needs to include the influences and effects of the following for each individual: the stage in the life cycle; the degree and impact of internalized homophobia; the stage in the coming-out process and the experience of coming out; the support and social network available; current relationship, if any, including spouses, and the history of past relationships; the relationship with the family of origin; comfort with sexuality and expression of sexual feelings; career and economic status; and health factors, including HIV or AIDS status.

Most clinicians working with addictions recognize that psychotherapy alone will not treat or cure substance abuse, and, in fact, may actually be harmful and not indicated (Vaillant 1983). Individual psychotherapy can be isolating and lonely and may create the false hope that understanding and insight will lead to recovery; often, the insights lead to an excuse to continue abusing substances. If a patient is already in therapy when recovery begins, the therapy need not stop, but the work will need to be much more supportive and focused on the here and now, while the emotional and neurological systems begin to heal. Once in solid recovery, the patient can deal with the grief and rage involved in mourning the loss of the "false self" and learn how to get his or her own real needs met. In most cases, a 12-step program such as Alcoholics Anonymous (AA) is a vital part of recovery and may well be essential for all substance-abusing patients in recovery who undertake psychotherapy.

■ Case Example 3

Mr. C had been in therapy for years. He drank heavily and frequently and had originally sought help years before for his self-perceived drinking problems. Over the years of treatment, he had explored the meaning of his homosexuality and his relationships with his mother, father, siblings, and series of short-term boyfriends. He continued, however, to drink large quantities of alcohol throughout the course of therapy. After Mr. C made a mild suicide gesture, his therapist abruptly terminated treatment and Mr. C sought a new therapist. The new treatment, with a therapist familiar with substance abuse, focused first on getting sober. The patient tried constantly to return to psychodynamic issues, denying the need to get sober. Finally, with persistent limit setting and refocusing on the part of the therapist, he agreed to enter a treatment program and was able to stop his alcohol use completely. He remained sober, attending predominately gay and lesbian AA meetings, and did not return to psychotherapy.

Often, staff at inpatient and outpatient detoxification and rehabilitation programs lack knowledge about homosexuality and are unaware that they have gay, lesbian, and bisexual patients, who may be too frightened to come out to the staff (Hellman et al. 1989). Many gay, lesbian, and bisexual staff are afraid to come out at work about their sexual orientation as well, because of administrative reaction, and are therefore not able to either serve as role models or provide a more open and relaxed treatment.

If treatment in a formal substance abuse program is indicated, the program should at least be gay-sensitive—aware of, knowledgeable about, and accepting of gay people in a nonprejudicial fashion. The ideal program would be gay-affirmative—actively promoting self-acceptance of a gay identity as a key part of recovery. One gay-affirmative treatment program, the PRIDE Institute (E. F. Ratner et al., unpublished observations, April 1991), reported in a 14-month follow-up study that 74% of all patients treated 5 or more days were continuously abstinent from alcohol use and 67% abstinent from all drugs compared with four gay-sensitive programs with recovery rates in 11- to 24-month follow-ups ranging from 43% to 63%.

Twelve-step recovery programs and philosophies are the mainstays in staying free from drug use and alcohol use (living clean and sober) for most substance abusers. Many larger communities now have gay and lesbian AA, Narcotics Anonymous (NA), and Al-Anon meetings; AA, as an organization, clearly embraces gay men and lesbians, as it embraces anyone concerned about a substance abuse problem (Kus 1987). Some groups parallel and similar to AA have formed to meet the needs of gay men, lesbians, and bisexual individuals, such as Alcoholics Together, and many big cities sponsor "round-ups"—large 3-day weekend gatherings focused on AA, NA, lectures, workshops, and drug- and alcohol-free socializing.

Although 12-step programs such as AA and NA recommend avoiding emotional stress and conflicts in the first 6 months of recovery, for the gay man, lesbian, or bisexual in such programs, relapse is almost certain if the gay or bisexual person cannot acknowledge and accept his or her sexual orientation. Discussion about the conflicts around acknowledging sexual orientation and ways to learn to live comfortably as a gay or bisexual person is essential for recovery, even if these topics are emotionally laden and stressful.

Many localities now have gay, lesbian, and bisexual health or mental health centers, almost all with a focus on recovery and substance abuse treatment. National organizations, such as the National Association of Lesbian and Gay Alcoholism Professionals, the National Gay and Lesbian Health Association, the Association of Gay and Lesbian Psychiatrists, the Gay and Lesbian Medical Association, the Association of Lesbian and Gay Psychologists, and the National Gay Social Workers, can help with appropriate referrals.

Some of the suggestions and guidelines of AA and NA and most treatment programs may be difficult for some gay men, lesbians, and bisexual individuals to follow; giving up or avoiding old friends, especially fellow substance users, may be difficult for a person who has limited contacts who relate to him as a gay person. Staying away from bars or parties may be difficult if they are the only available social outlets; special help on how to not drink or use drugs in such settings may be necessary. Many gay people mistakenly link AA and religion; because many religious institutions denounce or condemn homosexuality, gay men, lesbians, and bisexual individuals may be resistant to trying AA or NA.

■ Case Example 4

Mr. D learned he was HIV-infected and sought help in dealing with the emotional impact. In his first interview, he revealed that he used both intravenous amphetamines and alcohol. The patient acknowledged that his drug and alcohol use was out of control and that he knew he was an addict. He had tried both NA and AA and felt that they were "like cults" and that the groups did not want to hear about his HIV status. He reported wanting to use drugs more after he went to a meeting. In addition, when he went to a gay AA meeting, he felt it was nothing but a "pick-up place," just like a gay bar. Eventually, with the help of the therapist, he did find a support group for gay men that did not insist on total sobriety; there, he was able to discuss both being gay and being infected with HIV. Finally, he was able to use AA and NA when he saw he could get what he needed from the meetings and ignore what was not helpful.

Gay and lesbian adolescents as a group raise special concerns regarding substance abuse; many studies indicate a much higher suicide attempt rate in these youth, as well as a more volatile type of substance abuse, in contrast to other adolescents (Gibson 1989; Hetrick and Martin 1987; see Chapter 16 by D'Augelli and Chapter 49 by Hartstein). Older substance-abusing gay men and lesbians face the same problems other elderly people face (see Chapter by 18 Berger and Kelly), sometimes with added isolation and loneliness and a possible sense of hopelessness and resignation about substance abuse (Friend 1987). Gay men, lesbians, and, especially, bisexually identified people of color who abuse substances must deal with homophobia—often from within the same self-identified ethnic or cultural groups—in addition to possible racism and other prejudices in seeking recovery (see Chapter 35 by González and Espín; Chapter 33 by Jones and Hill; Chapter 34 by Nakajima, Chan, and Lee; and Chapter 36 by Tafoya).

As described above, the incidence of substance abuse is equally high for gay men and lesbians, but lesbians who abuse substances may have additional social struggles and concerns. Compared with gay men, lesbians are more likely to have lower incomes; lesbians are more likely to be parents—up to one-third of lesbians are biological parents (see Chapter 21 by Kirkpatrick); lesbians face the prejudices aimed at women as well as those for being gay, including the stronger reaction against and willingness to ignore female substance abusers (Gartrell 1983); lesbians are more likely to come out later in life (see Chapter 44 by Herbert); and lesbians more often have bisexual feelings or experiences (Bell and Weinberg 1978; Bell et al. 1981), and, as a result, are at greater risk for HIV infection via a heterosexual sexual route in addition to possible intravenous drug use and woman-to-woman transmission.

■ Case Example 5

Ms. E was referred by her primary care provider for assessment of depression. Ms. E had gone in for a routine examination; during the review of symptoms, she became tearful when she started to describe her daughter. During the physical exam, she became quiet and evasive when the provider asked her about some bruises on her arms and back.

In the mental health provider's office, Ms. E seemed frightened and became tearful during the initial questions. She described how she was in a long-term relationship with her female partner and that she was the mother of a child that they had planned to have together through impregnation by direct sexual experience with a gay male friend. Her lover was very loving with the daughter, but Ms. E described how the lover was increasingly irritable, angry, and jealous, even accusing Ms. E of having an ongoing sexual relationship with the child's father.

With further gentle questioning, Ms. E said that her lover was physically abusive, especially after drinking large quantities of alcohol. Ms. E said that she herself drank, at times heavily, to cope with the stress at home; her drinking was often used as the excuse for her lover's physical attacks. Ms. E did not wish to leave the relationship, stating she still very much loved her partner and needed the help with her daughter. Ms. E further described her own drinking, which was in fact daily and usually to the point of intoxication. She denied neglect or harm to the daughter.

Alarmed by the clinical picture, the mental health provider consulted with the primary care provider. A joint intervention was planned for Ms. E, who subsequently agreed to enter an inpatient substance abuse treatment program that had a reputation for working comfortably with gay men and lesbians, while her lover cared for the child. The lover was seen by the inpatient program staff and she too entered substance abuse treatment on an outpatient basis. The daughter was evaluated by the primary care provider and did not show any evidence of abuse or neglect; a protective services evaluation was determined not to be necessary.

On discharge, Ms. E returned home to the lover and daughter. Ms. E and her partner entered couples therapy, as well as using AA and a lesbian substance abuse recovery support group.

This case describes many of the problems lesbians may face in dealing with substance abuse. Child care issues are often very important and finding treatment that is accepting of women in general and lesbians in particular may be challenging.

Other factors affect the treatment of lesbians, gay men, and bisexual individuals. Many gay men, lesbians, and bisexual individuals are in long-term relationships, and treatment for these individuals must clearly focus on relationships and parenting and family concerns. Lesbians, gay men, and bisexual individuals are also subject to an increase in violent attacks, both verbal and physical, because of their sexual orientation (see Chapter 48 by Klinger and Stein); reaction to such an attack may include a relapse to drug or alcohol use in a person in recovery or an increase in use by someone currently using or abusing substances. In addition, many gay men, lesbians, and bisexual individuals are victims of domestic violence. This latter fact is often ignored by clinicians; however, because there are correlations with domestic violence and substance abuse, clinicians need to be aware of this possible combination (Schilit et al. 1990).

A brief list of additional treatment issues facing all people in recovery—with special impact on gay men and lesbians—includes learning how to have safer sex while clean and sober; learning how to adjust to clean and sober socializing, without the use of alcohol or drugs to hide social anxiety; dealing with employment problems and adjusting to the impact of being out as a gay person at work; working with the family of origin regarding their acceptance of the sexual orientation of their gay, lesbian, or bisexual child; helping couples adjust to the damaging effects substance use may have had over the years and embrace a recovery that will avoid the negative impact of codependent relationships; maintaining confidentiality in record keeping, especially around discussion in the medical record of sexual orientation or HIV status; dealing with child custody issues when necessary; diagnosing and treating additional medical problems; and coping with the effects of legal problems. Finnegan and McNally (1987) address most of these concerns.

Impact on the Clinician

Clinicians and counselors must be aware of their own personal attitudes regarding homosexuality. If a health care provider is homophobic and cannot get help in working through these attitudes with a supportive colleague or supervisor, such a provider should refer a gay, lesbian, or bisexual patient to a nonhomophobic provider for help (Cabaj 1988). Gay men and women facing recovery from substance abuse should not also have to fight homophobia in the health care system to get quality care.

If the psychotherapist working with a gay man, lesbian, or bisexual recognizes that the patient may also have the illness of substance abuse, that illness needs to be addressed at each visit in an attempt to break through the denial, "planting the seed" for recovery. Mental health and medical care should not be cut off if the patient refuses to get into recovery. An altered form of a full-scale intervention can be helpful—for example, listing the symptoms and evidence that the clinician sees to support the diagnosis of substance abuse and the probable problems ahead if something is not done to treat it. The persistent denial and avoidance of these problems by many substance abusers make providers frustrated and may lead to a wish to give up trying to help or intervene. The defenses most substance abusers have developed as a result of their substance abuse—projection, denial, manipulation, avoidance, isolation, dissociation—are challenging to work with as well. It is easy to collude with the patient's denial and frustration, and an attitude of "why bother" can easily develop. The clinician who does not recognize that relapse is part of the nature of the illness of substance abuse may feel personally offended or guilty if a patient relapses.

Conclusion

The growing literature on working with gay, lesbian, and bisexual substance abusers will help clinicians with the variety of situations and presentations described in this chapter (Cabaj 1992; Finnegan and McNally 1987; Gonsiorek 1985; Ziebold 1985). Substance use, especially alcohol, is woven into the fabric of the lives of many gay men, lesbians, and bisexual individuals. The use of substances can be associated with identity formation, coming out, and self-acceptance processes for many gay men, lesbians, and bisexual persons. The greater use and presence of alcohol and other drugs in settings where gay men, lesbians, and bisexual individuals socialize, combined with the dissociation and denial produced by the use of these substances, may help to explain a greater expression among homosexual people of a biological or genetic predisposition for substance abuse. Internalized homophobia and societal homophobia combine to reinforce the use of alcohol and drugs and may make the recognition and treatment of substance abuse in lesbians, gay men, and bisexual individuals more difficult. Extended recovery is more likely to happen—indeed, may only be possible—if a gay man, lesbian, or bisexual person is able to accept his or her sexual orientation, address internalized homophobia, and discover how to live clean and sober without fearing or hating his or her real self.

References

Beatty R: Alcoholism and Adult Gay Male Populations of Pennsylvania. Master's thesis, Pennsylvania State University, University Park, PA, 1983

Bell AP, Weinberg MS: Homosexualities: A Study of Diversities Among Men and Women. New York, Simon and Schuster, 1978

Bell AP, Weinberg MS, Hammersmith SK: Sexual Preference: Its Development in Men and Women. Bloomington, IN, Indiana University Press, 1981

Cabaj RP: Homosexuality and neurosis: Considerations for psychotherapy. J Homosex 15(1–2):13–23, 1988

Cabaj RP: Substance abuse in the gay and lesbian community, in Substance Abuse: A Comprehensive Textbook, 2nd Edition. Edited by Lowenson JH, Ruiz P, Millman RB. Baltimore, MD, Williams & Wilkins, 1992, pp 852–860

Cassel J: The contributions of the social environment to host resistance. Am J Epidemiol 104:107–123, 1976

Centers for Disease Control and Prevention: HIV/AIDS Surveillance Report, Year-End Edition 5(4):1–33, 1994

de Monteflores C: Notes on the management of difference, in Contemporary Perspectives on Psychotherapy with Lesbians and Gay Men. Edited by Stein TS, Cohen CC. New York, Plenum, 1986, pp 73–101

Diamond DL, Wilsnack SC: Alcohol abuse among lesbians: a descriptive study. J Homosex 4(2):123–142, 1978

Finnegan DG, McNally EB: Dual Identities: Counseling Chemically Dependent Gay Men and Lesbians. Center City, MN, Hazelden, 1987

Friend RA: The individual and social psychology of aging: clinical implications for lesbians and gay men. J Homosex 14(1–2):307–331, 1987

Gartrell N: Gay patients in the medical setting, in Treatment Interventions in Human Sexuality. Edited by Nadelson C, Marcotte D. New York, Plenum, 1983

Gibson P: Gay male and lesbian youth suicide, in Report of the Secretary of Health and Human Services' Task Force on Youth Suicide, Volume 3. Edited by Sullivan LW. Washington, DC, US Government Press, 1989, pp 110–142

Gonsiorek JC (ed): A Guide to Psychotherapy with Gay and Lesbian Clients. New York, Harrington Park Press, 1985

Hellman RE, Stanton M, Lee J, et al: Treatment of homosexual alcoholics in government-funded agencies: provider training and attitudes. Hosp Community Psychiatry 40(11):1163–1168, 1989

Hetrick ES, Martin AD: Developmental issues and their resolution for gay and lesbian adolescents. J Homosex 14(1/2):25–43, 1987

Isay RA: Being Homosexual: Gay Men and Their Development. New York, Farrar, Straus and Giroux, 1989

Israelstam S, Lambert S: Homosexuality as a cause of alcoholism: a historical review. Int J Addict 18(8):1085–1107, 1983

Israelstam S, Lambert S: Homosexuality and alcohol: observations and research after the psychoanalytic era. Int J Addict 21(4–5):509–537, 1986

Israelstam S, Lambert S: Homosexuals who indulge in excessive use of alcohol and drugs: psychosocial factors to be taken into account by community and intervention workers. Journal of Alcohol and Drug Education 34(3):54–69, 1989

Kus RJ: Alcoholics Anonymous and gay American men. J Homosex 14(1/2):253–276, 1987

Lewis CE, Saghir MT, Robins E: Drinking patterns in homosexual and heterosexual women. J Clin Psychiatry 43:277–279, 1982

Lohrenz L, Connelly J, Coyne L, et al: Alcohol problems in several midwestern homosexual communities. J Stud Alcohol 39(11):1959–1963, 1978

McKirman D, Peterson PL: Alcohol and drug abuse among homosexual men and women: epidemiology and population characteristics. Addict Behav 14:545–553, 1989a

McKirman D, Peterson PL: Psychological and cultural factors in alcohol and drug abuse: an analysis of a homosexual community. Addict Behav 14:555–563, 1989b

Miller A: The Drama of the Gifted Child. New York, Basic Books, 1981

Mosbacher D: Lesbian alcohol and substance abuse. Psychiatric Annals 18(1):47–50, 1988

Mosbacher D: Alcohol and other drug use in female medical students: a comparison of lesbians and heterosexuals. Journal of Gay and Lesbian Psychotherapy 2(1):37–48, 1993

Pillard RC: Sexual orientation and mental disorder. Psychiatric Annals 18(1):52–56, 1988

Pillard RC, Weinrich JD: Evidence of familial nature of male sexuality. Arch Gen Psychiatry 43:808–812, 1986

Pillard RC, Poumadere J, Carretta RA: A family study of sexual orientation. Arch Sex Behav 11(6):511–520, 1982

Saghir M, Robins E: Male and Female Homosexuality. Baltimore, MD, Williams and Wilkins, 1973

Schilit R, Lie GY, Montagne M: Substance use as a correlate of violence in intimate lesbian relationships. J Homosex 19(3):51–65, 1990

Stall R, Wiley J: A comparison of alcohol and drug use patterns of homosexual and heterosexual men: the San Francisco Men's Health Study. Drug Alcohol Depend 22:63 73, 1988

Vaillant GE: The Natural History of Alcoholism: Causes, Patterns, and Paths to Recovery. Cambridge, MA, Harvard University Press, 1983

Weinberg M, Williams C: Male Homosexuals: Their Problems and Adaptations. New York, Oxford University Press, 1974

Ziebold TO, Mongeon JE (eds): Gay and Sober: Directions for Counseling and Therapy. New York, Harrington Park Press, 1985

Impact of Violence, Childhood Sexual Abuse, and Domestic Violence and Abuse on Lesbians, Bisexuals, and Gay Men

Rochelle L. Klinger, M.D.
Terry S. Stein, M.D.

L esbians, bisexual persons, and gay men are victims of the same acts of violence as other individuals in our society. They also may be the objects of violence directed against them because of their sexual orientation—a form of violence that may be particularly vicious. Such violence may produce scars because of an interaction between the trauma resulting from violence and abuse and the sense of stigma associated with being lesbian, gay, or bisexual. This chapter explores three forms of violence that may have special rele-

This chapter is dedicated to the memory of Dr. Ilene M. Gold.

vance for these men and women: antigay and antilesbian violence, childhood sexual abuse, and domestic violence and abuse.

Antigay and Antilesbian Violence

Violence against lesbians and gay men is only one example of the larger problem of hate violence or "violence directly attributable to prejudice" (Center for Democratic Renewal and Education, 1992, p. 13). Only recently have acts of violence against gay men and lesbians been recognized as a form of hate violence. Throughout the 1980s, the National Gay and Lesbian Task Force, through its Anti-Violence Project, attempted to document the nature of the problem and lobbied to have acts of antigay and antilesbian violence covered by the Hate Crimes Statistics Act. Finally, after years of resistance from conservative members of Congress, the Hate Crimes Statistics Act (including reference to antigay and antilesbian violence) passed the U.S. Congress in 1990. Although antigay and antilesbian violence is the most recently recognized form of hate-based violence, gay men and lesbians were described in a report issued by the National Institute of Justice (P. Finn and T. McNeil, unpublished manuscript, October 7, 1987) as "probably the most frequent victims" (p. 2) of hate violence. A large and growing literature on antigay and antilesbian violence (Comstock 1991; Herek 1989; see Chapter 7 by Herek; Herek and Berrill 1992; Minkowitz 1992; Nardi and Bolton 1991) places the origins of these hate-based crimes in the broader context of cultural heterosexism and related ideologies of sexuality and gender.

Scope of the Problem

Thousands of incidents of violence, ranging from verbal abuse to homicide, are reported each year against lesbians and gay men. The categories of incidents recorded by the National Gay and Lesbian Task Force include murders, assaults, hate group activity, police abuse, arson and vandalism, threats and harassment, campus violence, acquired immunodeficiency syndrome (AIDS)-related violence, Colorado and Oregon incidents (added in 1993 because of the increase in incidents in these states associated with antigay ballot initiatives), military incidents, and defamation.

More incidents of violence against lesbians, gay men, and bisexual individuals are believed to go unreported than reported. In recent surveys of violence against lesbians, gay men, and bisexual individuals in urban areas, up to 28% of all respondents reported that they had been assaulted or physically abused during the previous 12 months because of their sexual orientation and up to 50% reported that they had been harassed (National Gay and Lesbians Task Force Policy Institute 1993).

Some gender differences in antigay and antilesbian violence have been documented (Berrill 1992). Gay men generally experience greater levels of antigay verbal harassment by nonfamily members, threats, victimization in school and by police, and most types of physical violence and intimidation. Lesbians generally experience higher rates of verbal harassment by family members and report greater fear of physical violence and a greater degree of discrimination. The small number of studies examining racial and ethnic differences in antigay violence show that gay men and lesbians of color, in particular blacks and Hispanics, are at increased risk for violent attacks and other forms of victimization because of their sexual orientation (Berrill 1992).

■ Description of Perpetrators

Antigay and antilesbian violence may be perpetrated by individuals, gangs, within families, and by authorities such as the police. The typical perpetrator of antigay and antilesbian violence tends to be a young white male, often acting together with other males, who are strangers to the victim (Comstock 1991). Almost half of the perpetrators reported in one study (Comstock 1991) are 21 or younger, and most are adolescents or in their 20s. In comparison with all crimes of violence, antigay and antilesbian violence tends to involve attacks on pairs and groups rather than lone victims and a higher percentage of groups of perpetrators than perpetrators acting alone.

■ Mental Health Consequences of Antigay and Antilesbian Violence

A significant proportion of lesbians and gay men have experienced verbal and physical abuse as a result of their sexual orientation; all experience the fear of such victimization. The consequences of this awareness of the potential for violence and oppression, whether the individual has been attacked or not, may include a heightened sense of vulnerability about and reluctance to disclose sexual orientation, depression, inappropriate denial, and a range of other psychological and emotional problems. Reactions to such victimization can include symptoms typical of posttraumatic stress disorder, including irritability, intrusive thoughts, sleep disturbances, nightmares, generalized signs of anxiety, and depression (Bohn 1984; Krupnick 1982).

Victimization creates psychological distress; in addition, particular psychological effects of antigay and antilesbian violence result from the pervasive heterosexism and stigmatization of homosexuality in our society (Garnets et al. 1992). The internalized homophobia of the gay, lesbian, or bisexual victim may be triggered and lead to the belief that being homosexual is the cause of the assault. Victims may feel inadequate and experience guilt, embarrassment, shame, depression, and loss of confidence. In some instances, because of the severity of the assault or the psychological characteristics of the victim, including the stage of coming out and degree of consolidation of a gay identity, a man or woman also may experience terror, paranoia, helplessness, and rage for months or years after the attack. As with the victim of rape, many survivors of antigay or antilesbian violence have trouble seeking help because of their embarrassment about the incident, possibly fearing mistreatment by caregivers or concerns about disclosure of their sexual orientation.

■ Treatment and Prevention

The mental health professional should be prepared to respond to the crisis that may immediately follow an incident of antigay or antilesbian violence, be aware of the long-term consequences of victimization on the survivor, and be sensitive to the effects of concern about such violence on all lesbians and gay men. Support for the appropriate expression of affect of the victim after an assault or violent incident can help in promoting resolution of the reaction to the event. Constructive channeling of concern into social activist involvement also can be beneficial.

Several levels of intervention are appropriate in responding to antigay and antilesbian violence, including provision of targeted health and mental health services; development of programs that will ensure adequate protection and safety for gay men, lesbians, and bisexual individuals; and creation of community-based initiatives for education about and prevention of these crimes. The health and mental health needs of gay men and lesbians are the same as those for victims of other types of violent crimes but must involve a sensitivity to the special needs of this population associated with their identities, communities, and nontraditional families. Specific preventive initiatives, such as improved collection of data about the crimes, widespread implementation of street patrols in urban settings with high concentrations of lesbians and gay men, attendance in self-defense classes, creation of liaisons between gay communities and police departments, court monitoring, increased legislative action, and education programs for youth and adolescents, can help in responding to the problem.

Childhood Sexual Abuse of Gay Men and Lesbians

Attention to childhood sexual abuse is part of the practice of most clinicians, regardless of specialty. Increased recognition of childhood sexual abuse of both men and women has occurred in the last two decades, primarily as a result of increased attention to this issue by both child welfare advocates and the women's movement. The authors address the issue of childhood sexual abuse in gay men, bisexual persons, and lesbians because of myths that homosexual orientation is caused by sexual abuse.

▮ Scope of the Problem

The prevalence of childhood sexual abuse is difficult to assess in the population in general, in part because of the stigma attached to it. For gay men, bisexual individuals, and lesbians, the stigma attached to being a member of a minority sexual orientation group and a survivor of sexual abuse may be additive and make prevalence of sexual abuse even more difficult to estimate.

Loulan (1988) surveyed 1,566 lesbians who attended her speaking engagements at conferences, workshops, women's bookstores, and other settings. She acknowledged that this method does not provide a representative sample but rather shows the difficulty of obtaining samples of lesbians or gay men in a random fashion. In her sample of primarily white and middle-class women age 25–60, 38% had been sexually abused before age 18. This finding was consistent with the findings of Russell (1986), who surveyed 930 women in San Francisco and found a rate of sexual abuse before age 18 of 38%.

The lesbian health survey of Bradford and Ryan (1988) sampled 1,917 lesbians of diverse geographic, class, and racial and ethnic backgrounds and is the most random large survey to date. Of their sample, 21% had been raped or sexually abused as children, which is consistent with estimates in heterosexual women; 19% of survey subjects reported that sexual abuse had been perpetrated by relatives.

A survey of 1,001 adult homosexual and bisexual men who attended sexually transmitted disease clinics in Chicago, Denver, and San Francisco in 1990 revealed that 37% had been forced or encouraged to have sexual contact before age 19 with an older or more powerful partner (Doll et al. 1992), an unusually high rate for males that may be attributable to the nonrepresentative nature of the sample in the study. In preliminary findings from a recent survey of gay male sexuality, Lever (1994) reported that 21% of gay or bisexual men surveyed had been sexually abused by men by age 15, which is within the 3%–31% estimates in the general male population (Finkelhor 1987).

These studies, although limited, reveal that sexual abuse is as common in gay men and lesbians as in the general population and may be slightly more common in gay than heterosexual men. Thus these surveys show that the theory that sexual abuse causes homosexual orientation cannot be substantiated.

▪ Description of Perpetrators

Both lesbians and gay men are abused primarily but not exclusively by men. In Loulan's survey (1988), 75% of women who said they were sexually abused were abused by their fathers, brothers, or older male relatives; 7% were abused by the male lover of the mother; and 20% by a male stranger. However, 8% were abused by their mothers and 2% by a female stranger. Some subjects were abused by more than one category of perpetrator. Bradford and Ryan (1988) reported that perpetrators were 98% male. The highest reported frequency was by males who were known by the victim but were not relatives (45%), followed by male strangers (33%) and male relatives (31%).

In the case of gay men, both Lever (1994) and Doll et al. (1992) examined only sexual abuse by males. In the survey of Doll et al., 68% of adult perpetrators were family members, 28% were other male ac-quaintances, and 4% were male strangers.

■ Mental Health Consequences of Childhood Sexual Abuse

Much of the literature on the mental health consequences of child sex-ual abuse focuses on clinical populations (i.e., individuals who seek mental health treatment and report a history of sexual abuse). How-ever, when nonclinical populations are reviewed, childhood sexual con-tact with adults still emerges as a significant trauma that is usually negative and may increase the risk of mental disorders later in life (Finkelhor 1984; Herman 1981). Browne and Finekelhor (1986) re-viewed the literature and found that sexual abuse survivors as a group show psychological impairment of some degree compared with non-victims and that 20% of adults who were sexually abused as children show serious psychopathology.

Reports of mental health consequences of childhood sexual abuse in gay men and lesbians are primarily anecdotal. Loulan (1988) re-ported that lesbian survivors are more likely to have difficulties with adult sexual relationships in terms of feeling vulnerable and having memories of sexual abuse reemerge during sexual contact. Loulan also reported a 27% incidence of adult rape among the lesbians who were abuse survivors versus 8% in those not sexually abused. This finding also has been reported in the general population and may be attribut-able to the difficulty of the survivor in recognizing and protecting themselves in potentially dangerous situations. A positive finding in Loulan's study was that women who were abused as children had the same level of sexual activity and enjoyment at the time of the survey as nonabused women.

Knisely (1992) surveyed 55 gay men (20 of whom had been sexually abused as children) and 25 heterosexual men as control subjects. He found no difference in self-esteem or depression between abused and nonabused males but internalized homophobia was increased in abused subjects. Gay men who had been abused had a significantly lower first age of sexual exposure than nonabused gay men (11 versus 15 years old). This finding may have significance in terms of safer sex education and HIV prevention. Childhood sexual victimization also has been suggested as a risk factor for suicide attempts in gay male and bisexual youth (Remafedi et al. 1991).

Male survivors of childhood sexual abuse may have more difficulty than women in coping with childhood trauma because of the hidden nature of the sexual abuse of boys in our society. The reality of rape and sexual abuse against boys and men is often not acknowledged. Therefore, gay men who had been sexually abused may have difficulty accepting that the abuse really happened. In addition, gay men may be unwilling to acknowledge sexual abuse, as they may expect (often realistically) that they, rather than the perpetrators, will be blamed.

■ Diagnosis and Treatment

Careful differential diagnosis is as essential when gay male and lesbian survivors of childhood sexual abuse seek treatment as with any other population. Some may suffer from serious Axis I or Axis II disorders caused or exacerbated by the abuse (e.g., posttraumatic stress disorder, major depression, or borderline personality disorder). Other patients may have unrelated psychiatric disorders, with the childhood sexual abuse being an incidental finding. Courtois (1988) listed depression, anxiety disorders, isolation, poor self-esteem, substance abuse, somatization disorders, eating disorders, and a tendency toward revictimization as common reasons to seek counseling. In addition, Courtois noted that, because the sexual abuse or incest occurs during the course of maturation and development, it can get integrated into the personality to cause maladaptive personality traits and personality disorders.

A full discussion of treatment of adult survivors of sexual abuse is beyond the scope of this chapter. Herman (1992) reviewed the literature and summarized three basic stages in treatment: establishing safety, remembrance of the events and mourning, and reconnection with ordinary life. Courtois (1988) emphasized the first step in particular, in which the therapist establishes a therapeutic relationship by believing the client and actively encouraging her or him to talk about the abuse. The therapist should be open and nonjudgmental, while at the same time maintaining proper boundaries. Courtois cautioned about the vissicitudes of transference and countertransference that often emerge. Survivors often initially seek individual therapy. As trust is built and the survivor becomes more comfortable talking about the abuse, group intervention can help. Lesbians may benefit from groups with women of any sexual orientation or lesbian-only groups, depending on the individual. Gay men are usually most comfortable in a group of gay male survivors.

Kirschner et al. (1993) suggested including the partner, if there is one, in therapy from the outset. The initial goals of treatment are usually symptom relief and memory retrieval. In midphase the therapy often deals with relationships in the here and now. Ideally, in the endphase the sexual abuse survivor is able to achieve a healthy relationship with a partner.

In the case of gay men and lesbians, internalized homophobia may complicate adult adjustment to childhood sexual abuse. This may come to the forefront when a crisis, such as HIV diagnosis, occurs.

■ **Case Example 1**

> Mr. A is a 28-year-old gay man who came to an HIV clinic immediately after finding out, during a routine insurance test, that he was infected with HIV. He was shocked, as he did not consider himself gay, despite having had only homosexual experiences in his life. He was distraught and attributed his homosexual behavior to being sexually abused at age 5 by a male relative. His large, close-knit family was religious and often attended a church where the evils of homosexuality were preached from the pulpit. Over the next 2 years, despite deteriorating health from his HIV infection, he was able to work through his self-hatred from internalized homophobia, come out to his family, and accept his gay male orientation. The childhood sexual abuse was of little import to the therapy except as a resistance to the real issue of internalized homophobia.

Domestic Violence and Abuse in Gay and Lesbian Relationships

Only recently has the problem of domestic violence and abuse been recognized in gay male and lesbian relationships. Domestic violence is defined as any pattern of behavior designed to coerce, dominate, isolate, or maintain control in a relationship via the threat of or actual violence (Walber 1988). Possible explanations for the lack of attention include the stereotypical belief that only men are batterers and only women are victims of domestic violence; beliefs within the lesbian and gay male culture that gay male and lesbian relationships are egalitarian and immune to domestic violence; homophobia in institutions such as the legal system and shelters for battered women that usually deal with domestic violence; and the desire of the gay male and lesbian community to keep its dirty laundry hidden to discourage additional stigma (Renzetti 1994). Although studies are recent and incomplete, in contrast to many other clinical phenomena discussed in this book, domestic violence has been studied more adequately in lesbian than in gay male couples.

Scope of the Problem

The incidence of violence in gay male and lesbian couples is difficult to gauge. Police statistics are not useful, as incidents are so rarely reported to the authorities. Prevalence studies in heterosexual couples estimate that battering occurs in 25%–33% of couples (Koss 1990). No systematic studies have been conducted of the rate of violence in gay male couples, although Island and Letellier (1991) estimate a 10%–20% anecdotal rate. Studies of violence in lesbian couples report that from 17% to 73% of lesbians have experienced violence in a relationship at some point (Bologna et al. 1987; Coleman 1990; Kelly and Warshafsky 1987; Lie and Gentlewarrier 1991; Lie et al. 1991; Loulan 1988). However, these studies are generally flawed by nonrandom self-selected samples (e.g., participants at women's festivals and self-definition of abuse). The survey of Brand and Kidd (1986) estimated that 25% of lesbians in committed relationships were physically abused, which is consistent with the rate of abuse in committed heterosexual relationships.

Description of the Problem

Domestic violence includes many forms of physical and psychological abuse, ranging from name calling to homicide. Leeder (1988) divides abusive lesbian dyads into those with situational, chronic physical, and chronic emotional battering. However, studies since that time negate the idea that abuse can be neatly divided into subtypes (Lie and Gentlewarrier 1991; Lie et al. 1991; Renzetti 1992). Lie et al. found that 50% of women who were victims of abuse also were perpetrators at times, challenging the notion that victims and abusers fall into clearly distinct categories.

Walker (1979, 1984) described a cycle of battering that is presumed to be identical for heterosexual and lesbian and gay male couples. Couples do not start out having an abusive relationship but at some point a recurring cycle of battering begins. The first stage is tension building, which leads to acute battering; next is a loving and contrite phase. A characteristic pattern of behavior, the "battered woman syndrome," is seen in victims who have decreased self-esteem and begin to focus their actions around trying to prevent battering incidents by their behavior. Such preventive behavior on the part of the victim is based on a fallacious belief that the victim can control the behavior of the batterer. While trying to prevent the battering, the victim becomes increasingly isolated, often because the batterer limits social contacts, and begins to feel less and less able to escape the violence. In addition, the batterer can be convincing, during the loving and contrite stage, that he or she really will stop the violence.

Because the question of etiology of abusive behavior is of great interest to clinicians, Renzetti (1992, 1993a, 1993b, 1994) examined the contribution of various correlates of abuse in lesbian couples, including 1) history of childhood abuse in the family of the victim or batterer; 2) substance abuse in victim or batterer; 3) balance of power in the relationship; 4) relative dependency of each partner on the other; and 5) jealousy.

The cyclical or intergenerational transmission hypothesis states that individuals who witnessed or who were victims of family violence as children are more likely as adults to be violent toward partners or children (Straus et al. 1980). Renzetti did not find a robust correlation in this area and concluded that a family history of violence is more likely to facilitate than cause domestic violence by giving the abuser and victim a rationalization to explain away the behavior. Substance abuse functioned in a similar way as a legitimization of violence by both the abuser and the victim.

Research on the relationship between balance of power and domestic violence is inconclusive. Bologna et al. (1987) found that the abuser tends to have a perceived deficit of power relative to the victim; Renzetti (1992) found the opposite. Whether the abuser is more powerful and manifesting his or her power by battering or less powerful and aware that he or she is losing power is not clear. The findings of Renzetti about dependency and jealousy are more clear. Renzetti found that the abusive partner tended to be overdependent and extremely jealous, pressuring the victim to be more and more isolated from other contacts.

As the victim tried to assert her independence, the abuse increased. Renzetti also found that the abuser threatened self-harm when the victim threatened to leave.

Mental Health Consequences of Partner Abuse

Domestic violence may have a range of consequences for the victim, including anxiety, affective, and somatoform disorders after victimization. Posttraumatic stress disorder is associated with victimization, but most victims do not develop the full clinical syndrome. Factors such as the quality of support, rapid debriefing, and nature of the trauma may influence whether posttraumatic stress disorder develops (Armstrong et al. 1991; Kemp et al. 1991). Even when posttraumatic stress disorder is not diagnosed, victims may have significant distress and subsyndromal anxiety and affective syndromes.

A controversial question in the treatment of victims of domestic violence is whether individuals become victims randomly or if persons are predisposed to become victims as a result of previous histories of trauma. Survivors of childhood trauma may be more prone to take risks and not to recognize danger and thus be more prone to revictimization (Courtois 1988). Horowitz et al. (1987) proposed the diagnosis of posttraumatic personality disorder to describe these individuals. Probably, victims of domestic violence comprise a heterogeneous group of individuals in terms of psychological health. Until more prospective data are obtained, clinicians treating victims of domestic violence should focus on the problem of domestic abuse, while addressing any preexisting or concomitant psychopathology as necessary in the treatment.

The mental health consequences for the perpetrators of domestic violence are poorly understood, because batterers do not often seek treatment and because of the stigma of being a batterer. Batterers may at times seek treatment on their own but usually seek treatment only when forced to do so by the legal system. Shame, anger, denial, and poor self-esteem are expected in this population (Klinger 1991).

Treatment and Prevention

Violent gay male and lesbian couples may seek the mental health clinician either individually or as a dyad. Violence often is not the initial complaint, and the clinician must specifically ask about it. The clinician should recognize that the risk of battering in gay male and lesbian couples is critical and ask routine questions about battering while taking the history. The first consideration of the therapist should be the safety of the victim. Batterers may be likely to abuse if they know the victim is seeking treatment, putting the victim at higher risk. The possibility of suicide or homicide also should be carefully evaluated.

In evaluating and treating a victim of domestic violence, the therapist should take a careful history of the circumstances and degree of abuse. The therapist should try to communicate his or her understanding of the risk to the victim. A safety plan in case of the need for escape and arrangement for between session contacts should be discussed. The victim often has significant ambivalence about leaving the abuser, even in the face of real danger. Forging a therapeutic alliance and keeping the victim in treatment can be difficult in the face of these complex issues. The following case is an example of failure to keep the patient in treatment, which is unfortunately not uncommon when working with domestic violence survivors.

■ Case Example 2

Ms. B is a 48-year-old bisexual who sought treatment with symptoms of generalized anxiety disorder. She was in her third lesbian relationship and had also had three serious heterosexual relationships with two marriages. She considered herself bisexual. All of her previous relationships with men and women had included verbal and physical abuse. In her first marriage, her husband went to prison for attempting to kill her. Ms. B's family history showed alcoholism in her father and male siblings and physical abuse of her mother and all of the children by her father. She had been sexually abused by an uncle. In her present relationship, some verbal outbursts by her partner but no physical abuse had occurred at the time of seeking counseling. However, her partner had become increasingly controlling, refusing to let her see either her lesbian friends (for fear that she would have affairs with them) or her heterosexual friends (for fear that they would "make her straight again"). Her partner also did not allow her to work outside the home to avoid contact with others and monitored all of her mail and telephone calls. The therapist pointed out to Ms. B that her partner's pattern of increasing control and verbal outbursts was abusive and a harbinger of possible physical violence to come. Ms. B recognized this but professed loyalty to her partner because of her financial support and feeling that she cared for her. A safety plan was discussed. Ms. B was unwilling to negotiate for between session contacts, saying she was unwilling to take the chance of her partner finding out that she was being discussed in therapy. Ms. B dropped out of treatment after three sessions and would not answer phone calls. It was not clear to the therapist whether it was Ms. B's own decision based on her ambivalence about confronting the abuse or whether her partner had intervened to stop the treatment. The therapist was reluctant to endanger her by continuing to attempt to contact her to encourage her to return to treatment.

Couples therapy is almost always contraindicated when domestic violence is occurring. Treatment for couples may increase the risk to the victim if he or she is perceived to be revealing information about the abuse (Frank and Houghton 1987). If battering is discovered during the course of treatment of couples, discontinuation and referral for individual treatment are usually indicated. Both victims and batterers benefit from careful assessment and targeted treatment. Modalities can include individual, group, pharmacological, and substance abuse treatment. Countertransference reactions should be carefully monitored and dealt with in supervision or consultation, particularly when working with batterers (Klinger 1991).

Prevention can be addressed by the individual clinician by incorporating discussion of domestic violence into routine interviewing (e.g., asking about previous victimization or abusive behavior when taking a history and by asking gay male and lesbian patients to examine how they would deal with abusive behavior if it occurred). At a systemic level, the existing legal and battering resources that are oriented toward heterosexuals need to increase their outreach to and inclusion of gay and lesbian domestic violence victims and perpetrators. Lesbian, bisexual, and gay male activists must sensitize the majority community to the problem and overcome their own denial and shame. Finally, research and clinical data need to be gathered to allow meaningful policy discussions of gay and lesbian domestic violence.

Conclusion

The effects of violence on lesbians, bisexual individuals, and gay men are largely the same as on other individuals. In addition, however, these men and women are often the objects of hate-based violence because of their sexual orientation and may show signs of exacerbated internalized homophobia after victimization. The clinician who provides counseling for the mental health consequences of violence and abuse in lesbians, bisexual individuals, and gay men should be informed about the general effects of trauma and violence and sensitive to the particular signs of trauma associated with a vulnerable and stigmatized sexual orientation.

References

Armstrong K, O'Callahan W, Marmar CR: Debriefing Red Cross disaster personnel: the multiple stressor debriefing model. J Trauma Stress 4:481–491, 1991

Berrill KT: Anti-gay violence and victimization in the United States: an overview, in Hate Crimes. Edited by Herek GM, Berrill KT. Newbury Park, CA, Sage, 1992, pp 19–45

Bohn TR: Homophobic violence: implications for social work practice, in With Compassion Toward Some: Homosexuality and Social Work in America. Edited by Schoenberg R, Goldberg RS. New York, Harrington Park Press, 1984, pp 91–112

Bologna MJ, Waterman CK, Dawson LJ: Violence in gay male and lesbian relationships: implications for practitioners and policy makers. Paper presented at the Third National Conference for Family Violence Researchers, Durham, New Hampshire, July 1987

Bradford J, Ryan C: The National Lesbian Health Care Survey, Washington, DC, National Lesbian and Gay Health Foundation, 1988, pp 76–85

Brand PA, Kidd AH: Frequency of physical aggression in heterosexual and female homosexual dyads. Psychol Rep 59:1307–1313, 1986

Browne A, Finkelhor D: Impact of child sexual abuse: a review of the literature. Psychol Bull 99:66–67, 1986

Center for Democratic Renewal and Education: A Handbook of Effective Community Responses, 2nd Edition: When Hate Groups Come to Town. Montgomery, AL, Black Belt Press, 1992

Coleman VE: Violence in lesbian couples: a between groups comparison. University Microfilms International, 9109022, 1990 (Unpublished doctoral dissertation)

Comstock GD: Violence Against Lesbians and Gay Men. New York, Columbia University Press, 1991

Courtois CA: Healing the Incest Wound. New York, WW Norton, 1988

Doll LS, Joy D, Bartholow BN, et al: Self-reported childhood and adolescent sexual abuse among adult homosexual and bisexual men. Child Abuse Negl 16:855–864, 1992

Finkelhor D: Child Sexual Abuse: New Theory and Research. New York, Free Press, 1984, p 16

Finkelhor D: The sexual abuse of children: current research reviewed. Psychiatric Annals 17:233–241, 1987

Frank P, Houghton B: Confronting the Batterer: A Guide to Creating the Spouse Abuse Educational Workshop. New City, Volunteer Counseling Service of Rockland County, 1987

Garnets L, Herek GM, Levy B: Violence and victimization of lesbians and gay men: mental health consequences, in Hate Crimes. Edited by Herek GM, Berrill KT. Newbury Park, CA, Sage, 1992, pp 207–226

Herek GM: Hate crimes against lesbians and gay men. American Psychologist 44:948–955, 1989

Herek GM, Berrill KT (eds): Hate Crimes. Newbury Park, CA, Sage, 1992

Herman JL: Father-Daughter Incest. Cambridge, MA, Harvard University Press, 1981, pp 34–35

Herman JL: Trauma and Recovery. New York, Basic Books, 1992

Horowitz MJ, Weiss DS, Marmar CR: Diagnosis of post-traumatic stress disorder. J Nerv Ment Dis 175:267–268, 1987

Island D, Letellier P: Men Who Beat the Men Who Love Them: Battered Gay Men and Domestic Violence. New York, Harrington Park Press, 1991

Kelly EE, Warshafsky L: Partner abuse in gay male and lesbian couples. Paper presented at the Third National Conference for Family Violence Researchers, Durham, North Carolina, July 1987

Kemp A, Rawlings EI, Green BL: Post-traumatic stress disorder (PTSD) in battered women: a shelter sample. Journal of Traumatic Stress 4:137–148, 1991

Kirschner S, Kirschner DA, Rappaport RL: Working With Adult Incest Survivors: The Healing Journey. New York, Brunner/Mazel, 1993

Klinger RL: Treatment of a lesbian batterer, in Gays, Lesbians and Their Therapists: Studies in Psychotherapy. Edited by Silverstein C. New York, WW Norton, 1991, pp 126–142

Knisely ER: Psychosocial factors relevant to homosexual men who were sexually abused as children and homosexual men who were not sexually abused as children: an exploratory-descriptive study. Dissertation Abstracts International 53(6): DA9227923, December 1992 (unpublished doctoral dissertation)

Koss MP: The women's mental health research agenda: violence against women. American Psychologist 45:374–380, 1990

Krupnick J: Brief psychotherapy with victims of violent crime. Victimology: An International Journal 5(2-4):347–354, 1982

Leeder E: Enmeshed in pain: counseling lesbian battering couples. Women and Therapy 7:81–89, 1988

Lever J: Sexual revelations: the 1994 Advocate survey of sexuality and relationships: the men. Advocate 661/662:16–24, 1994

Lie G, Gentlewarrier S: Intimate violence in lesbian relationships: discussion of survey findings and practice implications. Journal of Social Service Research 15:41–59, 1991

Lie G, Schlitt R, Bush J, et al: Lesbians in currently aggressive relationships: how frequently do they report aggressive past relationships? Violence and Victims 6:121–235, 1991

Loulan J: Research on the sex practices of 1566 lesbians and the clinical applications. Women and Therapy 7:221–234, 1988

Minkowitz D: It's still open season on gays. The Nation, March 23, 1992, pp 368–370

Nardi PM, Bolton R: Gay-bashing: violence and aggression against gay men and lesbians, in Targets of Violence and Aggression. Edited by Baenninger R. North-Holland, Elsevier Science Publishers, 1991, pp 349–401

National Gay and Lesbian Task Force Policy Institute: Anti-Gay/Lesbian Violence, Victimization and Defamation in 1992. Washington, DC, National Gay and Lesbian Task Force, 1993

Remafedi G, Farrow JA, Deischer RW: Risk factors for attempted suicide in gay and bisexual youth. Pediatrics 87:869–875, 1991

Renzetti CM: Violent Betrayal. Newbury Park, CA, Sage, 1992

Renzetti CM: Understanding and responding to violence in lesbian relationships: part I. Treating Abuse Today 3(5):10–12, 1993a

Renzetti CM: Understanding and responding to violence in lesbian relationships; part II: correlates of abuse. Treating Abuse Today 3(6):42–45, 1993b

Renzetti CM: Understanding and responding to violence in lesbian relationships: part III. Treating Abuse Today 4(1):20–24, 1994

Russell D: The Secret Trauma: Incest in the Lives of Girls and Women. New York, Basic Books, 1986

Straus MA, Gelles RJ, Steinmetz SK: Behind Closed Doors: Violence in the American Family. New York, Anchor/Doubleday, 1980

Walber E: Behind closed doors: battering and abuse in the lesbian and gay community, in the Sourcebook on Lesbian and Gay Health. Edited by Shernoff M, Scott W. Washington, DC, National Lesbian and Gay Health Foundation, 1988, pp 250–256

Walker LE: The Battered Woman. New York, Harper & Row, 1979

Walker LE: The Battered Woman Syndrome. New York, Springer, 1984

49

Suicide Risk in Lesbian, Gay, and Bisexual Youth

Norman B. Hartstein, M.D.

onsiderable controversy exists regarding the relationship between sexual orientation and suicide. Lesbians and gay men have often been portrayed in popular culture as victims of suicide (Russo 1987). Anecdotal case reports frequently associate suicidal behavior in the young with homosexuality and conflicts over sexual orientation (Asch 1980; Freud 1920/1955; McIntire 1977; O'Connor 1948; Spencer 1959; Tilton 1994). Although concern about the role of sexual orientation as a risk factor for suicide in youth has been voiced by members of the lesbian, gay, and bisexual communities, as well as by clinicians, parents, and advocacy organizations involved with bisexual, lesbian, and gay youth, the research necessary to clarify this issue has not been conducted. The major investigators of suicide in the young, such as Pfeffer (1989), Shafii et al. (1985), and Brent et al. (1993), have not reported on the sexual orientation of the children and adolescents whom they studied. Only recently has Shaffer (1993a) begun to report on the presumed sexual orientation of adolescents who committed suicide.

Rofes (1983), in his book *I Thought People Like That Killed Themselves: Lesbian, Gay Men, and Suicide,* observed,

> While suicide prevention workers targeted specific youth popula-
> tions—runaways, drug and alcohol abusers, emotionally disturbed
> youth—as risk groups requiring special attention, they avoided fac-
> ing the fact that lesbian and gay youth are also a population that
> greatly need special attention and services. (p. 36)

Rofes believed that taboos surrounding open discussion of lesbianism and male homosexuality were impeding research. Rubenstein et al.
(1989) acknowledged that when developing a questionnaire on suicidality for high school students, "questions about sensitive aspects of
sexual experience [i.e., sexual abuse, homosexuality] were deliberately
omitted to maximize participation" (p. 68).

In January 1989, a task force established by the Secretary of the
U.S. Department of Health and Human Services drafted a final report
that included chapters on "Sexual Identity Issues" by Joseph Harry
(1989) and "Gay Male and Lesbian Youth Suicide" by Paul Gibson.
Based on these presentations, the task force listed homosexuality as a
risk factor for youth suicide. The report was attacked by politicians who,
declaring its findings to be "anti-family" and "anti-Christian," prevailed in lobbying to have those chapters of the report at first suppressed and later included only as appendices.

In his chapter for the task force's report, Gibson (1989) noted that
although studies seemed to confirm a high rate of suicide attempts
among lesbians and gay males, particularly during their youth, uncertainty remained regarding the relationship between attempting suicide
and completing suicide. Nevertheless, Gibson did suggest that gay
youth may comprise up to 30% of completed youth suicides annually.
This estimate, although unsupported by research, has been cited repeatedly.

An increased risk for suicide among gay, lesbian, and bisexual
young people has not been generally recognized by clinicians and researchers. For instance, Blumenthal (1990a) did not discuss sexual orientation in her editorial on the physician's role in preventing youth
suicide. In response to a letter by Snelling (1991) that criticized this
omission, Blumenthal (1991) explained that the relationship of homosexuality to youth suicidal behavior has been inadequately studied.
Shaffer (1993b) argued,

> The lay public and special interest groups of all political hues regularly point to the prevalence of suicide or to individual case reports to support their particular cause, whether it be opposition to heavy metal music or to the fantasy game "Dungeons and Dragons" or support for greater tolerance of homosexual individuals. No matter how much merit these positions may have, their claims about the role of suicide are rarely established. (p. 172)

The National Institute of Mental Health has expressed an interest in funding studies on the relationship between emerging sexuality and suicide and convened a workshop in June 1994 to explore the research issues on suicide and sexual orientation. The proceedings and recommendations from this meeting were accepted for publication as a supplement to the 1995 volume of *Suicide and Life-Threatening Behavior.*

Much of the recent controversy over the role of sexual orientation in youth suicide has been reported in lay periodicals rather than in professional journals (Bull 1994; Shaffer 1993a). Shaffer's views appeared in *The New Yorker* (1993a) at the height of the controversy regarding the attempt by President Clinton to rescind the ban against lesbians, gay men, and bisexual individuals serving in the military. An increased risk for suicide had been cited by those on both sides of the dispute—either to justify excluding from the military those persons believed to be at increased risk for suicide or to argue for the end of discrimination and stigmatization, which might contribute to the increased rate of suicide.

Defining and Identifying the Population

The scientific study of the relationship of sexual orientation to youth suicide has been compromised by the lack of agreement as to the definitions of each of the following terms: "lesbian," "gay," "bisexual," "youth," and "suicide." The term "youth" eludes consistent definition. Although investigators working with children and adolescents generally refer to persons age 15–24 years as youth, subdivided further as adolescents (age 15–19 years) and young adults (age 19–24 years), investigators working primarily with adult populations define young people as those below an arbitrary age, such as 30 years (Rich et al. 1986).

It is difficult to identify those youth who are bisexual, lesbian, or gay; these youth are for the most part an invisible or, at least, an overlooked minority. Clinicians will address sexual orientation when evaluating a child or adolescent who manifests behaviors that do not conform to his or her biological sex, expresses concern about his or her sexual orientation, or has been known to engage in homosexual activities. However, in most cases, the issue of sexual orientation is ignored, and children and adolescents are presumed to be heterosexual.

Donovan (1992) commented that in order to randomly sample a population one must be able "first to define the boundaries of the category, and second to identify all members of the category" (p. 28). Donovan noted that this task was impeded when studying sexual orientation due to the hidden nature of the homosexual population and the lack of consensus as to the definition of gay, lesbian, and bisexual persons.

The Spectrum of Suicide

Although some researchers restrict the use of the term "suicide" to cases of completed suicide, others use the term to encompass the spectrum of suicide behaviors from deliberate self-harm, suicidal gesture, parasuicide, and attempted suicide to completed suicide. In many studies, self-reported suicide attempts are tallied without determination of the seriousness of the attempt by quantitative measures of intent and lethality. Moreover, whether the reported attempt was ever revealed or discovered and whether it received any form of treatment are seldom documented. It is estimated that fewer than one in eight reported suicide attempts ever come to medical attention (Smith and Crawford 1986).

Suicide attempts may occur up to 150 times more frequently than completed suicide (McIntire et al. 1977; Weissman 1974), depending on the definition of suicide attempt and the population being studied. Cohen-Sandler et al. (1982) viewed suicide attempts as active coping efforts as well as a means of interpersonal coercion and retaliation. Attempted suicide is generally recognized to be a major risk factor for subsequent completed suicide. Although some investigators see the populations of suicide attempters and completers as quite similar (Shafii et al. 1985), others believe that they are two distinct groups (Andrews and Lewinsohn 1992; Blumenthal 1990b; Brent and Kolko 1990). Suicide attempts are worthy of investigation regardless of their relationship to completed suicide, because they represent a "morbid health event that results in personal suffering and considerable economic cost" (Meehan et al. 1992, p. 41).

Risk Factors for Suicide

The identification of populations at risk for suicide has been a major focus of investigators of youth suicide because only after populations at risk are identified can interventions be developed to provide services to those youth who are most vulnerable. Suicide is not simply a response to the stresses and problems of adolescence (Schneider et al. 1989; Shaffer 1988). Hoberman and Garfinkel (1988), investigating completed suicide in persons under age 19 years, concluded that no single explanation of the nature of youth suicide will suffice. Blumenthal (1990a), who proposed that one consider several risk factor domains (sociodemographic variables; psychiatric diagnosis; psychosocial, personality, and environmental factors; genetic and familial variables; and biological correlates), suggested that "when a young person with these risk factors undergoes a humiliating life experience and when there is an available method for suicide, the threshold for suicidal behavior is lowered" (p. 3195). Brent and Kolko (1990) identified as common precipitants for youth suicide disciplinary or legal crisis, interpersonal loss, interpersonal conflict, exposure to suicide or suicidal behavior, and accumulation of life stressors.

Risk factors for suicide in the young include 1) mental illness; 2) history of suicide ideation and attempts; 3) drug and alcohol use; 4) sexual or physical abuse; 5) parental absence; 6) recent loss; 7) suicidality in the family; 8) disciplinary crisis; 9) impulsivity or antisocial behaviors; 10) a family environment that is less supportive, more conflicted, and characterized by hostility; 11) the availability of firearms; 12) exposure to suicide; and 13) sexual orientation (Adler and Jellinek 1990; Brent et al. 1987, 1993; Cohen-Sandler 1982; de Wilde et al. 1992; Gibson 1989; Gould and Davidson 1988; Hibbard et al. 1988; Hoberman and Garfinkel 1988; Hollinger et al. 1994; Kellerman et al. 1992; Kosky et al. 1990; Lewinsohn et al. 1993; Marttunen et al. 1992; Rich et al. 1988; Robbins and Conroy 1983; Runeson 1992; Shaffer 1988; Shaffer 1993b). Relatively little attention has been given to variables that might be protective against suicide. Rubenstein et al. (1989) cautioned that most studies examined correlates of adolescent suicidal behavior on a univariate basis, not controlling for the interrelationships among risk factors.

Studies of Suicidality and Gay Youth

■ Prevalence of Suicide Attempts

There are neither reliable estimates of the prevalence of lesbian, gay, and bisexual youth in the general population nor any large-scale population studies on the prevalence of attempted suicide or completed suicide among lesbian, gay, and bisexual youth. The available studies often survey only males, fail to use a commonly agreed-on method for assessing sexual orientation, and access only that population of youth who have already self-identified and come out before the end of adolescence. Many of the sampled gay youth might be categorized as "expendable children" (Sabbath 1969) or "throwaway children" (Richette 1969) whose sexual orientation had been revealed at a young age and who had been rejected by their families, or who had attempted to escape from family discord and abuse. These subjects cannot be assumed to represent either lesbian, gay, and bisexual youth in general or those youth who will only come to identify themselves as lesbian, gay, or bisexual as adults.

Roesler and Deisher (1972) interviewed young men age 16–22 years who had had at least one homosexual experience to orgasm. Nineteen of the 60 subjects (32%) stated that they had previously made a significant attempt on their lives. Remafedi (1987) surveyed 29 subjects age 15–19 years who were self-identified as homosexual, and all but one admitted to contemplating suicide. Of these subjects, 34% actually attempted suicide, and 80% of these attempts followed self-identification as homosexual.

Martin and Hetrick (1988), at the Institute for the Protection of Gay and Lesbian Youth, reported that 21% of their adolescent clients had attempted suicide before presenting for services. Gibson (1989) reported that at the Larkin Street Youth Center in San Francisco 65% of the homosexual or bisexual homeless youth, compared with only 19% of the heterosexual youth, reported ever being suicidal.

Schneider et al. (1989) studied 106 gay males age 16–24 years and reported high rates of suicide attempts (20%) and serious suicidal ideation (55%). The mean age of first attempt was 16.3 years, with the earliest reported attempt at age 12. The attempters reported being significantly younger than nonattempters when they first became aware of their attraction to members of the same sex. Twenty of 21 attempters were aware of being attracted to members of the same sex before their first attempt, but only 2 of the 21 attempters had disclosed their sexuality to any key support persons before their first attempt. Other factors cited by these authors as increasing the subjects' risk for suicide included paternal alcoholism, familial physical abuse, and ethnic minority—especially Latino.

Kruks (1991) reported that in Los Angeles an estimated 25%–30% of all street youth are gay and nearly all street youth have multiple problems. He observed that gay street youth exhibited many of the traits previously identified to have significant correlations with suicide attempts, including rejection by family or friends, awareness of being gay and first sexual experience at an earlier age, attempts to deal with the coming-out process at an earlier age, and ongoing substance abuse. Kruks concluded that 53% of gay street youth had attempted suicide at least once and 47% more than once.

Remafedi et al. (1991) reported on 137 males age 14–21 years who identified themselves as gay (88%) or bisexual (12%). Of these 137, 41 (30%) reported at least one suicide attempt. The mean age of the attempters was 15.5 years. Fifty of the 68 reported attempts did not come to medical attention, whereas 14 of the 68 attempts resulted in hospitalization. Three-fourths of the first suicide attempts followed self-labeling as gay or bisexual, but only one-third of the attempts were related by the subjects to turmoil regarding homosexuality.

Rotheram-Borus et al. (1994) found that attempted suicide was reported in 38.6% of a sample of 139 gay or bisexual males (mostly minority youth) age 14–19 years who presented to a social service agency. Gay-related stressors were significantly more common among suicide attempters compared with nonattempters, but general life stress was not higher.

None of these studies sampled unselected populations or included matched heterosexual control subjects. These reports also failed to compare youth who had multiple problems with lesbian, gay, and bisexual youth who did not have confounding risk factors for suicide. Correlations between suicide attempts and completed suicide were not demonstrated. Nevertheless, these studies consistently reported rates of suicide attempts among samples of gay, lesbian, and bisexual youth that were higher than the estimated 3.4%–15% prevalence of self-reported suicide attempts among adolescents in the general population (Meehan et al. 1992).

Sexual Orientation and Completed Suicide

Studies based on psychological autopsies, conducted by interviewing family and friends of the victims of suicide, are compromised by several limitations: retrospective distortion may occur; stigma, guilt, and shame may influence the information provided by informants close to a suicide victim; and some studies of suicides based on coroners' reports exclude the transient or street population for whom family informants may not be available to interview. In the only community-based study of completed suicide among adolescents that addressed sexual orientation, Shaffer (1993a) identified only 3 of 123 (2.5%) victims as homosexual; 4 others reportedly "showed behavior that could have been indicative of homosexuality" (p. 116). Informants were asked questions about gender-nonconforming behaviors and prior disclosure of sexual orientation by the adolescent.

Although self-reports and corroborating interviews remain the primary basis for assessing sexual orientation, these methods may be unreliable. Sexual orientation is frequently not recognized by youth before their twenties. Among those youth who identify themselves as homosexual before age 19 years, few will have come out to their family and friends (Schneider et al. 1989). It is likely that only a small percentage of parents of lesbian and gay youth accurately report the sexual orientation of their children when interviewed.

HIV and Suicide

The risk for suicide among lesbian, gay, and bisexual youth may increase because of the impact of HIV both on those infected and on survivors who have sustained multiple losses. Frances et al. (1985) and Flavin et al. (1986) suggested that a population of gay or bisexual youth who were depressed, alcoholic, and passively self-destructive or suicidal might be likely to seek multiple sexual partners with AIDS. Although Marzuk et al. (1988) argued that AIDS represented a significant risk factor for suicide, Starace (1993), studying suicidal behavior in people infected with HIV, concluded that belonging to specific populations at risk for HIV infection might be more important than actual serostatus in increasing the risk of suicide. Many of the patients infected with HIV who acknowledge attempting suicide report that the first suicide attempt preceded the diagnosis of AIDS or HIV positivity and often occurred during their youth. The growing rate of HIV infection among young gay males is of considerable concern, and Rotheram-Borus et al. (1994) predicted that a link between suicidality and testing HIV positive may be demonstrated in future studies of gay youth.

Studies of Suicidality and Young Gay Adults

■ Sexual Orientation and the Prevalence of Suicide Attempts

Several studies investigating prior suicide attempts as reported by community samples of gay, lesbian, or bisexual adults found higher rates of suicide attempts in young lesbians, bisexual individuals, and gay men. Saghir et al. (1970a, 1970b) and Saghir and Robins (1973) reported a higher rate of suicide attempts in gay males (7% of 89 gay males versus 0% of 35 control subjects) and in lesbians (23% of 57 lesbians versus 5% of 43 control subjects). It is noteworthy that most of the attempts reported by gay males were before age 20 years, whereas lesbians more often attempted suicide in their twenties.

Bell and Weinberg (1978) reported increased rates of suicide attempts in gay males (18% versus 3% for whites and 20% versus 2% for blacks) and in lesbians (25% versus 10% for whites and 17% versus 16% for blacks) compared with heterosexual control subjects. They also found that most of the reported attempts occurred before the age of 25 years. The gay men were more likely than the lesbians to report that their attempts were related to trying to deal with homosexuality; the lesbians' attempts were more often reported to be related to the breakup of their lesbian relationships.

In a study analyzing the Bell and Weinberg data, Harry (1983) found that among men of all sexual orientations, childhood cross-gender behaviors were related to an increased rate of suicide attempts. Harry also concluded that a large amount of the suicidality among the homosexual respondents occurred during late adolescence and early adulthood, when homosexual youth are very largely isolated from the adult gay movement.

Jay and Young (1979) noted that 40% of a nonrandom sample of 5,000 homosexual men and women admitted having seriously considered or attempted suicide. Hammelman (1993) reported that 29% of a sample of 48 lesbian, gay, and bisexual subjects age 15–32 years had attempted suicide, with 71% of these suicide attempts occurring by age 17. She also observed that concurrent risk factors for suicide were prevalent in the bisexual individuals, gay men, and lesbians surveyed. Of the respondents, 44% had been abused and 35% had an alcohol or drug problem. Muehrer (1994) questioned the reliability and validity of those studies that were not published in peer-reviewed scientific journals.

■ Sexual Orientation and Completed Suicide

Most studies of completed suicides in adults fail to report the sexual orientation of the victims (Apter et al. 1993; Barraclough et al. 1974; Dorpat and Ripley 1960; Marttunen et al. 1992; Robins et al. 1959; Runeson 1992). Robins (1981), in a book elaborating on his earlier study of 134 persons age 24 years and older who had completed suicide, concluded that the absence of a diagnosis of homosexuality among the 134 cases of completed suicide "is probably evidence of the relative rarity of homosexuals rather than a rarity of completed suicides among homosexuals" (p. 7). The failure to identify any of the subjects as homosexual might also have been a result of how successful gay, lesbian, and bisexual persons in the 1950s were in hiding their sexual orientation.

Beskow (1979), reporting on a series of 271 completed suicides among Swedish males older than 15 years, identified only 5 of 161 in the urban sample and 1 of 110 in the rural sample as homosexual. Rothberg et al. (1990), reporting on suicide in U.S. Army personnel, a population that had been screened to exclude lesbian, gay males, and bisexual individuals, identified problems with alleged sexual deviation in 1.7% of 212 suicides.

Only Rich et al. (1986), conducting a large-scale study of completed suicide in adults, compared gay males with straight males. They studied a series of 133 consecutive suicides in men under the age of 30 years and 150 suicides in men age 30 years or older. Thirteen (nine of whom were under age 30) were identified to be gay by histories obtained from a variety of informants. Thus, almost 7% of the men who completed suicide before age 30 were identified to be gay. Prior suicide attempts were as common in the gay group as in the comparison group. Of the 13 gay men who committed suicide, 12 had one or more DSM-III (American Psychiatric Association 1980) substance abuse diagnoses, and all but 2 also had a DSM-III diagnosis other than substance abuse. The authors commented that they discerned few, if any, differences between the young gay and straight males who committed suicide. Before generalizing this conclusion to all gay men, the authors acknowledged several limitations in their study: a sample size of 13 gay men is hardly adequate to justify highly sophisticated statistical analysis or any major conclusions; the true rate of homosexuality in the general population is unknown; and there was no way of knowing what the covert rate of homosexuality might have been in the study sample.

Clinical Issues

Clinicians need to appreciate that there are many gay, lesbian, and bisexual youth who are not readily recognized. There is a tendency to avoid questioning teenagers about their sexual orientation. When adolescents from unfamiliar cultures present for treatment, the clinician may be even more reluctant to inquire about sexual orientation. Direct questioning of a lesbian, gay, or bisexual teenager may result in denial and attempts to mislead the evaluator. When parents have brought the youngster for treatment and the patient has not as yet come out to the family, the patient may be reluctant to confide in the therapist. A youth who denies being gay, lesbian, or bisexual might still be conflicted about his or her sexual orientation and might benefit from having these issues discussed.

■ Case Example 1

Ms. A was 17 years old when she first presented with her family for evaluation. Her parents complained about her moodiness, anger, and inability to follow their rules. The elder of two children adopted by Japanese-American parents, Ms. A was of Asian-Pacific Island ancestry. Her temperament, energy level, and outspoken frankness did not fit well into this family. A series of family sessions proved only partially successful in improving communication and promoting a greater tolerance of difference. Two years later, Ms. A called the author for a consultation and revealed that she was depressed, suicidal, and abusing alcohol after a breakup with her lesbian lover. Only at follow-up did she reveal her sexual orientation, which had been overlooked previously.

■ Case Example 2

Mr. B was in his early 30s when he presented with complaints of depression. Mr. B identified himself as a gay man who was comfortable with his sexual identity. During the course of treatment, he revealed that he had been hospitalized after a suicide attempt while in college. He recalled concealing a history of homosexual activity and his conflict over his sexual orientation from the hospital staff. He had feared that the clinical staff might reveal his secret to his parents and the school administration. He chose instead to identify anxieties about his grades and rejection by a girlfriend as the precipitants of the suicide attempt.

■ Case Example 3

Mr. C was admitted to a psychiatric unit after a suicide attempt at age 17. On admission, he revealed to the evaluating psychiatrist that he had taken an overdose after he had seen a peer counselor at a local gay and lesbian social service agency because he thought he might be gay. When the counselor confirmed his fears by suggesting that he probably was gay, the patient felt confused, hopeless, and suicidal. The suicide attempt, which was of low lethality, brought his conflict into the open. Mr. C was recognized by the treatment team to be depressed; however, because his behavior was perceived to be gender appropriate, most of the staff felt he was not gay and should be encouraged to develop his heterosexual interests and dating skills. His concerns about being homosexual were minimized and not explored further during the hospitalization.

■ Case Example 4

Mr. D was a 17-year-old student in a Catholic high school. At age 14, he had revealed to his parents that he believed he was gay, and they had alternated between trying to ignore and accept his sexual orientation without talking about his feelings or his sexual experiences. The parents called the clinic when the patient appeared more depressed and less communicative. On evaluation, the patient was found to be dysthymic, and he also qualified for a diagnosis of borderline personality disorder. The patient had recurring suicidal ideation and was hospitalized briefly on two occasions. Mr. D was a very reluctant patient and was not able or willing to reveal much information about himself in therapy. The patient alluded to problems in a romantic relationship with an adult man but was ambivalent about discussing this relationship and possibly compromising his friend if he were to reveal his identity to the therapist. The patient discontinued therapy before he turned 18 years old.

These clinical examples are presented to portray only a few of the issues that are encountered when working with lesbian, gay, or bisexual youth. The patient's level of trust will be influenced by the perceived attitudes and comments of the clinician. A treatment milieu that seems intolerant or displays a heterosexist bias may be perceived as hostile and unsafe by the gay, lesbian, or bisexual youngster. Youth with adequate ego strength may choose to conceal their homosexuality while in treatment to avoid additional conflict and disapproval.

Conclusion

The available data support the conclusion that being lesbian, gay, or bisexual is associated with an increased risk for attempting suicide when young. We know that some youth who are lesbian, gay, or bisexual do commit suicide. We do not know the prevalence of lesbians, gay males, or bisexual individuals among youth who complete suicide. When comparing suicide rates of adolescents based on sex, females have been found to be at increased risk for suicide attempts, and males are at increased risk for completed suicide. It is possible that an increased risk for suicide attempts among lesbian, gay, and bisexual youth is not associated with an increased risk for completed suicide. It is likely that the rate of suicide among lesbian, gay, and bisexual youth varies among subgroups that are not yet unidentified, much as it does among Native American Indians, not all of whom share the same risk for suicide (Wyche and Rotheram-Borus 1990).

Because of changing political, social, and health factors, there is reason to expect that cohort specificity will limit the applicability of findings from research done in previous decades. The Stonewall revolution, removal of homosexuality as a mental disorder, the subsequent rise of a conservative political agenda challenging the acceptance of sexual orientations other than heterosexuality, and the effects of HIV infection may account for changes in the developmental experiences, attitudes, and self-esteem of bisexual individuals, gay men, and lesbians.

Factors that may increase a lesbian, gay, or bisexual youth's vulnerability for suicide include any of the known factors for youth suicide, such as mental disorder, substance abuse, a history of prior suicidal behavior, exposure to suicide, a history of abuse, and an available firearm. Gender nonconformity—especially when associated with isolation from peers, self-identification as homosexual at a young age, and rejection or condemnation by family and other significant sources of support because of sexual orientation—may be additional stressors unique to this population. Even when a patient does not self-identify as lesbian, gay, or bisexual, a clinician should explore the sexual orientation and sexual identity of the suicidal adolescent or young adult.

Understanding suicide and preventing suicide are important challenges for clinicians working with any group of youth, regardless of the relative risk for suicide of that specific group compared with other populations. In the final analysis, whether lesbian, gay, and bisexual youth are 7% or 30% of the total number of youth who attempt or commit suicide, the problems encountered by these youth warrant wider discussion, further investigation, and clearer understanding. One would hope that future studies of suicide will incorporate more effective methods of identifying gay, lesbian, and bisexual persons. Future research must try to access the large population of gay, lesbian, and bisexual youth who often seem to be invisible. It is especially important that populations of bisexual, lesbian, and gay youth who are not street youth, troubled youth seeking services in social service agencies, or psychiatric patients be included in such research. Accurate information must be made available to all—clinicians, researchers, families, teachers, clergy, politicians, the general public, and especially the youth themselves. Concerned professionals must also recognize that public policy determines both the research agenda and the information that is disseminated about both suicide and sexual orientation.

Blumenthal (1990a) suggested that "the presence of certain protective factors including cognitive flexibility, hopefulness, strong social supports, removal from stressors, and, importantly, receiving appropriate treatment for an associated psychiatric disorder contribute to maintaining a barrier to suicidal behavior" (p. 3195). By aggressively treating mental disorders and drug abuse in the young, diminishing stressors, and successfully promoting hopefulness, strong social supports, and cognitive flexibility among lesbian, gay, and bisexual youth, clinicians may be able to reduce the rate of suicide in this population. By protecting lesbian, gay, and bisexual youth from ignorance, intolerance, discrimination, abuse, and rejection that contribute to their despair and isolation, clinicians might further decrease their risk for suicide.

References

Adler RS, Jellinek MS: After teen suicide: issues for pediatricians who are asked to consult to schools. Pediatrics 86:982–987, 1990

American Psychiatric Association: Diagnostic and Statistical Manual of Mental Disorders, 3rd Edition. Washington, DC, American Psychiatric Association, 1980

Andrews JA, Lewinsohn PM: Suicidal attempts among older adolescents: prevalence and co-occurrence with psychiatric disorders. J Am Acad Child Adolesc Psychiatry 31:655–662, 1992

Apter A, Bleich A, King R, et al: Death without warning? A clinical postmortem study of suicide in 43 Israeli adolescent males. Arch Gen Psychiatry 50:138–142, 1993

Asch SS: Suicide and the hidden executioner. Int Rev Psychoanal 7:51–60, 1980

Barraclough B, Bunch J, Nelson B, et al: A hundred cases of suicide: clinical aspects. Br J Psychiatry 125:355–377, 1974

Bell A, Weinberg M: Homosexualities. New York, Simon and Schuster, 1978

Beskow J: Suicide and mental disorder in Swedish men. Acta Psychiatr Scand Suppl 277:1–138, 1979

Blumenthal SJ: Youth suicide: the physician's role in suicide prevention. JAMA 264:3194–3196, 1990a

Blumenthal SJ: Youth suicide: risk factors, assessment and treatment of adolescent and young adult suicidal patients. Psychiatr Clin North Am 13:511–555, 1990b

Blumenthal SJ: In reply. JAMA 265:2806–2807, 1991

Brent DA, Kolko DJ: Suicide and suicidal behavior in children and adolescents, in Psychiatric Disorders in Children and Adolescents. Edited by Garfinkel BD, Carlson GA, Weller EB. Philadelphia, PA, WB Saunders, 1990, pp 372–391

Brent DA, Perper JA, Allman CJ: Alcohol, firearms, and suicide among youth. JAMA 257:3369–3372, 1987

Brent DA, Perper JA, Moritz G, et al: Psychiatric risk factors for adolescent suicide: a case-control study. J Am Acad Child Adolesc Psychiatry 32:521–529, 1993

Bull C: Suicidal tendencies. The Advocate, April 5, 1994, pp 35–42

Cohen-Sandler R, Berman AL, King RA: Life stress and symptomatology: determinants of suicidal behavior in children. Journal of the American Academy of Child Psychiatry 21:178–186, 1982

de Wilde EJ, Kienhorst ICWM, Diekstra RFW, et al: The relationship between adolescent suicidal behavior and life events in childhood and adolescence. Am J Psychiatry 149:45–51, 1992

Donovan JM: Homosexual, gay, and lesbian: defining the words and sampling the population. J Homosex 24:27–42, 1992

Dorpat TL, Ripley HS: A study of suicide in the Seattle area. Compr Psychiatry 1:349–359, 1960

Flavin DK, Franklin JE, Frances RJ: The AIDS and suicidal behavior in alcohol-dependent homosexual men. Am J Psychiatry 143:1440–1442, 1986

Frances RJ, Wikstrom T, Alcena V: Contacting AIDS as a means of committing suicide (letter). Am J Psychiatry 142:656, 1985

Freud S: Psychogenesis of a case of homosexuality in a woman (1920), in The Standard Edition of the Complete Psychological Works of Sigmund Freud, Vol 18. Translated and edited by Strachey J. London, Hogarth Press, 1955, pp 145–172

Gibson P: Gay male and lesbian youth suicide, in Report of the Secretary's Task Force on Youth Suicide, Vol 3: Prevention and Interventions in Youth Suicide. Washington, DC, U.S. Department of Health and Human Services, 1989, pp 110–142

Gould MS, Davidson L: Suicide contagion among adolescents, in Advances in Adolescent Mental Health, Vol III: Depression and Suicide. Edited by Stillman AR, Feldman RA. Greenwich, CT, JAI Press, 1988

Hammelman TL: Gay and lesbian youth: contributing factors to serious attempts or considerations of suicide. Journal of Gay and Lesbian Psychotherapy 2:77–89, 1993

Harry J: Parasuicide, gender, and gender deviance. J Health Soc Behav 24:350–361, 1983

Harry J: Sexual identity issues, in Report of the Secretary's Task Force on Youth Suicide, Vol 2: Risk Factors of Youth Suicide. Washington, DC, U.S. Department of Health and Human Services, 1989, pp 131–142

Hibbard RA, Brack CJ, Rauch S, et al: Abuse, feelings, and health behaviors in a student population. Am J Dis Child 142:326–330, 1988

Hoberman HM, Garfinkel BD: Completed suicide in children and adolescents. J Am Acad Child Adolesc Psychiatry 27:689–695, 1988

Hollinger PC, Offer D, Barber JT, et al: Suicide and Homicide Among Adolescents. New York, Guilford, 1994

Jay K, Young A: The Gay Report: Lesbians and Gay Men Speak Out About Sexual Experiences and Lifestyles. New York, Summit, 1979

Kellerman AL, Rivara FP, Somes G, et al: Suicide in the home in relation to gun ownership. New Engl J Med 327:467–472, 1992

Kosky R, Silburn S, Zubric KS: Are children and adolescents who have suicidal thoughts different from those who attempted suicide? J Nerv Ment Dis 178:38–43, 1990

Kruks G: Gay and lesbian homeless/street youth: special issues and concerns. J Adolesc Health 12:515–518, 1991

Lewinsohn PM, Rohde P, Seeley JR: Psychosocial characteristics of adolescents with a history of suicide attempt. J Am Acad Child Adolesc Psychiatry 32:60–68, 1993

Martin AD, Hetrick ES: The stigmatization of the gay and lesbian adolescent. J Homosex 15:163–183, 1988

Marttunen MJ, Aro HM, Lönnquist JK: Adolescent suicide: endpoint of long-term difficulties. J Am Acad Child Adolesc Psychiatry 31:649–654, 1992

Marzuk PM, Tierney H, Tardiff K, et al: Increased risk of suicide in persons with AIDS. JAMA 259:1333–1337, 1988

McIntire MS, Angle OR, Wikoff RL, et al: Recurrent adolescent suicidal behavior. Pediatrics 60:605–608, 1977

Meehan PJ, Lamb JA, Saltzman LE, et al: Attempted suicide among young adults: progress toward a meaningful estimate of prevalence. Am J Psychiatry 149:41–49, 1992

Muehrer P: Suicide and sexual orientation: a critical summary of recent research and direction for future research. Address presented at the American Association of Suicidology convention, New York, NY, April 8, 1994

O'Connor WA: Some notes on suicide. Br J Med Psychol 21:222–228, 1948

Pfeffer CR: Studies of suicidal preadolescent and adolescent inpatients: a critique of research methods. Suicide Life Threat Behav 19:58–77, 1989

Remafedi G: Male homosexuality: the adolescent's perspective. Pediatrics 79:326–330, 1987

Remafedi G, Farrow JA, Deisher RW: Risk factors for attempted suicide in gay and bisexual youth. Pediatrics 87:869–875, 1991

Rich CL, Fowler RC, Young D, et al: San Diego suicide study: comparison of gay to straight males. Suicide Life Threat Behav 16:448–457, 1986

Rich CL, Fowler RC, Fogarty LA, et al: San Diego suicide study, III: relationships between diagnoses and stressors. Arch Gen Psychiatry 45:589–592, 1988

Richette LA: The Throwaway Children. New York, Dell Publishing, 1969

Robbins D, Conroy RC: A cluster of adolescent suicide attempts: is suicide contagious? J Adolesc Health Care 3:253–255, 1983

Robins E: The Final Months. New York, Oxford University Press, 1981

Robins E, Murphy GE, Wilkinson RH, et al: Some clinical considerations in the prevention of suicide based on a study of 134 successful suicides. Am J Public Health 49:888–899, 1959

Roesler T, Deisher RW: Youthful male homosexuality. JAMA 219:1018–1023, 1972

Rofes EE: I Thought People Like That Killed Themselves: Lesbians, Gay Men, and Suicide. San Francisco, CA, Grey Fox Press, 1983

Rothberg JM, Fagan J, Shaw J: Suicide in United States Army personnel, 1985–1986. Mil Med 155:452–456, 1990

Rotheram-Borus MJ, Hunter J, Rosario M: Suicidal behavior and gay-related stress among gay and bisexual male adolescents. Journal of Adolescent Research 9:498–508, 1994

Rubenstein JL, Heeren T, Housman D, et al: Suicidal behavior in "normal" adolescents: risk and protective factors. Am J Orthopsychiatry 59:59-71, 1989

Runeson BS: Youth suicides unknown to psychiatric care providers. Suicide Life Threat Behav 22:494–503, 1992

Russo V: The Celluloid Closet: Homosexuality in the Movies, Revised Edition. New York, Harper and Row, 1987

Sabbath JC: The suicidal adolescent: the expendable child. Am Acad Child Psychiatry 8:272–289, 1969

Saghir MT, Robins E: Male and Female Homosexuality. Baltimore, MD, Williams and Wilkins, 1973

Saghir MT, Robins E, Walbran B, et al: Homosexuality, III: psychiatric disorders and disability in the male homosexual. Am J Psychiatry 126:1079–1086, 1970a

Saghir MT, Robins E, Walbran B, et al: Homosexuality, IV: psychiatric disorders and disability in the female homosexual. Am J Psychiatry 127:147–154, 1970b

Schneider SG, Farberow NL, Kruks GN: Suicidal behavior in adolescent and young adult gay men. Suicide Life Threat Behav 19:381–393, 1989

Shaffer D: The epidemiology of teen suicide: an examination of risk factors. J Clin Psychiatry 49(suppl):36–41, 1988

Shaffer D: Political science. The New Yorker, May 3, 1993a, p 116

Shaffer D: Suicide: risk factors and the public health. Am J Public Health 83:171–172, 1993b

Shafii M, Carrigan S, Whittinghill JR, et al: Psychological autopsy of completed suicide in children and adolescents. Am J Psychiatry 142:1061–1064, 1985

Smith K, Crawford S: Suicidal behavior among "normal" high school students. Suicide Life Threat Behav 16:313–325, 1986

Snelling LK: Adolescents who attempt suicide (letter). JAMA 265:2806, 1991

Spencer SJG: Homosexuality among Oxford undergraduates. Journal of Mental Science 105:395–405, 1959

Starace F: Suicidal behaviour in people infected with human immunodeficiency virus: a literature review. Int J Psychiatry 39:164–170, 1993

Tilton P: Religion and psychiatry. Clinical Psychiatric News 22:17, 1994

Weissman MM: The epidemiology of suicide attempts. Arch Gen Psychiatry 30:737–746, 1974

Wyche KF, Rotheram-Borus MJ: Suicidal behavior among minority youth in the United States, in Ethnic Issues in Adolescent Mental Health. Edited by Stiffman AR, Davis LE. Newbury Park, CA, Sage, 1990, pp 323–338

50

Mental Health Care Providers Working With HIV

Avoiding Stress and Burnout

J. Stephen McDaniel, M.D.
Eugene W. Farber, Ph.D.
Mary B. Summerville, Ph.D.

Rabkin et al. (1993) called living with AIDS one of the most stressful of human experiences. Intense painful emotions, including grief, accompany the HIV epidemic for patients, loved ones, and health care providers. Such feelings result from the physical and emotional demands that HIV and AIDS place on affected individuals. Through 1995, over 300,000 individuals have died from AIDS in this country (Centers for Disease Control and Prevention 1995). Although the demography of HIV is slowly changing as a result of increased heterosexual transmission, the gay and bisexual male community has continued to be hardest hit by AIDS, representing over 50% of AIDS cases (Centers for Disease Control and Prevention 1995). In this regard, reports of entire gay social networks decimated by AIDS in the first decade of the epidemic remain common today (Shilts 1987).

As HIV infection has spread and the incidence of AIDS cases has grown, the adverse psychological impact on health care professionals working with AIDS patients has become increasingly apparent (Silverman 1993). Adapting to the pressures of front-line AIDS involvement requires that individuals who work with individuals with AIDS balance their commitment and motivation with the stresses inherent in their work. Difficulty in managing this balance has resulted in the onset of a constellation of symptoms suggestive of burnout in some health care providers caring for persons with HIV (Macks and Abrams 1992). Mental health care providers in particular are prone to burnout as they struggle to assist their patients with often overwhelming anger, sadness, and hopelessness by employing a range of intervention strategies (Robinson 1994).

Definition of Burnout

The term "burnout" first appeared in the health care literature in the mid-1970s (Freudenberger 1974; Maslach 1976) and refers broadly to the response of an individual to work-related stressors that have not been successfully managed or resolved (Macks and Abrams 1992). Pines and Aronson (1988) describe burnout as "a state of physical, emotional, and mental exhaustion caused by long-term involvement in situations that are emotionally demanding" (p. 9). Similarly, Scott and Jaffe (1989) summarized the literature by describing burnout as "the end-stage result of the inability to manage work stress" (p. 86). These definitions share a common reference to the potential complications of ineffective efforts to cope with overwhelming work-related stress.

Burnout may be expressed in varied ways in affected individuals, organizations, and communities (Grosch and Olson 1994). These symptoms may range from physical to emotional or behavioral difficulty and may result in an array of costly consequences (Table 50–1). Individuals with burnout have difficulty functioning both in the workplace and in their personal lives and are at risk for a decline in health and an increase in psychological distress. Generally, where burnout is high, organizations experience increased staff conflict, tardiness, absenteeism, higher turnover rates, and lower productivity (Macks and Abrams 1992). When providers with burnout withdraw from their patients, become cynical, and begin to feel demoralized themselves, the quality of care they provide to their patients diminishes. For these reasons, recognizing these symptoms and understanding their consequences are essential for care providers. To understand this issue, the authors describe factors that heighten the risks for burnout in those affected by the AIDS epidemic.

Table 50–1.   Manifestations of burnout

Physical symptoms

Chronic fatigue	Somatic complaints
Changes in appetite	Tension headaches
Gastrointestinal problems	Ulcers
Sleep disturbance	Vulnerability to illness

Psychological symptoms

Alienation	Loss of concern
Anger toward patients	Loss of meaning
Anxiety	Negativism about self and others
Apathy	Obsessions, phobias about HIV
Black humor	Posttraumatic stress syndrome
Cynicism	Paranoia
Depression	Repression of feeling
Disillusionment	Sense of omnipotence
Emotional liability	Suicidal ideation
Helplessness, hopelessness	Unrealistic expectations

Behavioral symptoms

Avoiding responsibilities	Increased alcohol or drug use
Anger directed at patients	Interpersonal conflict
Criticism of co-workers	Lethargy
Chronic tardiness for work	Missed appointments
Decreased contact with clients	Neglect of personal hygiene
Decreased productivity	Under/Overeating
Distraction, irritation, resentfulness	Withdrawal and isolation
Disorganization	Overreaction

Source.   Adapted from Macks and Abrams 1992.

The Multilayered Context of AIDS Burnout

■ Responses of Health Care Providers to the Stresses of AIDS

The process of burnout of health care providers has become increasingly complex because of the multilayered context of AIDS care, including the sociocultural, medical, and psychological dimensions that come into play. Previous studies of stress and physical illness, including terminal illness, do not adequately capture the stresses involved in AIDS care, as these complicating factors are unique to the AIDS phenomenon (Fawzy et al. 1991).

Sociocultural context.   Examinations of cultural responses to infectious disease epidemics have shown that fear of contagion often precipitates discrimination of those afflicted (Kain 1994; McCombie 1990). The epidemic of HIV and AIDS has unfolded in a cultural context of fear and stigma, as many persons with AIDS have been shunned and rejected, isolated from others, terminated from places of employment, and blamed for being ill (Cadwell 1994a; Herek 1990; Quam 1990). The intensity of this social stigma has been attributed to the synergistic impact of the medical aspects of AIDS and the emergence of AIDS first from culturally marginalized communities, including gay and bisexual men, injection drug users, and ethnic minority groups (Herek 1990; Quam 1990). Perceptions of AIDS as characterized by a degenerative course, the low physical concealability of many AIDS symptoms that routinely may be perceived by others as repulsive or disturbing, and the potential for AIDS to disrupt the ordinary flow of social discourse in those afflicted with the disease also may heighten AIDS stigma (Herek 1990).

Health care providers working with HIV and AIDS patients must conduct their professional activities within this broad cultural context of stigma and fear. Their work involves treating a complicated and fatal disease and assisting patients with the cultural fallout of the illness, including feelings of shame, guilt, anger, frustration, and demoralization. In many cases, the effects of social stigma may contribute to the onset of generalized malaise and apathy in patients, thereby compromising motivation to participate in treatment and prompting heightened treatment noncompliance. In this way, the effects of social stigma may complicate the treatment of a disease that presents formidable medical challenges and may compound work-related stress in the care provider.

Additionally, the social and political environment surrounding the AIDS epidemic is such that care providers often find that their work moves beyond the role of health care provider into unfamiliar and often stressful advocacy roles. These roles may include pursuit of health and social support services for patients, participation in public education programs to enhance understanding and prevention, and involvement in policy discussions and ethical debates regarding management of the AIDS epidemic. Although these are important contributions for those health care providers, they are likely to add stress to the daily health care practice of the provider.

Finally, cultural fear and stigma regarding HIV and AIDS also may result in a pattern of stigma by association for those who are care providers for AIDS patients. For example, reports exist of ostracism of some care providers by professional colleagues not involved in AIDS care (Lessor and Jurich 1986). At the least, fear about the disease and misunderstanding about how HIV is transmitted may prompt some to question why anyone would work with such patients. These effects may spill over into the private lives of some care providers who may find themselves in a position of having to explain their professional decision to work with AIDS patients to family and friends (Lessor and Jurich 1986).

Medical context.   The medical aspects of HIV also contribute to the risk of burnout in care providers. Because AIDS is fatal, an obvious source of stress is created for care providers working in the AIDS community. In the course of their work, providers experience repeated losses, which naturally heightens the stress of the work, often bringing to mind the cumulative toll of past losses. In this regard, although AIDS issues are unique, much can be learned about the experience of managing and reducing burnout in care providers working with cancer patients or persons with other terminal illnesses.

The medical severity of AIDS is compounded by the complex history of the search for a cure for AIDS, with earlier proclamations of rapid progress giving way to repeated frustrations. Now, more than 14 years since the disease was first identified, there remains little hope of a cure soon, a realization that has resulted in frustration and disappointment in the community of AIDS care providers, as during the 1993 International Conference on AIDS in Berlin. This lack of medical progress is apt to lower morale for some providers on the front lines of AIDS treatment.

The course of AIDS is such that it consists of multiple paths of suffering that are not easily predicted. There are discontinuous periods of stable health followed by sharp declines, with care providers often reduced to the role of witness to the complex physical and emotional pain of AIDS. In addition, many of the medications used to treat AIDS-related ailments are themselves prone to generating a large number of side effects, a state of affairs that may lower the morale of patient and care provider alike.

Finally, AIDS is an infectious disease, and care providers (specifically those providing direct medical care that could result in exposure to blood products) must live with the knowledge that procedural errors could result in their being infected with the virus. Although the disease is not easily transmitted and the likelihood is small that a care provider might be infected by a patient in the course of daily clinical activity, the knowledge of such a possibility has been documented as a source of stress for care providers directly involved in the provision of medical treatment (Silverman 1993).

Psychological context.   Ongoing exposure to the complicated bio-psychosocial factors of HIV and AIDS may create a heightened psychological vulnerability to the emergence of burnout symptoms in the care provider. Specifically, when confronted with the sometimes overwhelming aspects of the work, some care providers may experience loss of a sense of control and increased futility and professional impotence. Increased vulnerability to this type of stress is expected because laboratory research has demonstrated that repeated inability to control aversive circumstances may result in passive tolerance of negative events (Seligman 1975). The growing epidemic, the increase of HIV-related problems on individual and societal levels, the difficulties in finding adequate solutions to the problems, and the irreversibility of the disease may contribute to the adoption of attributions of the problem as temporally stable and global in its adverse influence. Consistent with recent research findings regarding attributional processes and mood or outlook (Burns and Seligman 1991), this set of attributions may lead to increased feelings of helplessness and hopelessness.

Although working with dying individuals can be personally and professionally enriching and meaningful for care providers, in some instances continual confrontation with death and dying is apt to contribute to burnout. One reason for this is the activation of death anxiety (Yalom 1980), the awareness of which typically is steadfastly defended against in everyday life (Becker 1973). As such, some dimensions of burnout in the care provider may be understood as a response to heightened death anxiety that is likely to be elicited not only because their patients are dying but also because the tangible limits in available resources serve as reminders of their capacity to help. This may involve being confronted with awareness of one's limits and the realization that one is unable to stop the suffering in these patients.

In a related vein, some care providers who witness the suffering of their patients may wonder about the meaning of such experiences and engage in self-reflective challenges of their existing world views. Although this process can be psychologically and emotionally productive, a risk exists that it may precipitate a crisis of meaning if such feelings remain unresolved. This may include the emergence of a paralyzing cynicism regarding the meaning and value of their professional roles as caregivers, and the ultimate usefulness of their craft. To the extent that they remain entangled in such a crisis of meaning and are unable to resolve such questions, manifestations of burnout are likely to ensue.

In summary, care providers on the front lines of the HIV and AIDS epidemic operate within a multilayered context that spans broad sociocultural issues, specific medical realities, and specific psychological vulnerabilities that they may be exposed to in their work. An understanding of burnout may be enhanced by considering the collective impact of these intertwined psychosocial domains on the work of the health care provider.

■ Gay, Lesbian, and Bisexual Health Care Providers

The AIDS epidemic has taken on special meaning to those providers who are gay, lesbian, or bisexual. Because the gay and bisexual male community was the first group affected by HIV and because the lesbian community has long been active in providing HIV-related health care, these communities have experienced myriad adversities as a result of the AIDS epidemic. Gay, lesbian, and bisexual providers grieve not only their personal losses but also the losses of their culture and community (Schwartzberg 1992). Three types of stressors to which these care providers may be susceptible are multiple losses, overidentification, and survivor guilt.

The stresses of bereavement for these providers are compounded by multiple losses on multiple levels. Kastenbaum (1977) coined the phrase "bereavement overload" in reference to elderly individuals who experience the deaths of many friends within a short time, and Lehman and Russell (1985) applied this concept to those people dealing with the multiple losses of persons with AIDS. Gay, lesbian, and bisexual health care providers are apt to experience this bereavement overload more deeply than providers who identify less with affected communities. In this regard, Carmack (1992) conducted interviews with gay and lesbian individuals to gain understanding about their management of multiple AIDS-related losses. Carmack found that a key to managing their overwhelming losses was how well an individual managed the continuum of engaging and detaching with both patients and fellow staff.

Biller and Rice (1990) have explained that for members of the gay, lesbian, and bisexual community experiencing multiple losses of friends with AIDS, the issue of resolving grief is complicated by two factors. The first relates to the unwillingness of society to fully accept the gay identity and the importance of the loss of a gay friend or significant other. The second factor relates to the exacerbation of grief induced by repetitive loss over a brief time. A common belief (Di Angi 1982) is that loss reminds people of other losses; thus, when gay people deal with the grief of someone dying, they may be reminded of the grief of coming to terms with their own self-identity (Siegal and Haefer 1988).

Gay and lesbian physicians working with AIDS patients tend to have strong feelings of identification with their patient populations and occasionally experience irrational fears of vulnerability to the disease (Goldblum 1986). These physicians also have been found to be more likely to experience psychological stress as their percentage of time spent with AIDS patients increases (Goldblum 1986). Cadwell (1994b) recently studied the concept of overidentification with patients in a sample of gay psychotherapists working with gay AIDS patients. Cadwell found that several themes emerged related to the therapists' identifications with their patients, including concerns about contagion, vulnerability to death and grief, and concerns about homophobia. Providers also may lose perspective on the severity of illness in their patients and may minimize observed symptoms (Cabaj 1991).

Other investigators, including McKusick (1992), have studied the concept of survivor guilt, particularly in gay male health care providers. The term "survivor guilt," initially coined to describe some survivors of the Holocaust, refers to the manifestations of symptoms such as depression, anxiety, and somatic complaints that may arise when pervasive feelings of guilt result from the phenomenon of survival when loved ones do not survive (McKusick 1992). For mental health care providers offering treatment to other clinicians in the AIDS arena, survivor guilt may frequently manifest within psychotherapy. Such guilt is largely unconscious, is generally denied or rationalized, and is virtually never an explicit part of the presenting complaint (Odets 1994). The following case study describes the impact of survivor guilt:

■ Case Example 1

> Dr. A was a young, gay, HIV-seronegative, male mental health care provider who sought individual psychotherapy to facilitate his dealing with AIDS-related burnout. He worked primarily in the

AIDS clinic of a large public hospital with a patient population consisting largely of young, gay, HIV-seropositive men. He presented with symptoms of feelings of being overwhelmed, irritability, intermittent insomnia, nightmares, and "difficulty maintaining a sense of life's meaning." He was concerned because he felt himself withdrawing from his patients and fellow staff. He also described the odd phenomenon on two occasions of mistaking the identity of strangers on the street for deceased patients. During the initial course of psychotherapy, Dr. A described the following dreams:

1. Dr. A was walking across the parking lot of a local convenience store located near the AIDS clinic. A frenzy of activity occurred with many people scurrying about. One by one, the people in the parking lot were shot by what appeared to be distant but invisible sharpshooters. Suddenly, Dr. A was the only person left standing, and gunfire stopped. He stood physically immobilized and confused as to why he was not also killed.

2. Dr. A was in a large group of gay, lesbian, and bisexual people marching in a gay pride parade. There was an air of proud community spirit and excitement associated with the festivities. Suddenly, the group began marching into a crowd of Ku Klux Klan members armed with firearms. The Ku Klux Klan members subsequently began shooting the gay pride marchers. As friends and acquaintances began falling around Dr. A, he continued to march through the Ku Klux Klan group without receiving even a scratch. He realized he was the only survivor and was left standing confused and guilty.

Dr. A's dream content expressed an identification, probably an overidentification, with his patients—clearly seeing himself as a member of a community being devastated. Survivor guilt was a central theme in both dreams as Dr. A was the lone survivor in each scenario. His affect of bewilderment over his surviving suggests guilt, implying that perhaps he should have been among the dead. These themes reappeared in various ways, throughout the course of his therapy rekindling earlier childhood experiences of guilt and responsibility related to the death of his father when Dr. A was a child, and the multiple personal and family losses related to this event. His nightmares, preoccupation with his deceased patients, and mistaking the identity of strangers (reexperiencing patients) were symptoms of posttraumatic stress, suggesting the severity of the personal traumatic impact of his work.

His psychotherapy focused on finding meaning in loss through relating his current experiences and symptoms to earlier but similar life events and on catharsis through retelling and reexperiencing the feelings of his traumas. Strategies were implemented to facilitate a sense of finality with regard to the deaths Dr. A continued to experience. For example, he was encouraged to continue providing therapy for some gravely ill patients even when they were too sick to come to his office. He conducted psychotherapy by telephone and at the bedside, and, when appropriate, he continued his relationships with patients until their death. Moreover, he made attempts to attend memorial services and ritualized the planting of flowers each time a patient died. He also had the occasion to hold family therapy sessions for the families of some deceased patients as a way of bringing about family and personal closure. These therapeutic activities, which brought some resolution to his work, provided the energy to reinvest in relationships with friends and family. Ultimately, as Dr. A proceeded to work on these issues of survivor guilt and multiple loss throughout therapy, he was able to find strength by learning effective ways to grieve his losses while maintaining his strong desire to contribute to his community.

The stressors of some gay, lesbian, and bisexual care providers are exemplified in the content of Dr. A's dream and therapeutic process. Survivor guilt is now a well-recognized complication of AIDS care, particularly prevalent in seronegative gay male providers (Odets 1994). In some instances, burnout symptoms brought on by multiple losses and overidentification can progress to symptoms of posttraumatic stress disorder (McKusick 1992; Schoen 1992). Martin (1989) has characterized the multiple and continuing deaths associated with the AIDS epidemic as traumatic events outside the range of usual human experience for those who witness these losses. Martin (1989) and Trice (1988) have documented the emergence of chronic posttraumatic stress disorder in the gay, lesbian, and bisexual community and the general AIDS caregiver community as a consequence of the need to deal with multiple losses.

■ Seropositive Health Care Providers

For HIV-seropositive health care providers, both the rewards and stresses of working in the AIDS arena are more complex than for any other providers. Although the literature contains a few articles about the imminent death of the provider, particularly in the case of providers who are therapists, literature on the therapist and patient sharing the same life-threatening condition has emerged only recently (Shernoff 1994). Clearly, each new death is experienced within the context of previous deaths and the fear of future deaths, including one's own demise (Carmack 1992). The experience of multiple losses is compounded by the multiple personal lifestyle losses that are inevitable for HIV-seropositive patients and providers, for example, loss of employment and role or professional status, alterations in physical functioning, and significant changes in sexual patterns of relating (Lennon et al. 1990).

Several additional issues are apt to be of special significance in the daily work of the HIV-seropositive care provider. For example, these providers may be at particular risk of overidentifying with their patients. Alternatively, they may become excessively distant emotionally from patients as they struggle to maintain distance from their own feelings and conflicts regarding their disease process. Their work also presents these care providers with multiple living examples of how the disease progression could occur for them, a state of affairs that might heighten worries about what their future has in store with regard to HIV disease progression. Finally, unlike HIV-seronegative providers, HIV-seropositive providers are never able to take a break from HIV disease. When they are not at work, they must manage their own health care as well as their psychological responses to their disease process. These and other factors create a unique set of stressors for HIV-seropositive providers.

The decision of whether or not to disclose their HIV status to patients and colleagues and its accompanying stress becomes a major factor in the relationship between HIV-seropositive providers and their patients and co-workers. For many patients, the fantasy that their provider will not die before them provides a safe environment for their health care, perhaps prompting some providers to hesitate about disclosing their HIV status. However, because some patients may feel a sense of betrayal if providers do not disclose their health status, such conflicts must be carefully figured into each individual decision of whether and how to disclose. Phillip (1994) described how the benefits of disclosing her terminal diagnosis to patients promoted both patient and therapist growth. Philip found that disclosure brought about rich opportunities to explore universal life and death issues and the particular meaningful losses of each patient. Furthermore, Philip described the inherent therapeutic effect of allowing patients to work with their therapists around the timing of termination related to illness.

Eventually, HIV-seropositive health care providers must become caregivers to themselves as they give up aspects of their professional life (Hutton 1994). This stressful transition may be best facilitated through professional supervision and psychotherapy. Rosner (1986) has addressed the importance of direct practice alternatives, suggesting pursuits such as writing, teaching, lecturing, or consulting for such providers. These alternatives may provide the necessary buffers to combat the stress of losing or altering one's professional role.

Recommendations for Coping

Strategies to prevent burnout symptoms in the workplace have been discussed in the literature, and for the most part, such strategies are applicable to AIDS mental health care providers (Marks and Abrams 1992). However, the unique combination of stressors associated with AIDS health care necessitates consideration of strategies for the management of burnout at the level of the individual, the organization, and the community at large. Table 50–2 provides a detailed list of strategies.

■ Individual Strategies

Cadwell (1994b) recently described specific strategies for managing the vulnerability of therapists to identify with AIDS patients. These strategies include behavioral management such as limiting numbers of patients, affiliating with peers, choosing other means of community involvement, and maintaining a personal life; ego supportive resources through such actions as supervision and collegial support; supportive friendships; political and community involvement; management through personal growth; and maintaining or developing a spiritual life. Cognitive management skills include clarifying one's role as a therapist, for example, by understanding the need for multiple interventions such as social casework and education; time frame change with the understanding that AIDS work has become oriented less toward crisis care and more toward long-term care; specialization or focusing on specific interventions for some patients such as diagnostic consul-

Table 50–2.   Strategies for managing burnout

Individual interventions
  Allow oneself to grieve openly rather than withdraw
  Altruism—volunteering, activism
  Attend grieving rituals: funerals, wakes, memorial services
  Desensitize and reframe survivor's guilt
  Development of a heightened spiritual identity
  Develop new hobbies and interests
  Find ways to appropriately use humor
  Health care provider support groups
  Journal writing
  Participate in forums that focus on rewards of AIDS work such as AIDS
    Walks or fundraisers
  Physical exercise
  Periodic getaways or vacations
  Psychotherapy
  Reach out to available support systems
  Supervision and collegial support
  Take time to visit patients in their support systems

Organizational interventions
  Appreciation mechanisms
  Celebration of significant life events of staff such as birthdays,
    anniversaries, and achievements
  Enhancing communication systems
  Formal support
  Honoring of cultural diversity
  Informal communication

Issues related to different HIV statuses of staff
  Acknowledgment of staff appreciation
  Supportive personnel policies, such as bereavement leave
  Job structure and workload
  Ongoing acknowledgment of losses
  Policies and benefits
  Role of management
  Staff development

Community interventions
  Celebrate significant community anniversaries, for example, the 25th
    anniversary Stonewall celebration
  Participate in community-wide memorial services, such as World AIDS Day
  Maintain camaraderie between community service organizations through
    efforts such as joint fundraisers

tation, pharmacotherapy, or behavioral management; and the finding of meaning in work, conceptualizing the special significance of AIDS work. In one survey of AIDS providers (Hortsman and McKusick 1986), respondents identified talking with a friend, lover, or family member; teaching others about AIDS; remaining objective; and getting support from other providers as effective coping strategies.

Macks and Abrams (1992) describe the importance of separating one's work from home life through the use of techniques that punctuate the work day with an activity that separates it from one's home life. Physical exercise, one such activity, allows one the time to disengage from the details of the workday while promoting a sense of well-being. Periodic getaways, for example, non-work-related vacations, have been suggested to combat burnout as the change of scenery may break the insulating effect of working in the epidemic by providing psychological diversions that facilitate a freshening of emotional resources (Hortsman and McKusick 1986).

Psychotherapy and related mental health interventions can have a significant impact on ameliorating the burnout symptoms of providers (Winiarski 1991). A large literature exists describing the benefits of support groups for providers (Biller and Rice 1990; Feingold 1994; Frost et al. 1991). Such therapeutic modalities can alleviate many of the symptoms and consequences of burnout, and they can facilitate the search of providers for meaning in the suffering of the AIDS epidemic, a task that has been described as vital for optimal human functioning in adversity (Frankl 1946). Psychotherapy, while not a cure for the devastation of the epidemic, is a powerful tool to facilitate working through the complex grief brought on by the toll of AIDS work, particularly for the unique toll of gay, lesbian, and bisexual providers. Psychotherapy may facilitate mourning, thus facilitating a successful grief resolution, an important psychological task for AIDS care providers (Schwartzberg 1992; Shelby 1994).

■ Organizational Strategies

Strategies targeted at an organizational level are often necessary adjuvants for managing the HIV-related stresses of health care staff. For example, Schoen (1992) has described specific strategies for addressing grief within AIDS organizations that include acknowledging loss or finding sensitive ways to disclose deaths to staff such as personal notes, staff journals, or periodic memorials; finding informal and formal ways to provide staff support; assessing personnel policies and benefits such as bereavement leave, dependent care leave, or "mental health days"; and formalizing staff appreciation through such avenues as staff lunches, outings, or retreats. Addressing work-related stress at an organizational level can be thought of as a measure for preventing individual stress and as an investment in patient care and work productivity.

■ Community Strategies

Although AIDS has now crossed all demographic barriers, the gay, lesbian, and bisexual community has struggled the longest to cope with the stresses of the epidemic. This community, which has been beset by AIDS since the beginning of the epidemic, has struggled to make sense of and stem the suffering by turning to activities such as political activism, community involvement, caring for the ill, and spirituality (Schwartzberg 1992). Such involvements have contributed to the resiliency of the gay, lesbian, and bisexual community. In this regard, although earlier studies have shown that members of the at-risk gay and bisexual male community are experiencing significant distress levels (Holland and Tross 1986; Martin 1988; Ostrow et al. 1986; Tross 1986), more recent investigations have documented a community with significant resiliency. For example, Rabkin et al. (1990) investigated psychiatric and psychosocial variables thought to be related to level of hope in a large cohort of HIV-positive and -negative gay men in New York City and found that the men had high levels of hope and low levels of psychiatric disorders, including symptoms of depression. Similarly, in an investigation of the extent to which deaths of lovers and close friends from AIDS increased the frequency of symptoms of depression and depressive disorders in a group of gay men in New York City, Neugebauer et al. (1992) found that the level of symptoms of depressions, the presence of specific symptom clusters, and the presence of diagnosed depressive disorder were unrelated to the number of AIDS deaths a subject reported. These investigators theorized that changes in normative expectations of AIDS deaths and mobilization against AIDS within the gay community probably explained their results.

Interpretation of studies such as these must include consideration of the duration of the AIDS epidemic. These investigations were carried out in the late 1980s when a multitude of community agencies were organized in the midst of community-motivated AIDS activism. It remains difficult to predict how AIDS will continue to impact the gay, lesbian, and bisexual community. Some researchers have documented increases in unsafe sexual practices in the gay male community, particularly among gay male youth in recent years (Lemp et al. 1994; Shafer et al. 1993). A key contributing factor to this behavior has been the phenomenon of growing up and "coming out" during an era of fatalism in the community and massive loss and sorrow (Munzell 1992). Whether the hopefulness and positive coping strategies of the gay, lesbian, and bisexual community of the first decade of AIDS can continue may in large part depend on the extent of individual and community psychosocial interventions aimed at reducing the impact of chronic stress.

A major implication of these studies with regard to managing stress and burnout is the importance of engaging members of the affected AIDS community in creative efforts to organize a community response to the epidemic. These findings suggest that such a process can empower community members faced with adversity as severe as AIDS.

Conclusion

Burnout as it pertains to the AIDS epidemic is a complex but often transient phenomenon that must be understood in the context of complex sociocultural, medical, and psychological factors, particularly as these factors affect the gay, lesbian, and bisexual community. Recognition of burnout symptoms is a key to implementing timely, effective interventions at the individual, organizational, and community levels.

References

Becker E: The Denial of Death. New York, Free Press, 1973
Biller R, Rice S: Experiencing multiple loss of persons with AIDS: grief and bereavement issues. Health Soc Work 15:283–290, 1990

Burns MO, Seligman MEP: Explanatory style, helplessness, and depression, in Handbook of Social and Clinical Psychology: The Health Perspective. Edited by Snyder CR, Forsyth DR. New York, Pergamon, 1991, pp 267–284

Cabaj RP: Overidentification with a patient, in Gays, Lesbians, and Their Therapists: Studies in Psychotherapy. Edited by Silverstein C. New York, WW Norton, 1991, pp 31–39

Cadwell SA: Twice removed: the stigma suffered by gay men with AIDS, in Therapists on the Front Lines: Psychotherapy with Gay Men in the Age of AIDS. Edited by Cadwell SA, Burnham RA, Forstein M. Washington, DC, American Psychiatric Press, 1994a, pp 3–24

Cadwell SA: Overindentification with HIV clients. Journal of Gay and Lesbian Psychotherapy 2:77–99, 1994b

Carmack BJ: Balancing engagement/detachment in AIDS-related multiple losses. J Nurs Scholarship 24:9–14, 1992

Centers for Disease Control and Prevention: HIV/AIDS Surveillance Report 7:1–18, 1995

Di Angi P: Grieving and the acceptance of the homosexual identity. Issues in Mental Health Nursing 4:101–113, 1982

Fawzy FI, Fawzy NW, Pasnau RO: Bereavement in AIDS. Psychiatr Med 9:469–482, 1991

Feingold A: Peer supervision and HIV: one group's process, in Therapists on the Front Line: Psychotherapy with Gay Men in the Age of AIDS. Edited by Cadwell SA, Burnham RA, Forstein M. Washington, DC, American Psychiatric Press, 1994, pp 517–534

Frankl V: From Death Camp to Existentialism. Boston, MA, Beacon Press, 1946/1959

Freudenberger JH: Staff burnout. J Social Issues 30:159–165, 1974

Frost JC, Makadon HJ, Judd D, et al: Care for caregivers: a support group for staff caring for AIDS patients in a hospital-based primary care practice. J Gen Int Med 6:162–167, 1991

Goldblum PB: Professionals facing the AIDS epidemic: who helps the helpers? Paper presented at the annual meeting of the American Psychological Association, Washington, DC, August 1986

Grosch WN, Olson DC: When Helping Starts to Hurt: A New Look at Burnout Among Psychotherapists. New York, WW Norton, 1994

Herek GM: Illness, stigma, and AIDS, in Psychological Aspects of Serious Illness: Chronic Conditions, Fatal Diseases, and Clinical Care. Edited by Costa PT, VandenBos GR. Washington, DC, American Psychological Association, 1990, pp 105–149

Hortsman W, McKusick L: The impact of AIDS on the physician, in What To Do About AIDS. Edited by McKusick L. Berkeley, CA, University of California Press, 1986, pp 23–35

Hutton LE: The process of closing a practice when the therapist has AIDS: a case study, in Therapists on the Front Line: Psychotherapy with Gay Men in the Age of AIDS. Edited by Cadwell SA, Burnham RA, Forstein M. Washington, DC, American Psychiatric Press, 1994, pp 561–582

Kain EL: Some sociological aspects of HIV disease, in Sociological Footprints. Edited by Cargan L, Ballantine JH. Belmont, CA, Wadsworth Publishing, 1994, pp 27–32

Kastenbaum RJ: Death and development through the life span, in New Meanings of Life. Edited by Feigel H. New York, McGraw-Hill, 1977, pp 35–47

Lehman V, Russel N: Psychological and social issues of AIDS, in Understanding AIDS. Edited by Gong V. New Brunswick, NJ, Rutgers University Press, 1985, pp 177–182

Lemp GF, Hirozawa AM, Givertz D, et al: Seroprevalence of HIV and risk behaviors among young homosexual and bisexual men. JAMA 272:449–454, 1994

Lennon MC, Martin JL, Dean L: The influence of social support on AIDS-related grief reactions among gay men. Soc Sci Med 31:477–484, 1990

Lessor R, Jurich K: Ideology and politics in the control of contagion: the social organization of AIDS care, in The Social Dimensions of AIDS: Method and Theory. Edited by Feldman DA, Johnson TM. New York, Praeger, 1986, pp 245–259

Macks JA, Abrams DI: Burnout among HIV/AIDS health care providers, in AIDS Clinical Review. Edited by Volberding P, Jacobson M. New York, Marcel Dekker, 1992, pp 283–299

Martin JL: Psychological consequences of AIDS-related bereavement among gay men. J Consult Clin Psychol 56:856–862, 1988

Martin JL: Human immunodeficiency virus infection and the gay community: counseling and clinical issues. Journal of Counseling Development 68:67–72, 1989

Maslach C: Burned-out. Hum Behav 5:16–22, 1976

McCombie SC: AIDS in cultural, historic, and epidemiologic context, in Culture and AIDS. Edited by Feldman DA. New York, Praeger, 1990, pp 9–27

McKusick L: Meeting the challenges of grief and multiple loss. HIV Frontline 6, February 1992

Munzell M: Dancing with death. San Francisco Chronicle Image August 23:23–27, 1992

Neugebauer R, Rabkin JG, Williams JBW, et al: Bereavement reactions among homosexual men experiencing multiple losses in the AIDS epidemic. Am J Psychiatry 149:1374–1379, 1992

Odets W: Survivor guilt in seronegative gay men, in Therapists on the Front Line: Psychotherapy with Gay Men in the Age of AIDS. Edited by Cadwell SA, Burnham RA, Forstein M. Washington, DC, American Psychiatric Press, 1994, pp 453–474

Ostrow DG, O'Brien K, Emmons CA, et al: Sexual practices and mental health in a cohort of homosexual men. Paper presented at the Second International Conference on AIDS, Paris, France, June 1986

Phillip CE: Necessary and unnecessary disclosure: a therapist's life-threatening illness, in Therapists on the Front Line: Psychotherapy with Gay Men in the Age of AIDS. Edited by Cadwell SA, Burnham RA, Forstein M. Washington, DC, American Psychiatric Press, 1994, pp 535–548

Pines A, Aronson E: Career Burnout. New York, The Free Press, 1988

Quam MD: The sick role, stigma, and pollution: the case of AIDS, in Culture and AIDS. Edited by Feldman DA. New York, Praeger, 1990, pp 29–44

Rabkin GR, Remien R, Katoff L, et al: Resilience in adversity among long-term survivors of AIDS. Hosp Community Psychiatry 44:162–167, 1993

Rabkin JG, Williams JBW, Neugebauer R, et al: Maintenance of hope in HIV-spectrum homosexual men. Am J Psychiatry 147:1322–1326, 1990

Robinson CS: Counseling gay males with AIDS: psychosocial perspectives. Journal of Gay and Lesbian Social Services 1:15–32, 1994

Rosner S: The seriously ill or dying analyst and the limits of neutrality. Psychology 4:357–371, 1986

Schoen K: Managing grief in AIDS organizations. Focus 7:1–4, May 1992

Schwartzberg SS: AIDS-related bereavement among gay men: the inadequacy of current theories of grief. Psychotherapy 29:422–429, 1992

Scott CD, Jaffe DT: Managing occupational stress associated with HIV infection. Occup Med 4:85–93, 1989

Seligman MEP: Helplessness: On Depression, Development, and Death. San Francisco, CA, Freeman, 1975

Shafer MA, Hilton JF, Ekstrand M, et al: Relationship between drug use and sexual behaviors and the occurrence of sexually transmitted diseases among high-risk male youth. Sex Transm Dis 20:307–313, 1993

Shelby RD: Mourning within a culture of mourning, in Therapists on the Front Line: Psychotherapy with Gay Men in the Age of AIDS. Edited by Cadwell SA, Burnham RA, Forstein M. Washington, DC, American Psychiatric Press, 1994, pp 53–80

Shernoff M: Therapists' disclosure of HIV status and the decision to stop practicing: an HIV-positive therapist responds, in Therapists on the Front Line: Psychotherapy with Gay Men in the Age of AIDS. Edited by Cadwell SA, Burnham RA, Forstein M. Washington, DC, American Psychiatric Press, 1994, pp 549–560

Shilts R: And the Band Played On. New York, St. Martin's Press, 1987

Siegal R, Haefer D: Bereavement counseling for gay individuals. Am J Psychotherapy 35:517–525, 1988

Silverman DC: Psychosocial impact of HIV-related caregiving on health providers: a review and recommendations for the role of psychiatry. Am J Psychiatry 150:705–712, 1993

Trice AD: Posttraumatic stress syndrome-like symptoms among AIDS caregivers. Psychol Rep 63:656–658, 1988

Tross S: Psychological impact of AIDS-spectrum disorders in New York City. Paper presented at the annual meeting of the American Psychological Association, Washington, DC, May 1986

Winiarski MG: Caring for ourselves, in AIDS-Related Psychotherapy. Edited by Winiarski MG. New York, Pergamon, 1991, pp 134–143

Yalom ID: Existential Psychotherapy. New York, Basic Books, 1980

51

Mental Health Issues Across the HIV-1 Spectrum for Gay and Bisexual Men

David G. Ostrow, M.D., Ph.D.

The increasingly chronic nature of infection with human immunodeficiency virus-1 (HIV-1) and the increasing risk of contracting HIV-1 create a natural history of mental health functioning and coping that parallels the physiological effects of HIV-1 across a spectrum, ranging from preoccupations about risk of becoming infected (the "worried well"), to initial infection, through asymptomatic and symptomatic infection, to AIDS and terminal illness. As individuals move through the physiological course of HIV-1, they experience a range of psychological reactions to the disease, social attitudes, and the threats of illness and death; in this chapter, the author focuses on the psychological challenges and adaptation of gay and bisexual men with HIV-1 infection. Long-term prospective cohort studies of gay and bisexual men at risk for HIV-1 infection have provided an opportunity to study mental health functioning across this spectrum, beginning with risk behaviors and seroconversion, antibody testing and disclosure, long-term asymptomatic infection, the likely eventual AIDS diagnosis, and ending with the terminal phase of HIV-1–related illnesses (Table 51–1).

The mental health natural history of HIV-1 infection also may be divided into sequential phases (see Table 51–1; Ostrow and Wren 1993). In the first phase, the at-risk gay or bisexual man is engaging in sexual or drug use behaviors that place him at significant risk for acquiring primary HIV infection. The second phase encompasses the period of time between primary infection—exposure—and the emergence of antibodies to HIV-1—seroconversion. This period may range from a few weeks to months and usually occurs within 6 months of exposure. The third phase is known as the "asymptomatic phase," or that period between when a person first seroconverts and develops serious symptoms. This period may last from months to years, averaging 9–10 years for adult gay white men (Bacchetti and Moss 1989). Although an individual may not experience severe life-threatening disease during this phase, he may experience intermittent symptoms such as night sweats, rashes, or diarrhea. Some men may experience more serious physiological symptoms, such as fatigue, which can be incapacitating at times. The fourth phase begins with symptoms of severe immunosuppression or the diagnosis of significant neurological impairment, a life-threatening opportunistic infection, a secondary neoplasm, debilitating wasting syndrome, or a CD4 lymphocyte count below $200/mm^3$. At this point a person is diagnosed as having AIDS according to specific criteria developed by the Centers for Disease Control (1993). During each of these stages, an individual may experience a variety of mental health problems; when specific problems are more likely to occur at a particular stage of HIV-1 infection, they are indicated in Table 51–1.

The biopsychosocial conceptualization of HIV-1 disease means that mental health, well-being, and cognitive functioning become the ultimate determinants of the quality of life. Furthermore, many of the proponents of holistic health would argue that mental health influences physical health, measured in terms of length of survival (long-term survival), rate of immunological deterioration (psychoimmunology), and neurological functioning (psychoneuroimmunology). Thus, if mental disorders are properly detected and treated among individuals infected with HIV-1, not only would quality of life improve, but quite possibly, also immune functioning and length of survival. Although this is still an area of considerable debate and controversy, several recent studies of gay or bisexual cohorts have suggested that, at least among men in the

Table 51–1. Overview of individual and family psychosocial issues in relation to stage in spectrum of HIV infection

Stage in spectrum of HIV-1 infection	Time	Developing psychosocial issues	
		Infected individual	Family
Exposure	0 years	High-risk behaviors, denial, fear	Possible high-risk behaviors, denial, secrecy, concern, fear
I. Testing HIV positive		Crisis reaction, shock, denial, depression, suicidal thoughts, guilt, withdrawal, anger, relief	Crisis reaction, shock, denial, depression, uncertainty
		Disclosure—fear	Disclosure—fear
II. Symptom-free period		Reestablish equilibrium, search for meaning, restore self-esteem, try to gain control, uncertainty	Reestablish equilibrium, search for meaning, uncertainty
		Changes in lifestyle	Possible changes in lifestyle
III. Signs and symptoms		Loss of control and independence, guilt, anger, depression, suicidal thoughts, support, reciprocity, disfigurement, treatment decisions, bargaining	Caregiving support, reciprocity, treatment decisions, bargaining
IV. AIDS		Grief, possible relief at diagnosis, depression	Anticipatory grief, depression
Terminal stage		Preparation for death, depression, acceptance, final treatment decisions, assisted suicide	Preparation for death, caregiver burnout, final treatment decisions, depression, acceptance, requests for suicide assistance
Death	2–10+ years		Bereavement, recovery

Note. Adapted from Adelman 1989, Kubler-Ross 1987, and Wadland and Gleeson 1991.

earlier stages of HIV-1 infection, depression is associated with faster rates of immunological decline (Burack et al. 1993; Caumartin et al. 1991).

As has been found in most chronic illnesses, relationships exist between levels of stress experienced by gay and bisexual men with HIV-1 infection and levels of mental health functioning, but resulting levels of distress and psychopathology vary widely among persons suffering equivalent levels of stress (Folkman et al. 1993; Lackner et al. 1993). Both coping styles and social support can mediate the relationship between stress and distress, with the ability to both positively and negatively affect outcomes. In addition, several studies have indicated that familial or prior history of mental illness is an additional strong predictor of mental dysfunction among gay and bisexual men with HIV-1 or AIDS (Atkinson et al. 1988; O'Dowd et al. 1993; Perkins et al. 1994; Perry et al. 1993). Premorbid substance abuse or dependence—problems that are highly prevalent among at-risk gay and bisexual men (Stall and Wiley 1988)—can also seriously compromise mental health and behavioral functioning at any stage of the HIV-1 spectrum (see Chapter 47 by Cabaj).

Sources of distress for gay and bisexual men with HIV-1 include the knowledge that they carry a lethal infectious virus; have a highly stigmatized disease that the larger society associates with an equally stigmatized lifestyle; may be socially ostracized with significant risk of loss of job, income, housing, family, and other support; and may eventually suffer from a disfiguring, painful, and terminal illness. Bisexual men may be at even greater risk of suffering depression and isolation than self-identified gay men (Ostrow et al. 1989), perhaps because gay men are more connected to supportive networks in their community while bisexual men fear rejection from their heterosexual friends and may not readily identify with the gay community (Dew et al. 1990).

Several studies have demonstrated that specific coping mechanisms, such as active appraisal and adaptation, and supportive social interactions can contribute to well-being and improved quality of life for men with HIV-1 (Folkman et al. 1993; Halman et al. 1994; Hays et al. 1992; Wolf et al. 1991). Conversely, maladaptive coping strategies—such as denial or passive fatalism; use of alcohol, recreational drugs, or casual sex as distraction coping responses; and conflict with one's social network—can all contribute negatively to well-being and have a significant impact on the quality of life. Gay and bisexual men experience social conflict not only as a result of others' responses to their being infected but also because of societal reactions to their homosexuality (Holland and Tross 1985; Nichols 1985). Some men may have kept their homosexuality hidden from their family and work environment. With a diagnosis of HIV-1 infection or AIDS, they may no longer want to, or be capable of, keeping this secret. This social conflict may be compounded by fear of eviction from their housing, termination from their place of employment, and loss of their health insurance, all in reaction to their diagnosis (Cassens 1985). Social conflict has been found to increase the symptoms of depression among men at risk for AIDS (O'Brien et al. 1993). Not surprisingly, peer-led social support groups have proven to be effective in ameliorating distress and isolation experienced by gay and bisexual men living with HIV-1 (Kelly et al. 1993b). The earliest community support programs, such as Shanti and Gay Mens Health Crisis, were based on a social support and coping model.

Intervention Issues for the At-Risk Gay or Bisexual Man

Psychological reactions to the threat of HIV-1 or AIDS itself are varied. Prior to seroconversion, gay and bisexual men may begin to manifest psychological symptoms from the stress of potentially becoming HIV-1 infected (Joseph et al. 1990). These men have been described as the "worried well" (Faulstich 1987; Jenike and Pato 1986; Morin et al. 1984). Their psychological distress may take the form of generalized or AIDS-specific anxieties, panic attacks, hypochondriasis, or obsessive-compulsive disorders (Faulstich 1987). In addition, gay and bisexual men at risk for HIV-1 illness may be experiencing the illness or death of friends and lovers, which in turn may cause depression both directly and through the loss of their significant social supports or the threat of their own premature mortality (Holland and Tross 1985; Nichols 1985). While observing these reactions, it is important for clinicians to account for preexisting psychiatric disorders (including substance abuse or dependency) that may become exacerbated by the threat of HIV-1 illness but are not directly caused by HIV-1.

■ HIV-1 Antibody Testing Issues

Counseling related to HIV antibody testing is often the first contact that HIV-infected men will have with mental health caregivers. According to the Centers for Disease Control (1993):

Successful HIV prevention counseling involves four essential components: 1) personalized risk assessment to facilitate a realistic self perception of risk; 2) identification and discussion of barriers to behavior change and reinforcement of behavior change already initiated by the client; 3) negotiation between the counselor and the client of a realistic and incremental risk reduction plan; and 4) establishment of a specific plan to receive test results and post-test counseling. (p. 23)

In addition, prevention requires the need for the strictest confidentiality to develop trust and protect clients from possible discrimination. Of paramount importance is the evaluation of all patients for possible adverse behavioral or mental health consequences of testing and provision of psychological therapies aimed at ameliorating those responses. Often, this will mean referring a patient to one or more gay-sensitive community-based AIDS service organizations (ASOs) that provide HIV-1 psychosocial and case management services.

■ Case Example 1

Scott is a 28-year-old white, bisexual male who comes to see you with the complaint of increasing anxiety, insomnia, poor appetite with 10-pound weight loss over the past month, and fatigue. The precipitant appears to be his recent break-up with a male lover of 5 years and the ex-lover's informing Scott that he had tested positive for HIV-1 antibodies. Scott reports frequent nightmares and daytime anxiety attacks, all focusing on fears that he has AIDS and will soon die, alone and disfigured. At times, suicidal thoughts occupy his thinking, and he is unable to concentrate on his work or household chores. He has withdrawn from friends and his female lover, Brenda, for fear that they will notice his illness and react negatively. He was referred to you for psychiatric evaluation by his internist, who found mildly swollen axillary lymph glands on examination of this otherwise healthy appearing but extremely anxious patient.

During Scott's first visit, you listen to his concerns and provide reassurance and factual information regarding the natural history of HIV-1 infection, the signs and symptoms of AIDS, and the practical aspects of HIV-1 antibody testing. After discussing his anxiety attacks, you decide to prescribe an anxiolytic medication. You then take a detailed sexual behavior history, noting Scott's significant potential exposure history and his continuing sexual activities with

Brenda. After discussing the pros and cons of HIV-1 antibody testing, you and Scott agree that a test is indicated and blood is drawn for the enzyme-linked immunosorbent assay (ELISA) and confirmatory Western blot analyses. You schedule a follow-up appointment for 1 week later, at which time you will evaluate Scott's response to anxiolytic therapy and the result of his HIV-1 antibody test. You provide him with some written materials about HIV-1 testing and encourage him to call you if he experiences any anxiety attacks or problems with the medication. On leaving your office, Scott informs you that he feels relieved at having finally been tested and discussing his fears with you.

A realistic personalized plan for behavior modification based on the client's own risk behavior history needs to be developed during the pretest counseling session. It is important that both counselor and client agree on the feasibility of this plan and that possible barriers to the suggested changes are discussed and reactions to them anticipated. Although behavioral risk assessment and planning for behavioral change are of the utmost importance, it is also important that the therapist take into account the psychological needs and state of the person seeking the test. For gay or bisexual men requesting testing, there are a number of highly emotionally charged issues: feelings that they may have put themselves or partners at risk for HIV-1 and may actually soon learn that they are HIV-1 seropositive; thoughts about the possible consequences of a positive test and fears of having to disclose the result (and related indiscretions) to loved ones; and the associated fears of abandonment. In anticipation of these fears, the therapist should walk the client through different scenarios by asking, for instance, "What may you feel like and what will you subsequently do if you find out that you are HIV-1 positive?" or "What if you are negative?" A counselor or therapist can and should be as helpful as possible in pointing out behavioral, emotional, societal, legal, and psychological consequences of both scenarios. Finally, sufficient time should be spent discussing the test procedures, the meaning and limitations of the laboratory findings, and the recommended follow-up procedures for each individual. There are, in addition, many ethical and legal issues that complicate the patient–therapist relationship when HIV-1 testing or treatment is involved (Wren 1993). Many states have passed legislation or public health regulations that define the therapist's obligations and the conditions under which patient privacy may be breached for public health considerations. Mental health practitioners need to be familiar with their local laws and regulations related to patient confidentiality and HIV-1 testing and discuss their implications with all new gay and bisexual patients.

■ Seroconversion and Disclosure Issues

Varied and conflicting reports have been made about the impact of testing and disclosure of serostatus for those who are at risk for HIV-1. Possible impacts include depression, suicidal ideation or suicidal attempts, anxiety and somatic preoccupations, an increased sense of isolation, anger, substance abuse or other forms of distraction coping, symptoms of adjustment disorder, and mild transient patterns of psychological distress (Holland and Tross 1985; Jacobsen et al. 1990; Kelly et al. 1993a; Kelly and St. Lawrence 1988; Ostrow et al. 1988; Perry et al. 1990). Some researchers have reported a sharp rise in anxiety and depression for some individuals at the time of diagnosis of HIV-1 infection but also found that these states dissipated with time (Ostrow et al. 1992). However, specific concerns about AIDS and the long-term impact of being HIV-1 seropositive will significantly increase after learning that one is infected; dealing with these "AIDS worries" is often a major goal of therapy for HIV-1-seropositive gay or bisexual men. Substance abuse and other forms of maladaptive coping may increase or recur, and issues of informing sexual partners and other significant persons are frequently central to therapy in the postdisclosure period.

> Scott returns for his posttest counseling appointment, at which time he reports a significant decrease in his anxiety, with no incapacitating attacks or suicidal ideation during the past week. However, he reports significant increased anxiety this morning, focusing on his reaction to an expected positive test result. He appears somewhat relieved when you tell him that his test was, indeed, positive but that he is in the earliest stage of infection. Scott's anxiety returns when the issue of informing his girlfriend, Brenda, about his HIV-1 seropositivity is raised. Although she has always been aware of his bisexuality and Scott expects her to be supportive of him, he feels extreme embarrassment and guilt over the thought that he might have infected her. You reassure Scott and counsel him about the importance of HIV-1 testing for Brenda and any other unprotected sexual contacts he might have had in the past year. You

and Scott agree on the need to continue the anxiolytic therapy and weekly psychotherapy with you, focusing on his anxiety and AIDS-specific worries. As Scott expresses a preference for seeing a gay physician specializing in HIV and AIDS care, you refer him to the infectious disease practitioner you work closest with and also provide him with a list of local ASOs.

◼ Social Support Issues and Interventions for Gay or Bisexual Men Recently Diagnosed as Seropositive

In addition to the psychological impact of HIV-1 infection, there are also social effects, both positive and negative. Researchers have speculated on the occurrence of depression and suicidal ideation among men at the time of HIV-1 antibody testing and again at the time of an AIDS diagnosis. Most clinicians believe that gay and bisexual men who have recently been diagnosed as HIV-1 positive need to be watched closely for suicidality. Although Marzuk et al. (1988) reported a relative risk for suicide in men between the ages of 20 and 59 to be 36 times greater in those with AIDS than in men without the diagnosis, Perry et al. (1990) found that the increased risk for suicide dissipated 2 months after diagnosis. Less reassuring, Perry et al. found that suicidal ideation persisted after notification for 15% of both seropositive and seronegative gay men. Regardless of the initial psychological reaction at the time of a seropositive test notification, it is important to perform a suicide potential assessment (Beckett and Shenson 1993) and begin appropriate intervention if indicated. The usual risk factors for serious suicide potential also apply to gay or bisexual patients recently diagnosed as HIV-1 seropositive, including preexisting affective illness, prior suicidality, substance abuse, social isolation and conflict, extreme hopelessness, and impulsivity. These issues may be difficult to assess during the immediate posttest counseling period, because the patient may be in a state of acute shock (Ostrow 1992). Therefore, after immediate attention has been paid to the acute psychological reaction, a follow-up session should be arranged, at which time further assessment and initiation of appropriate treatment can take place. Often, individual psychotherapy and social support group interventions are sufficient to reduce suicidal ideation. However, if serious suicidality persists, it may be necessary to consider more intense intervention, including possible inpatient treatment.

Issues for Seropositive Gay and Bisexual Men

During Stages II and III (Table 51–1), patients may experience a wide range of intermittent physiological symptoms, such as thrush, diarrhea, or night sweats. These symptoms vary in both magnitude and frequency among all HIV-1-seropositive individuals but will generally not be serious or meet the criteria for AIDS until several to 10 or more years after the initial infection. For those who experience minor symptoms, the symptoms serve as frequent reminders that indeed they are ill, and for those who do not experience symptoms or are unaware that their symptoms are related to HIV-1, the lack of symptoms may add to the denial that they are infected. Psychological reactions, such as depression, may take the form of sadness, hopelessness, or anticipatory grief. Some authors have reported difficulty differentiating between depression as a reaction to HIV-1 infection, demoralization, and hopelessness and as symptoms of HIV-1 infection, which may be similar to depression, such as difficulty sleeping, poor concentration, and fatigue (Ostrow et al. 1991). In addition, multiple AIDS-related bereavements are related to increased levels of hopelessness, depression, and symptoms related to HIV-1 infection (Kessler et al. 1991; Martin 1988; Neugebauer et al. 1992; Rabkin et al. 1990).

◾ Depression: Prevalence, Diagnosis, and Treatment Issues

Scott returns quarterly after the resolution of his initial anxiety attacks at the time of his HIV-1 diagnosis. He has done well for the past 4 years, both in terms of physical and mental health. He has continued working as a massage therapist, stayed active in his support group, and has not needed any antiretroviral or prophylactic medications. His CD4 cell counts have fluctuated between 1,000 and 600 cells/mm^3 but more recently have been in the 500–650 range. When you see him on the fifth anniversary of his initial positive antibody test, he complains of feeling depressed, frequently tired and unable to get out of bed, poor appetite, loss of interest in social activities, and occasionally being tearful. He reports first noticing these symptoms after Tim, one of the long-term members of his support group and Scott's "buddy" when he first joined the group, died from an opportunistic infection. Aside from fatigue, he denies difficulties in his work as a massage therapist but does complain of occasional forgetfulness, which is unusual for him.

You and Scott decide that even if his depressive symptoms are in reaction to Tim's death, a trial of an antidepressant medication that may restore his energy, concentration, and mood is warranted given the degree of discomfort he is feeling. You start him on a low dose of an activating antidepressant medication, and he reports an immediate improvement in sleep, appetite, and energy levels. Over the next several weeks, you gradually increase his dosage as his mood returns to normal. You keep him on a maintenance dose of the antidepressant for 6 months while continuing psychotherapy focusing on the issues of loss and coping with physical deterioration of oneself and close friends. Scott eventually volunteers to be a "buddy" for someone else in the group and volunteers one evening per week in the HIV clinic of the local medical center.

This case illustrates a common difficulty in the management of depressive symptoms in an otherwise asymptomatic person with >500 CD4 cells. Although the likelihood that the symptoms are organic in origin is exceedingly small, it may be extremely difficult to differentiate symptoms that are reactive to HIV-related losses from "pseudodepression" resulting directly from HIV-1 infection of the brain. The situation is made even more difficult if typical vegetative signs and symptoms are not present, yet the person appears to be significantly impaired in work or social performance. Experts are still divided over whether to be aggressive in treatment of what may be reactive or subsyndromal depression in such patients. Although prospective cohort studies of largely asymptomatic gay men have indicated low current rates of major depression (Kalichman and Sikkema 1994; Markowitz et al. 1994; Williams et al. 1991), clinicians frequently see varying levels of depression in patients infected with HIV-1. Many have also described the effects in gay or bisexual men infected with HIV-1 of living with a chronic disease (Holland and Tross 1985; Faulstich 1987). Several of the symptoms of depression seen with HIV-1 infection are similar to those seen with other chronic diseases, such as cancer, heart disease, or Alzheimer's disease. Although gay or bisexual men affected by these diseases may share some of the same concerns—such as the prospect of debilitating disease, loss of financial resources, or early death—conditions that are related to HIV-1 additionally elicit fear and stigma from the community at large (Kelly et al. 1993a).

African American gay or bisexual men with HIV-1 infection may be at even greater risk of depression and suicide than their white counterparts; Cochran and Mays (1994) found that one-third to almost one-half of HIV-1-positive African American gay or bisexual men reported elevated levels of depression symptoms compared with 10%–20% of white gay or bisexual men in most studies (Kalichman and Sikkema 1994; Markowitz et al. 1994). Given the theorized contributions of social stigma and isolation to distress related to HIV-1 infection, it is likely that racial or ethnic minority gay or bisexual men in general are at increased risk of depression.

Depression occurring in gay or bisexual men with HIV-1 infection can be treated with the usual spectrum of antidepressants regardless of the underlying cause as long as the medications are chosen carefully in terms of side effect profiles and are given in judicious doses for HIV-infected persons (Fernandez 1989; Markowitz et al. 1994; Rabkin et al. 1994a, 1994b). Furthermore, there appear to be no untoward immunological effects of antidepressant treatment in HIV-1 infection (Rabkin et al. 1994a, 1994b). In fact, one recent study of HIV-infected gay and bisexual men suggests that depressed individuals suffer more accelerated deterioration of their immune systems than do nondepressed individuals (Burack et al. 1993), although this finding remains controversial (Kessler et al. 1991; Lyketsos et al. 1993; Perry and Fishman 1993), and the converse—that treatment of depression leads to slower progression of immunodeficiency in HIV-1—has not been demonstrated. The emphasis should be on maximizing the quality of life, and aggressive treatment of depression in men with HIV-1 infection has been shown to markedly improve their quality of life and preference for life-sustaining treatments (Fogel and Mor 1993).

■ Anxiety: Differential Diagnosis and Treatment

Most gay or bisexual men with adverse reactions to their initial HIV-1 diagnosis will experience a decrease in anxiety symptoms upon acceptance into psychosocial treatment; some, as in the case study, respond well to a combination of acceptance, reassurance, and brief anxiolytic therapy. However, a careful evaluation of anxiety symptoms is necessary before beginning treatment to determine the underlying causes and type of disorder. The differential diagnosis of anxiety in HIV-infected gay and bisexual patients is similar to that for any person facing a life-threatening chronic illness complicated by concerns about loss of social support as a result of the stigmatization of AIDS and homosexuality. In addition, assessment is also necessary of possible underlying medical disorders (such as hyperthyroidism), excess caffeine consumption, stimulant drug usage or withdrawal, and medications used in the treatment of AIDS that can also have anxiety-producing side effects. Evaluation of any patient presenting with excess anxiety should also include consideration of possible depression or panic disorder, both of which may present with prominent anxiety symptoms. Given the relatively high degree of overlap between anxiety, depression, and somatic symptoms frequently observed in patients infected with HIV-1, diagnoses of "subsyndromal" anxiety or "mixed anxiety–depression" may be relatively common among HIV-1-seropositive gay or bisexual men (Hintz et al. 1990).

Supportive or cognitive psychotherapy is the first-line treatment for anxiety and often includes referral to ASOs offering support group services. Counseling of a patient's partners, close friends, and family members can often be of benefit in relieving social conflict or fears of abandonment. Anxiolytic treatment should be considered if the anxiety is severe and disabling or is accompanied by panic attacks or if a diagnosis of generalized anxiety disorder or posttraumatic stress disorder is made. There is an increasing spectrum of anxiolytic medications available, and nonbenzodiazepine medications should be considered for all patients not previously treated chronically with a benzodiazepine compound as well as those who can be successfully tapered off of benzodiazepines.

■ Neuropsychology

Both anxiety and depression can be accompanied by mild cognitive deficits such as poor concentration or short-term memory difficulty. For the person with HIV-1 infection, these symptoms can themselves be stressful, because they may be experienced as indicators of early HIV-1 brain involvement. If the cognitive symptoms are mild and in keeping with the degree of affective dysfunction, the patient should be counseled that the symptoms will probably disappear when the anxiety or depression is adequately treated. However, if the cognitive symptoms appear to be out of proportion to the degree of affective involvement or they do not respond to adequate antidepressant or anxiolytic treatment, then a neuropsychological evaluation is indicated, even in patients with >500 CD4 cells.

In terms of HIV-1 and mental functioning, it is not clear whether significant central nervous system (CNS) involvement precedes the development of full-blown AIDS (Grant et al. 1987; Levy and Bredeson 1989; Selnes et al. 1990; Ostrow 1990). In part, this controversy reflects our lack of knowledge about the highly variable natural history of HIV-1 infection of the CNS and the etiopathogenesis of HIV-1–related cognitive and motor disease. Further complicating the picture are the myriad factors that may have an impact on neuropsychological functioning of the gay or bisexual man living with HIV: prescribed and recreational drug side effects, the stresses of living with HIV and its manifest social consequences, nutritional deficiencies, CNS opportunistic infections and neoplasms, and altered affective states. Again, careful assessment, which may include formal neuropsychological testing, and treatment of any underlying conditions that may be contributing to cognitive dysfunction are essential before a diagnosis of HIV-1–associated cognitive/motor syndrome is made. Psychostimulant treatment has been shown to be particularly useful in ameliorating mixed affective and cognitive symptoms in persons with later stage HIV-1 illness (Fernandez et al. 1988).

Symptomatic Infection, AIDS, and Terminal Illness

After almost 10 years of living and working with HIV-1 infection, Scott learns that his CD4 cell count has gone below 200 cells/mm^3, qualifying him for the diagnosis of AIDS according to current criteria (Centers for Disease Control 1992). Through his work with you and the support group, he has prepared himself for this eventuality. This preparation has included writing a living will and formally designating his long-term female partner as the person responsible for medical and financial decisions were he to become incapacitated. When you next see him, he is somewhat sad, having just retired from work and applied for Social Security Insurance disability and Medicaid coverage. You discuss the plans he has made for this, the fourth and final stage of his HIV-1 natural history. In response to your questions about suicidal ideation, Scott tells you that he has decided to end his life if and when he becomes mentally incapacitated. You suggest a group counseling session with Scott, his long-term partner (Brenda), his support "buddy," and other members of his immediate support network. That session is very emotional but provides an opportunity for Scott to make his terminal care preferences known to his support network and for them to reaffirm their support for him.

Grief over receiving a diagnosis of AIDS may begin with an acute response of shock and denial, which may then be followed by guilt, anger, or sadness. This is frequently followed by a transitional state during which individuals may alternate between anger, guilt, self-pity, anxiety, and denial (Nichols 1985). These feelings can be particularly distressing and confusing, with men experiencing changes in self-esteem, identity, and considerations of suicide. New symptoms or events may precipitate new crises for the individual. This scenario has caused some to describe the uncertainty of HIV-1 illness as an "emotional roller coaster" (Nichols 1985). Many will find reinforcement for their denial through recurring reports in the press and popular media about the myth of HIV-1 being the cause of AIDS, whereas others will be forced to acknowledge the life-threatening nature of AIDS when hearing media accounts of disappointments in antiviral drug development.

Inevitably, issues of loss reemerge at the time of an AIDS diagnosis and complicate the management of end-of-life issues. Psychological treatment must usually be refocused on helping clients adapt to changes in their levels of mental and physical functioning and associated fears of debilitation and dependency on others, management of pain, maximizing quality of life, and terminal care preferences. It may be particularly difficult for psychotherapists who have worked with patients across multiple stages of HIV-1 infection to discuss those patients' fears and wishes about terminal care, especially plans for assisted suicide. The involvement of spiritual and palliative care can be extremely important for both improving the quality of life of the terminal patient and preventing depression and burnout among mental health and informal caregivers.

Summary and Conclusion

Consideration in this chapter of the complex interrelations among the various goals in treating HIV-1 illness in gay and bisexual men—physical health, immunocompetence, mental health, social and functional well-being, and overall quality of life—and the accompanying case study have emphasized the importance of an integrated biopsychosocial treatment approach. Given the central role of quality of life issues in the treatment of any person living with HIV, the coordinating role of the mental health care provider has been emphasized. An integrated holistic or biopsychosocial treatment approach works best when it is applied to the full range of problems experienced by HIV-infected persons and includes all the diverse elements of health care required. For this reason, many communities have established central HIV/AIDS care coordinating organizations, which, in turn, either provide or contract for comprehensive HIV case management services. Given the complexity and multidisciplinary nature of coordinated biopsychosocial HIV-1 care, frequently involving, in addition to medical and mental health services, a host of education and support services for patients and their families, it is extremely important that a case management model of care be used whenever possible.

The establishment of interdisciplinary care teams, AIDS task forces, and HIV case management systems does not automatically solve the major problems inherent in the delivery of such care for gay and bisexual men. For example, programs that provide comprehensive long-term care need to minimize actions that will isolate patients from mainstream society while maximizing the availability of specialized services. The intense stigma and discrimination to which HIV-infected patients are still subject require extraordinary attention to the confidentiality of medical records, while at the same time ensuring adequate communication among the diverse care team members. The frequent prevalence of dually or triply diagnosed patients—most usually a combination of a functional mental health disorder, a substance use disorder, and organic illness—means that already limited treatment facilities for such patients are oftentimes unavailable, and specific efforts have to be made to create appropriate treatment options. The occurrence of cognitive deficits in late-stage HIV-1 illness means that patients may have difficulty with the complicated diagnostic and treatment regimens made necessary by the nature of their illness. The close involvement of ASOs able to provide in-home assistance, support "buddies," and transportation can frequently make outpatient treatment possible across the full spectrum of HIV-1 infection.

The daily stresses of working in the HIV/AIDS health care arena, combined with the experience of seeing relatively young patients deteriorate and die despite one's best efforts, are a formula for burnout

(Fawzi et al. 1994; Ostrow and Gayle 1986; see Chapter 50 by McDaniel, Farber, and Summerville). Any viable AIDS/HIV treatment program must, therefore, provide adequate education, emotional support, and counseling not only for patients but also for those who care for them. In achieving this goal, mental health caregivers can contribute enormously to the compassionate care of gay and bisexual men living with HIV-1 infection, improving the quality of life of their patients while setting a leadership example for the practice of holistic health care.

References

Adelman M: Social support and AIDS. AIDS and Public Policy Journal 4:31–39, 1989

Atkinson H, Grant I, Kennedy CJ, et al: Prevalence of psychiatric disorders among men infected with human immunodeficiency virus. Arch Gen Psychiatry 45:859–864, 1988

Bacchetti P, Moss AR: Incubation period of AIDS in San Francisco. Nature 338:251–253, 1989

Beckett A, Shenson D: Suicide risk in patients with human immunodeficiency virus infection and acquired immunodeficiency syndrome. Harvard Review of Psychiatry 1:27–35, 1993

Burack JH, Barrett RD, Stall MA, et al: Depressive symptoms and CD4 lymphocyte decline among HIV-infected men. JAMA 270:2568–2573, 1993

Cassens BJ: Social consequences of the acquired immunodeficiency syndrome. Ann Intern Med 103:768–771, 1985

Caumartin S, Joseph JG, Chmiel J: Premorbid psychosical factors associated with differentiated survival time in AIDS patients. Paper presented at VII International AIDS Conference, Florence, Italy, June 1991

Centers for Disease Control: 1993 revised classification system for HIV infection and expanded surveillance case definition for AIDS among adolescents and adults. MMWR 41:1–19, 1992

Centers for Disease Control: Technical guidance on HIV counseling. MMWR 42:11–17, 1993

Cochran S, Mays V: Depressive distress among homosexually active African-American men and women. Am J Psychiatry 151:524–529, 1994

Dew MA, Ragni MV, Nimorwica P: Infection with human immunodeficiency virus and vulnerability to psychiatric distress. Arch Gen Psychiatry 47:737–744, 1990

Faulstich ME: Psychiatric aspects of AIDS. Am J Psychiatry 144:551–555, 1987

Fawzi FI, Fawzy NW, Pasnau RO: Bereavement in AIDS. Psychiatric Med 1994

Fernandez F: Anxiety and the neuropsychiatry of AIDS. J Clin Psychiatry 50 (suppl):9–14, 1989

Fernandez F, Adams F, Levy JK: Cognitive impairment due to AIDS-related complex and its response to psychostimulants. Psychosomatics 29:38–46, 1988

Fogel BS, Mor V: Depressed mood and care preferences in patients with AIDS. Gen Hosp Psychiatry 15:203–207, 1993

Folkman S, Chesney MA, Pollack L, et al: Stress, control, coping and depressive mood in human immunodeficiency virus-positive and -negative gay men in San Francisco. J Nerv Mental Dis 181:409–416, 1993

Grant I, Atkinson JH, Hesselink JR, et al: Evidence for early central nervous system involvement in the acquired immunodeficiency virus (HIV) infections. Ann Intern Med 107:823–836, 1987

Halman LJ, Ostrow DG, Eshleman S, et al: Structure of coping in a gay cohort at risk for AIDS. Presented at AIDS' Impact: 2nd International Conference on Biopsychosocial Aspects of HIV Infection, Brighton, England, July 1994

Hays RB, Turner H, Coates TJ: Social support, AIDS-related symptoms and depression among gay men. J Consult Clin Psychol 60:463–469, 1992

Hintz S, Kuck J, Peterkin JJ, et al: Depression in the context of human immunodeficiency virus infection: implications for treatment. J Clin Psychiatry 51:497–501, 1990

Holland JC, Tross S: The psychosocial and neuropsychiatric sequelae of the acquired immunodeficiency syndrome and related disorders. Ann Intern Med 103:760–764, 1985

Jacobsen PB, Perry SW, Hirsch DA: Responses to HIV antibody testing: behavioral and psychological responses to HIV antibody testing. J Consult Clin Psychology 58:31–37, 1990

Jenike M, Pato C: Disabling fear of AIDS responsive to imipramine. Psychosomatics 27:143–144, 1986

Joseph J, Caumartin S, Tal M, et al: Psychological functioning in a cohort of gay men at risk for AIDS. J Nerv Mental Dis 178:607–615, 1990

Kalichman SC, Sikkema KJ: Psychological sequelae of HIV infection and AIDS: review of empirical findings. Clinical Psychology Review 14:611–632, 1994

Kelly JA, St. Lawrence JS: The AIDS Health Crisis: Psychological and Social Interventions. New York, Plenum, 1988

Kelly JA, Murphy DA, Bahr GR, et al: Factors associated with severity of depression and high-risk behavior among persons diagnosed with immunodeficiency virus (HIV) infection. Health Psychology 12:215–219, 1993a

Kelly JA, Murphy DA, Bahr GR, et al: Outcome of cognitive-behavioral and support group brief therapies for depressed, HIV-infected persons. Am J Psychiatry 150:1671–1686, 1993b

Kessler RC, Foster C, Joseph J, et al: Stressful life events and symptom onset in HIV infection. Am J Psychiatry 148:733–738, 1991

Kubler-Ross E: AIDS: The Ultimate Challenge. New York, McMillan, 1987

Lackner JB, Joseph JG, Ostrow DG, et al: A longitudinal study of psychological distress in a cohort of gay men: effects of social support and coping strategies. J Nerv Mental Disord 181:4–12, 1993

Levy RM, Bredesen DE: Central nervous system dysfunction in acquired immunodeficiency syndrome. Journal of AIDS 1:13–17, 1988

Lyketsos CG, Hoover DR, Guccione M, et al: Depressive symptoms as predictors of medical outcomes in HIV infection. JAMA 270:2563–2567, 1993

Markowitz JC, Rabkin JG, Perry SW: Treating depression in HIV-positive patients. AIDS 8:403–412, 1994

Martin JL: Psychological consequences of AIDS-related bereavement among gay men. J Consult Clin Psychol 56:856–862, 1988

Marzuk PM, Tierney H, Tardiff K, et al: Increased risk of suicide in persons with AIDS. JAMA 259:1333–1337, 1988

Morin SF, Charles KA, Mayon AK: The psychological impact of AIDS on gay men. Am Psychologist 39:1288–1293, 1984

Neugebauer R, Rabkin J, Williams J, et al: Bereavement reactions among homosexual men experiencing multiple losses in the AIDS epidemic. Am J Psychiatry 149:1374–1379, 1992

Nichols SE: Psychosocial reactions of persons with the acquired immunodeficiency syndrome. Ann Intern Med 103:765–767, 1985

O'Brien K, Wortman CB, Kessler RC, et al: Social relationships of men at risk for AIDS. Soc Sci Med 36:1161–1167, 1993

O'Dowd MA, Biderman DJ, McKegney FP: Incidence of suicidality in AIDS and HIV-positive patients attending a psychiatry outpatient program. Psychosomatics 34:33–40, 1993

Ostrow DG: Psychiatric Aspects of Human Immunodeficiency Virus Infection. Kalamazoo, MI, Scope Publications, 1990

Ostrow DG, Gayle TC: Psychosocial and ethical issues of AIDS health care programs. Quality Review Bulletin 12:284–293, 1986

Ostrow DG, Wren PA: Mental Health Aspects of HIV/AIDS. Ann Arbor, University of Michigan Comprehensive HIV and AIDS Mental Health Education Program (CHAMHEP), 1993

Ostrow DG, Joseph JG, Kessler R, et al: Disclosure of HIV antibody status: behavioral and mental health correlates. AIDS Prevention Education 1:1–11, 1988

Ostrow DG, Monjan A, Joseph J, et al: HIV-related symptoms and psychological functioning in a cohort of homosexual men. Am J Psychiatry 146:737–742, 1989

Ostrow D, Grant I, Atkinson H: Assessment and management of AIDS patients with neuropsychiatric disturbances. J Clin Psychiatry 49:14–22, 1991

Ostrow DG, Leite MC, Lackner J, et al: Time course, mental health, and social support changes after learning HIV serostatus in the Chicago MACS/CCS cohort. Presented at the Neuroscience of HIV Satellite Meeting, Amsterdam, June 1992

Perkins DO, Stern RA, Golden RN, et al: Mood disorders in HIV infection: prevalence and risk factors in a nonepicenter of the AIDS epidemic. Am J Psychiatry 151:233–236, 1994

Perry S, Jacobsberg L, Card CA, et al: Severity of psychiatric symptoms after HIV testing. Am J Psychiatry 150:775–779, 1993

Perry S, Jacobsberg L, Fishman B: Suicidal ideation and HIV testing. JAMA 263:679–682, 1990

Perry S, Fishman B: Depression and HIV: how does one affect the other? JAMA 270:2609–2610, 1993

Rabkin JG, Williams JB, Neugebauer R, et al: Maintenance of hope in HIV-spectrum homosexual men. Am J Psychiatry 147:1322–1326, 1990

Rabkin JG, Rabkin R, Harrison W, et al: Imipramine effects on mood and enumerative measures of immune status in depressed patients with HIV illness. Am J Psychiatry 151:516–523, 1994a

Rabkin JG, Rabkin R, Wagner G: Fluoxetine effects on mood and immune status in depressed patients with HIV illness. J Clin Psychiatry 55:92–97, 1994b

Selnes OA, Miller E, McArthur J, et al: HIV-1 infection: no evidence of cognitive decline during the asymptomatic stages. Neurology 40:204–208, 1990

Stall R, Wiley J: A comparison of alcohol and drug use patterns of homosexual and heterosexual men: the San Francisco Men's Health Study. Drug Alcohol Depend 22:63–73, 1988

Wadland WC, Gleeson CJ: A model for psychosocial issues in HIV disease. J Fam Pract 33:82–86, 1991

Williams JBW, Rabkin JG, Remien RH, et al: Multidisciplinary baseline assessment of homosexual men with and without human immunodeficiency virus infection. Arch Gen Psychiatry 48:124–130, 1991

Wolf TM, Galson PM, Morse EV, et al: Relationship of coping style to affective state and perceived social support in asymptomatic and symptomatic HIV-infected persons: implications for clinical management. J Clin Psychiatry 52:171–173, 1991

Wren PW: Legal and ethical issues, in Mental Health Aspects of HIV/AIDS. Edited by Ostrow DG, Wren PA. Ann Arbor, University of Michigan Comprehensive HIV and AIDS Mental Health Education Program (CHAMHEP), 1993, pp 227–286

52

Spirituality and Religion in the Lives of Lesbians and Gay Men

Douglas C. Haldeman, Ph.D.

A t a San Francisco inn that caters to a primarily gay clientele, breakfast table conversation on a recent Easter morning centered around the guests' plans for the day. Most of the eight guests described their plans to sightsee, shop, or take in cultural events. But when one guest said that he intended to attend an Easter service at a nearby church, another of the guests thundered, "Why would you do that? They don't want you!" This guest then proceeded to describe his chronic sense of disaffection with his (Catholic) religious upbringing; to share his belief that the church has historically been a powerful agent in the institutionalization of homophobia; and to state that until the church was willing to acknowledge him, he would have nothing to do with it. He likened continued church membership on the part of lesbians and gay men as tantamount to remaining in an abusive relationship. After a long (and uncomfortable) pause, the first guest stated that he wished the issue could be that black and white for him, but that his religious and spiritual practices were as intrinsic to his sense of identity as was his sexual orientation. For him, leaving the church was no more an option than changing his sexual orientation—neither of which he was inclined to attempt.

Such is the dilemma experienced by many lesbians and gay men around the meaning and import of religion in their lives. In this chapter, the ways in which these meanings are constructed and assessed are examined. The response of organized religion to visible lesbians and gay men is discussed, with an explanation of the history of the conversion (or "reparative") therapy movement. The psychological importance of separation from hostile institutions is considered, as well as the needs of individuals whose sense of identity rests in part on the ability to integrate religious practice into their lives. Finally, clinical implications of spiritual issues for lesbians and gay men are discussed. This chapter reflects the fact that the bulk of the writing in this area is directly related to positions taken by the Christian churches. Nevertheless, in a number of instances, much of this writing is also applicable to non-Christian viewpoints.

Spirituality and Gay Identity

The psychological components of identity development for lesbians and gay men have been well documented (Gonsiorek and Rudolph 1991). The spiritual components of identity development, however, have scarcely been mentioned in the mental health literature. The subject often invites skepticism from social scientists, because dimensions of the human experience that are commonly associated with spirituality are difficult to quantify. Further, the history of institutional antipathy on the part of organized religion toward lesbians and gay men has alienated some of the gay community, including the lesbian and gay mental health sector. Nevertheless, spiritual experience and practice are important aspects of the lives of many lesbians and gay men, despite the position taken by most organized religions. To fully understand many lesbians and gay men, their spiritual lives and the meanings thereof must be considered.

Writer Mark Thompson (1994) described spiritual meaning in the lives of gay men as proceeding from the nature of soul. He characterized soul as "the repository of all that I feel: my appetites and ambitions, sadness and joy. It is the place where inspiration germinates and from which vitality grows. . . . Somewhere in this great container of ceaseless death and rebirth lies, too, the mystery of my being gay" (p. 1). The soul then becomes the foundation for spiritual, affective, and moral experience, thereby becoming a primary organizing force in the psyche. By extension, such centrality in the individual's identity accords it a similarly central role in the process of psychotherapy. Thus, many gay men would consider the soul to be the locus of both celebration and grief with respect to gayness.

Thompson's description may seem universally applicable in that many nongay persons would characterize the concept of soul in a similar way. But what is different about the soul of the lesbian or gay man is that it is forged out of pain and struggle. New Age theologian Andrew Harvey (1992) described the wound experienced by lesbians and gay men as a result of stigmatization and its consequent role in spiritual development. In Harvey's view, examination of the wound leads to a confrontation with all of its elements: shame, terror of abandonment, rage, and self-loathing. Embracing and reexperiencing these emotional elements become a mystical journey that purifies the soul, ultimately leading to a transcendent state. Harvey theorized that this mystical journey is the means by which the psychic wounds of lesbians and gay men become healed.

Theologians from a more traditional Christian context have presented a similar view, though in different language. Generally speaking, it has been noted that the lack of connectedness to a supportive or relevant external world experienced by many gay men and lesbians can, of necessity, turn the individual's attention inward. This may have the beneficial effect of enhancing the individual's spiritual self. It may also account for a greater development of spiritual qualities, such as sensitivity, compassion, and service to others, in gay men and lesbians (Boyd 1994).

Fortunato (1982) observed that the psychotherapeutic journey involves an ultimate "self to self" enlightenment, whereas the spiritual journey involves transcendence and an eventual "openness to God or the Mystery of the cosmos" (p. 22). Social rejection and hostility, according to Fortunato, create a rift for gay men and lesbians that can only be healed through spiritual experience. From a Christian perspective, Fortunato considered the ability to love in the presence of hatred and to maintain a sense of wholeness where one is unwanted as exemplary of the ultimate in Christ-like behavior and as healing the schism between spirituality and sexuality.

In a similar vein, Matthew Fox (1984) presented a fourfold path of spiritual development for gay men and lesbians. This path takes the individual through 1) creation, in which the gay self is truly embraced; 2) letting go, in which the pain of rejection is acknowledged and released; 3) creativity, leading to a rebirth of the soul; and 4) transformation, in which the individual extends compassion and a sense of celebration to others. These steps, along with the views of the author previously cited, provide a model for resolving the conflict and healing the wounds inflicted on lesbians and gay men by a homophobic society. Presumably, there are other ways to resolve the conflict; one may actively reject religion and spirituality or deny their importance. But what is significant in the work of these gay-affirmative spiritualists are the assumptions that all gay men and lesbians have a need to resolve in some way soul-based injuries and that healing is derived from spiritual process. Thus, spirituality assumes an important function in overall identity for lesbians and gay men.

The work of gay-affirmative theologians has paralleled psychological theories about gay identity development. Malyon (1982) described the psychological impact of internalized homophobia on gay identity development. In his view, the social devaluation accorded homosexual orientation becomes internalized in the lesbian or gay man, contaminating psychosexual development with shame and self-negation. Although other aspects of the self may continue to develop normally, the sexual self becomes truncated. The therapist assists the individual in confronting these internalized messages and provides both rational and emotional support to correct the harmful experiences of biased socialization. This corrective experience facilitates the individual's integration of sexual orientation into his or her identity.

In many ways, the tasks of spiritual identity development outlined by Fox, Fortunato, Harvey, and others parallel the tasks of identity development presented in gay-affirmative psychotherapy. The former seeks to heal the wounded spirit, permitting the individual to move forward in whatever spiritual path seems appropriate. The latter seeks to soothe the effects of sociocultural injuries, enabling the individual to release the pain and move on. Obviously, the two are not mutually exclusive. Quite the opposite is true: attentiveness to both of these overlapping processes facilitates the repair and growth of the whole person.

It should also be noted that spiritual healing may not always lead an individual to a reconciliation with theism. To the contrary, alternative paths—to atheism, paganism, or animism, for example—may be as well reasoned and emotionally meaningful as a reconnection with one's original religious practices. The therapist's task, overall, is not to develop an agenda to guide the process, but to accompany the individual on a journey. For many, a purely psychological approach may omit a significant component of the healing process. The experience of social stigma can lead to enlightenment, as evidenced by the work of numerous gay-affirmative theologians. It may also lead to social, psychological, and spiritual alienation. The spiritual aspect of identity can only be healed if it is addressed directly.

For reasons unclear, the spiritual aspect of identity has minimal impact on some lesbians and gay men. For others, spiritual experience and expression are intrinsic and essential elements of identity, as is sexual orientation; neglecting or rejecting spirituality may be inappropriate and impossible. Ways in which the clinician may facilitate the integration of spiritual experience into overall identity are discussed in the "Clinical Implications of Spirituality" section of this chapter.

Lesbians, Gay Men, and Organized Religion

As noted in the previous section, Harvey (1992) and others alluded to wounds that are universally experienced by lesbians and gay men in a homophobic world. Organized religion has contributed significantly to the wounding of gay men and lesbians, through a long history of negative bias that has been extensively documented (Blumenfeld and Raymond 1988; Goss 1993; Scanzoni and Mollenkott 1978). Blumenfeld and Raymond distinguished the views of various church bodies on homosexuality in three categories: those viewing homosexuality as sinful and unnatural, those viewing homosexuality as imperfect, and those upholding it as natural and good. The first perspective is best summarized by the "Letter to the Bishops of the Catholic Church on the Pastoral Care of Homosexual Persons." This letter was written by Cardinal Ratzinger in 1986 and addresses the church position on homosexuality in response to an increasingly visible group of gay Catholics seeking dialogue with the hierarchy. It states, in part,

> Although the particular inclination of the homosexual person is not a sin, it is more or less a strong tendency ordered toward an intrinsic moral evil. . . . It is only in the marital relationship that the use of sexual faculty can be morally good.

> A person engaging in homosexual behavior therefore acts immorally. . . . Homosexual activity is not a complimentary union, able to transmit life, and so it thwarts the call to a life to that form of self-giving which the Gospel says is the essence of Christian living. This does not mean that homosexual persons are not often generous and giving of themselves, but when they engage in homosexual activity they confirm within themselves a disordered sexual inclination which is essentially self-indulgent. (Blumenfeld and Raymond 1988, p. 206)

This perspective is founded on a scriptural interpretation of homosexuality—and, by implication, any sexual activity purely intended for pleasure—as sinful and damnable. Critics of this position have argued that the New Testament does not mention homosexuality per se and that those who argue otherwise have accepted mistranslated material as God's word. It has been further argued that those Bible passages that have been used to condemn homosexuality in general have been semantically distorted and that they actually address homosexual rape (Scanzoni and Mollenkott 1978). Still others have found inconsistencies in singling out homosexuality for scorn when the Bible appears to condemn a whole host of sexual practices (masturbation, oral sex, intercourse during menstruation) in its generally sex-negative perspective. Certainly, the arbitrary use of scriptural passages to justify devaluation of a particular group is suspect. Boswell (1980) addressed this issue:

> Careful analysis can almost always differentiate between conscientious application of religious ethics and the use of religious precepts as justification for personal animosity or prejudice. If religious structures are used to justify oppression by people who regularly disregard precepts of equal gravity from the same moral code, or if prohibitions which restrain a disliked minority are upheld in their most literal sense as absolutely inviolable while comparable precepts affecting the majority are relaxed or reinterpreted, one must suspect something other than religious belief as the motivating cause of the oppression. (p. 7)

A number of Protestant denominations maintain the stance that homosexuality is "imperfect" (Blumenfeld and Raymond 1988). While devaluing the status of homosexuality in contrast to heterosexuality, this perspective holds that the homosexual is not responsible for his or her condition and should not be viewed as sinful, providing that the individual is seeking help for his or her "condition." This is not to say that homosexual individuals should be in any way encouraged to adapt to their sexual orientation, that their relationships should be sanctioned by the church, or that their members should be ordained as priests or ministers. Rather, a distinction is made between sinful choices (as in the first perspective) and the individual's condition. This perspective allows for individuals with disordered conditions to remain in a state of grace providing that they do not engage in behaviors that may be the natural result of such conditions. In other words, homosexual persons may be tolerated provided that they maintain celibacy.

Both of the aforementioned perspectives are based on subjective interpretations of a series of Biblical passages that have undergone numerous translative iterations throughout the centuries. An individual or institutional belief in the literal truth of such tracts is driven entirely by subjective experience. As a result, it is difficult to assess these issues from a scientific perspective, partly because the process through which these beliefs are adopted is so personal and idiosyncratic and partly because vocabularies of religion and science are so different. As is the case in the debate between creationism and evolution, the underlying assumptions of the two points of view—a theology that would devalue homosexuality on scriptural grounds and a psychology that would uphold it on scientific grounds—are incompatible. Perhaps that is why so little research has been done to investigate why church membership is so central to the identities of many lesbians and gay men and what makes them cling to institutions that are openly hostile to them. Although homosexuality was long ago depathologized by organized mental health based on compelling scientific grounds (Gonsiorek 1991), empirical arguments do not penetrate the inner sanctum of church law—particularly when, as Boswell suggests, such law may itself be motivated by prejudice.

Two Protestant denominations, however, have gone on record as being gay affirmative. The Quakers and the congregations of the United Church of Christ have argued for interpreting scriptural condemnation of all nonprocreative sexual behavior in a historical context. As such, they acknowledge the parallel worth and validity of gay men and lesbians as church members and leaders, permit the use of church property by gay and lesbian groups, and even sanction gay and lesbian relationships in nonlegally binding ceremonies of Holy Union. These churches, along with the gay Metropolitan Community Church and numerous independent gay churches across the country, have become an alternative for many gay and lesbian Christians seeking a church home in a nonhomophobic environment.

The social climate in different churches with respect to lesbians and gay men can be as variable as church doctrine itself. Some churches at present openly offer reconciliation to lesbians and gay men, and many offer tolerance, making them hospitable spiritual homes for the self-affirming. The more fundamentalist Christian churches, however, have used antigay Biblical interpretations to stigmatize and exclude lesbians and gay men and to support the mounting of aggressive campaigns to deny them protection from discrimination. Self-affirmation and dignity are, for many lesbians and gay men, irreconcilable with membership in homophobic religious institutions whose tenets are used in an ongoing effort to delimit civil rights based on sexual orientation.

The notion that homosexuality is freely chosen behavior serves as the foundation for the church's condemnation of lesbians and gay men. This unproven hypothesis has in turn become the principal argument of those working against antidiscrimination protection for lesbians and gay men. These individuals claim that since gay men and lesbians freely chose their sexual behavior, it can also be avoided, and, therefore, does not entitle them to true minority group status. Based on this line of reasoning, these individuals also argue that antidiscrimination statutes for gay men and lesbians are unnecessary because they constitute special protection. For some lesbians and gay men who seek to maintain a relationship with their denominations, this attitude becomes the salt that is rubbed into the wound.

"Ex-Gay" Conversion Therapies

Despite the harm homophobic religious arguments do to all lesbians and gay men, some would sooner reject themselves than their churches. There is a sizable group of gay men and lesbians who, despite having been scorned by the churches in which they were raised, seek to remain members in good standing. Many of these people experience their religious affiliation so intensely that they may perceive their sexual orientation as being of secondary importance. Their struggle may be likened to a person whose individuation process from family of origin is so arrested that they will do anything to retain group approval.

That an institution could hold such sway over a person's psyche is explicable when the institution performs a surrogate parental function. For many distressed homosexual individuals, who may be socially marginalized and experiencing difficulties at home, the church assumes monolithic importance for its presumed ability to comfort and reassure. Furthermore, many who have attempted to come out have discovered the gay social world to be insular and often hostile to religion. The initial experience of sociosexual relating in a gay context is fraught with difficulties for many; the church, by contrast, seems familiar and reassuring. Therefore, given the tremendous value associated with church acceptance, the logical solution for many unhappy lesbians and gay men is to change their sexual orientation.

To attempt to change their sexual orientation, many religiously affected gay men and lesbians turn to the ex-gay ministries or to the programs offered by professional mental health workers who offer to treat homosexual orientation through conversion or reparative therapy. Journalist Patrick Clements (1994) reported that most of the participants in ex-gay programs that he investigated came from fundamentalist religious backgrounds and sought to secure a place in their church home. This place was so valuable to them that they were willing to attempt to give up their sexual orientation.

The strength of this desire was illustrated by one panelist at a recent symposium on Christian approaches to the treatment of lesbians and gay men, who said of his numerous unsuccessful attempts at sexual reorientation: "I felt it was what I had to do in order to gain a right to live on the planet." This statement reflects the depth of the conflict experienced by many lesbians and gay men between their homoerotic feelings and their need for acceptance by a homophobic religious community.

This conflict causes such individuals to seek the guidance of pastoral care providers or Christian support groups whose aim is to sexually reorient gay men and lesbians. Such programs seek to divest the individual of his or her "sinful" feelings or at least to make the pursuit of a heterosexual or celibate lifestyle possible. Their theoretical base is always founded on subjective scriptural interpretations, their often-unspecified treatment methods rely on prayer, and their outcome measures are generally limited to testimonials in a context heavily laden with social demand influences. Nonetheless, these programs bear examination because of the mental and emotional impact they have on the unhappy gay men and lesbians who seek their services and because of some mental health workers' willingness to refer clients to them. Lastly, many such programs have been associated with serious ethical problems, including sexual exploitation of clients.

Gay men who are more likely to be inclined toward doctrinaire religious practice are also likely to have generally lower self-concepts, to see homosexuality as sinful, to feel a greater sense of apprehension about negative responses from others, and to be more depressed in general (Weinberg and Williams 1974). Such individuals make vulnerable targets for the ex-gay ministries. Fundamentalist Christian groups, such as Homosexuals Anonymous, Metanoia Ministries, Love In Action, Exodus International, and EXIT of Melodyland, are the most visible purveyors of conversion therapy. The workings of these groups are well documented by Blair (1982), who stated that although many of these practitioners publicly promise a change in sexual orientation, they privately acknowledge that celibacy is the realistic goal to which gay men and lesbians must aspire. He further characterized many religious conversionists as individuals who are deeply troubled about their sexual orientation or whose sexual conversion is incomplete. Blair reported a host of problems with such counselors, including the sexual abuse of clients.

The most notorious of such ministers is Colin Cook. Cook's counseling program, Quest, led to the development of Homosexuals Anonymous, the largest antigay fundamentalist counseling organization in the world. The work of Cook, his ultimate demise, and the subsequent cover-up of his activities by the Seventh Day Adventist Church were described by sociologist Ronald Lawson (1987). Over the course of 7 years, approximately 200 people received reorientation counseling from Cook, his wife, and an associate. From this ministry sprang Homosexuals Anonymous, a 14-step program modeled after Alcoholics Anonymous.

Lawson, in attempting to research the efficacy of Cook's program, was denied access to counselees on the basis of confidentiality. Nonetheless, he managed to interview 14 clients. None reported any change in sexual orientation, but 12 reported that Cook had been sexual with them during the course of treatment. Interestingly, Lawson reported that the survivors of this program, in developing an informal support group to deal with Cook's abuses, became more self-affirming and better adjusted as gay people. The men attributed this outcome to mutual support from other gay men who had been victimized in similar ways. According to Blair, another homosexual pastor who used his ministry to gain sexual access to vulnerable gay people was Guy Charles, foun-der of Liberation in Jesus Christ. Charles was a homosexual who had claimed a heterosexual conversion subsequent to his acceptance of Jesus Christ. Like Cook, Charles was ultimately disavowed by the Chris-tian organization that sponsored him after charges of sexual miscon-duct were raised.

To date, the only study of a spiritually based sexual orientation conversion program to appear in the professional literature was done by Pattison and Pattison (1980). These authors described a supernatu-ral healing approach in the treatment of 30 individuals culled from a group of 300 who sought sexual reorientation counseling at EXIT of Melodyland, a charismatic ex-gay ministry affiliated with a Christian amusement park. The Pattisons did not explain their sampling criteria, nor did they explain why 19 of their 30 subjects refused follow-up in-terviews. Their data indicated that only 3 of the 11 subjects (out of a total of 300) reported no current homosexual desires, fantasies, or im-pulses and that 1 of the 3 subjects was listed as still being "incidentally homosexual." Several of the other eight subjects indicated ongoing neurotic conflict about their homosexual impulses. Although six of these men married heterosexually, two admitted to more than inciden-tal homosexual ideation as an ongoing issue. In defending these re-sults, Dr. Pattison explained that he thought homosexual ideation could be considered normal, "especially after a fight with one's wife" (Blair 1982).

Recently, founders of another prominent ex-gay ministry, Exodus International, an umbrella organization for over 100 ex-gay groups, denounced their own program as ineffective. Michael Busse and Gary Cooper, cofounders of Exodus and lovers for 13 years, were involved with the organization from 1976 through 1981. The program was de-scribed by these men as "ineffective . . . not one person was healed" ("Newswatch Briefs" 1990, p. 43). They stated that the program often exacerbated already prominent feelings of guilt and personal failure among the counselees; many were driven to suicidal thoughts as a result of the failed reparative therapy. Clements (1994) reported that Cooper later characterized other ex-gay leaders as "sincere . . . just sincerely wrong."

The fundamentalist ex-gay programs possess enormous symbolic power because they hold out the promise of a "normal" life to many naive, shame-ridden, frightened counselees. They operate outside the jurisdiction of any professional organizations that may impose ethical standards of practice and accountability on them. Increasingly, these programs are seeking to legitimize themselves with mental health professionals as affiliates and referral sources.

It is nearly impossible to assess the outcomes of the ex-gay programs due to the suspect nature of self-report testimonials. Conversion therapy programs of all varieties are doomed to failure because of the immutable properties of sexual orientation. There is anecdotal information, however, to suggest that they may cause harm in some cases. Individuals undergoing conversion treatment are not likely to emerge as heterosexually inclined, but often they do become shamed, conflicted, and fearful about their homoerotic feelings. It is not uncommon for gay men who have undergone conversion therapy to notice a temporary or even chronic decline in libido. They often also report increased guilt and anxiety and lowered self-esteem (Haldeman 1993). Some flee into heterosexual marriages that are doomed to problems inevitably involving spouses and often children as well.

However, not one investigator, particularly those affiliated with the ex-gay ministries, has ever raised the possibility that conversion treatments may harm some participants, even in a field where a 30% "success rate" is seen as high. The fundamentalist purveyors of conversion treatments have yet to offer proof of any real efficacy, and their programs are often fraught with ethical problems. To enroll in a "reparative" program implies a self-designation of "broken," which is neither scientifically defensible nor in the best interest of any client's mental health. Other aspects of secular conversion therapy programs are reviewed by Stein in Chapter 6.

Clinical Implications of Spirituality

Incorporating spirituality into an overall treatment plan for a gay man or lesbian is based on careful assessment. First, spirituality should not be avoided or ignored, as it often is, in taking a history and conceptualizing the individual. It is an area to which significant meaning may be attached, and thus it deserves inclusion in an overall conceptual framework. Understanding the importance of spirituality in a person's life and investigating the underlying meanings of religious attachments help to create a context in which the individual may fully integrate spirituality into the gestalt of identity.

This investigation starts with the therapist's attentiveness to certain spiritual concerns and the possible ways in which they may impact the lesbian or gay patient.

For instance, what is the nature of the individual's psychic wounds around spirituality, and what remains unhealed or incomplete? Many of these wounds occur early in life and may require some persistence to uncover. For some patients, an optimal sense of well-being cannot be restored if these issues are not addressed.

How do family attachments affect spiritual issues? One patient was intensely enmeshed with his fundamentalist Christian mother, which complicated his coming-out process, making it both more prolonged and fraught with anxiety. Working on separation from his mother was met with significant resistance until he began to separate from his fundamentalist denomination. As he began to study the subjective, arbitrary basis for the church's position against homosexuality, he was able to activate a rational, critical view that he was unable to achieve when focused exclusively on his mother. Developing this individuated stance from the church served as a model for how he might view his mother, which greatly enhanced his level of self-acceptance and reduced his level of shame.

Ultimately, the therapist must be able to facilitate the patient's ability to discern the function of spirituality in identity and thus its appropriate place in his or her life. Lesbian and gay psychotherapy patients with spiritual concerns need to be treated with the respect they often do not receive, either in their churches or in the gay community. A patient recently stated, "I feel judged at church for being gay and judged by other gay people for being religious. I feel as though therapy is the only place I can speak without being judged at all."

The profound emotional and existential meanings associated with religious issues for many gay men and lesbians mandate that these issues be taken seriously and that therapists (particularly gay therapists, who may often be negative about religion) facilitate a value-neutral process of exploration. Spirituality is complex and requires attentiveness to affective, cognitive, and existential features. The therapist must also be willing to include observations about the patient's daily spiritual process as an ongoing part of therapy. This is particularly important with the large number of lesbians and gay men involved in spiritually based addiction recovery programs. The therapist need not adopt or even be intimately conversant with a wide range of spiritual beliefs and practices to do effective therapy, but he or she must demonstrate a basic openness to and understanding of the dimensions of spirituality, a general vocabulary for such experience, and an appreciation for the particular functions of spirituality in the patient's life.

Although certain homophobic religious doctrines are clearly incompatible with a healthy self-concept for lesbians and gay men, the answer for everyone is not a wholesale rejection of religion. The work of numerous gay-affirmative theologians speaks to the creativity involved in living a life that includes a full expression of both sexuality and spirituality. What kind of support system does the individual have around his or her spiritual experience? Although conversion therapies seem to be gaining more visibility at present, so too are gay-affirmative spiritual groups and programs that are intended to harmonize with a positive gay identity.

Goss (1993) cited a variety of ways in which gay men and lesbians can retain their self-respect and their church connectedness at the same time. First, individuals are encouraged to be as out as possible with regard to their sexual orientation. This is important from an overall mental health standpoint, because the degree of openness about sexual orientation correlates with the perceived level of psychological functioning (Weinberg and Williams 1974). Further, for gay men and lesbians to be out in their religious communities is the only way to confront what Goss called "ecclesial homophobia" and all of its manifestations.

Second, the experience of being gay and religious can be doubly isolating, leaving people with a sense of living between two worlds. To affiliate with other like-minded people offers the normalizing experience of solidarity, as well as increasing the chance for proactive work within the particular denomination or institution. Most mainstream Protestant denominations, the Roman Catholic church, and numerous Jewish congregations have gay-affirmative religious groups associated with them. Though the official sanction of the parent denomination varies from case to case, these groups, as well as the Metropolitan Community Church and other independent gay churches, are excellent ways for gay people to connect with one another in a religious context. Goss further recommended the establishment of "Queer Christian base communities," which serve as activist organizations.

For others, the healing journey may lead away from institutional religion toward atheism and humanism, paganism and goddess worship, witchcraft, New Age metaphysical practice, Buddhism, or some combination of perspectives. It is not for the therapist to evaluate the path itself, but to consider its function in the individual's life. All varieties of spiritual practice may serve to strengthen a positive sense of self. It is when spiritual practice engenders shame, fear, and self-loathing, or when it leads to a fragmentation of identity, that the therapist needs to consider the patient's spiritual path critically and assist her or him in loosening bonds that may be tied to the past.

Spirituality has not historically been familiar terrain for mental health researchers, nor has it been friendly terrain for gay men and lesbians. It is time, however, to recognize its potential import in psychotherapy with lesbians and gay men. For the patient who has been abused by his or her religious background, the therapist can provide support, information, and emotional sustenance. At the point where the pain has been embraced and resolved, the individual can then decide what role spirituality will assume in her or his life. It is natural for us to seek ways to make sense of our lives on this planet and our relative place in the cosmos. In this regard, spirituality offers a vehicle for transcendence that may lead to a special kind of healing for lesbians, gay men, and bisexual individuals.

References

Blair R: Ex-Gay. New York, Homosexual Counseling Center, 1982

Blumenfeld W, Raymond D: Looking at Gay and Lesbian Life. New York, Philosophical Press, 1988

Boswell J: Christianity, Social Tolerance, and Homosexuality: Gay People in Western Europe from the Beginning of the Christian Era to the Fourteenth Century. Chicago, IL, University of Chicago Press, 1980

Boyd M: Survival with grace, in Gay Soul: Finding the Heart of Gay Spirit and Nature. Interviews by Thompson M. San Francisco, CA, Harper, 1994, pp 233–245

Clements P: From gay to ex-gay, part I: the ex-gays. The Stonewall News (Tampa, FL), April 22, 1994, pp 5–8

Fortunato J: Embracing the Exile: Healing Journeys for Gay Christians. New York, Seabury Press, 1982

Fox M: The spiritual journey of the homosexual . . . and just about everyone else, in A Challenge to Love: Gay and Lesbian Catholics in the Church. Edited by Nugent R. New York, Crossroad Publishing, 1984, pp 189–204

Gonsiorek J: The empirical basis for the demise of the pathology model of homosexuality, in Homosexuality: Research Issues for Public Policy. Edited by Gonsiorek J, Weinrich J. Newbury Park, CA, Sage, 1991, pp 115–136

Gonsiorek J, Rudolph J: Homosexual identity: coming out and other events, in Homosexuality: Research Issues for Public Policy. Edited by Gonsiorek J, Weinrich J. Newbury Park, CA, Sage, 1991, pp 161–176

Goss R: Jesus Acted Up: A Gay and Lesbian Manifesto. San Francisco, CA, Harper, 1993

Haldeman D: The practice and ethics of sexual orientation conversion therapy. J Consult Clin Psychol 62:221–227, 1994

Harvey A: Hidden Journey: A Spiritual Awakening. New York, Arkana/Penguin Books, 1992

Lawson R: Scandal in the Adventist-funded program to "heal" homosexuals: failure, sexual exploitation, official silence and attempts to rehabilitate the exploiter and his methods. Paper presented at the annual convention of the American Sociological Association, Chicago, IL, June 1987

Malyon A: Psychotherapeutic implications of internalized homophobia in gay men. J Homosex 7:59–70, 1982

Newswatch briefs. Gay Chicago Magazine, February 22, 1990, p 43

Pattison E, Pattison M: "Ex-gays": religiously mediated change in homosexuals. Am J Psychiatry 137:1553–1562, 1980

Scanzoni L, Mollenkott VR: Is the Homosexual My Neighbor? Another Christian View. New York, Harper & Row, 1978

Thompson M: Gay Soul: Finding the Heart of Gay Spirit and Nature. San Francisco, CA, Harper, 1994

Weinberg M, Williams C: Male Homosexuals: Their Problems and Adaptations. New York, Penguin Books, 1974

53

Ethical Concerns With Sexual Minority Patients

Laura S. Brown, Ph.D., A.B.P.P.

To practice ethically is a goal for most mental health care providers. This chapter explores some of the ethical dilemmas that can arise when a patient of a mental health professional is gay, lesbian, bisexual, or transgendered (a sexual minority). These special ethical considerations emerge from the bias in society, in the mental health professional, and in the sexual minority patient, against persons of other than heterosexual orientation. Such bias can affect the judgment of the mental health professional and interfere with the delivery of competent services to patients or their families. This chapter explores potential risks to ethical practice and suggests ways in which mental health professionals can become more aware of those risks and engage in corrective strategies, thus ensuring ethical delivery of services.

What Is Ethical Practice?

All of the mental health and helping professions define certain behaviors as ethical (good or acceptable) or unethical (bad or unacceptable) in codes and sets of principles that are assumed to guide and regulate the practice of psychotherapists and other mental health care providers (Gabbard 1989). The creation of a code of ethics implies a special relationship known as a "fiduciary relationship" (Feldman-Summers 1989) between the professional and the public that receives professional services, in which the professional has the goals of avoiding harm to the recipient of services and taking steps to ensure the well-being of those being served. Practicing ethically for mental health professionals requires that professionals be familiar with and apply the codes of their discipline toward the goals of protecting patients from harm. Such practice also rests on the development by each individual professional of a personal code of conduct that derives from the formal standards promulgated by the profession (Keith-Spiegel and Koocher 1985).

The manner in which a psychotherapist or other mental health professional ensures ethical practice is often not clear when the ethics codes encounter practice. Although the ethical codes and standards of the mental health disciplines delineate specific acts that are proscribed and define in broad terms the parameters of minimally ethical practice, many of the dilemmas that arise in the every day work of a mental health professional are invisible, ignored, or ambiguously addressed. Often, professionals are left to make their own interpretations of the meaning of a particular statement in the formal code and to feel uncertain as to what constitutes an ethical course of action. When what will harm or protect a patient is unclear and when bias on the part of the professional can distort decision making, ethical risks arise.

Additionally, as the boundaries of the legal and ethical worlds begin to blur and intersect, ethics standards are being revised by professional organizations to constitute legalistic documents defining minimally acceptable activities by the professional, the goals of which are as much to protect professionals from litigation as they are to inspire practitioners to an ideal of ethical practice (Payton 1994). As feminist therapy ethicists Lerman and Porter (1990) noted, current ethics codes tell us a great deal about what we ought not to do but little about an affirmative, proactive stance for therapists in which ethics is integrated into every aspect of the practice of the therapist.

The special ethical issues of working with sexual minority patients frequently fall within gray areas of ethics codes. Ethical practice with lesbians, gay men, and bisexual and transgendered individuals is not a simple matter of following the general rules. Rather, affirmative ethical mental health practice with sexual minority individuals requires the professional to make careful interpretations of ethical standards and concepts to uncover the most ethical path to be taken and to be an active ethical decision maker rather than a passive recipient of sets of rules. Ethical clinical practice with sexual minority patients also calls for a consideration of the manners in which ethics and politics blend into the mental health treatment of the group of sexual minority patients, people who are still in many parts of society stigmatized, discriminated against, and ill-treated simply because of their sexual orientations, often as a result of the prior actions of mental health professionals.

One of the best examples of such institutional discrimination arising from the actions of mental health professions has been the treatment of sexual minority individuals by the United States military (see Chapter 46 by Purcell and Hicks). Until the early 1970s, homosexuality (and by implication any other sexual minority status) was defined as psychopathology. With the use of this mental health definition as a rationale, gay and lesbian service members were persecuted, imprisoned, and dishonorably discharged. As Jones and Koshes (1995) noted in their review, the military relied heavily on the authority of the mental health definition, quoting one U.S. Army document that stated, "Homosexuality is a manifestation of a severe personality defect which appreciably limits the ability of such individuals to function effectively in a military environment" (Personnel Separations 1966). The distress suffered by sexual minority individuals in the services, as well as the permanent stigma attached to those less than honorably discharged, has been documented in first-person accounts (Berube 1990; Humphrey 1990); the role of mental health professionals in both establishing and implementing this distress and stigma is apparent throughout these histories.

Any mental health professional working with sexual minorities thus inherits this history of collaboration between the mental health professions and oppression of individuals who are sexual minorities. Doing the ethical thing with a patient who has been directly or indirectly affected by this historical context is likely to necessitate a different and more fully developed notion of what constitutes ethical practice, with possible social and legal implications for the patient taken carefully into account.

Even when the mental health professional is not intending to reinforce bias, the outcome can be devastating. Karen Thompson described how a naively helpful liaison consultation psychologist urged her to reveal her lesbian relationship to the parents of her partner after the latter suffered a traumatic brain injury (Thompson and Andrzejewski 1988). This course of action was the catalyst for many years of biased treatment of Thompson and Sharon Kowalski (her partner) by the family and by other health professionals, treatment that impeded Kowalski's recovery from her injury and that confined her to a care facility to prevent her from returning home with Thompson.

At the core of pursuing ethical practice with individuals who are sexual minorities is an understanding of how two related forms of bias—heterosexism and antihomosexual bias (or homophobia)—can influence the application of ethical standards by mental health professionals (see Chapter 7 by Herek). Heterosexism is defined as the institutionalized cultural privilege given to heterosexual persons, which leads to the invisibility and marginality of individuals who are sexual minorities even in the absence of overt hatred and persecution. Homophobia is the fear and hatred of nonheterosexual individuals and includes intentional persecution of and violence against people assumed to be gay, lesbian, bisexual, or transgendered. These two forms of bias affect the attitudes and values of mental health professionals, their access to useful information, and their intellectual and emotional competence to work with this population. All mental health professionals, regardless of their sexual orientations, have some degree of both of these forms of bias, because personal and professional development in the pervasively antihomosexual and heterosexist environments of our culture ensures that no one remains unaffected. The differences will emerge in the degree to which a clinician is aware of and has responded to the presence of these biases, which can otherwise appear as unworked-through countertransference that may steer a mental health professional toward ethically problematic behavior (Gartrell 1984; Isay 1989).

Additionally, for sexual minority therapists living and working within the same community as their patients, ethical practice requires an attention to questions of how boundaries are defined and managed within the de facto small towns of sexual minority subcultures. Such therapists encounter special ethical dilemmas that often fall outside of the relatively separated therapist-patient relationships envisioned by standard ethical guidelines (Brown 1989).

Social and Historical Contexts

Many of the matters described here as of ethical concern might be redefined by other commentators as aspects of what constitutes good practice in mental health care. Others would argue that the issues identified in this chapter are political, not ethical. However, it seems impossible to make these divisions when speaking of mental health treatment, particularly psychotherapy of sexual minority patients. Individuals who are sexual minorities have a unique relationship to the mental health professions, because the defining characteristic of minority status, erotic and emotional attractions to individuals of the same sex, has long been a target of attempts at psychopathologizing by all of the established mental health disciplines. Mental health professions have not treated this supposed pathology as equal to others but have held it out as extreme and disturbed behavior. A long and sordid history of alliances exists between these disciplines and legal authorities for the purposes of banning sexual minority individuals from jobs, immigration, military service, and parenthood and restricting personal freedom in a manner that can be seen in the history of mental health response to almost no other group of diagnoses. Although in the past decade we have seen some reversals of these trends by the official organizations representing mental health professions, the slate does not appear to be cleared.

Even after the removal, first of homosexuality and then of egodystonic homosexuality from formal diagnostic manuals, this collusion between mental health and political entities to oppress people simply for being a sexual minority continued and forms the foundation for many ethical problems in clinical practice with sexual minority individuals. For example, in a study recently conducted by the Committee on Lesbian and Gay Concerns (1990) of the American Psychological Association, numerous examples of contemporaneous discriminatory practice with sexual minority patients were uncovered. Several of the therapists surveyed in this study expressed strong views that whether or not homosexuality was included in the diagnostic manuals, it was psychopathology and would be treated as such. Anecdotal evidence also continues to abound in examples arising from custody cases in which parents who are sexual minorities are stigmatized by mental health evaluators and denied access to children.

As a consequence of this historical (as well as present day) situation that serves to create the social context of clinical practice with patients who are sexual minorities, ethical issues must be more broadly defined to include questions of quality of care and the political implications of diagnostic or therapeutic decisions. The ethical questions are not simply about equitably treating patients who are sexual minorities. Rather, they are inquiries into how and if the treatment and the professional administering the intervention, be it assessment, medication management, psychotherapy, or liaison consultation, collude with, worsen, or resist the ways in which society continues to legally discriminate against members of this minority group. Ethical practice with sexual minority patients thus begins with the awareness of the mental health professional that this treatment does not take place in a vacuum but that mental health professional and patient alike are affected by these social forces and must take them into account in the way in which services are delivered.

Antihomosexual Bias as an Ethical Problem

The effects of antihomosexual bias (referred to in most previous literature as "homophobia," a term that is falling into disuse because of its imprecision) are a frequent source of ethical challenges for the therapist working with patients who are sexual minorities. Antihomosexual bias can be defined as fear and hatred of sexual minority individuals; it is overt and can be more readily observed and confronted in oneself and others than is the companion bias of heterosexism. The latter is more subtle and likely to be present in supportive, well-meaning allies of sexual minority individuals but who are not especially homophobic. Both can be ethically problematic for mental health professionals because, as forms of bias, they skew perspectives on the assessment and treatment of sexual minority patients in ways that can lead to harm through either action or neglect.

Antihomosexual bias in mental health is most commonly expressed through the assessment of sexual minority status as a form of mental illness, developmental arrest, or other problem diagnosis and through the delivery of treatments aimed at the conversion of minority sexual orientation to heterosexuality. Although overt antihomosexual bias once was a normative characteristic of mental health practitioners in the United States, the outpouring of data over the past 25 years regarding the mental health status of sexual minority individuals has led to a transformation in the presentation of this bias by mental health professionals.

Because of changes in the official approach to homosexuality stemming from its removal in 1973 as a diagnostic classification from the *Diagnostic and Statistical Manual of Mental Disorders* (American Psychiatric Association 1968), overt antihomosexual bias in mental health has gone underground. Instead of some of the negative descriptions of homosexuals that can be found in research published from the 1940s to the late 1960s, antihomosexual bias is now more commonly framed in current discourse as an expression of concern for patients who will purportedly be denied adequate treatment if their sexual minority status is not pathologized. For example, a therapist may inform a patient seeking treatment for depression that the "real" problem is his or her homosexuality and insist on "treating" this problem rather than directly addressing the depression through more conventional means such as medication or cognitive or interpersonal therapy, thereby potentially prolonging the depression in the service of this inaccurate and biased assessment. This sort of misdiagnosis and deferral of treatment is ethically problematic, as it places the need of the practitioner to uphold antihomosexual beliefs over the need of the patient for adequate and equal care.

Professional antihomosexual bias may manifest itself through a presentation of apparent correlations between homosexuality and a mental illness diagnostic entity, suggesting that sexual minority status is somehow either cause or cognate of the psychopathology. One anonymous responder to a survey conducted by the Task Force on Bias in Psychotherapy with Lesbians and Gay Men (Committee on Lesbian and Gay Concerns 1990) of the American Psychological Association who represents this latter trend wrote,

> I'm convinced that homosexuality is a genuine personality disorder and not merely a different way of life. Everyone that I have known socially or as a client has been a complete mess psychologically. I think they are simply narcissistic personality disorders—see the description in the DSM III—that's what they have looked and acted like—all of them. (pp. 12–13)

Such impressions, however derived, are refuted by extensive empirical data regarding the mental health of sexual minority individuals; most commonly, these anecdotal observations reflect a post hoc diagnosis informed by an already extant set of biased beliefs. Haldeman (1991) reviewed the sexual orientation conversion therapy literature and documented both the abuses perpetrated by practitioners of these models, as well as their consistent failure to change the sexual orientations of their patients. Haldeman and other earlier commentators (Davison 1976, 1991) questioned whether it is ethical to define sexual minority status as a form of pathology (even if listed in the official diagnostic manuals) and argues that attempts to do what is now called "reparative therapy" (Nicolosi 1991) are ethically problematic because they are known to be patently inefficacious. Few other groups of people, aside from sexual minorities, have been consistently offered clearly inefficacious and often harmful treatments. Consequently, for a psychotherapist to persist with this approach to treatment, given the strong data regarding lack of successful outcome for the so-called conversion therapies, would constitute ethically problematic action.

In addition, the ethically problematic nature of expression of overt antihomosexual bias couched in mental health terminology is greater than that resulting from the negative effects on individual patients who are sexual minorities. Such antihomosexual bias promulgated by mental health professionals supports and enables bias against sexual minority individuals in the larger societal milieu and serves to justify the passage and enforcement of laws discriminating against sexual minority individuals, denial of child custody to parents who are sexual minorities, and the criminalization of forms of sexual expression that are most closely identified with sexual minority practices. Antihomosexual bias within the mental health field constitutes an ethical problem because it harms patients directly and because it encourages other forms of direct discrimination against sexual minority individuals by lending a pseudoscientific respectability to discrimination against sexual minority individuals in legal and legislative arenas. For example, in 1992, Joseph Nicolosi, a leading reparative therapist, appeared at hearings to testify in support of Colorado Amendment 2, the ballot measure that, had it not been ruled unconstitutional, would have banned laws protecting the civil rights of sexual minority individuals in that state. In Oregon and Washington, Paul Cameron, a social psychologist who publishes antihomosexual material under the banner of supposed science, provided "research" underpinnings for antigay civil rights initiatives in both of those states.

The mental health professional who feels strongly that, despite the evidence, sexual minority individuals have a form of psychopathology or the mental health professional whose religious convictions generate a belief that being a sexual minority is a sin in need of psychotherapeutic intervention would be ethically well advised to abstain from working with any sexual minority patient because such beliefs are likely to harm the patient. Such professionals also should consider abstaining from public promulgation of their beliefs, because of the risk that the professional will contribute to broader forms of social harm. Although therapists are entitled to their personal prejudices, the dangers to patients of mixing this sort of bias with treatment can be serious. The personal testimonies of survivors of reparative therapies (Duberman 1991; Haldeman 1991) bear witness to the pain and damage created by these expressions of professional antihomosexual bias—clear violations of the ethic of doing no harm. The harm caused to the mental health of sexual minority persons in Oregon and Colorado by these ballot initiatives also has been considerable, to judge by accounts given by mental health professionals who work with the sexual minority communities in those states.

However, being a member of a sexual minority group does not exempt one from holding antihomosexual sentiments. The sexual minority mental health professional who is dealing with strong feelings of internalized self-hatred regarding sexual orientation is at a particular sort of ethical as well as personal risk from this form of bias.

First, this self-directed bias may become a source of distress or impairment; a number of sexual minority writers have given personal testimonies about the depression, substance abuse, and self-destructive risky behaviors that resulted from their inability to embrace their sexual minority status (Duberman 1991; Grahn 1984). Although these are not accounts published by mental health professionals, the available anecdotal data from discussions with sexual minority colleagues suggest that as a group, we have not been spared the problems arising from self-hatred. Professionals who are impaired for whatever reason are at increased risk for malpractice because of deficits in judgment or patterns of self-defeating behavior arising from their impairment (Kilburg et al. 1986). The ethical choice, when impaired, is to refrain from practice and seek treatment aimed at resolving the impairment; in this instance, to work through and reduce internalized feelings of antihomosexual bias.

Second, the self-hating sexual minority mental health professional may engage in countertransference acting out with sexual minority patients. These actions may reflect efforts by the mental health professional to work through the self-hatred via interactions with patients in which the latter become the surrogate for the psychotherapist in confronting antihomosexual bias. The psychotherapist unable to come out on the job or to family may urge or insist on such actions by patients, without regard to whether the patient is ready for self-disclosure or the actual risks to the patient of such a course of action. Such acting out allows the psychotherapist to vicariously experience this aspect of coming out without the attendant personal risk; when the consequences to the patient are negative, self-hating sexual minority psychotherapists are then affirmed in their antihomosexual beliefs. Because this course of action places the needs of the therapist over and above the well-being of the patient and actual treatment considerations, it is an ethically problematic direction for a therapist to take.

Because such struggles with internalized self-hatred are often a normative aspect of the coming-out process, Brown (1989) and Gonsiorek (1994) have proposed that the mental health professional who is currently coming out should abstain from working with sexual minority patients until the crisis of self-acceptance has been adequately resolved and that this issue should be addressed in both personal psychotherapy and supervision for the sexual minority mental health professional. Both Brown and Gonsiorek have suggested a 2-year period for this process. Such abstinence from working with sexual minority patients also is important for mental health professionals to establish their own personal and social support network in a sexual minority community rather than having their entire known complement of sexual minority individuals coming from their patient population. This latter concern, regarding social role overlap, will be addressed at greater length below.

Heterosexism and Mental Health Ethics

Heterosexism is a more thorny ethical dilemma for mental health practitioners. Heterosexist attitudes and values pervade the training and practice of even the most well-meaning mental health professionals, often even those who are members of sexual minority groups. Heterosexism is more subtle and ubiquitous among well-intentioned practitioners because it functions more as a mechanism of invisibility and diminishment for sexual minority individuals. Heterosexism constitutes oppression via marginalization and minimization, rather than oppression through the more obvious means of harm and stigma. Expression of heterosexist attitudes serves to diminish the importance of the unique life experiences that sexual minority status confers and enables ignorance of the contribution of oppression and discrimination to mental health problems. Heterosexism is based on the assumption that sexual minority individuals wish to emulate the attitudes and values of the dominant culture, leading to curious and inaccurate beliefs among some heterosexual practitioners about the lives of sexual minorities. Heterosexist bias leads to minimizing the meanings and worth of sexual minority experience. An absence of course content on working with sexual minority patients, invisibility of sexual minority staff or faculty in training programs, and a lack of knowledge regarding sexual minority individuals on the part of the average well-intended mental health practitioner are all manifestations of heterosexism in mental health practice.

Heterosexism becomes ethically problematic in several ways. First, it affects the competency of the practitioner. Practicing with a special patient population without adequate knowledge gained via course work and supervised practice with that group can be a violation of ethics because it may lead to harm that could have been averted by adequate training. This failure to obtain knowledge regarding minority groups is not isolated to the sexual minority patient; indeed, this sort of damage by default through the actions of well-intended but ignorant therapists has been a shared experience of most minority groups in the mental health setting.

Failures of competency can manifest in a variety of ways. For example, a mental health practitioner can make errors that will harm the patient by assuming that all patients are heterosexual and fail to take an adequate history regarding nonheterosexual feelings, fantasies, and experiences. For a highly closeted patient or for one who is just beginning to address the coming-out process, this assumption may lead to a failure of treatment as a result of the silencing of the patient, who receives the meta-message that this evaluator or psychotherapist or consultant does not want to know about sexual minority experiences. A mental health professional in a consultation liaison position can mislabel a partnered person as single if the sexual minority patient is not yet comfortable with coming out to the professional, and thereby ignore important aspects of psychosocial care for a medically ill individual.

Mental health professionals also can have distorted notions, because of lack of information, about what it means to be a member of a sexual minority group. The therapist who reassures patients that they cannot really be gay or lesbian because of a history of heterosexual behavior is reflecting the erroneous belief that patients will be reassured by having their sexual orientation denied and that only heterosexual experiences are defining and of value. A variation on this theme occurs when sexual minority adolescents are perceived as incapable of knowing their sexual orientation and defined as acting out, oppositional, or "going through a phase" when asserting that they know themselves to be other than heterosexual. The heterosexist therapist who assumes that sexual minority lives are isomorphic with heterosexual lives or who perceives the former to be of lesser value than the latter also places patients at risk from this failure of competence arising from bias.

Heterosexism also may lead to ethically questionable practices when the mental health professional does not sufficiently account for the extent to which sexual minority identity development is complicated by the encounters of a patient with real societal discrimination and oppression. Lacking data on normative aspects of sexual minority experience, a mental health professional may ignore or misunderstand the impact of oppression or trauma, thus leading to misdiagnosis and inefficacious treatment. For example, because confusion and questioning regarding sexual orientation might be defined by a clinician as the sort of "identity disturbance," which is among the diagnostic criteria for borderline personality disorder, there may be an increased risk that a sexual minority patient who is in the normative questioning and experimenting stage of identity development will be mislabeled as borderline by a mental health professional who cannot place this behavior into the appropriate social and developmental framework, with potentially disastrous consequences for the treatment alliance and the course of psychotherapy. Similarly, a sexual minority patient who is having panic episodes after being the target of violence needs a therapist who will address this anxiety as a response to a dangerous situation that may recur, not a mental health professional who treats all anxiety symptoms as equivalent in meaning and prescribes anxiolytics as the sole treatment of choice.

The ethically affirmative stance for mental health practitioners to take in regard to sexual minority patients is to assume the presence in themselves of both antihomosexual bias and heterosexism and then to seek to discover and disengage from these biases. Given the conflation of sexual minority status with psychopathology in stereotypes held by the larger society, all mental health professionals are at some degree of risk of ethically problematic practice with sexual minority patients if this sort of active quest for biased beliefs is not engaged. Herek (1994) suggests that the best predictor of a lack of bias regarding sexual minority persons is personal contact with them. However, often the entire conscious personal contact between a heterosexual mental health professional and sexual minority individuals may be limited to the consulting room; the ongoing stigma in mental health training as well as in society in general frequently results in a social segregation between persons who are members of sexual minority groups and the heterosexual majority. Such skewed contact is likely to produce reinforcement of bias regarding the poor mental health of sexual minority individuals, as no one enters the office of a mental health professional because he or she is feeling emotionally sound. This unfortunate reality heightens the responsibility incumbent on ethical mental health professionals to pursue experiences and contact with sexual minorities who are not patients, as well to obtain accurate, scientifically sound professional training. It is easier to imagine mentally healthy sexual minority individuals when they are colleagues or acquaintances and to develop a more sophisticated and differentiated comprehension of the effects of oppression when learning about them from well-functioning peers than when all of these data of experience derive from patient contact.

The Sexual Minority Therapist and the Small Community Problem

Sexual minority mental health professionals, particularly psychotherapists, often live and work within the same social circles as many of their sexual minority patients. Although some sexual minority mental health professionals treat a more general patient population, it is common for sexual minority psychotherapists to have a large percentage of their patients come from their own social group for a number of reasons. First, sexual minority persons, particularly lesbians, are active consumers of psychotherapy (Ryan and Bradford 1988; Shannon and Woods 1991). Psychotherapy serves the function of a secular religion in many sexual minority communities in which antihomosexual bias, not homo-

sexuality, is the sin and in which the priests and priestesses are psychotherapists (Brown 1989). Sexual minority individuals are also constantly exposed to the insidious traumata of oppression, raising the risk
of bias-caused mental health problems and need for treatment. Finally,
many sexual minority psychotherapists, particularly those from the age
cohort who came out after the beginning of the gay liberation movement at Stonewall in 1969, entered their disciplines with a goal of serving their own communities and offering nonbiased, sexual
minority-affirmative treatment. Because the mental health disciplines
(despite lingering prejudices) have after some struggles become among
the most receptive of the professions to sexual minority individuals,
many sexual minority psychotherapists also have been in the position
of being able to be out and active in their professions and to serve as
pillars of the sexual minority communities, bringing them into contact
with many people who might one day become patients.

This overlap of personal and professional life creates unique ethical challenges for sexual minority mental health professionals, of a sort
also commonly found in other small social groups and in rural areas.
These problems result from the role overlap between professionals and
patients. In a survey of lesbian, gay, and bisexual psychologists, Lynn
(1994) found that it was common for these therapists to encounter
clients accidentally in social situations ranging from locker rooms at
health clubs, to community events such as concerts or political activities, to more intimate settings such as social gatherings with friends.
Some therapists in this study also reported intentional creation of role
overlap with patients, rationalizing this as eventually inevitable, given
the smallness of a sexual minority community, and therefore acceptable. Many of the respondents to this study spoke of their struggles to
maintain the boundaries between professional and personal life, particularly when the psychologist in question was identified as the sole
mental health care provider in a particular locale.

Should there be a different, lower standard of boundary maintenance for sexual minority therapists? No lesser standard is acceptable,
because it would reflect a heterosexist devaluation of the needs of sexual
minority patients to receive mental health services competently and
ethically delivered. However, ethical practice by sexual minority psychotherapists living and working in the same community requires a
constant attention to issues of boundaries and dual relationships. Berman (1985), attempting to address this sort of dilemma, has proposed
the concept of "overlapping" as delineated from "dual" roles between

therapists and patients. Dual roles are defined as multiple relationships between psychotherapist and patient in which the patient is exploited to meet the emotional, financial, sexual, or other personal needs of the psychotherapist. Overlapping roles are defined as unintentional and inevitable crossings of boundaries between the lives of therapists and patients that occur in small communities, roles that are not created to exploit the patient but instead reflect life in a socially small setting. Such overlapping relationships are not ethically problematic, because of their unintended character. However, they carry the potential seeds of ethical problems for the sexual minority mental health professional. Smith (1990) and Brown (1989) have addressed the issue of ethical practice in role overlap situations for sexual minority psychotherapists.

Psychotherapists and other mental health professionals who find themselves facing situations of role overlap must be attentive to issues related to boundary violations such as breaks in confidentiality. What are the risks to confidentiality of an extended conversation with a patient accidentally encountered in public? If patients befriend their psychotherapist's friend because both of them happen to belong to a local lesbian and gay choral group and form their relationship before the shared connection to the psychotherapist is known, how does the mental health professional manage the entry of the patient into a preexisting social circle? If a person known socially to a mental health professional is admitted to the inpatient service where the professional is employed, how do professionals ethically respond to this change in status, particularly if they are the sole providers of service to the sexual minority individuals?

Because situations like these are common for sexual minority psychotherapists and other mental health professionals living and working in the same communities as patients, proactive and affirmatively ethical practice necessitates conscious attention to the possibility of role overlap. The professional must take responsibility to initiate conversations with patients about role overlap possibilities and make the needs of the patient and the protection of the frame of treatment paramount to avoid ethically problematic practice. Regular and frequent consultation with colleagues in similar situations also is a necessary aspect of self-care for the sexual minority mental health professional to avoid unnecessarily self-sacrificing solutions to this kind of ethical dilemma.

The problems that do emerge for sexual minority psychotherapists in this type of situation often arise not from this unintended overlap (no matter how trying it may become) but from the intentional creation of exploitive dual roles. Because the psychotherapists accidentally run into a patient at a party is not a rationale for inviting patients to their own parties. However, both the anecdotal and empirical data on non-sexual dual relationships in sexual minority communities indicate that some mental health professionals, confused about the difference in meaning and ethical valence between overlapping and dual roles, do pursue such courses of action, which are inherently ethically problematic because of the risk that the professional will then exploit patients to meet social, emotional, or sexual needs (Benowitz 1994; Gartrell and Sanderson 1994).

Ethically sound practice for sexual minority psychotherapists working in their community requires that the therapist have a solid and well-defined social network composed primarily of people who have no relationship to the patients of the professional. One problem that has been observed for coming-out therapists is the risk that such therapists may create a social network consisting of their patients (Brown 1989; Gartrell 1994; Gonsiorek 1994). The 2-year abstinence from working with sexual minority patients suggested earlier for the therapist who is coming out can serve as a protection against such an outcome. Otherwise serious risk of ethically problematic behaviors and potential for harm to patients may arise. A particular risk is that of sexual boundary violations by a psychotherapist who has patients as a primary social network and thus a major source of potential sexual partners. Because sexual contact between a provider and a patient is always unethical (and harmful) and frequently signals the end of the career of the mental health professional, prevention of the behaviors potentially leading to this outcome is important for the well-being of all parties.

Ethically effective practice for sexual minority mental health professionals cannot and should not require separation from sexual minority communities, because this deprives both elements of the equation of benefits necessary for both individual and culture to thrive. Consequently, sexual minority psychotherapists like other practitioners in small communities must remain alert to the possibility of breaks in the therapeutic frame deriving from unavoidable role overlap. Such attention often has, as its ultimate consequence, a higher standard for ethical practice among communities of sexual minority practitioners, evidenced by the strong interest shown by such professionals in ethics education that is specifically targeted at dealing with the small-community ethical problem (Brown 1989, 1991).

Summary and Conclusion

Ethical mental health practice with sexual minority patients requires practitioners to pay conscious and continuous attention to the emotional and intellectual effects of antihomosexual bias and heterosexism. The pursuit of an actively ethical stance, rather than the passive acceptance of a minimal standard of following the rules, can lead the mental health practitioner toward incorporation of ethical questions into all facets of practice. Ethics thus becomes no longer simply a set of rules added on to the practice of mental health care. Instead, ethical and clinical questions become entwined, increasing the complexity of the dilemmas, and potentially enriching the quality of ethical decision making. Good clinical practice with sexual minority patients calls for the consistent integration of ethics into practice, because ethically problematic practice also is likely to be biased and thus inefficacious and often harmful.

Because the formal training of most mental health professionals leaves large gaps in teaching about sexual minorities, ethical practice with this population almost always requires continuing professional education. Directed continuing education is as necessary for sexual minority therapists as for heterosexual therapists; simply living as a lesbian, gay man, bisexual, or transgendered person does not provide adequate information and training for ethically sound and effective practice with sexual minority patients. Such continuing education must address both cognitive and affective learning (with special emphasis on the latter), given the intense affect that attaches itself to questions of sexuality in society and to the personal development of mental health professionals as well. Although much of the data on bias in psychotherapy with sexual minority individuals indicate that we have far to go, some of this research also tells us that education to eradicate antihomosexual bias and heterosexism among mental health professionals is effective (Buhrke and Douce 1991) and contributes significantly to the development of ethically sound practice with sexual minority patients.

References

American Psychiatric Association: Diagnostic and Statistical Manual of Mental Disorders, 2nd Edition. Washington, DC, American Psychiatric Association, 1968

Benowitz M: Comparing the experiences of women clients sexually exploited by female versus male psychotherapists. Women and Therapy 15:69–84,1994

Berman JS: Ethical feminist perspectives on dual relationships with clients, in Handbook of Feminist Therapy: Women's Issues in Psychotherapy. Edited by Rosewater LB, Walker LEA. New York, Springer, 1985, pp 287–296

Berube A: Coming Out Under Fire: The History of Gay Men and Women in World War Two. New York, Free Press, 1990

Brown LS: Beyond thou shalt not: thinking about ethics in the lesbian therapy community. Women and Therapy 10:13–25, 1989

Brown LS: Ethical issues in feminist therapy. Psychology of Women Quarterly 15: 323–336, 1991

Buhrke RA, Douce LA: Training issues for counseling psychologists in working with lesbian women and gay men. Counseling Psychologist 19:216–234, 1991

Committee on Lesbian and Gay Concerns: Bias in Psychotherapy with Lesbians and Gay Men. Washington, DC, American Psychological Association, 1990

Davison GC: Homosexuality: the ethical challenge. J Consult Clin Psychol 44:157–162, 1976

Davison GC: Constructionism and morality in therapy for homosexuality, in Homosexuality: Research Implications for Public Policy. Edited by Gonsiorek JC, Weinrich JD. Newbury Park, CA, Sage, 1991, pp 137–148

Duberman M: Cures: A Gay Man's Odyssey. New York, Dutton, 1991

Feldman-Summers S: Sexual contact in fiduciary relationships, in Sexual Exploitation in Professional Relationships. Edited by Gabbard GO. Washington, DC, American Psychiatric Press, 1991, pp 193–210

Gabbard GO (ed): Sexual Exploitation in Professional Relationships. Washington, DC, American Psychiatric Press, 1989

Gartrell NK: Combating homophobia in the psychotherapy of lesbians. Women and Therapy 3:13–30, 1984

Gartrell NK: Boundaries in lesbian therapist-client relationships, in Lesbian and Gay Psychology: Theory, Research and Clinical Applications. Edited by Greene B, Herek GM. Newbury Park, CA, Sage, 1994, pp 98–117

Gartrell NK, Sanderson BE: Sexual abuse of women by women in psychotherapy: counseling and advocacy. Women and Therapy, 15: 39–54, 1994

Gonsiorek JC: Boundary challenges when both therapist and client are gay males, in Breach of Trust. Edited by Gonsiorek JC. Newbury Park, CA, Sage, 1994, pp 225–234

Grahn J: Another Mother Tongue: Gay Words, Gay Worlds. Boston, MA, Beacon Press, 1984

Haldeman DC: Sexual orientation conversion therapy for gay men and lesbians: a scientific examination, in Homosexuality: Research Implications for Public Policy. Edited by Gonsiorek JC, Weinrich JD. Newbury Park, CA, Sage, 1991, pp 149–160

Herek GM: Assessing heterosexuals' attitudes towards lesbians and gay men: a review of empirical research with the ATLG scale, in Lesbian and Gay Psychology: Theory, Research and Clinical Applications. Edited by Greene B, Herek GM. Newbury Park, CA, Sage, 1994, pp 206–228

Humphrey MA: My Country, My Right to Serve. New York, HarperCollins, 1990

Isay RA: Becoming Homosexual: Gay Men and Their Development. New York, Farrar Straus Giroux, 1989

Jones FD, Koshes RJ: Homosexuality and the military. Am J Psychiatry 152: 16–21, 1995

Keith-Spiegel P, Koocher GP: Ethics in Psychology: Professional Standards and Cases. New York, Random House, 1985

Kilburg RR, Nathan PE, Thoreson RW (eds): Professionals in Distress: Issues, Syndromes and Solutions in Psychology. Washington, DC, American Psychological Association, 1986

Lerman H, Porter N: The contribution of feminism to ethics in psychotherapy, in Feminist Ethics in Psychotherapy. Edited by Lerman H, Porter N. New York, Springer, 1990, pp 5–13

Lynn L: Lesbian, gay and bisexual therapists' social and sexual interactions with clients, in Breach of Trust. Edited by Gonsiorek JC. Newbury Park, CA, Sage, 1994, pp 193–212

Nicolosi J: Reparative Therapy of Male Homosexuality. Northvale, NJ, Jason Aronson, 1991

Payton CR: Implications of the 1992 ethics code for diverse groups. Professional Psychology: Research and Practice 25:317–320, 1994

Personnel Separations—Homosexuality. Army Regulations 635-89 Washington, DC, Department of the Army, Headquarters, July 15, 1966

Ryan C, Bradford J: The national lesbian health care survey: an overview, in The Sourcebook on Lesbian/Gay Healthcare. Edited by Shernoff M, Scott WA. Washington, DC, National Lesbian and Gay Health Foundation, 1988, pp 30–40

Shannon JW, Woods WJ: Affirmative psychotherapy for gay men. Counseling Psychologist 19:197–215, 1991

Smith AJ: Working within the lesbian community: the dilemma of overlapping relationships, in Feminist Ethics in Psychotherapy. Edited by Lerman H, Porter N. New York, Springer, 1990, pp 92–96

Thompson K, Andrzejewski J: Why Can't Sharon Kowalski Come Home? San Francisco, CA, Spinsters/Aunt Lute, 1988

Epilogue

Evelyn Hooker, Ph.D.

T hat the American Psychiatric Press would publish this book is extraordinary. A lot of energy went into the diagnostic changes in 1973, and this edition must indicate at least a grudging acceptance, or even outright approval, of the legitimacy of gay and lesbian studies. If this book reaches medical schools and other graduate training programs—and especially practitioners—much will be accomplished, but I suspect it will not be easy. Important research is also being conducted by gay and lesbian psychiatrists, psychologists, and other mental and medical health professionals. The scientific view of homosexuality is thus coming to prevail.

What was taught in the 1950s about homosexuality was different. When I first applied to the National Institute of Mental Health (NIMH) for my study of gay men I was told I needed a psychiatric consultant because what I was going to study was looked on as psychopathology.

Editors' note. The work of Evelyn Hooker, Ph.D., has been featured prominently throughout this text. Her studies, beginning in the 1950s, were the first to indicate that gay men were as psychologically healthy as their heterosexual matches. This research started the cascade of material now available on homosexuality, gay men, lesbians, bisexuals, and transgendered persons. Honored in many ways throughout the years, most recently at the dedication of the Evelyn Hooker Center for Gay and Lesbian Mental Health at the University of Chicago, she has been the subject of an award-winning documentary. Dr. Hooker now lives in quiet but active retirement in Santa Monica, California. In March 1994, she welcomed Drs. Robert Cabaj, David McWhirter, and Andrew Mattison to spend a morning with her in her apartment, reviewing the table of contents for this volume, and discussing the future of gay and lesbian studies. Highlights of that conversation form this epilogue.

When I then sought help from the chairman of the Psychiatry Department, and told him that I was going to study "normal male homosexuals," he literally gripped the arms of his chair and said, "What do you think you are talking about; there is no such person!" However, he did agree to let me spend time with one of his psychiatric staff who said, "I've never met a homosexual man like this, but I sure would like to!" I said, "You're my man!" He was amazing; he had obviously not been ruined by his education.

Many must question if I am lesbian, but only gay and lesbian people asked if I am. No, I am not, but I am interested in prejudice and fighting stigma. When I taught about prejudice and Jews, Jewish students would come up after class and ask, "You are Jewish, aren't you?" And I would say, "No, you honor me by thinking that I am, but no, I am not." I guess they could not figure out why I would do this type of teaching if I were not myself Jewish.

I came from a poor background. I remember that early in my childhood I knew I was going to get away from the farm and do something about people who are victims. After finishing my training, it had never occurred to me to do research about gay issues. I had been through a lot of personal and professional changes, and when I was back in California, a gay male friend, a former student, insisted I study gay men. He said, "We have let you see us as we are, and now it is your scientific duty to study people like us." I said I could not be objective because they were my friends, but he promised to find a hundred gay men I did not know if I needed them. I realized I needed a control group, and that is what led to the NIMH application. My first study called, "A Preliminary Analysis of Group Behavior of Homosexuals"—a terrible title!—did present normal, walking-around gay people, with no real pathology, but also showed the effects of stigmatization. NIMH kept renewing my funds, even when I said I did not want them any more. Site visitors and other people would invent reasons to come to visit me; I think all they wanted to see was who was that crazy lady studying gay men. I was told my research was making a difference and filling a need. I gave the first report in August of 1956 in Chicago, and the report was published in April of 1957 (Hooker 1957).

I did more work and study into the 1960s and chaired a task force for the NIMH starting in 1969. A lot of the changes made would not have been possible without Dr. Judd Marmor. That man is marvelous; without him, we might as well have folded our tents. I am surprised to learn that my work did lead to the 1973 change in diagnosis by the

American Psychiatric Association; I did not realize the information really had been used for that purpose!

Currently, I do a lot of reading and follow reports as much as I can. Many researchers and investigators have come to talk with me and get advice over these last 40 years. Friendship has been my favorite thing to offer. I am so pleased with the plaque that you gave me: "The Association of Gay and Lesbian Psychiatrists honors Dr. Evelyn Hooker in recognition of her pioneering research, courageous advocacy, and enduring friendship. May 16, 1990."

If I could still be doing research, one of the first things to come to mind is studying homophobia and heterosexism. Bias still affects research. Civil rights and the gay liberation movement have made changes and could themselves be studied. When we think how different things are from what they were 10 or 20 years ago, we owe that to gay people themselves. The fact that gay people were willing to conceive that they could make a difference if they came out in the open and demanded a place in society was terribly important. There is still a lot to do: equal treatment for gay and lesbian people; the military issues; the impact of AIDS.

Money for research will be hard to come by, but necessary. Medical and political groups will need to change and adjust to openly gay people. People can open up to new ideas and can change their opinions. I am sure that your book will play an important role in this process.

Reference

Hooker E: The adjustment of the male overt homosexual. J Projective Techniques 21:18–31, 1957

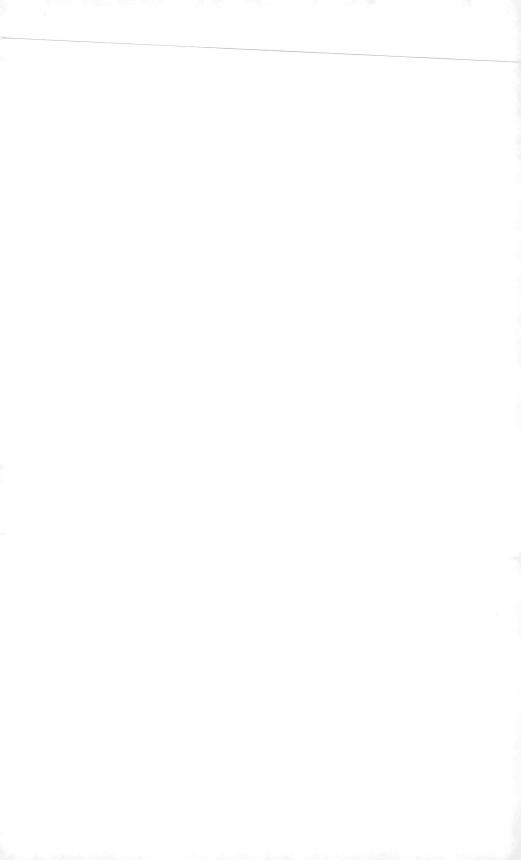

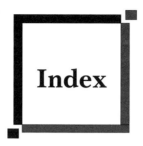

Index

Page numbers printed in **boldface** type refer to tables or figures.

DATE DUE

OCT 2 2 1997			
JUN 0 6 1999			
4/11/00			
APR 1 3			
DE 04 '05			

Demco, Inc. 38-293